BREAST CANCER SCREENING

VOLUME 15

This publication represents the views and expert opinions of an IARC Working Group on the Evaluation of Cancer-Preventive Strategies, which met in Lyon, 11–18 November 2014

LYON, FRANCE - 2016

IARC HANDBOOKS OF CANCER PREVENTION

International Agency for Research on Cancer

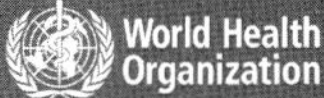

Published by the International Agency for Research on Cancer, 150 cours Albert Thomas, 69372 Lyon Cedex 08, France

Distributed by WHO Press, World Health Organization, 20 Avenue Appia, 1211 Geneva 27, Switzerland (tel.: +41 22 791 3264; fax: +41 22 791 4857; email: bookorders@who.int).

This book is also available in electronic format from http://publications.iarc.fr/.

Corrigenda to the *IARC Handbooks* are published online at http://handbooks.iarc.fr/publications/corrigenda.php.

To report an error, please contact editimo@iarc.fr.

IARC Library Cataloguing in Publication Data

Breast cancer screening / IARC Working Group on the Evaluation of Cancer-Preventive Interventions, 2014. – 2nd edition.

(IARC Handbooks of Cancer Prevention ; Volume 15)

1. Breast Neoplasms – prevention and control 2. Mass Screening 3. Early Detection of Cancer 4. Cost-Benefit Analysis

I. International Agency for Research on Cancer II. Series

ISBN 978-92-832-3015-1
ISSN 1027-5622

(NLM Classification: W1)

PRINTED IN FRANCE

International Agency for Research on Cancer

The International Agency for Research on Cancer (IARC) was established in 1965 by the World Health Assembly, as an independently funded organization within the framework of the World Health Organization. The headquarters of the Agency are in Lyon, France.

The Agency has as its mission to reduce the cancer burden worldwide through promoting international collaboration in research. The Agency addresses this mission through conducting cancer research for cancer prevention in three main areas: describing the occurrence of cancer; identifying the causes of cancer, and evaluating preventive interventions and their implementation. Each of these areas is a vital contribution to the spectrum of cancer prevention.

The publications of the Agency contribute to the dissemination of authoritative information on different aspects of cancer research. Information about IARC publications, and how to order them, is available at http://publications.iarc.fr/.

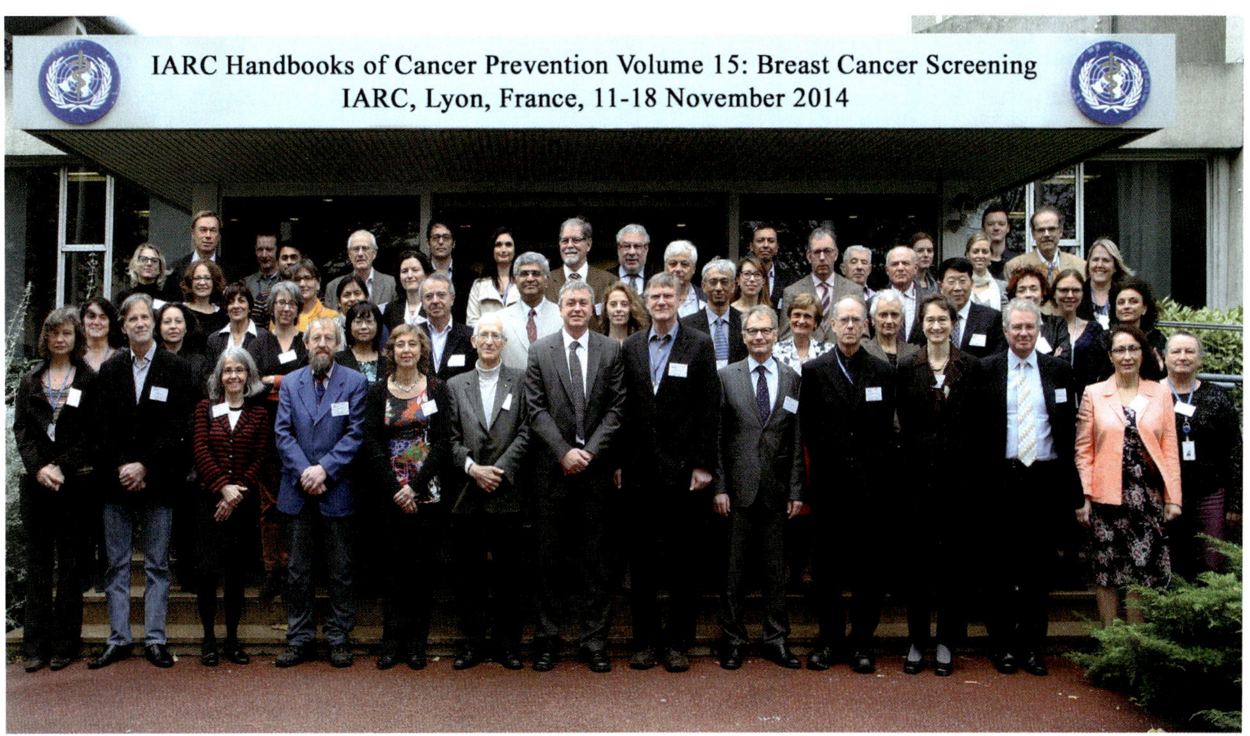

IARC Handbooks of Cancer Prevention

In 1969, the International Agency for Research on Cancer (IARC) initiated a programme on the evaluation of the carcinogenic risk of chemicals to humans involving the production of critically evaluated monographs on individual chemicals.

The *IARC Handbooks of Cancer Prevention* complement the *IARC Monographs*' evaluations of carcinogenic hazards. The objective of the programme is to produce and publish a series of critical reviews of data on the cancer-preventive effects of primary or secondary interventions, to evaluate these data in terms of cancer prevention with the help of international working groups of experts in prevention and related fields, and to indicate where additional research efforts are needed. The lists of evaluations are regularly updated and are available at http://handbooks.iarc.fr/.

This *IARC Handbook of Cancer Prevention* is partly funded by the French Institut National du Cancer (INCa) by Convention N° 2013-219 (HAP Dépistage 2013 - K sein).

Cover image: An oblique view mammogram of the left breast of an asymptomatic 57-year-old woman. The arrow points to a small invasive cancer detected at screening. This cancer could not be detected with palpation even after it had been detected with mammography. Photograph courtesy of Peter Dean.

CONTENTS

NOTE TO THE READER 1

LIST OF PARTICIPANTS 3

WORKING PROCEDURES 7

A. GENERAL PRINCIPLES AND PROCEDURES 7
1. Background 7
2. Scope 7
3. Objectives 8
4. Meeting participants 8
5. Working procedures 9
6. Inclusion criteria for data for the *Handbooks* 10

B. SCIENTIFIC REVIEW AND EVALUATION 11
1. Global burden and disease characteristics 11
2. Screening techniques 11
3. Availability and use of screening programmes 11
4. Efficacy of screening tests 12
5. Effectiveness of population-based screening 12
6. Summary 13
7. Evaluation 13

References 14

GENERAL REMARKS 15

LIST OF ABBREVIATIONS 17

GLOSSARY 19

1. BREAST CANCER 23

1.1 The global burden of breast cancer: incidence, mortality, survival, and prevalence 23
1.1.1 Global burden 23
1.1.2 International variation 24
1.1.3 Incidence and mortality in relation to level of development 28
1.1.4 Time trends 28
1.1.5 Time trends by age 29
1.1.6 Projection to 2025 32

1.2 Classification and natural history 33
1.2.1 Benign breast disease 33
1.2.2 Breast carcinoma in situ 44
1.2.3 Invasive breast carcinoma 47
1.2.4 Breast cancer with hereditary and somatic mutations 51
1.2.5 Summary 52
1.3 Risk factors 53
1.3.1 Hormonal and reproductive factors 54
1.3.2 Lifestyle factors and environmental exposures 58
1.3.3 Non-modifiable risk factors 59
1.3.4 Ionizing radiation 61
1.3.5 Women at high genetic risk of breast cancer 69
1.3.6 Attributable burden to known risk factors 73
1.4 Stage at diagnosis, survival, and management 74
1.4.1 Stage at diagnosis and survival 75
1.4.2 Management 79
1.5 Breast awareness, early detection and diagnosis, and screening 84
1.5.1 Breast awareness 85
1.5.2 Early diagnosis of symptomatic breast cancer 85
1.5.3 Screening asymptomatic women 87
References 90

2. SCREENING TECHNIQUES 113
2.1 X-ray techniques 113
2.1.1 X-ray equipment 113
2.1.2 Screen-film mammography 116
2.1.3 Digital mammography 119
2.1.4 Digital breast tomosynthesis 123
2.1.5 Breast computed tomography 124
2.1.6 Radiation dose 125
2.1.7 Quality assurance and quality control in mammography 126
2.1.8 Mammography screening performance 129
2.1.9 Host factors that affect performance 135
2.2 Non-mammographic imaging techniques 138
2.2.1 Ultrasonography 138
2.2.2 Magnetic resonance imaging 143
2.2.3 Positron emission tomography/mammography 146
2.2.4 Scintimammography 147
2.2.5 Electrical impedance imaging 148
2.2.6 Other techniques 149
2.3 Clinical breast examination 149
2.3.1 Technique 149
2.3.2 Training 151
2.3.3 Quality control 151
2.3.4 Screening performance 151
2.3.5 Host factors that affect performance 152

2.4 Breast self-examination 152
2.4.1 Technique 152
2.4.2 Training 152
2.4.3 Quality control 153
2.4.4 Screening performance 153
2.4.5 Host factors that affect performance 154
References 154

3. SCREENING PROGRAMMES 165
3.1 Determinants of participation in screening 165
3.1.1 Personal and socioeconomic factors 165
3.1.2 Cultural factors 168
3.1.3 Information and understanding 169
3.1.4 Psychological consequences of mammography screening 172
3.2 Availability and use of screening programmes 174
3.2.1 Europe 174
3.2.2 North America 181
3.2.3 Latin America 187
3.2.4 Sub-Saharan Africa 193
3.2.5 Central and West Asia and North Africa 199
3.2.6 South-East Asia 206
3.2.7 Oceania 214
References 217

4. EFFICACY OF BREAST CANCER SCREENING 237
4.1 Methodological and analytical issues 237
4.1.1 Efficacy versus effectiveness 237
4.1.2 Primary outcome measures 237
4.1.3 Biases 238
4.1.4 Use of randomized controlled trials 239
4.1.5 Use of observational studies in assessing efficacy 241
4.2 Mammography 241
4.2.1 Description of randomized trials 241
4.2.2 Beneficial effects 247
4.2.3 Performance indicators 254
4.3 Clinical breast examination 260
4.3.1 Randomized clinical trials 260
4.3.2 Nested case–control study 262
4.3.3 Observational studies 265
4.4 Breast self-examination 267
4.4.1 Randomized trials 267
4.4.2 Observational studies 269
References 274

5. EFFECTIVENESS OF BREAST CANCER SCREENING 281
5.1 Indicators for monitoring and evaluating effectiveness 281
5.1.1 Performance indicators 281

5.1.2 Study designs to assess the effectiveness of screening . . . 287
5.1.3 Surrogate indicators of effect on mortality . . . 295
5.2 Preventive effects of mammography . . . 295
5.2.1 Incidence-based cohort mortality studies. . . . 295
5.2.2 Case–control studies . . . 328
5.2.3 Ecological studies . . . 346
5.2.4 Other measures of screening performance . . . 348
5.3 Adverse effects of mammography . . . 363
5.3.1 False-positive rates . . . 363
5.3.2 Overdiagnosis . . . 364
5.3.3 Overtreatment . . . 378
5.3.4 Risk of breast cancer induced by radiation . . . 379
5.3.5 Psychological consequences of mammography screening . . . 384
5.4 Cost–effectiveness and balance of harms and benefits . . . 388
5.4.1 Mammography screening programmes in developed countries. . . . 390
5.4.2 Screening in low- and middle-income countries. . . . 391
5.4.3 Harm–benefit ratio and generalizability. . . . 392
5.4.4 Lower age limit for screening . . . 392
5.4.5 Upper age limit for screening . . . 393
5.4.6 Digital mammography . . . 394
5.4.7 Impact of individual risk factors. . . . 394
5.4.8 Quality of life . . . 395
5.5 Other imaging techniques . . . 395
5.5.1 Preventive effects. . . . 396
5.5.2 Adverse effects . . . 406
5.5.3 Cost–effectiveness analysis . . . 407
5.5.4 Other techniques. . . . 408
5.5.5 Psychosocial harm. . . . 409
5.6 Screening of women at an increased risk. . . . 410
5.6.1 High familial risk, with or without a *BRCA1* or *BRCA2* mutation . . . 410
5.6.2 Personal history of invasive breast cancer or DCIS. . . . 418
5.6.3 Lobular neoplasia or atypical proliferations. . . . 422
5.7 Clinical breast examination. . . . 422
5.7.1 Preventive effects of clinical breast examination . . . 422
5.7.2 Adverse effects . . . 423
5.7.3 Cost–effectiveness analysis . . . 423
5.8 Breast self-examination . . . 423
5.8.1 Preventive effects of teaching breast self-examination. . . . 423
5.8.2 Adverse effects . . . 425
5.8.3 Cost–effectiveness analysis . . . 425
References. . . . 426

6. SUMMARY . . . 451
6.1 Breast cancer . . . 451
6.2 Implementation of breast cancer screening worldwide . . . 452
6.2.1 Europe . . . 452

6.2.2 North America.....453
6.2.3 Latin America.....453
6.2.4 Sub-Saharan Africa.....453
6.2.5 Central and West Asia and North Africa.....453
6.2.6 South-East Asia.....454
6.2.7 Oceania.....454
6.3 Mammography screening.....454
6.3.1 Efficacy of mammography screening from randomized controlled trials.....454
6.3.2 Effectiveness of mammography screening.....456
6.3.3 Adverse effects of mammography screening.....459
6.3.4 Cost–effectiveness of mammography screening.....461
6.4 Other imaging techniques.....461
6.4.1 Techniques.....461
6.4.2 Effectiveness in screening.....462
6.5 Screening of women at an increased risk.....463
6.5.1 Women with a *BRCA1/2* mutation.....463
6.5.2 Women with a high familial risk without a *BRCA1/2* mutation.....464
6.5.3 Women with a high familial risk with or without a *BRCA1/2* mutation.....464
6.5.4 Women with a personal history of breast cancer (invasive or in situ).....464
6.5.5 Women with lobular neoplasia or atypical proliferations.....464
6.6 Clinical breast examination.....465
6.7 Breast self-examination.....465

7. EVALUATION.....467
7.1 Mammography screening.....467
7.1.1 Mammography screening: preventive effects.....467
7.1.2 Mammography screening: adverse effects.....467
7.1.3 Mammography screening: cost–effectiveness.....468
7.2 Other imaging techniques.....468
7.2.1 Breast ultrasonography.....468
7.2.2 Digital breast tomosynthesis/three-dimensional mammography.....468
7.3 Screening of women at an increased risk.....468
7.4 Clinical breast examination.....469
7.5 Breast self-examination.....469

NOTE TO THE READER

The *IARC Handbooks of Cancer Prevention* series was launched in 1995 to complement the *IARC Monographs'* evaluations of carcinogenic hazards. The *IARC Handbooks of Cancer Prevention* evaluate the published scientific evidence of cancer-preventive interventions.

Inclusion of an intervention in the *Handbooks* does not imply that it is cancer-preventive, only that the published data have been examined. Equally, the fact that an intervention has not yet been evaluated in a *Handbook* does not mean that it may not prevent cancer. Similarly, identification of organ sites with *sufficient evidence* or *limited evidence* of cancer-preventive activity in humans should not be viewed as precluding the possibility that an intervention may prevent cancer at other sites.

The evaluations of cancer prevention strategies are made by international Working Groups of independent scientists and are qualitative in nature. No recommendation is given for regulation or legislation.

Anyone who is aware of published data that may alter the evaluation of cancer-preventive interventions is encouraged to make this information available to the Section of IARC Monographs, International Agency for Research on Cancer, 150 cours Albert Thomas, 69372 Lyon Cedex 08, France, or by email to imo@iarc.fr, in order that these data may be considered for re-evaluation by a future Working Group.

Although every effort is made to prepare the *Handbooks* as accurately as possible, mistakes may occur. Readers are requested to communicate any errors to the Section of IARC Monographs at imo@iarc.fr.

LIST OF PARTICIPANTS

Members [1]

Ahti Anttila (Co-Meeting Chair)

Finnish Cancer Registry
Institute for Statistical and Epidemiological Cancer Research
Helsinki
Finland

Bruce Armstrong (Meeting Co-Chair; Senior Visiting Scientist at IARC)

Cancer Epidemiology and Control Department
Sydney School of Public Health
Camperdown
Australia

Rajendra A. Badwe

Department of Surgical Oncology
Tata Memorial Centre
Mumbai
India

Ronaldo Corrêa Ferreira da Silva

National Cancer Institute
Rio de Janeiro
Brazil

Geertruida H. de Bock

University Medical Center Groningen
University of Groningen
Groningen
The Netherlands

[1] Working Group Members and Invited Specialists serve in their individual capacities as scientists and not as representatives of their government or any organization with which they are affiliated. Affiliations are provided for identification purposes only.
Each participant was asked to disclose pertinent research, employment, and financial interests. Current financial interests and research and employment interests during the past 4 years or anticipated in the future are identified here. Minor pertinent interests are not listed and include stock valued at no more than US$ 1000 overall, grants that provide no more than 5% of the research budget of the expert's organization and that do not support the expert's research or position, and consulting or speaking on matters not before a court or government agency that does not exceed 2% of total professional time or compensation. All grants that support the expert's research or position and all consulting or speaking on behalf of an interested party on matters before a court or government agency are listed as significant pertinent interests.

Harry J. de Koning (Subgroup Chair, Mammography Screening)

Department of Public Health
Erasmus University Medical Center
Rotterdam
The Netherlands

Stephen W. Duffy

Cancer Research UK
Centre for Cancer Prevention
London
United Kingdom

Ian Ellis

Faculty of Medicine and Health Sciences
Department of Histopathology
Nottingham
United Kingdom

Chisato Hamashima

Centre for Cancer Prevention and Screening
National Cancer Centre
Tokyo
Japan

Nehmat Houssami

School of Public Health
The University of Sydney
Sydney
Australia

Vessela Kristensen

Department of Genetics
Oslo University Hospital Radiumhospitalet
Oslo
Norway

Anthony B. Miller

Dalla Lana School of Public Health
University of Toronto
Toronto, ON
Canada

Raul Murillo

Instituto Nacional de Cancerología
Subdirección General de Investigaciones, Vigilancia Epidemiológica, Promoción y Prevención
Bogotá
Colombia

Eugenio Paci [retired]

Cancer Prevention and Research Institute
Florence
Italy

Julietta Patnick

Public Health England
NHS Cancer Screening Programmes
Sheffield
United Kingdom

You-Lin Qiao

Department of Cancer Epidemiology
Chinese Academy of Medical Sciences and Peking Union Medical College
Beijing
China

Agnès Rogel

Department of Chronic Diseases and Injuries
French Institute for Public Health Surveillance
Saint-Maurice
France

Nereo Segnan

Visiting Scientist at IARC
Department of Cancer Screening and Unit of Cancer Epidemiology
Piedmont University Hospital
Turin
Italy

Surendra S. Shastri

Department of Preventive Oncology
WHO Collaborating Centre for Cancer Prevention
Mumbai
India

Robert A. Smith (Subgroup Chair, Screening Programmes)

Cancer Control Science Department
American Cancer Society
Atlanta, GA
USA

Marit Solbjør

Department of Social Work and Health Science
Norwegian University of Science and Technology
Trondheim
Norway

David B. Thomas (Subgroup Chair, Clinical Breast Examination, Breast Self-Examination, Women at Increased Risk)

Fred Hutchinson Cancer Research Center
Epidemiology Research Unit
Seattle, WA
USA

Elisabete Weiderpass Vainio (Subgroup Chair, Breast Cancer)

Department of Etiological Research
The Cancer Registry of Norway
Oslo
Norway

Invited specialists

Sylvia H. Heywang-Köbrunner[2]

Munich Mammography Reference Centre
Munich
Germany

Martin J. Yaffe[3]

Imaging Research Program,
University of Toronto
Toronto, ON
Canada

[2] Sylvia H. Heywang-Köbrunner works part-time in private practice, where 70% of her work is related to mammography screening.

[3] Martin J. Yaffe has significant research funding from GE Healthcare, a manufacturer of mammography systems. Further, he holds significant shares of Matakina Ltd., a manufacturer of software for measuring breast density. He is also a principal of a private company, Mammographic Physics Inc. (MPI). His wife's retirement account includes shares of a company that makes mammography systems.

Representatives

Frederic de Bels

Cancer Screening Department
French National Cancer Institute (INCa)
Boulogne-Billancourt
France

Solveig Hofvind

The Cancer Registry of Norway
Oslo
Norway

Mary White

Division of Cancer Prevention and Control
Centers for Disease Control and Prevention
Atlanta, GA
USA

Observers

Hans-Werner Hense [unable to attend]

University of Münster
Münster
Germany

Jessica Kirby

Cancer Research UK
London
United Kingdom

IARC/WHO Secretariat

Maribel Almonte
Srikant Ambatipudi
Franca Bianchini *(Rapporteur)*
Veronique Bouvard *(Rapporteur)*
Anya Burton
Graham Byrnes
Peter Dean *(Senior Visiting Scientist)*
Carolina Espina Garcia
David Forman *(with writing assignment)*
Silvia Franceschi
Béatrice Lauby-Secretan *(Responsible Officer, Rapporteur)*
Dana Loomis *(Rapporteur)*
Valerie McCormack
Karen Müller *(Editor)*
Sandra Perdomo
Isabelle Romieu
Rengaswamy Sankaranarayanan (*with writing assignment)*
Catherine Sauvaget
Chiara Scoccianti (*Co-Responsible Officer, Rapporteur)*
Kurt Straif *(Head of Programme)*
Eero Suonio
Lamia Tallaa *(Rapporteur)*
Isabelle Thierry-Chef
Andreas Ullrich *(WHO Geneva)*
Diama Vale
Lawrence von Karsa *(with writing assignment)*

Administrative Assistance

Marieke Dusenberg
Sandrine Egraz
Michel Javin
Brigitte Kajo
Annick Leroux
Helene Lorenzen-Augros

Production Team

Elisabeth Elbers
Solène Quennehen

WORKING PROCEDURES

The Working Procedures of the *IARC Handbooks of Cancer Prevention* describe the objective and scope of the programme, the scientific principles and procedures used in developing a *Handbook*, the types of evidence considered, and the scientific criteria that guide the evaluations.

A. GENERAL PRINCIPLES AND PROCEDURES

1. Background

The global burden of cancer is high and continues to increase: the annual number of new cases was estimated at 14.1 million in 2012 and is expected to reach 22.2 million by 2030 (Ferlay et al., 2014). With current trends in demographics and exposure, the cancer burden has been shifting from high-resource countries to low- and medium-resource countries.

Prevention of cancer is one of the key objectives of the International Agency for Research on Cancer (IARC). Cancer prevention can be achieved by primary prevention – aimed at preventing the occurrence of cancer – or by secondary prevention – aimed at diagnosing cancer sufficiently early to reduce related mortality and suffering.

Screening and early clinical diagnosis are the principal instruments of secondary prevention of cancer and a fundamental component of any cancer control programme. Screening may enable detection of cancer sufficiently early that cure and resulting reduction in mortality and having the disease are realistic possibilities given suitable treatment. Screening for some cancers, such as cervical cancer, may also detect precancerous lesions, effective treatment of which can prevent occurrence of cancer.

When screening is planned as part of a cancer control programme, only strategies proved to be effective should be proposed to the general population. Screening usually requires repeated interactions between "healthy" individuals and health-care providers, which can be inconvenient and costly. Furthermore, screening requires an ongoing commitment between the public and health-care providers.

2. Scope

Cochrane (1972) first discussed the concepts of efficacy and effectiveness in the context of health interventions. "Efficacy" was recently defined by Porta (2008) as "the extent to which a specific intervention, procedure, regimen or service produces a beneficial result under ideal conditions; the benefit or utility to the individual or the population of the service, treatment regimen, or intervention. Ideally, the determination of efficacy is based on the results of a randomized controlled trial." In contrast, the related term "effectiveness" is defined by the same author as "a measure of the extent to which a specific intervention, procedure, regimen or service, when deployed in the field in routine circumstances, does what it is intended to do for a specific population; a measure of the extent to which a health care intervention fulfils its objectives in practice." The distinction between efficacy as measured in experimental studies and the effectiveness of a mass population intervention is a crucial one for public health decision-making. In particular, the fact that the effectiveness of a screening procedure may be different in different populations is often overlooked. A mass programme of screening must satisfy certain minimal requirements (e.g. acceptability, availability of relevant personnel, facilities for screening, and access to pertinent health services) if it is to achieve the results that have been documented in epidemiological studies.

The acceptance and use of screening services may vary from one population to another, implying that a given screening procedure is not universally effective. Even when a screening procedure is effective as a mass intervention, other outcomes, such as harm and costs and the potential for other interventions to achieve equivalent benefits, must be considered. Efficacy is a necessary but not sufficient basis for recommending screening. The efficacy of a screening procedure can be inferred if effectiveness can be proven. Screening has sometimes been implemented by a given procedure on the assumption that "earlier is better," even when no evidence of efficacy was available. If such interventions result in a significant reduction in mortality that cannot otherwise be explained, it can be inferred that the procedure is effective. However, uncontrolled interventions in which individuals are exposed to unknown risks and benefits should be avoided.

3. Objectives

The objectives of the Working Group are:

1. To evaluate the strength of the evidence for the preventive efficacy of a screening procedure;
2. To assess the effectiveness of defined screening interventions in defined populations;
3. To assess the balance of benefit and harm in target populations.

The conclusions of the Working Group are published as a volume in the *IARC Handbooks of Cancer Prevention* series.

4. Meeting participants

Five categories of participant can be present at a *Handbook* meeting:

1. The Working Group is responsible for the critical reviews and evaluations. The tasks of *Working Group Members* are described in detail below. Working Group Members are selected on the basis of: (i) knowledge and experience; and (ii) absence of real or apparent conflicts of interests. They have often published significant research related to the intervention being reviewed, and IARC uses literature searches to identify such experts. Experts in the general subject matter or methodology who have not published on the subject of the evaluation may also be included. Consideration is also given to demographic diversity and balance of scientific findings and views.
2. *Invited Specialists* are experts who also have important knowledge and experience, but have a real or apparent conflict of interests. These experts are invited when necessary to assist the Working Group by contributing technical knowledge and experience during subgroup and plenary discussions. They may also review text prepared by the Working Group and contribute text on issues that

do not influence the final evaluation, for example, description of the agent evaluated (for chemicals) or techniques (for screening) (see Part B, Section 2). Invited Specialists do not serve as meeting chair or subgroup chair, and do not participate in the evaluations.

3. *Representatives* of national and international health agencies often attend meetings because their agencies are sponsors of the programme or are interested in the subject of a meeting. Representatives do not serve as meeting chair or subgroup chair, do not draft any part of a *Handbook*, and do not participate in the evaluations.
4. *Observers* with relevant scientific credentials may be admitted to a meeting in limited numbers. Attention will be given to achieving a balance of Observers from constituencies with differing perspectives. They are invited to observe the meeting and should not attempt to influence it. At the meeting, the meeting chair and subgroup chairs may grant Observers an opportunity to speak, generally after they have observed a discussion. Observers agree to respect the Guidelines for Observers at Meetings of the *IARC Handbooks of Cancer Prevention* (available at http://handbooks.iarc.fr).
5. The *IARC Secretariat* consists of IARC scientists who have relevant expertise. They serve as rapporteurs and participate in all discussions. When requested by the meeting chair or subgroup chair, they may also draft text or prepare tables and analyses. They do not participate in evaluations.

Before an invitation is extended, each potential participant, including the IARC Secretariat, completes the "Declaration of Interests for IARC/WHO Experts" form to report financial interests, employment and consulting, and individual and institutional research support related to the subject of the meeting. IARC assesses these interests to determine whether there is a real or apparent conflict that warrants some limitation on participation. The declarations are updated and reviewed again at the opening of the meeting. Interests related to the subject of the meeting are disclosed to the meeting participants and in the published volume.

The names and principal affiliations of participants are available on the website of the *IARC Handbooks of Cancer Prevention* (http://handbooks.iarc.fr) approximately two months before each meeting. It is not acceptable for Observers or third parties to contact other participants before a meeting or to lobby them at any time. Meeting participants are asked to report all such contacts to IARC.

All participants are listed, with their principal affiliations, at the beginning of each volume. Each participant who is a Working Group Member serves as an individual scientist and not as a representative of any organization, government, or industry.

5. Working procedures

A separate Working Group is responsible for developing each volume of the *Handbooks*. Approximately one year before the Working Group meeting, the agents to be reviewed are announced on the *Handbooks* website (http://handbooks.iarc.fr) and participants are selected by IARC staff in consultation with other experts. Subsequently, IARC performs literature searches of recognized sources of information on cancer prevention. Meeting participants are expected to supplement the IARC literature searches with their own searches.

The relevant articles are made available to meeting participants, who prepare preliminary drafts of the sections assigned to them. The preliminary drafts are sent to Working Group Members and Invited Specialists for peer review, and the peer-review comments are sent to the original author, who revises the draft before the meeting.

The Working Group meets at IARC for eight days to discuss and review the text and to formulate the evaluations. The objectives of the meeting are peer review, evaluation, and consensus. During the first few days, the participants meet in subgroups to review the drafts of their subgroup, develop a joint draft, and write summaries. Care is taken to ensure that each study summary is written or reviewed by someone not associated with the study being considered. During the last few days, the Working Group meets in plenary session to review the subgroup drafts and develop the evaluations. As a result, the entire volume is the joint product of the Working Group, and there are no individually authored sections.

IARC Working Groups strive to achieve a consensus evaluation. Consensus reflects broad agreement among Working Group Members, but not necessarily unanimity. The chair may elect to poll Working Group Members to determine the diversity of scientific opinion on issues where consensus is not readily apparent.

Thus, the tasks of the Working Group are as follows:

1. Ascertain that all appropriate data have been retrieved;
2. Select the data relevant for evaluation on the basis of scientific merit;
3. Prepare summaries of the data that will allow the reader to follow the reasoning of the Working Group;
4. Evaluate separately the efficacy and the effectiveness of the screening procedure;
5. Summarize the potential adverse consequences of screening;
6. Prepare an overall evaluation of the screening procedure at the population level, combining all lines of evidence.

A summary of the outcome is published on the *Handbooks* programme website and as a short report in the *New England Journal of Medicine* shortly after the meeting. Subsequently, the accuracy of the final draft ("master") is verified by consulting the original literature, and the volume is edited and prepared for publication. The aim is to publish the volume within 12 months after the Working Group meeting.

6. Inclusion criteria for data for the *Handbooks*

The *Handbooks* do not necessarily summarize or even cite the entire literature on the intervention being evaluated. Only those data considered by the Working Group to be relevant to making the evaluation are included. Data judged to be inadequate or irrelevant to the evaluation may, at the discretion of the Working Group, be cited but not summarized. If a group of similar studies is not reviewed, the reasons are indicated (see Part B for details). Meeting abstracts and other reports that do not provide sufficient detail upon which to base an assessment of their quality are generally not considered. With regard to reports of basic scientific research, epidemiological studies, clinical trials, and meta-analyses, only those that have been published or accepted for publication in the openly available scientific literature are reviewed by the Working Group. The same publication requirement applies to meta-analyses or pooled analyses commissioned by IARC in advance of a meeting (see Part B). Government agency reports that have undergone peer review and that are publicly available are considered. Exceptionally, doctoral theses and other materials that are in their final form and publicly available may be reviewed if their inclusion is considered pertinent to making a final evaluation.

B. SCIENTIFIC REVIEW AND EVALUATION

The available studies are summarized by the Working Group, with particular regard to the qualitative aspects discussed below.

Inclusion of a study does not imply acceptance of the adequacy of the study design or of the analysis and interpretation of the results. Major limitations, important aspects of a study that directly impinge on its interpretation, or reasons for not giving further consideration to an individual study are brought to the attention of the reader by the addition of square bracket comments.

Studies that are judged to be inadequate or irrelevant to the evaluation are generally omitted. They may be mentioned briefly: (i) when the information is considered to be a useful supplement to that in other reports; (ii) if they provide the only data available; or (iii) in exceptional cases, if they have been perceived as being pertinent by the scientific community but are deemed otherwise by the Working Group.

The Working Group may conduct additional analyses of the published data and use these in their assessment of the evidence. They are usually identified by square bracket comments.

The framework of a *Handbook* on screening includes the following sections.

1. Global burden and disease characteristics

Descriptive epidemiology

The purpose of this section is to document the importance of the disease in terms of the worldwide burden of the cancer described (mortality, incidence, prevalence, and survival rates), including regional differences and time trends. Expected trends in the absence of screening are a relevant component of this section.

Natural history of the disease, risk factors, treatment, and survival

In this section, the natural history of the disease of interest and the established risk factors are briefly described. Information on treatment and survival in different settings is reviewed, with a worldwide perspective.

2. Screening techniques

It is important to distinguish between screening techniques and screening procedures, i.e. between the technique itself and the way in which it is administered. The two merit separate, detailed evaluation. Each of the screening techniques to be considered is described. The ability of each test to detect cancer and to distinguish cancer from non-cancer conditions is assessed:

- Technique of screening test;
- Technical quality control;
- Screening performance;
- Host factors affecting screening performance;
- Cost of the test when implemented in mass screening programmes.

3. Availability and use of screening programmes

Information on how screening is delivered in different countries is reviewed in this section, with emphasis on the following aspects:

- Infrastructure for diagnosis and treatment: standard diagnostic procedures and treatment regimens and their availability to the target population;
- Extent of population coverage and participation rates;
- Equity, as defined by the extent to which access to the procedure (including diagnostic investigation and treatment) is ensured for

all eligible individuals, irrespective of any personal characteristics;

- Informed decision and informed consent: the extent to which individual values are respected when information on potential benefit and harm is conveyed and recommendations for screening made;
- Behavioural and demographic considerations that affect participation in screening.

4. Efficacy of screening tests

In this section, evidence from efficacy studies is reviewed, and aspects of study design and analysis are critically discussed. The *Handbooks* are not intended to summarize all published studies (see Part A). The Working Group considers the following aspects:

- Relevance of the study;
- Appropriateness of the design and analysis to the question being asked;
- Adequacy and completeness of the presentation of the data;
- Degree to which chance, bias, and confounding may have affected the results.

The appropriate outcomes (mortality or incidence) of a given procedure, for example the detectable phases of the natural history of the disease, are also defined.

Aspects that are particularly important in evaluating randomized controlled trials are: the selection of participants, the nature and adequacy of the randomization procedure, evidence that randomization achieved an adequate balance between the groups, exclusion criteria used before and after randomization, compliance with the intervention in the screened group, and "contamination" of the control group with the intervention. Other considerations are the means by which the end-point was determined and validated (either by screening or by other means of detection of the disease), the length and completeness of follow-up of the groups, and the adequacy of the analysis.

When randomized controlled trials are lacking, relevant observational studies should be considered and similar criteria used for their evaluation. In evaluating case–control and cohort studies, particular attention is paid to the definition of cases, controls, and exposure and, for cohort studies, to the length and completeness of follow-up. Potential bias, especially selection bias, is carefully examined in all observational studies.

5. Effectiveness of population-based screening

The impact of the screening procedure when implemented in defined populations is examined in this section. Indicators used to monitor effectiveness, such as positive and negative predictive values, detection rate, rates of interval cancers, and the number of tests performed, are reported. Time trends before and after implementation of screening as well as comparisons, including geographical comparisons, of the occurrence of the disease and death from the disease in populations exposed and not exposed to screening are reviewed and interpreted. In doing this, the Working Group takes into account differences in screening procedures (e.g. frequency and the age of the target population) and of participation rates.

An integral component of this section is an evaluation of the expected benefit or harm of the screening procedure to the population. Reductions in mortality from and/or incidence of invasive disease are fundamental indicators of benefit. An additional benefit is that more cases may be treated initially by less aggressive, less invasive procedures, thus improving quality of life.

The spectrum of health care is dynamic, and a screening procedure should not be viewed in isolation. Greater awareness of the disease, brought about by publicity about screening that may result in early diagnosis, could be regarded as another benefit of a screening programme. Also, in this section the possibility should be considered that there might have been a change in treatment of the cancer, which even in the absence of screening would have resulted in a substantial decrease in mortality. As far as possible, an evaluation should be made of the extent to which improved treatment has been responsible for any changes seen in mortality from the specific disease. Estimates of rates of false-positive and false-negative findings in screened individuals and their consequences (false sense of security with false-negatives, and false alarm and consequent diagnostic and sometimes therapeutic intervention with false-positives) are an integral part of this section. The rates of short- and long-term side-effects of the screening procedure and the likelihood of unnecessary treatment are discussed.

Management procedures for lesions detected at screening are reviewed. Psychological factors, such as anxiety induced by undergoing the test procedure, are also considered. Finally, the cost–effectiveness of various modalities of test administration in various settings is considered. The discussion takes into account the costs per case detected and per death prevented.

6. Summary

In this section, the relevant data from each of the previous sections are summarized. Inadequate studies identified in the preceding text are not included.

7. Evaluation

Evaluations of the screening procedures

An evaluation of the degree of evidence of the efficacy and of the effectiveness of each screening procedure is formulated according to the following definitions.

Sufficient evidence for the efficacy and effectiveness of a cancer-preventive effect will apply when screening interventions by a defined procedure are consistently associated with a reduction in mortality from the cancer and/or a reduction in the incidence of invasive cancer, and chance and bias can be ruled out with reasonable confidence.

Limited evidence for the efficacy and effectiveness of a cancer-preventive effect will apply when screening interventions by a defined procedure are associated with a reduction in mortality from the cancer and/or a reduction in the incidence of invasive cancer, or a reduction in the incidence of clinically advanced cancer, but bias or confounding cannot be ruled out with reasonable confidence as alternative explanations for these associations.

Inadequate evidence for the efficacy and effectiveness of a cancer-preventive effect will apply when data are lacking, or when the available information is insufficient or too heterogeneous to allow an evaluation.

Sufficient evidence that the screening procedure is not efficacious in cancer prevention will apply when any of the following cases hold:

- The procedure does not result in earlier diagnosis than with standard methods already in use;
- The survival of cases detected at screening is no better than that of cases diagnosed routinely;
- The screening interventions are consistently associated with no reduction in mortality from or incidence of invasive cancer, and bias can be ruled out with reasonable confidence.

In the case of *limited* or *inadequate* evidence, the Working Group should highlight those aspects of the procedure for which information is lacking, and which led to the uncertainty in evaluation. This will provide indications of research priorities.

Overall evaluation

The body of evidence for each screening procedure is considered as a whole, and summary statements are made about the cancer-preventive effects of the screening intervention and other beneficial or adverse effects, as appropriate. The overall evaluation is usually in the form of a narrative. The data on the effectiveness of the screening intervention are summarized, including the factors that determine its success and failure under routine conditions. Finally, the balance between expected benefit and harm is described.

References

Cochrane AL (1972). Effectiveness and efficiency: random reflections on health services. Oxford: Nuffield Provincial Hospitals Trust.

Ferlay J, Soerjomataram I, Dikshit R, Eser S, Mathers C, Rebelo M et al. (2015). Cancer incidence and mortality worldwide: sources, methods and major patterns in GLOBOCAN 2012. *Int J Cancer*, 136(5):E359–86. doi:10.1002/ijc.29210 PMID:25220842

Porta M, editor (2008). A dictionary of epidemiology, 5th edition. Oxford: Oxford University Press.

GENERAL REMARKS

This fifteenth Volume of the *IARC Handbooks of Cancer Prevention* series evaluates the beneficial and adverse effects of various modalities of breast cancer screening. It is the first Volume since the relaunch of the series in 2014; the fourteenth Volume was published in 2011 (IARC, 2011).

The *IARC Handbooks of Cancer Prevention* have had a major impact on WHO global cancer policies. The previous *Handbook* on breast cancer screening, published in 2002 (IARC, 2002a), was for more than a decade the reference for governments when deciding on a national breast cancer screening programme.

Breast cancer has become the most common cancer in women worldwide, in both developed and developing countries. Primary prevention can be achieved by reducing exposure to preventable risk factors, such as excess body fatness (IARC, 2002b) and consumption of alcoholic beverages (IARC, 2012), and by increasing physical activity (IARC, 2002b); secondary prevention provides important additional options for breast cancer control.

In 2002, a Working Group of international experts developed Volume 7 of the *IARC Handbooks*, on breast cancer screening (IARC, 2002a). The resulting consensus evaluations are presented in Table 1.

Recent improvements in treatment outcomes for late-stage breast cancer, and renewed concerns about overdiagnosis, call for an up-to-date, systematic, transparent, and independent evaluation of the benefits and harms of mammography screening. The definition of what constitutes the best implementation of mammography screening programmes (e.g. which age groups should be screened and with what frequency) needs to be revisited in the light of the results of recent studies. In addition, new studies on clinical breast examination and breast self-examination warrant a re-evaluation of their efficacy and effectiveness in reducing mortality from breast cancer.

Furthermore, imaging techniques other than mammography need a rigorous scientific evaluation of their usefulness for breast cancer screening. These include: adjunct ultrasonography for women with dense breasts; digital tomosynthesis; magnetic resonance imaging, either as adjunct to mammography or as a stand-alone technique; and positron emission tomography.

Finally, the screening of women at increased risk of breast cancer requires a thorough reassessment, particularly in the context of better data now available on adjunct or alternative screening modalities.

After a review of the available literature, the Working Group made evaluations for different outcomes and variables, including age group, screening interval, adverse effects, and cost–effectiveness. For the screening of women at increased risk, evaluations were made for four different risk categories (*BRCA* mutations, family history of breast cancer without known mutations, personal history of breast cancer, and

Table 1 Evaluations of breast cancer screening, *IARC Handbooks* Volume 7 (2002)

Type of evaluation	Strength of evidence
Effect of screening with mammography in reducing mortality from breast cancer for women aged 50–69 years	*Sufficient evidence*
Effect of screening with mammography in reducing mortality from breast cancer for women aged 40–49 years	*Limited evidence*
Effect of screening with mammography in reducing mortality from breast cancer for women younger than 40 years or older than 69 years	*Inadequate evidence*
Effect of breast cancer screening by clinical breast examination in reducing mortality from breast cancer	*Inadequate evidence*
Effect of breast cancer screening by breast self-examination in reducing mortality from breast cancer	*Inadequate evidence*

personal history of breast lesions) and various screening modalities and combinations thereof.

The aim of breast cancer awareness programmes is to educate women about the signs and symptoms of breast cancer and the importance of seeking early diagnosis and treatment. Overall, these steps aim at promoting the early diagnosis of the disease, for better treatment and prognosis; they are not considered as *screening* activities and are therefore not included in the evaluation.

While this Volume does not provide public health recommendations regarding implementation of breast cancer screening or recommendations for future research, it may serve as the scientific evidence base for implementation of national breast cancer screening programmes.

A summary of the findings of this Volume has appeared in *The New England Journal of Medicine* (Lauby-Secretan et al., 2015).

References

IARC (2002a). Breast cancer screening. *IARC Handb Cancer Prev*, 7:1–229. Available from: http://www.iarc.fr/en/publications/pdfs-online/prev/handbook7/Handbook7_Breast.pdf.

IARC (2002b). Weight control and physical activity. *IARC Handb Cancer Prev*, 6:1–315. Available from: http://www.iarc.fr/en/publications/pdfs-online/prev/handbook6/Handbook6.pdf.

IARC (2011). Effectiveness of tax and price policies for tobacco control. *IARC Handb Cancer Prev*, 14:1–366. Available from: http://www.iarc.fr/en/publications/pdfs-online/prev/handbook14/handbook14.pdf.

IARC (2012). Personal habits and indoor combustions. *IARC Monogr Eval Carcinog Risks Hum*, 100E:1–575. Available from: http://monographs.iarc.fr/ENG/Monographs/vol100E/index.php. PMID:23193840

Lauby-Secretan B, Scoccianti C, Loomis D, Benbrahim-Tallaa L, Bouvard V, Bianchini F et al.; International Agency for Research on Cancer Handbook Working Group (2015). Breast-cancer screening – viewpoint of the IARC Working Group. *N Engl J Med*, 372(24):2353–8. doi:10.1056/NEJMsr1504363 PMID:26039523

LIST OF ABBREVIATIONS

ABUS	automated breast ultrasonography
ACR	American College of Radiology
ACS	American Cancer Society
ADH	atypical ductal hyperplasia
AJCC	American Joint Committee on Cancer
ALH	atypical lobular hyperplasia
APC	annual percentage change
ASP	active study population
BI-RADS	Breast Imaging Reporting and Data System
BMI	body mass index
BSE	breast self-examination
BSGI	breast-specific gamma imaging
CANSA	Cancer Association of South Africa
CBCSI	Canadian Breast Cancer Screening Initiative
CBE	clinical breast examination
cDNA	complementary DNA
CI	confidence interval
CMF	cyclophosphamide, methotrexate, and 5-fluorouracil
CNBSS	Canadian National Breast Screening Study
2D	two-dimensional
3D	three-dimensional
DALY	disability-adjusted life year
DCIS	ductal carcinoma in situ
DWI	diffusion-weighted imaging
EBSN	European Breast Screening Network
ER	estrogen receptor
EU	European Union
FDG	fluorodeoxyglucose
GDP	gross domestic product
HDI	Human Development Index
HER2	human epidermal growth factor receptor 2
HHUS	handheld ultrasonography
HR	hazard ratio
HRT	hormone replacement therapy

IBM	incidence-based mortality
ICER	incremental cost–effectiveness ratio
JRC	European Commission Joint Research Centre
LCIS	lobular carcinoma in situ
LFS	Li–Fraumeni syndrome
LMICs	low- and middle-income countries
MISCAN	Microsimulation Screening Analysis
MQSA	Mammography Quality Standards Act
MRI	magnetic resonance imaging
mRNA	messenger RNA
NGOs	nongovernmental organizations
NHS	National Health Service
OMIM	Online Mendelian Inheritance in Man
OR	odds ratio
PBCR	population-based cancer registry
PEM	positron emission mammography
PET	positron emission tomography
PPV	positive predictive value
PR	progesterone receptor
PSP	passive study population
QALY	quality-adjusted life year
RCT	randomized controlled trial
RR	relative risk
SBCN	Swaziland Breast Cancer Network
SEER	Surveillance, Epidemiology, and End Results
STORM	Screening with Tomosynthesis or Standard Mammography
TNM	tumour–node–metastasis
UICC	Union for International Cancer Control
USPSTF	United States Preventive Services Task Force
WHO	World Health Organization

GLOSSARY

Background incidence rate	The breast cancer incidence rate expected in the absence of screening.
Breast awareness	Breast awareness programmes are intended to encourage women to be conscious of how their breasts normally look and feel, so that they can recognize and report any abnormality, with the goal of improving breast cancer survival by detecting breast cancer at an early stage.
Breast cancer detection rate	The number of histologically proven malignant lesions of the breast, in situ (ductal only, not lobular) and invasive, detected at screening per 1000 women.
Breast cancer incidence rate	The rate at which new cases of breast cancer occur in a population. The numerator is the number of newly diagnosed cases of breast cancer that occur in a defined period. The denominator is the population at risk of a diagnosis of breast cancer during this defined period, sometimes expressed as person–time at risk during that period.
Breast cancer mortality rate	The rate at which deaths from breast cancer occur in a population. The numerator is the number of breast cancer deaths that occur in a defined time period. The denominator is the population at risk of dying from breast cancer during this defined period, sometimes expressed as person–time at risk during that period.
Breast cancer register	A record of information on all new cases of breast cancer and deaths from breast cancer that occur in a defined population.
Breast cancer survival rate	The percentage of women in a study group who are still alive for a certain period of time after they were diagnosed with breast cancer. The survival rate is often stated as the 5-year survival rate, which is the percentage of women in a study who are alive 5 years after their diagnosis.
Breast density	The relative proportion of radiodense mammary collagen-rich stromal tissues in the breast, as opposed to the lower-density adipose tissue. Commonly referred to as "mammographic density".
Breast self-examination	An examination of a woman's breasts by the woman herself, purportedly for early detection of breast cancer.
Clinical breast examination	A detailed examination of a woman's breasts by a health-care professional (i.e. nurse, physician, or surgeon) for early detection of breast cancer. (See also "Physical breast examination".)
Effectiveness	A measure of the extent to which screening, when deployed in the field under real conditions, does what it is intended to do for a specified population. The most important indicator of the effectiveness of a screening programme is its effect in reducing breast cancer mortality.
Efficacy	The extent to which screening produces a beneficial result under ideal conditions. Randomized controlled trials, which are conducted to initially assess whether screening works, assess efficacy by estimating a primary outcome, such as reduction in breast cancer mortality in the study arm compared with the control arm.
Eligible population	The adjusted target population, i.e. the target population minus those women who are excluded according to screening policy on the basis of eligibility criteria other than age, sex, and geographical location.

False positive	A test result indicating that a person has breast cancer when the person does not have breast cancer.
Incremental cancer detection rate	The number of additional cancers detected at screening with a particular modality relative to another. This is often stated as a percentage of screens or as a rate per 1000 screens.
Interval cancer	A primary breast cancer diagnosed in a woman who had a result in a screening test, with or without further assessment, that was negative for malignancy, either (i) before the next invitation to screening was due or (ii) within a period equal to a screening interval for a woman who has reached the upper age limit for screening.
Interval cancer rate	The number of interval cancers diagnosed within a defined period since the last negative result in a screening examination, per 1000 women with negative results.
Invasive breast cancer	Invasive carcinoma of the breast is a malignant tumour, commonly adenocarcinoma, part or all of which penetrates the basement membrane of the mammary epithelial site of origin, particularly from the terminal duct lobular unit.
Lead time	The period between when a cancer is found by screening and when it would have been detected from clinical signs and symptoms (not directly observable) in the absence of screening.
Length bias	The bias towards detection of cancers with longer sojourn times, and therefore a better prognosis, by screening.
Opportunistic screening	Screening outside an organized or population-based screening programme, as a result of, for example, a recommendation made during a routine medical consultation, a consultation for an unrelated condition, on the basis of a possibly increased risk of developing breast cancer (family history or other known risk factor), or by self-referral. Opportunistic screening relies on individual health-care providers taking the initiative to offer screening or to encourage individuals to participate in a screening programme, or to undertake screening outside the context of any programme.
Organized screening	Screening programmes organized at national or regional level, with an explicit policy, a team responsible for organization and for health care, and a structure for quality assurance.
Overdiagnosis	The diagnosis of a breast cancer as a result of screening that would not have been diagnosed in the patient's lifetime if screening had not taken place.
Participation rate	The number of women who have a screening test as a proportion of all women who are invited to attend screening.
Physical breast examination	An examination of the breast performed to differentiate normal breast tissue from possibly cancerous breast tissue. The term is often used to mean specifically "clinical breast examination" (see this term).
Positive predictive value	The proportion of all positive results at screening that lead to a diagnosis of cancer.
Prevalence	The proportion of a population that exhibits a disease (classified as cases) at a single point in time. Approximately the product of the incidence and the average duration of the disease.
Recall	The physical recall of women to the screening unit, as a consequence of the screening examination, for (i) a repeat mammogram because of technical inadequacy of the screening mammogram (technical recall) or (ii) clarification of a perceived abnormality detected at screening, by performance of an additional procedure (recall for further assessment).
Recall rate	The number of women recalled for further assessment as a proportion of all women who were screened.
Refined mortality	The breast cancer mortality rate ascertained specific to the diagnostic period, excluding women in whom breast cancer was diagnosed before screening began.
Screening interval	The fixed interval between routine screenings decided upon in each programme, depending on screening policy.
Screening policy	A policy for a specific screening programme that defines the targeted age and sex group, the geographical area, and other eligibility criteria; the screening test and interval (usually 2 or 3 years); and requirements for payment or co-payment, if applicable. As a minimum, the screening protocol and repeat interval and determinants of eligibility for screening are stated.
Screening test	A test applied to all women participating in a programme. In mammography screening, it usually consists of a bilateral, two-view mammogram with or without clinical examination.

Sensitivity	The proportion of truly diseased persons in the screened population who are identified as diseased by the screening test. The more general expression for "sensitivity of the screening programme" refers to the ratio of true positives (breast cancers correctly identified at the screening examination) / [true positives + false negatives (breast cancers not identified at the screening examination, detected as interval cases)].
Sojourn time	The preclinical detectable phase; the duration during which a tumour is detectable by screening but before clinical signs and symptoms appear (not directly observable).
Specificity	The proportion of truly non-diseased persons in the screened population who are identified as non-diseased by the screening test (i.e. true negatives / [true negatives + false positives]).
Stage shift	A shift of the stage distribution of the tumours detected towards a lower stage.
Target population	The age-eligible population for screening, for example all women offered screening according to the policy.
Unrefined mortality	The breast cancer mortality rate regardless of the time of diagnosis.

1. BREAST CANCER

1.1 The global burden of breast cancer: incidence, mortality, survival, and prevalence

1.1.1 Global burden

Breast cancer is the most commonly diagnosed cancer in women and the most common cause of cancer death in women worldwide. Globally, it is estimated that in 2012 there were 1.68 million new diagnoses (25% of all new cancer diagnoses in women) and 0.52 million deaths (15% of all cancer deaths in women) from invasive breast cancer, corresponding to age-standardized incidence and mortality rates of 43.3 and 12.9 per 100 000, respectively (Ferlay et al., 2013, 2014a). Unless otherwise stated, all further references in Section 1 to breast cancer refer to invasive breast cancer in women.

Before age 75 years, 1 in 22 women will be diagnosed with breast cancer and 1 in 73 women will die from breast cancer, worldwide. Breast cancer in men is a very rare disease, with incidence rates of about 1% of those for women and with little evidence for changes over time (Ly et al., 2013). Male breast cancer is not considered further in this Handbook.

The estimated global incidence of breast cancer in 2012 was 3 times that of the next most common types of cancer in women: cancers of the colorectum (0.61 million new cases, 14.3 per 100 000), lung (0.58 million, 13.6 per 100 000), and cervix (0.53 million, 14.0 per 100 000) (Fig. 1.1; Ferlay et al., 2013, 2014a). Mortality from breast cancer was broadly similar to that from lung cancer in women (0.49 million deaths, 11.1 per 100 000) and substantially greater than that from the next most common causes of cancer death in women: cancers of the colorectum (0.32 million, 6.9 per 100 000) and cervix (0.27 million, 6.8 per 100 000) (Fig. 1.1; Ferlay et al., 2013, 2014a).

About one quarter of the breast cancer cases and deaths in the world in 2012 occurred in Europe, and approximately 15% of the cases and 9% of the deaths occurred in North America (Fig. 1.2; Ferlay et al., 2013, 2014a). However, the largest contributor to the global burden was East and Central Asia, where 36.3% of the cases and 41.5% of the deaths occurred. Within East and Central Asia, China and India contributed substantially to the global burden, with 11.2% and 8.6% of the cases, respectively, and 9.2% and 13.5% of the deaths, respectively. Latin America and the Caribbean contributed 9.1% of the cases and 8.3% of the deaths, whereas sub-Saharan Africa was estimated to contribute 5.6% of the cases and 9.1% of the deaths (Fig. 1.2).

For women diagnosed in 2005–2009, 5-year net survival rates from breast cancer generally exceeded 80% in Europe (excluding eastern Europe), in Australia and New Zealand, and in some countries in South America and Asia, and reached almost 90% in the USA (Allemani et al., 2014). High 10-year relative survival rates have also been reported in the more-developed regions of the world, such as 71.0% in Europe (Fig. 1.3; Allemani et al., 2013) and 82.7% in the

Fig. 1.1 Estimated age-standardized (World) cancer incidence and mortality rates (ASR) per 100 000, for 10 major sites, in men and women, 2012

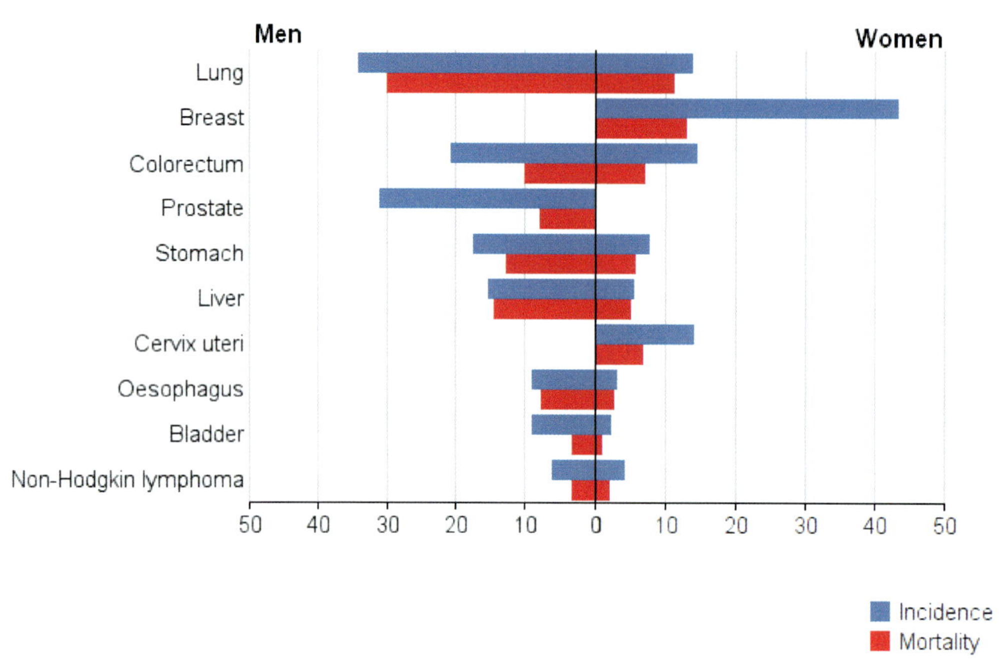

From GLOBOCAN 2012 (Ferlay et al., 2013).
Male breast cancer rates not available.

USA (SEER, 2014a). A combination of this level of survival with high incidence rates results in a high global prevalence of breast cancer. Thus, in 2012 there were an estimated 6.3 million women alive who had had a diagnosis of breast cancer in the previous 5 years (Ferlay et al., 2013). This represents more than one third (36.4%) of all 5-year prevalent cancer cases in women and almost one fifth (19.2%) of those in both sexes combined. There are many more women living with a history of breast cancer than there are people living with a history of any other type of cancer (excluding non-melanoma skin cancer); the next highest estimated 5-year prevalence rates are for prostate cancer (3.9 million) and colorectal cancer (3.5 million in both sexes combined) (Fig. 1.4; Ferlay et al., 2013).

Similarly to most cancer types, both incidence and mortality rates of breast cancer increase with increasing age (Fig. 1.5), although (in the absence of screening) not as rapidly as for most other cancers; the majority of breast cancer cases and deaths occur in women older than 50 years. Of the worldwide burden of 1.68 million incident cases in 2012, 0.55 million (33%) were estimated to occur in women younger than 50 years, 0.91 million (54%) in women aged 50–74 years, and 0.22 million (13%) in women aged 75 years and older. Of the 0.52 million deaths in 2012, 0.13 million (25%) were estimated to occur in women younger than 50 years, 0.27 million (52%) in women aged 50–74 years, and 0.12 million (23%) in women aged 75 years and older (Ferlay et al., 2013).

1.1.2 International variation

Breast cancer was the most frequently diagnosed cancer among women in 140 (76%) of the 184 major countries included in the GLOBOCAN database (Ferlay et al., 2013). In most of the remaining countries, breast cancer was the

Fig. 1.2 Estimated global number of new cases and deaths with proportions by major world regions for breast cancer in women, 2012

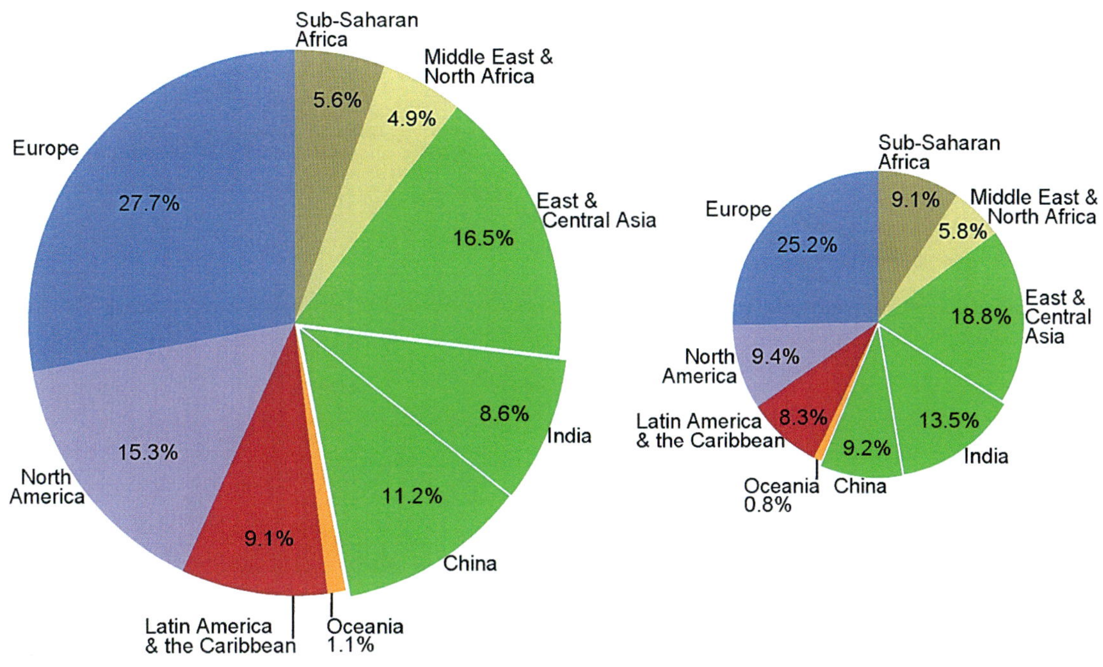

From GLOBOCAN 2012 (Ferlay et al., 2013).

second most frequently diagnosed cancer, after cervical cancer. However, there are substantial regional variations in breast cancer incidence rates worldwide (Fig. 1.6). In 2012, more than a 3-fold variation in the age-standardized breast cancer incidence rates was recorded between North America and western Europe (rates > 90 per 100 000) and Central Africa and East and South-Central Asia (rates < 30 per 100 000) (Fig. 1.7).

At the country level, data from Volume X of *Cancer Incidence in Five Continents* for 2003–2007 showed an approximately 5-fold variation in risk, which can reach 10-fold at the extremes (Fig. 1.8; Forman et al., 2013). In populations with incidence rates higher than 90 per 100 000, such as USA SEER, US Non-Hispanic White (92.5), the Netherlands (93.5), and Belgium (110.8), the risk of a woman being diagnosed with breast cancer before age 75 years is about 1 in 10, whereas in populations with rates lower than 20 per 100 000, such as Thailand, Khon Kaen (18.6), Malawi, Blantyre (14.3), and India, Dindigul (12.0), this risk is less than 1 in 50. Between these extremes, a gradient in risk is observed, including within the same continent. For example, within Europe, rates per 100 000 in Latvia (48.4), Bulgaria (52.7), and Spain, Granada (54.8) were less than half those in Belgium (110.8); similarly, within South America, rates in Ecuador, Quito (38.0) were about half those in Argentina, Córdoba (78.1).

The general shape of the age–incidence curve (Fig. 1.5) – a rapid rate of increase before age 50 years and a general flattening in later years – is observed in many populations. However, there is some variation between countries in the shape after age 50 years. Some populations show a plateau (e.g. Tunisia, North), whereas others show a decline

Fig. 1.3 10-Year age-standardized relative survival (age at diagnosis, 0–89 years) for breast cancer in Nordic countries, 1964–2011

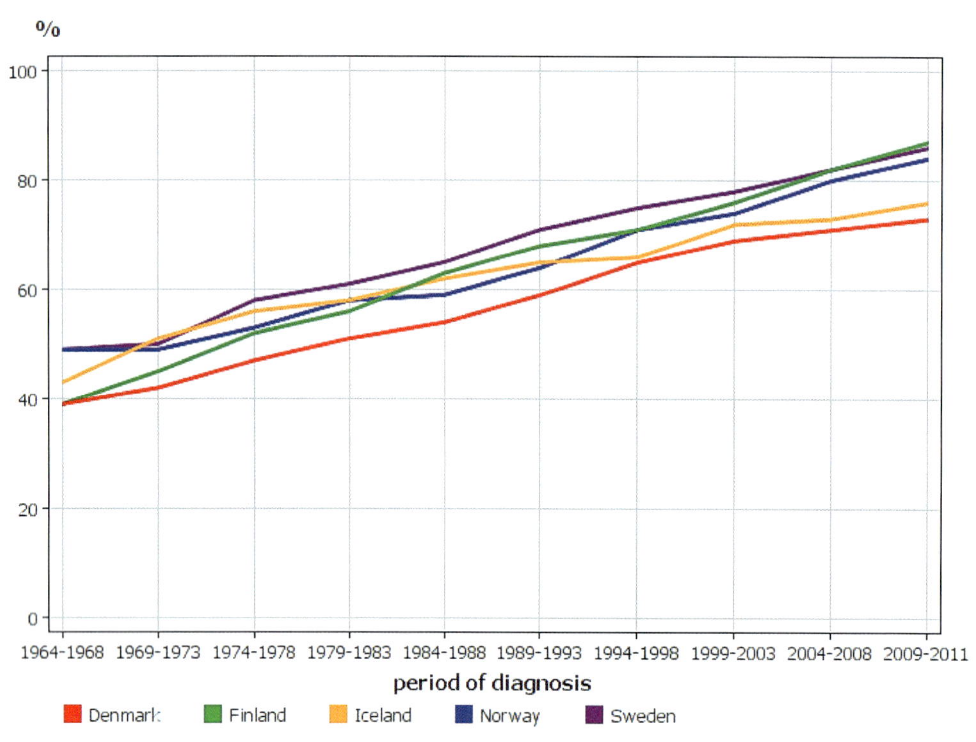

From Engholm et al. (2014). NORDCAN: Cancer Incidence, Mortality, Prevalence and Survival in the Nordic Countries, Version 7.0 (17.12.2014). Association of the Nordic Cancer Registries. Danish Cancer Society. Available from: http://www.ancr.nu, accessed 5 December 2014.

(e.g. Thailand, Khon Kaen), which may be due to an increasing risk of occurrence in successive generations rather than to a real decline in risk with age (Moolgavkar et al., 1979). In less-developed countries, which are characterized by both a generally young age structure and a flat age–incidence curve, the increasing occurrence translates to a considerably lower mean age at diagnosis compared with more-developed countries. Although it has been suggested that this indicates different biological characteristics of breast cancer in women in less-developed countries, the evidence does not generally support such an interpretation (McCormack et al., 2013). Nevertheless, the existing variations in mean age at diagnosis can have important implications for early detection strategies (Harford, 2011; Corbex et al., 2012).

International variation in breast cancer mortality is also evident, although considerably less so than for incidence (Fig. 1.9). Regions with the highest age-standardized mortality rates (> 17 per 100 000) were Melanesia, North Africa, and West Africa; the lowest rates (< 10 per 100 000) were seen in East Asia and Central America (Fig. 1.10). At the country level, selected results from the World Health Organization (WHO) Mortality Database for the period 2003–2007 showed the highest age-standardized mortality rates (~20 per 100 000) in Denmark (21.6), the Netherlands (20.8), Argentina (19.3), and the United Kingdom (19.3); the lowest rates (≤ 6 per 100 000) were seen in Ecuador (6.0), Egypt (5.6), and the Republic of Korea (4.9) (Fig. 1.11; WHO, 2014).

Fig. 1.4 Estimated global number of 5-year prevalent cancer cases in the adult population (total: 32 544 633 for all sites combined) with proportions by major sites for both sexes, 2012

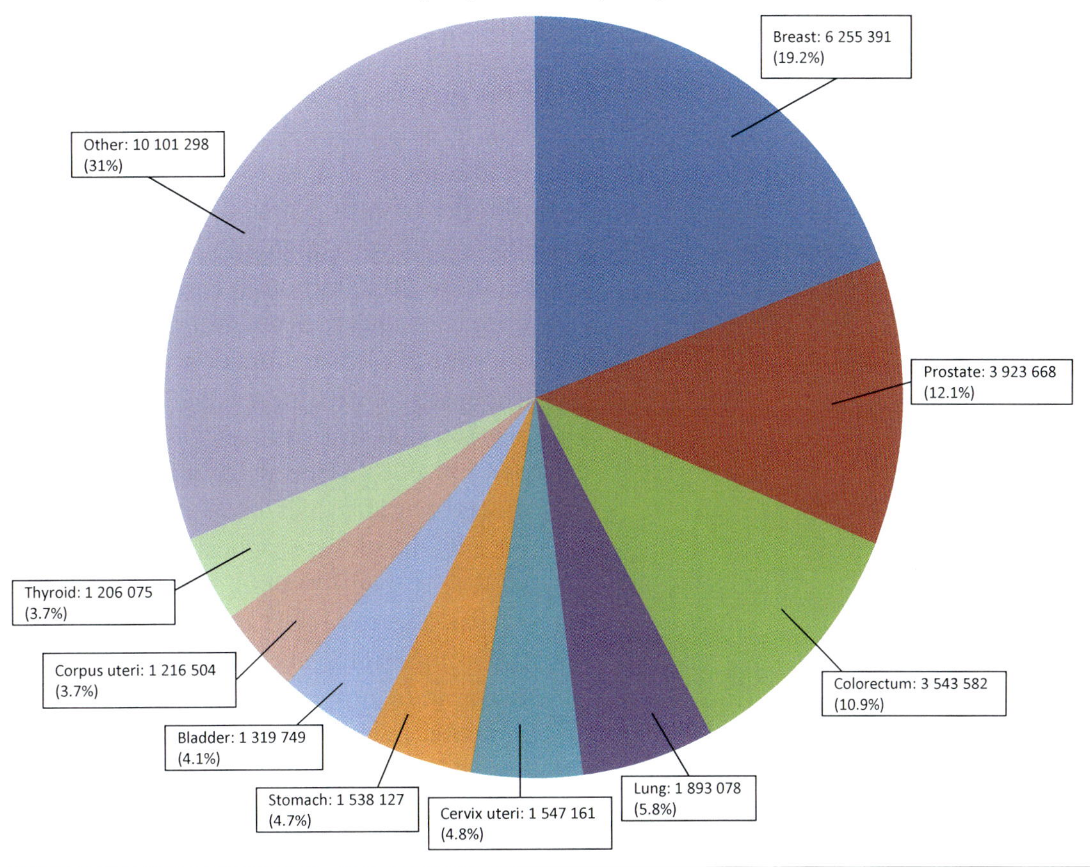

From GLOBOCAN 2012 (Ferlay et al., 2013).
Excluding non-melanoma skin cancer.

This observed smaller variation in mortality rates than in incidence rates is mainly a consequence of the relatively improved survival and lower case fatality rates that are seen in high-incidence, high-income countries and are not generally seen in lower-incidence, lower-income countries. Thus, as stated above, whereas the 5-year survival rate is usually more than 80% in high-income countries, it is about 60% in countries such as Algeria and India (Allemani et al., 2014). Within Europe, 5-year survival ranges from 71% in Latvia to 87% in Finland (Allemani et al., 2014), and 10-year survival ranges from 54% in eastern Europe to 75% in northern Europe (Allemani et al., 2013). In another international comparative study, of women mainly diagnosed in the mid-1990s, the 5-year relative survival rate varied from 82% in China to 47% in the Philippines, 46% in Uganda, and 12% in The Gambia (Sankaranarayanan et al., 2010). Lower relative survival rates are explained largely by lower proportions of women presenting with localized disease, within both high-resource settings (Walters et al., 2013a) and low-resource settings (Sankaranarayanan et al., 2010). Comparable differences can also be observed within countries, among different socioeconomic, racial, or ethnic groups. For example, within the USA in 2011, White women had a slightly higher age-standardized breast cancer incidence rate compared with Black women (127.2 vs 122.7 per 100 000, respectively) and a lower

Fig. 1.5 Age-specific incidence rates per 100 000 for breast cancer in women in selected cancer registry populations, 2003–2007

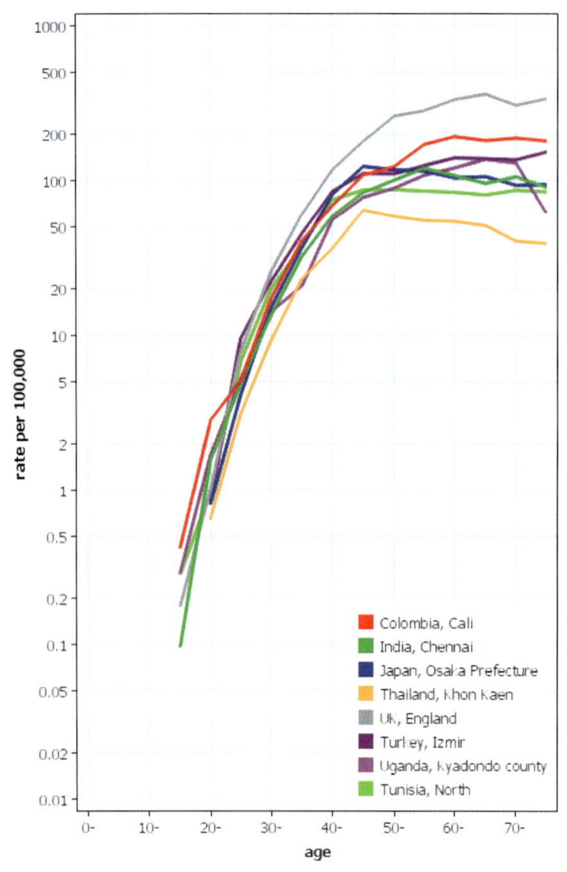

From *Cancer Incidence in Five Continents*, Volume X (Forman et al., 2013).

age-standardized mortality rate (20.9 vs 30.2 per 100 000, respectively) (SEER, 2014a). This finding reflects substantially different survival rates (90.0% vs 77.3% at 5 years and 84.3% vs 68.4% at 10 years, respectively) (SEER, 2014a).

1.1.3 Incidence and mortality in relation to level of development

Table 1.1 compares incidence and mortality estimates for breast cancer among countries aggregated according to four different levels of the Human Development Index (HDI) in 2012 (UNDP, 2012). The HDI is a composite index based on life expectancy at birth, adult literacy rate, education enrolment rate, and gross domestic product (GDP) per capita. In 2012, almost half of the global breast cancer burden (45%; 0.75 million cases) and one third of the breast cancer deaths (33%; 0.17 million) occurred in countries with very high HDI. A substantial number of cases (29%; 0.49 million) and deaths (35%; 0.18 million) occurred in countries with medium HDI, although this includes the highly populous countries of China and India. Whereas age-standardized incidence rates broadly increased with increasing HDI (from 32.6 per 100 000 in countries with low HDI to 79.0 per 100 000 in countries with very high HDI), mortality rates had no equivalent relationship with HDI and were highest in countries with low HDI (17.0 per 100 000), largely in sub-Saharan Africa. The net effect of this is that the ratio of the number of deaths to the number of cases (a crude indicator of survival), by HDI category, increases from 23% for very high HDI to 36% for high HDI, 37% for medium HDI, and 47% for low HDI. Breast cancer was the most commonly diagnosed cancer within all four HDI levels, the most common cause of cancer death within the very high and low HDI levels, and the second most common cause of cancer death (after lung cancer) within the high and medium HDI levels.

1.1.4 Time trends

Figs. 1.11–1.14 show the annual age-standardized breast cancer incidence and mortality trends by year, for all ages and for the age group 50–74 years (which is the age group most likely to have received breast cancer screening), for several representative populations.

The incidence graphs make use of data provided by population-based cancer registries and published in successive volumes of *Cancer Incidence in Five Continents* (Ferlay et al., 2014b). Registries have been selected that represent different world regions and for which

Table 1.1 Breast cancer in women: estimated annual number of cases, age-standardized incidence rate, number of deaths, age-standardized mortality rate, and number of deaths as a percentage of number of cases, by HDI ranking and for the world, in 2012

Level of HDI[a]	Number of cases (millions)	ASIR per 100 000	Number of deaths (millions)	ASMR per 100 000	Number of deaths/ number of cases (%)
Very high	0.75	79.0	0.17	14.1	23
High	0.28	45.2	0.10	14.6	36
Medium	0.49	26.5	0.18	9.8	37
Low	0.15	32.6	0.07	17.0	47
World	**1.68**	**43.3**	**0.52**	**12.9**	**31**

[a] The HDI is a composite index based on life expectancy at birth, adult literacy rate, education enrolment rate, and gross domestic product (GDP) per capita. Predefined categories of the distribution of HDI by country have been used: low (HDI < 0.55), medium (0.55 ≤ HDI < 0.7), high (0.7 ≤ HDI < 0.8), and very high (HDI ≥ 0.8) (UNDP, 2012).
ASIR, age-standardized incidence rate; ASMR, age-standardized mortality rate; HDI, Human Development Index.
Derived from GLOBOCAN 2012 (Ferlay et al., 2013).

comparatively long time series were available. In general, all-age incidence rates, although variable between populations, have consistently increased over the five decades considered, although without ever exceeding 100 per 100 000. There are signs of the rate of increase slowing down and the incidence rates reaching a plateau since the late 1990s, noticeably in the higher-incidence countries (Australia, Denmark, Finland, Israel, the United Kingdom, and the USA), whereas the lower-incidence countries tend to show ongoing increases and less of an evident plateau effect in the most recent 10 years (Fig. 1.11). A detailed study from India shows that the recent increase in female breast cancer incidence rates is one of the most important secular trends in the overall pattern of cancer applying to both urban and rural populations (Badwe et al., 2014). Incidence trends for the age group 50–74 years are broadly similar to those for all ages, with some evidence of a downtrend beginning in the late 1990s to early 2000s in the higher-incidence countries (Fig. 1.12).

The mortality data are from the WHO Mortality Database (WHO, 2014), and countries were selected according to the same criteria as for the incidence graphs (different world regions and comparatively long time series). All-age mortality rates increased modestly in most populations until the mid-1980s and have since declined in the higher-mortality countries (Fig. 1.13). Data from Japan singularly show a consistent increase since the mid-1960s. The highest mortality rates were observed in Denmark and the United Kingdom, where they approached 30 per 100 000 in the early 1980s (Fig. 1.13). Mortality trends for the age group 50–74 years are, overall, similar to those for all ages, with a decline in mortality rates over the most recent two decades especially notable in the higher-mortality countries (Fig. 1.14). The start of the period of decline in mortality rates varies between countries (the mid-1980s in the United Kingdom and the USA, the early to mid-1990s in Australia, Denmark, and Israel, and the early 2000s in Estonia).

1.1.5 Time trends by age

Using the same sources as for Figs. 1.11–1.14, a more detailed consideration of time trends for selected individual countries is provided in Fig. 1.15 and Fig. 1.16. Each graph shows time trends for age-standardized breast cancer incidence and mortality, within the age groups 25–49 years, 50–74 years, and 75 years and older. Where possible, these figures are based entirely on national data, but for some (Japan

Fig. 1.6 Global distribution of estimated age-standardized (World) incidence rates (ASR) per 100 000 for breast cancer in women, 2012

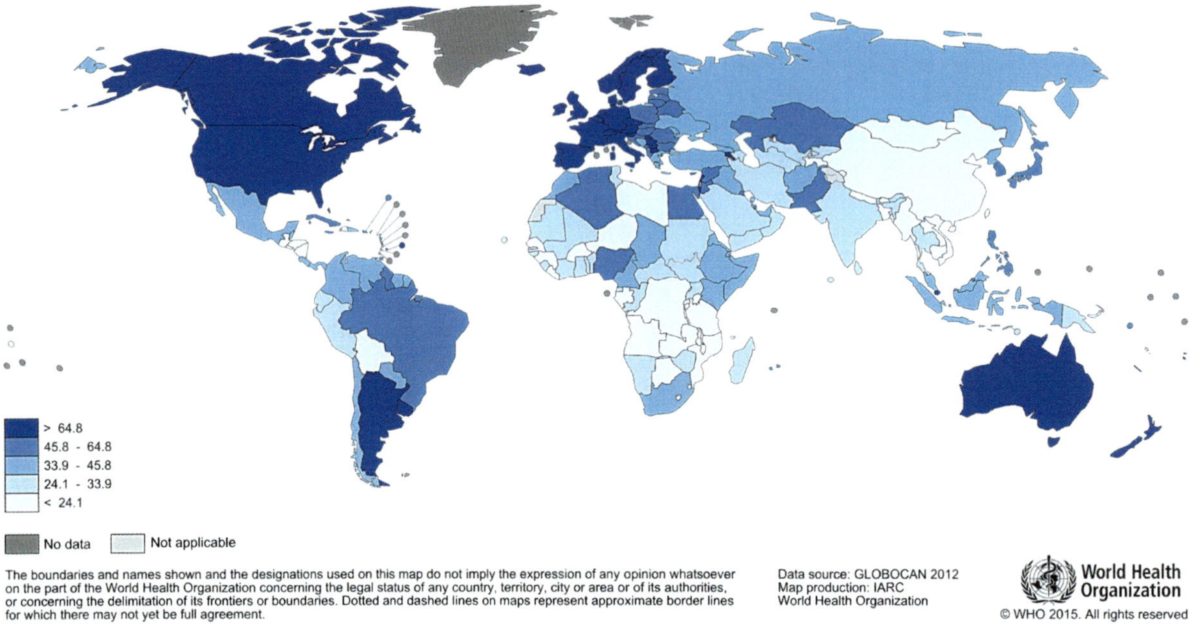

From GLOBOCAN 2012 (Ferlay et al., 2013).

and the USA), regional cancer registry data for incidence and national data for mortality were used. For each country, an indication is provided (by shading) of the period within which population-based breast screening programmes were operational within the age group offered screening (usually the age group 50–69 years) (see Section 3.2). It should be noted that before the implementation of a programme, opportunistic screening would usually have been taking place for subsets of the population, and that after a screening service became operational, full roll-out to eligible women may have taken at least 10 years. In addition, due to the relatively high breast cancer survival rates, several years are required before the impact of a service screening programme becomes discernible in routine cancer statistics. Thus, the time trends shown here are presented to provide context for the incidence and mortality trends, but they do not allow conclusions to be drawn about the impact of breast cancer screening programmes (see Section 5.2.1c for further discussion).

Fig. 1.15 shows trends in countries where national or regional mammography screening services were introduced during the 1980s or the 1990s. An increase in incidence rates in the two younger age groups (25–49 years and 50–74 years) was evident before the introduction of screening; in general, this increase continued after the introduction of screening, but the rate of increase was greater in the age group 50–74 years. Such an increase was generally less evident in the age group 75 years and older, and in Sweden and New Zealand it was hardly evident at all. The introduction of screening tended to coincide with (or to just follow) the beginning of a period of decline in mortality rates in all three age groups. In Denmark, no such decline was apparent in the age group 75 years and older.

Fig. 1.16 shows trends in countries where screening services were introduced after 2000

Fig. 1.7 Estimated age-standardized incidence and mortality rates (ASR) per 100 000 for breast cancer in women, for major world regions, 2012

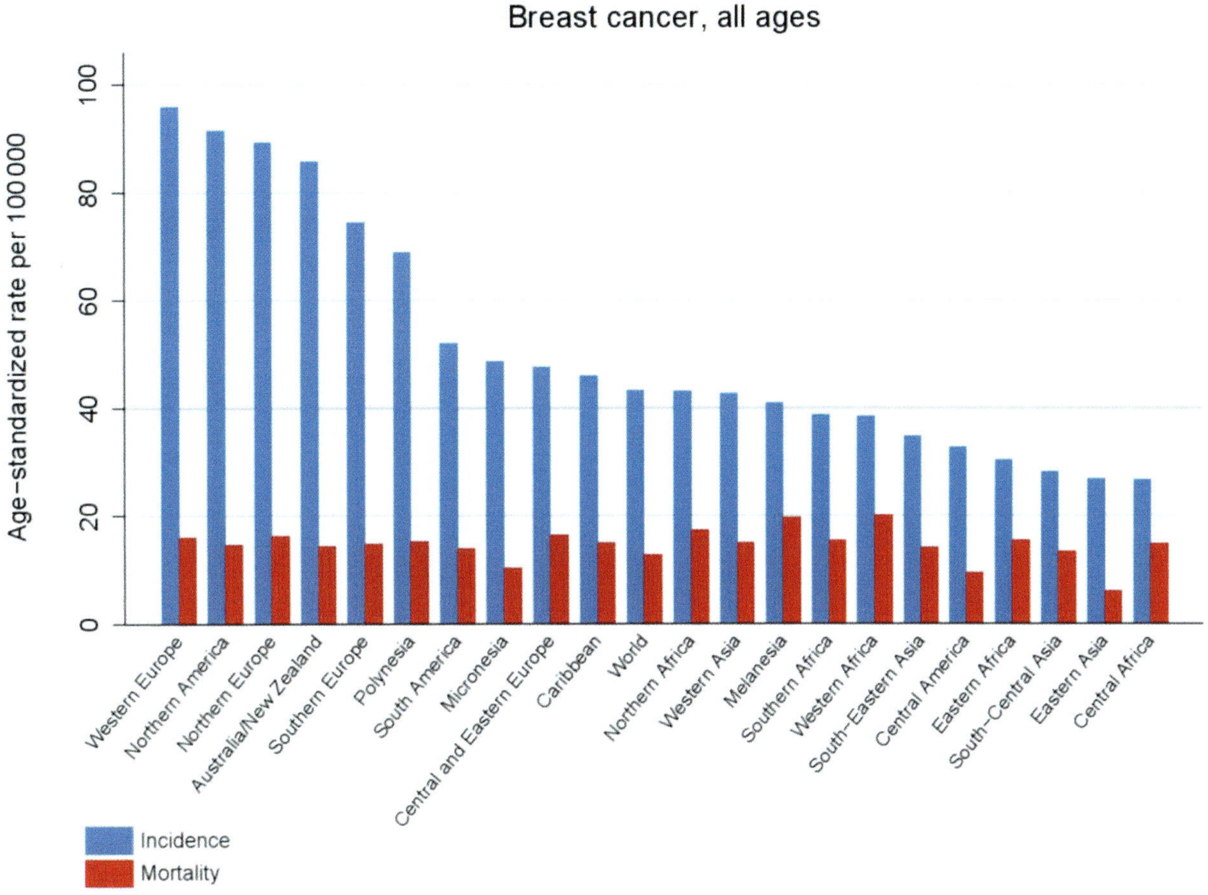

From GLOBOCAN 2012 (Ferlay et al., 2013).

or have never been introduced. In all of these countries, incidence rates increased consistently over time in each of the three age groups. In the Czech Republic, Ireland, Slovakia, and Slovenia, mortality rates declined in the two younger age groups; this decline started before the onset of screening and was less apparent in the age group 75 years and older. In Bulgaria, Costa Rica, Japan, and Singapore, there is evidence of a decline in mortality rates, although this is confined to the age group 25–49 years. In Bulgaria, Japan, and Singapore, mortality rates continued to increase in the two older age groups, whereas in Costa Rica mortality rates increased in the age group 75 years and older but remained stable for the age group 50–74 years.

Overall, Fig. 1.15 and Fig. 1.16 show a general increase in incidence and a general decrease in mortality in all three age groups starting before the introduction of screening programmes. In those countries where screening services were introduced in the 1980s or the 1990s (Fig. 1.15), the increase in incidence was most rapid in the age group 50–74 years. In Bulgaria, Costa Rica, Japan, and Singapore, no decrease in mortality rates was seen in women older than 50 years. It is noteworthy that breast cancer incidence and mortality rates have been changing in different

Fig. 1.8 Age-standardized incidence rates (ASR) per 100 000 for breast cancer in women, in selected cancer registry populations, 2003–2007

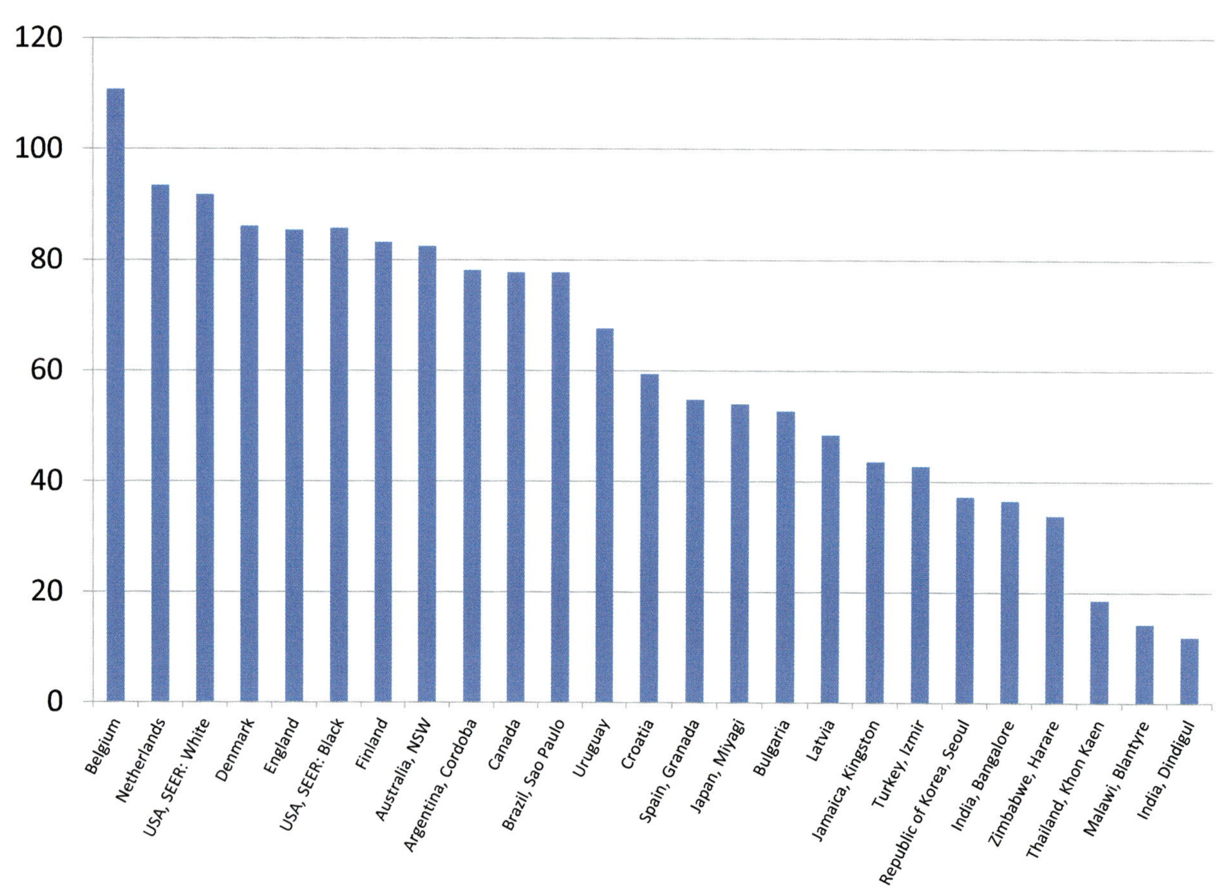

Created by the Working Group using data from Forman et al. (2013).

ways during the recent decades, during which national mammography screening programmes have been established.

1.1.6 Projection to 2025

Table 1.2 shows the estimated global burden of incidence and mortality from breast cancer in 2012 projected to 2025, overall and by HDI category. Overall, a 30% increase in the estimated number of new cases (from 1.68 million to 2.19 million) and a 33% increase in the number of deaths (from 0.52 million to 0.69 million) is projected by 2025. Because of differential population growth levels among different HDI categories, the numbers of cases and deaths are projected to increase most rapidly in countries with low HDI. The number of deaths is also projected to increase more rapidly in countries with medium HDI.

It is important to note that these projections only take account of global demographic changes in population structure and growth based on United Nations estimates (United Nations, 2012). The risk of developing or of dying from breast cancer is assumed to remain constant at 2012 levels, and no allowance is made for changes in screening intensity. At least in more-developed countries, the projections in Table 1.2 may well underestimate incidence and overestimate mortality.

Fig. 1.9 Global distribution of estimated age-standardized mortality rates (ASR) per 100 000 for breast cancer in women, 2012

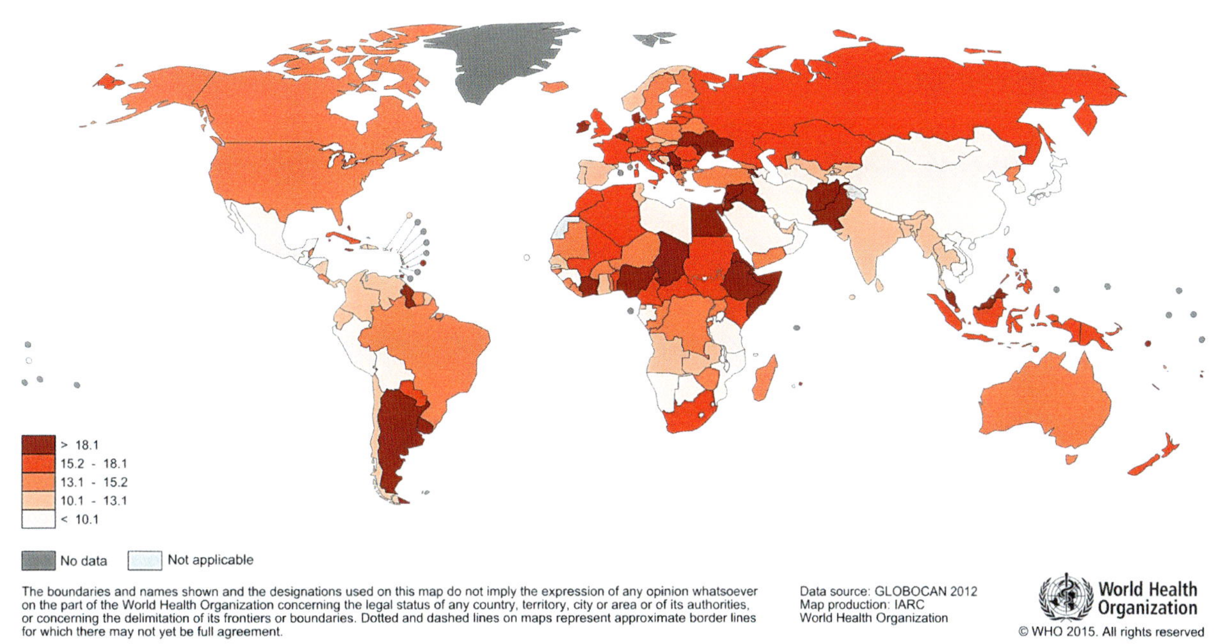

From GLOBOCAN 2012 (Ferlay et al., 2013).

1.2 Classification and natural history

Several guidelines on breast disease classification and on diagnostic criteria with respect to mammography screening are available (NHSBSP, 2005; Perry et al., 2006; Lakhani et al., 2012; Table 1.3). This section highlights areas of relevance to the different forms of breast screening, i.e. all forms of imaging and of palpation. The section on benign breast disease (Section 1.2.1) describes common breast conditions that may be indistinguishable from invasive ones by palpation and/or imaging, and lesions that may exhibit microcalcifications similar to those seen in some forms of carcinoma in situ. The section on breast carcinoma in situ (Section 1.2.2) provides an overview of those lesions that are found at a higher frequency in mammography screen-detected breast cancers than in symptomatic breast cancers, and may thus contribute to overdiagnosis and overtreatment. The section on invasive breast carcinoma (Section 1.2.3) provides a concise summary of the detailed classification and current understanding of the underlying molecular genetic basis (provided in detail elsewhere; Dixon & Sainsbury, 1998; Lakhani et al., 2012). Section 1.2.4 provides an overview of hereditary and somatic mutations in breast cancers.

1.2.1 Benign breast disease

Benign breast conditions constitute a heterogeneous group of lesions, presenting a wide range of symptoms and leading to mammographic abnormalities or incidentally detected microscopic findings. The frequency of presentation of symptomatic palpable benign lesions and invasive lesions differs according to a woman's age. Fibroadenomas are most frequently observed in women younger than 20 years, representing more than 50% of presentations of women in this age group. Women aged 20–50 years generally present with localized benign lesions, and

Table 1.2 Breast cancer in women: estimated annual number of cases and deaths, by HDI ranking and for the world, 2012 and 2025 projection

Level of HDI[a]	Number of cases (millions)			Number of deaths (millions)		
	2012	2025	Increase (%)	2012	2025	Increase (%)
Very high	0.75	0.87	16	0.17	0.21	24
High	0.28	0.37	32	0.10	0.13	30
Medium	0.49	0.64	31	0.18	0.25	39
Low	0.15	0.22	47	0.07	0.11	57
World	**1.68**	**2.19**	**30**	**0.52**	**0.69**	**33**

[a] The HDI is a composite index based on life expectancy at birth, adult literacy rate, education enrolment rate, and gross domestic product (GDP) per capita. Predefined categories of the distribution of HDI by country have been used: low (HDI < 0.55), medium (0.55 ≤ HDI < 0.7), high (0.7 ≤ HDI < 0.8), and very high (HDI ≥ 0.8) (UNDP, 2012).
HDI, Human Development Index.
Derived from GLOBOCAN 2012 (Ferlay et al., 2013).
The 2025 projection is based on demographic change and constant risk.

only about 20% have invasive breast cancer. In contrast, more than 40% of women aged 51–60 years and more than 80% of women aged 60 years and older present with invasive lesions (Lakhani et al., 2012). A similar age-related pattern of palpable symptomatic lesions is usually detected by breast self-examination (BSE). Most benign breast lesions have no known relationship to the development of breast cancer and merit treatment by excision only if causing symptoms, otherwise requiring no intervention.

(a) Histopathological classification of benign breast disease and molecular genetic characteristics

The current WHO classification of tumours of the breast (Lakhani et al., 2012) categorizes benign breast lesions under the categories shown in Table 1.3. Alternative systems of classification essentially use identical terminology and definitions but classify according to specific entity, associations, or clinical relevance. The European Union and the United Kingdom guidelines for classification of common benign breast lesions in the context of breast screening (NHSBSP, 2005; Perry et al., 2006) use the definitions detailed below.

The majority of benign conditions are masses that may be indistinguishable from an invasive breast lesion by palpation or imaging. Some other conditions, particularly forms of benign and neoplastic epithelial proliferations, are also discussed below. These may occur in conjunction with some benign mass-forming entities, for example fibrocystic change, papilloma, and sclerosing lesions, and may present symptomatically or through palpation. In more recent years, they have increasingly been identified (alone or in combination with more subtle forms of related benign breast disease) using mammography, due to their ability to form microcalcifications, particularly of the low-risk clustered type, which can also be associated with low- and intermediate-grade forms of ductal carcinoma in situ (DCIS).

(b) Pathology and molecular genetics of common benign breast conditions

(i) Solitary cyst

This term describes a dilated space with a benign epithelial lining, usually larger than 10 mm and usually attenuated or apocrine in type. No specific molecular genetic changes are associated with this pathology.

Fig. 1.10 Age-standardized mortality rates (ASR) per 100 000 for breast cancer in women, in selected populations, 2003–2007

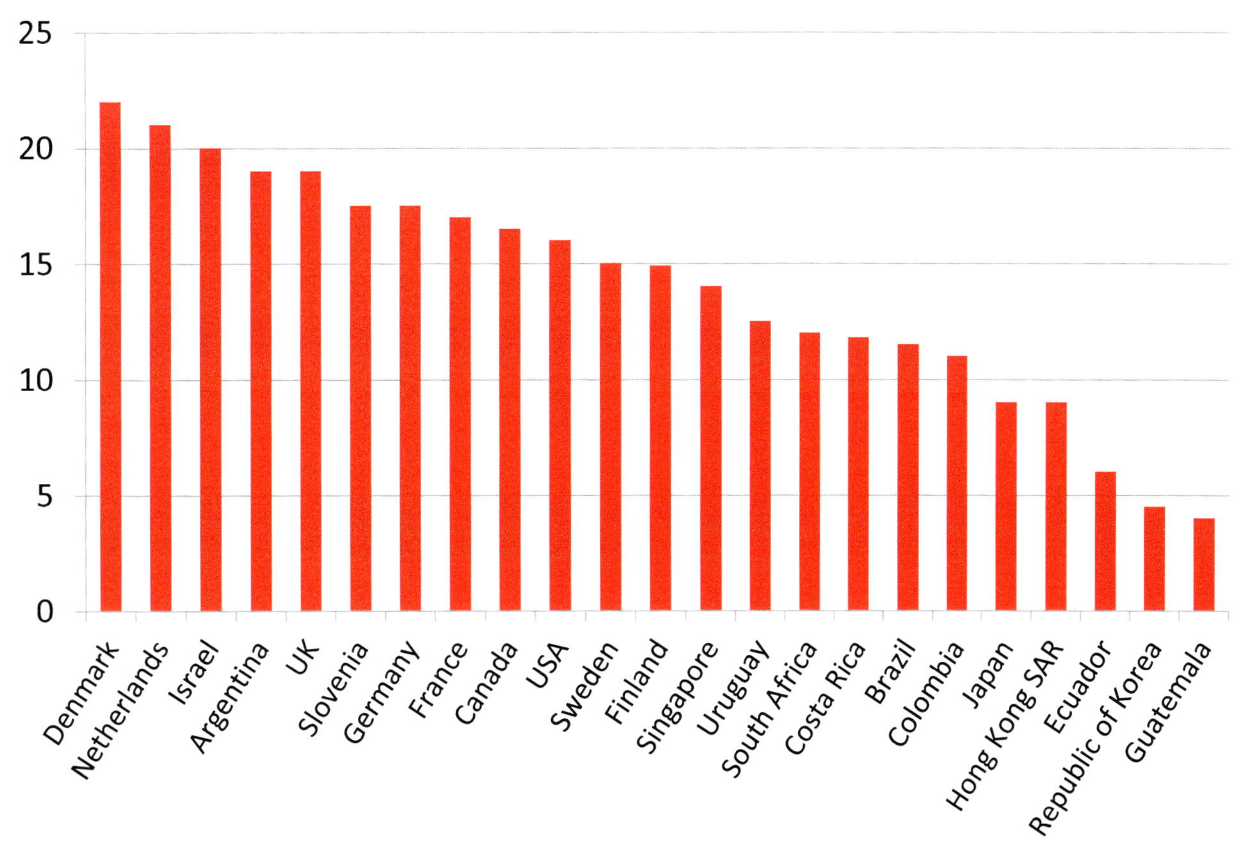

Created by the Working Group using data from WHO (2014).

(ii) Fibrocystic change

This term describes a variety of benign features, including cysts (some of which may be lined by apocrine epithelium), fibrosis, usual epithelial hyperplasia, and columnar cell change. No specific molecular genetic changes are associated with this pathology (see also epithelial hyperplasia below).

(iii) Fibroadenoma

This term describes connective tissue and epithelium exhibiting a pericanalicular and/or intracanalicular growth pattern. The connective tissue is generally composed of spindle-like cells and may rarely also contain other mesenchymal elements such as fat, smooth muscle, osteoid, or bone. The epithelium is characteristically bilayered, but some of the changes commonly seen in lobular breast epithelium (e.g. apocrine metaplasia, sclerosing adenosis, blunt duct adenosis, and hyperplasia of usual type) may also occur in fibroadenomas. Sometimes individual lobules may exhibit increased stroma, producing a fibroadenomatous appearance, and occasionally such lobules may be loosely coalescent. These changes are often called fibroadenomatoid hyperplasia. Consequently, fibroadenomas do not need to be perfectly circumscribed. Old lesions may show hyalinization and calcification (and, less frequently, ossification) of the stroma and atrophy of the epithelium. Calcified fibroadenomas may present as areas of indeterminate calcification, which are detectable by mammography. Fibroadenomas are occasionally multiple.

Fig. 1.11 Age-standardized incidence rates per 100 000 by year in selected populations for breast cancer in women of all ages

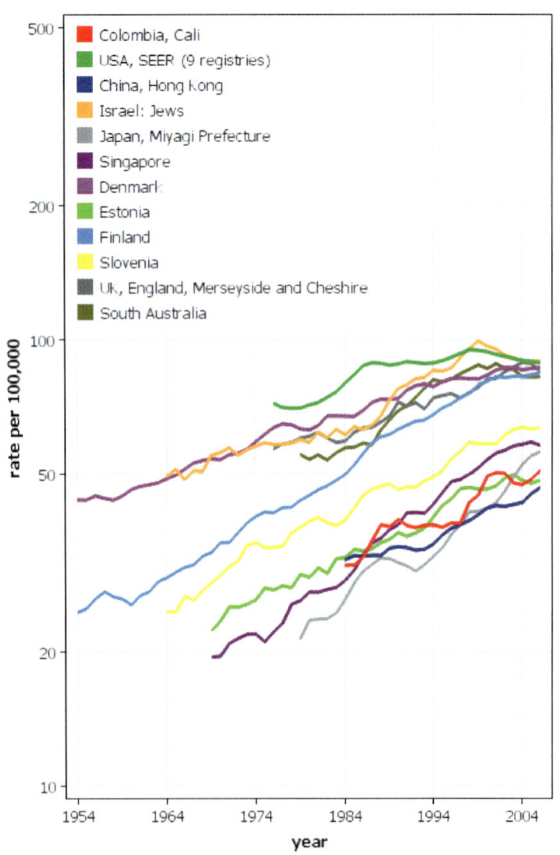

From Ferlay et al. (2014b).

Fig. 1.12 Age-standardized incidence rates per 100 000 by year in selected populations for breast cancer in women aged 50–74 years

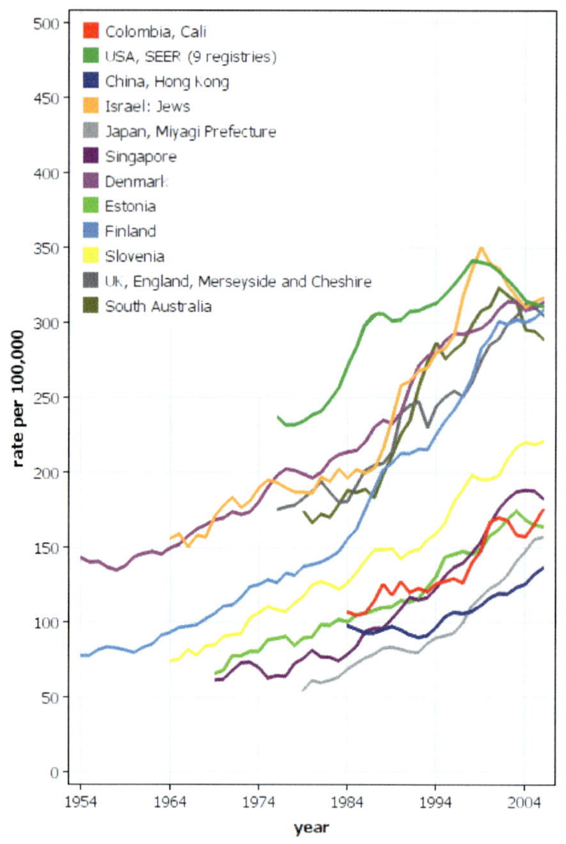

From Ferlay et al. (2014b).

Malignant changes are very rare in the epithelial component, and usually take the form of carcinoma in situ, more frequently lobular carcinoma in situ (LCIS) than DCIS. Fibroadenomas should be distinguished from phyllodes tumours, which are characterized by the presence of increased stromal cellularity and epithelium-lined cleft spaces.

Fibroadenomas have been associated predominantly with polyclonality, although numerical aberrations of chromosomes 16, 17, 18, and 21 have also been described. Phyllodes tumours have been associated with monoclonality, DNA methylation, and alternations of the Wnt signalling pathway.

(iv) *Papilloma*

This term describes an arborescent, fibrovascular stroma covered by an inner myoepithelial layer and an outer epithelial layer. Epithelial hyperplasia without cytological atypia is often present, whereas atypical hyperplasia is rarely seen. Solitary papillomas usually occur centrally in subareolar ducts and are associated with low-grade tumours. Multiple papillomas are more likely to be peripheral and to involve terminal duct lobular units, and are frequently associated with atypical hyperplasia and DCIS.

Fig. 1.13 Age-standardized mortality rates per 100 000 by year in selected populations for breast cancer in women of all ages

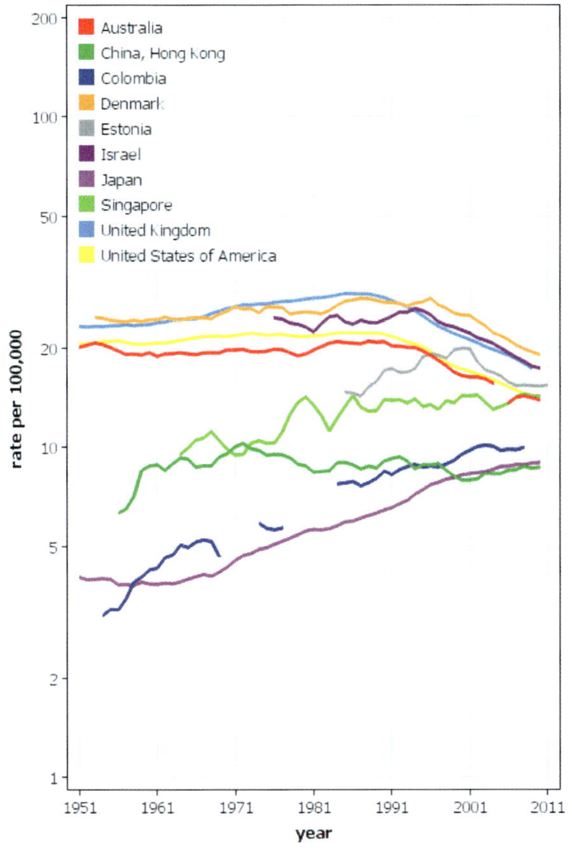

From WHO (2014).

Fig. 1.14 Age-standardized mortality rates per 100 000 by year in selected populations for breast cancer in women aged 50–74 years

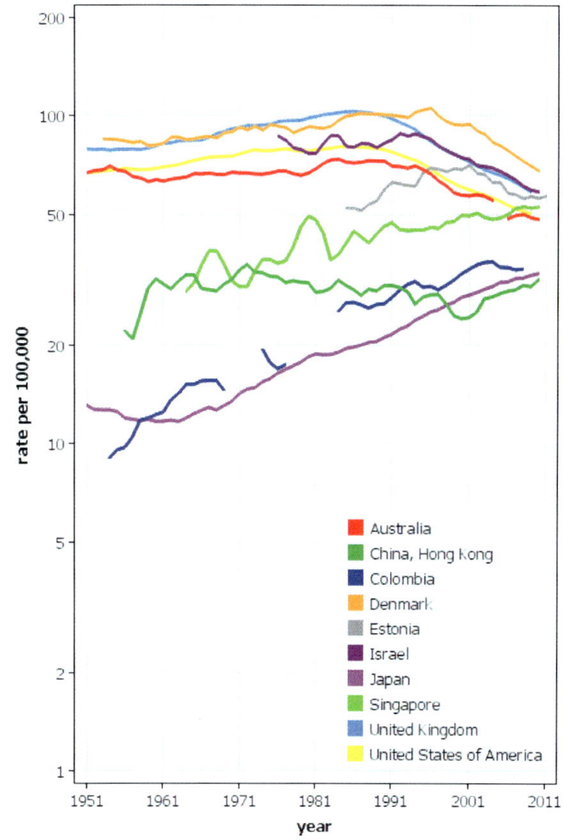

From WHO (2014).

Benign papillomas are monoclonal proliferations characterized by somatic point mutations in the *PIK3CA*, *AKT1*, and *RAS* genes. Alterations of chromosome 16 have been described in both benign and malignant papillary lesions.

Lesions termed ductal adenoma (sclerosing duct papilloma) exhibit a variable appearance, similar to a certain extent to other benign breast lesions. They may resemble papillomas, although they exhibit a growth pattern that is adenomatous rather than papillary.

(v) Sclerosing adenosis

This term describes an organoid lobular enlargement in which increased numbers of acinar structures exhibit elongation and distortion. The normal two-cell lining is retained, but there is myoepithelial and stromal hyperplasia. The acinar structures may infiltrate the adjacent connective tissue and occasionally the nerves and blood vessels, thus possibly leading to an erroneous diagnosis of malignancy. Early lesions of sclerosing adenosis are more cellular-like, and later ones are more sclerotic-like. Calcification may be present. A coalescence of adjacent lobules of sclerosing adenosis may form a mass,

Fig. 1.15 Age-standardized incidence rates (solid lines) and mortality rates (dashed lines) per 100 000 by year in selected countries for breast cancer in women

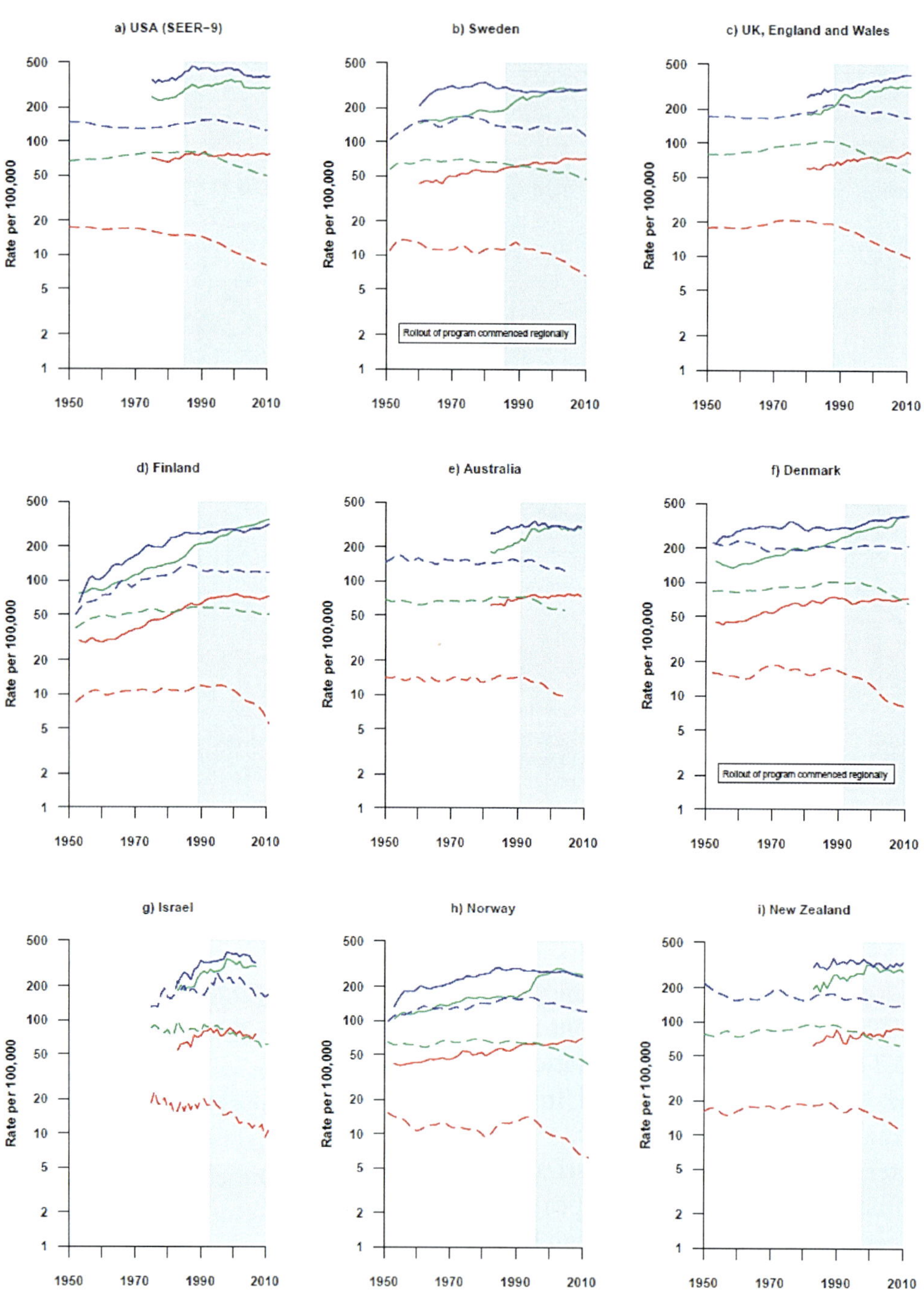

25–49 years (red), 50–74 years (green), and 75 years and older (blue).
Selected countries in which population-based or opportunistic breast cancer screening programmes using mammography were initiated during the 1980s or 1990s. Shading indicates the period within which screening programmes were operational. In Sweden and Denmark, the start of the shaded period indicates the year when pilot screening programmes were implemented in a region of the country before national adoption.
Created by the Working Group using incidence data from Ferlay et al. (2014b) and mortality data from WHO (2014). All data are national, except for incidence data for the USA, which are for the SEER-9 group of cancer registries (Atlanta, Connecticut, Detroit, Hawaii, Iowa, New Mexico, San Francisco-Oakland, Seattle-Puget Sound, and Utah).

Fig. 1.16 Age-standardized incidence rates (solid lines) and mortality rates (dashed lines) per 100 000 by year in selected countries for breast cancer in women

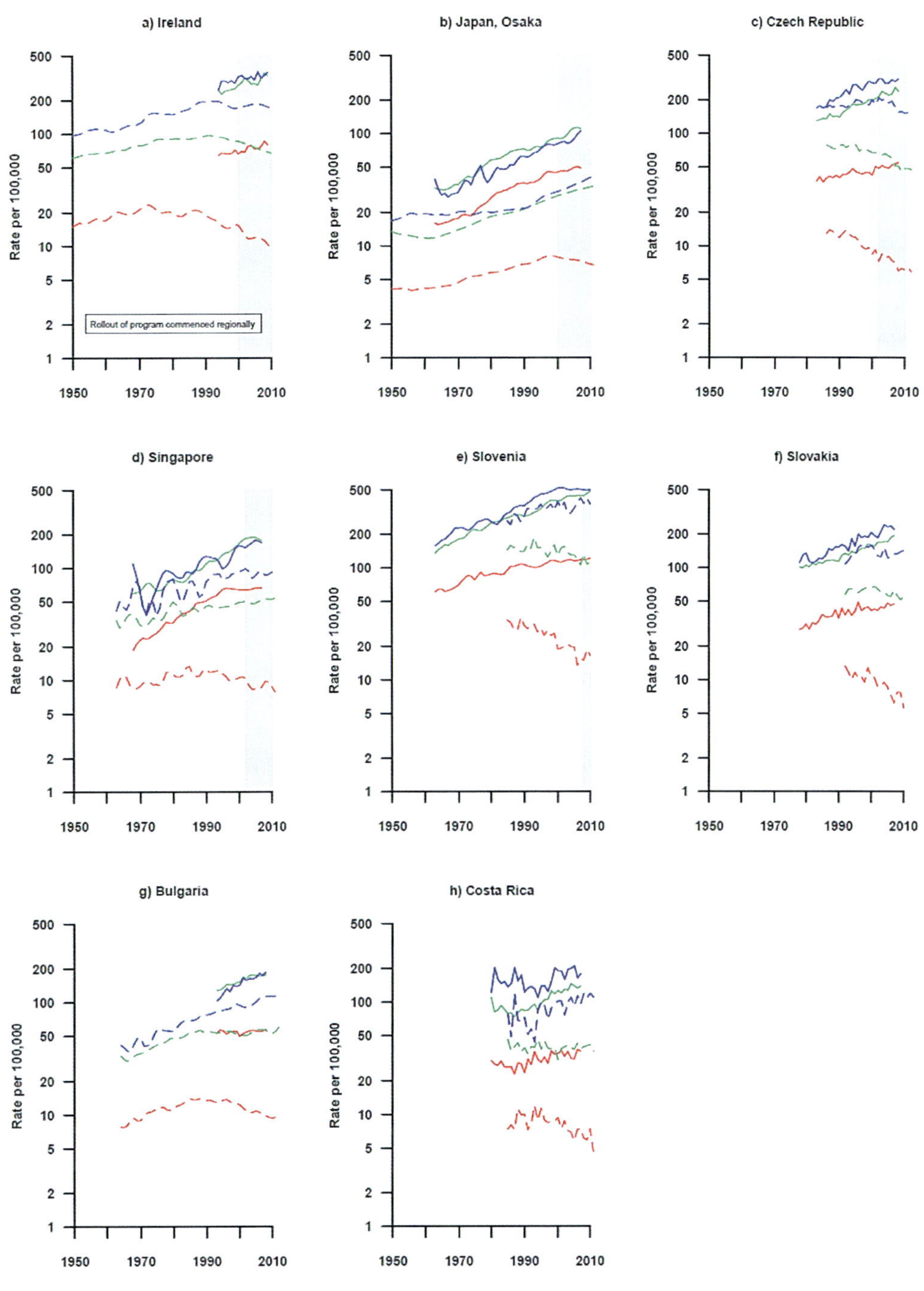

25–49 years (red), 50–74 years (green), and 75 years and older (blue).

Selected countries in which population-based or opportunistic breast cancer screening programmes using mammography were initiated after 2000 or have never been implemented. Shading indicates the period within which screening programmes were operational. In Ireland, the start of the shaded period indicates the year when a pilot screening programme was implemented in a region of the country before national adoption. Created by the Working Group using incidence data from Ferlay et al. (2014b) and mortality data from WHO (2014). All data are national, except for incidence data for Japan, which are for the Osaka Cancer Registry.

Table 1.3 Benign and malignant breast tumours recognized in the current WHO classification of tumours of the breast

EPITHELIAL TUMOURS	
Microinvasive carcinoma	
Invasive breast carcinoma	
Invasive carcinoma of no special type (NST)	8500/3
Pleomorphic carcinoma	8022/3
Carcinoma with osteoclast-like stromal giant cells	8035/3
Carcinoma with choriocarcinomatous features	—
Carcinoma with melanotic features	—
Invasive lobular carcinoma	8520/3
Tubular carcinoma	8211/3
Cribriform carcinoma	8201/3
Mucinous carcinoma	8480/3
Carcinoma with medullary features	
Medullary carcinoma	8510/3
Atypical medullary carcinoma	8513/3
Invasive carcinoma NST with medullary features	8500/3
Carcinoma with apocrine differentiation	—
Carcinoma with signet-ring-cell differentiation	—
Invasive micropapillary carcinoma	8507/3*
Metaplastic carcinoma of no special type (NST)	8575/3
Low-grade adenosquamous carcinoma	8570/3
Fibromatosis-like metaplastic carcinoma	8572/3
Squamous cell carcinoma	8070/3
Spindle cell carcinoma	8032/3
Metaplastic carcinoma with mesenchymal differentiation	8571/3
Mixed metaplastic carcinoma	8575/3
Myoepithelial carcinoma	8982/3
Rare types	
Carcinoma with neuroendocrine features	
Neuroendocrine tumour, well-differentiated	8246/3
Neuroendocrine carcinoma, poorly differentiated (small cell carcinoma)	8041/3
Carcinoma with neuroendocrine differentiation	8574/3
Secretory carcinoma	8502/3
Invasive papillary carcinoma	8503/3
Acinic cell carcinoma	8550/3
Mucoepidermoid carcinoma	8430/3
Polymorphous carcinoma	8525/3
Oncocytic carcinoma	8290/3
Lipid-rich carcinoma	8314/3
Glycogen-rich clear cell carcinoma	8315/3
Sebaceous carcinoma	8410/3
Salivary gland/skin adnexal type tumours	
Cylindroma	8200/0
Clear cell hidradenoma	8402/0*

Table 1.3 (continued)

Epithelial–myoepithelial tumours	
Pleomorphic adenoma	8940/0
Adenomyoepithelioma	8983/0
Adenomyoepithelioma with carcinoma	8983/3*
Adenoid cystic carcinoma	8200/3
Precursor lesions	
Ductal carcinoma in situ	8500/2
Lobular neoplasia	
Lobular carcinoma in situ	
Classic lobular carcinoma in situ	8520/2
Pleomorphic lobular carcinoma in situ	8519/2*
Atypical lobular hyperplasia	—
Intraductal proliferative lesions	
Usual ductal hyperplasia	—
Columnar cell lesions including flat epithelial atypia	—
Atypical ductal hyperplasia	—
Papillary lesions	
Intraductal papilloma	8503/0
Intraductal papilloma with atypical hyperplasia	8503/0
Intraductal papilloma with ductal carcinoma in situ	8503/2*
Intraductal papilloma with lobular carcinoma in situ	8520/2
Intraductal papillary carcinoma	8503/2
Encapsulated papillary carcinoma	8504/2
Encapsulated papillary carcinoma with invasion	8504/3
Solid papillary carcinoma	
In situ	8509/2
Invasive	8509/3
Benign epithelial proliferations	
Sclerosing adenosis	—
Apocrine adenosis	—
Microglandular adenosis	—
Radial scar/complex sclerosing lesion	—
Adenomas	
Tubular adenoma	8211/0
Lactating adenoma	8204/0
Apocrine adenoma	8401/0
Ductal adenoma	8503/0
MESENCHYMAL TUMOURS	
Nodular fasciitis	8828/0*
Myofibroblastoma	8825/0
Desmoid-type fibromatosis	8821/1
Inflammatory myofibroblastic tumour	8825/1
Benign vascular lesions	
Haemangioma	9120/0
Angiomatosis	—
Atypical vascular lesions	—
Pseudoangiomatous stromal hyperplasia	—

Table 1.3 (continued)

Granular cell tumour	9580/0
Benign peripheral nerve-sheath tumours	
Neurofibroma	9540/0
Schwannoma	9560/0
Lipoma	8850/0
Angiolipoma	8861/0
Liposarcoma	8850/3
Angiosarcoma	9120/3
Rhabdomyosarcoma	8900/3
Osteosarcoma	9180/3
Leiomyoma	8890/0
Leiomyosarcoma	8890/3
FIBROEPITHELIAL TUMOURS	
Fibroadenoma	9010/0
Phyllodes tumour	9020/1
Benign	9020/0
Borderline	9020/1
Malignant	9020/3
Periductal stromal tumour, low grade	9020/3
Hamartoma	
TUMOURS OF THE NIPPLE	
Nipple adenoma	8506/0
Syringomatous tumour	8407/0
Paget disease of the nipple	8540/3
MALIGNANT LYMPHOMA	
Diffuse large B-cell lymphoma	9680/3
Burkitt lymphoma	9687/3
T-cell lymphoma	
Anaplastic large cell lymphoma, ALK-negative	9702/3
Extranodal marginal-zone B-cell lymphoma of MALT type	9699/3
Follicular lymphoma	9690/3
METASTATIC TUMOURS	
TUMOURS OF THE MALE BREAST	
Gynaecomastia	
Carcinoma	
Invasive carcinoma	8500/3
In situ carcinoma	8500/2
CLINICAL PATTERNS	
Inflammatory carcinoma	8530/3
Bilateral breast carcinoma	

[a] The morphology codes are from the International Classification of Diseases for Oncology (ICD-O). Behaviour is coded /0 for benign tumours, /1 for unspecified, borderline, or uncertain behaviour, /2 for carcinoma in situ and grade 3 intraepithelial neoplasia, and /3 for malignant tumours.

[b] The classification is modified from the previous WHO histological classification of tumours (2003), taking into account changes in our understanding of these lesions. In the case of neuroendocrine neoplasms, the classification has been simplified to be of more practical utility in morphological classification.

* These new codes were approved by the IARC/WHO Committee for ICD-O in 2013.

Source: Adapted from Lakhani et al. (2012).

detectable by mammography or by macroscopic examination, which is termed "nodular sclerosing adenosis" or "adenosis tumour". Occasionally, apocrine metaplasia is seen in areas of sclerosing adenosis (termed "apocrine adenosis"), with or without cytological atypia. Rarely, the epithelium in sclerosing adenosis may show atypical hyperplasia or carcinoma in situ. No specific molecular genetic changes are associated with this pathology.

(vi) Complex sclerosing lesions and radial scars

This term describes sclerosing lesions with a pseudo-infiltrative growth pattern. A radial scar is characterized by a diameter of 10 mm or less and by a central fibro-elastic zone from which radiate out tubular bilayered structures, which may exhibit intraluminal proliferation. Lesions larger than 10 mm are generally termed complex sclerosing lesions; they have the same features as radial scars but a larger size and more disturbance of structure, often with nodular masses around the periphery. Changes such as papilloma formation, apocrine metaplasia, and sclerosing adenosis may be superimposed on the main lesion, thus giving rise to complex sclerosing lesions. Atypia or a noticeable quantity of carcinoma in situ may also be present. No specific molecular genetic changes are associated with this pathology.

(vii) Periductal mastitis/duct ectasia

This process involves larger and intermediate-size ducts, generally in a subareolar location. The ducts are lined by normal or attenuated epithelium, are filled with amorphous, eosinophilic material and/or foam cells, and exhibit marked periductal chronic inflammation, often with large numbers of plasma cells (periductal mastitis). There may be pronounced periductal fibrosis. Calcification may be present. The process may ultimately lead to obliteration of ducts (duct ectasia), leaving dense fibrous masses, often associated with nipple discharge or retraction. No specific molecular genetic changes are associated with this pathology.

(viii) Inflammatory breast conditions

This term refers to mastitis, mammary duct fistula, lymphocytic lobulitis, specific infections, and granulomatous mastitis. No specific molecular genetic changes are associated with this pathology.

(c) Pathology and molecular genetics of benign epithelial proliferations

(i) Usual epithelial hyperplasia

This term describes the proliferation of a mixed cell population comprising (luminal) epithelial cells and basal/myoepithelial cells with a streaming epithelial architecture, with formation of irregular, slit-like, and peripheral luminal spaces. Most studies have found no consistent molecular genetic alterations associated with this pathology.

(ii) Columnar cell lesions

This term describes blunt duct adenosis, columnar cell change, columnar cell hyperplasia, unfolded lobule, and columnar alteration with prominent apical snouts and secretions. In broad terms, these lesions cover a spectrum of changes, ranging from bland columnar cell change to columnar cell hyperplasia (piling up of several layers) to flat epithelial atypia (superimposed mild atypia). These lesions have become increasingly identified by clinical examination as a consequence of more rigorous investigations of radiological calcifications. Lobular acini are commonly formed and are lined by tall and snouted epithelial cells, similar to those observed in tubular carcinoma. Commonly, this is associated with luminal secretions and/or microcalcifications. As well as atypical ductal hyperplasia (ADH)/low-grade DCIS, other epithelial proliferations may merge or be associated with columnar cell hyperplasia, including atypical lobular hyperplasia (ALH), LCIS, and invasive carcinoma, often of low-grade tubular or tubulolobular type. There is limited information about the molecular genetic alterations associated with this pathology; loss of chromosome 16q is the most frequently described (Moinfar et al., 2000; Simpson et al., 2005; Abdel-Fatah et al., 2008; Go et al., 2012).

(iii) Atypical ductal hyperplasia

ADH is a rare lesion, which is identified based on some but not all features of DCIS. Difficulties are encountered mainly in distinguishing ADH from the low-grade variants of DCIS. Areas of ADH usually do not exceed 2–3 mm in size, with less than two complete membrane-bound spaces. Loss of heterozygosity on chromosomes 16q, 17p, and 11q13 is a common feature of ADH, low-grade DCIS, and low-grade invasive breast cancer, implying that these lesions belong to a precursor progression pathway (Lopez-Garcia et al., 2010; Bombonati & Sgroi, 2011; Lakhani et al., 2012).

(iv) Atypical lobular hyperplasia

ALH and LCIS have traditionally been separated as distinct lesions, based on cytological and quantitative features relating to the extent of lobular involvement and on different risks of subsequent invasive breast cancer. However, the two lesions have similar molecular profiles. It has been suggested that ALH and LCIS should be grouped together as in situ lobular neoplasia, except when their degree and extent can be assessed to estimate the risk of subsequent invasive carcinoma. In situ lobular neoplasia is characterized by the proliferation within the terminal duct lobular units of discohesive round, cuboidal, or polygonal cells with clear or light cytoplasm. The distension of lobular units may vary from patent lumina to complete obliteration. In ALH, there is minimal extension of less than half of the acini, whereas in LCIS more than half of the acini within the terminal duct lobular unit are distended by an expansion of the typical cells (≥ 8 cells across each acinus). ALH and LCIS are clonal lesions and share the same abnormalities, indicating that they are part of a precursor progression pathway. Loss of chromosomes 11q13, 16q, and 17p and alterations of the E-Cadherin *CCND1* locus have been reported (Simpson et al., 2003; Lopez-Garcia et al., 2010; Bombonati & Sgroi, 2011; Lakhani et al., 2012).

(d) Natural history of benign lesions associated with increased risk of breast cancer

See Lakhani et al. (2012) for review.

Various forms of breast epithelial proliferation have been associated with an increased risk of invasive breast cancer (Lopez-Garcia et al., 2010; Bombonati & Sgroi, 2011; Lakhani et al., 2012), both ipsilateral and contralateral. A 1.5–2.0-fold increased risk for usual epithelial hyperplasia, a 2.5–4.0-fold increased risk for ADH, and a 4.0–5.0-fold increased risk for ALH have been reported. Other forms of benign breast disease, such as sclerosing adenosis, fibroadenoma, and papillary apocrine change, appear not to alter the risk of breast cancer or to have a risk equivalent to that for any coexisting epithelial proliferation. All of these epithelial proliferative lesions may be detected by breast screening and excised.

1.2.2 Breast carcinoma in situ

The two non-invasive forms of breast carcinoma in situ are DCIS and LCIS, each with distinctive morphological and behavioural characteristics. The neoplastic cell populations are confined within the parenchymal site of origin without stromal invasion across the basement membrane. DCIS, but rarely LCIS, may harbour calcifications that give rise to mammographic abnormalities.

(a) Pathological classification of DCIS

See NHSBSP (2005), Perry et al. (2006), and Lakhani et al. (2012) for review.

DCIS is, in most cases, a unicentric (involving a single duct system) proliferation of epithelial cells with malignant cytological features within the parenchymal structures of the breast. Most DCIS lesions arise from the terminal duct lobular units.

The classification of DCIS is evolving, and it is now considered to represent a heterogeneous group of in situ neoplastic processes. The cytonuclear features of DCIS are less frequently variable within a lesion, and lesions of high nuclear grade are more clinically aggressive. There is less heterogeneity in nuclear grade characteristics, and most of the contemporary histological classification systems are based on a three-tier grading or differentiation system with nuclear grade: high, intermediate, and low nuclear grades (NHSBSP, 2005; Perry et al., 2006; Lakhani et al., 2012).

High-nuclear-grade DCIS cells have pleomorphic, irregularly spaced, and (usually) large nuclei exhibiting marked variation in size. Mitoses are usually frequent, and abnormal forms may be seen. High-grade DCIS may exhibit several growth patterns, often solid with comedo-type central necrosis, frequently containing deposits of amorphous calcification. Sometimes a solid proliferation of malignant cells fills the duct without necrosis, and is confined to nipple/lactiferous ducts in cases presenting with Paget disease of the nipple. High-nuclear-grade DCIS may also exhibit micropapillary and cribriform patterns, frequently associated with central comedo-type necrosis. A high-grade flat form of DCIS is also recognized, although it is infrequent. These lesions are usually human epidermal growth factor receptor 2 (HER2)-positive.

Intermediate-grade DCIS cells show moderate pleomorphism of the nuclei, which lack the monotony of the low-grade cell type, with nuclei that are typically larger. The growth pattern may be solid, cribriform, or micropapillary, and clear cell or apocrine types often fall into this category.

Low-nuclear-grade DCIS is composed of monomorphic, evenly spaced cells with usually, but not invariably, rounded small nuclei, and rare individual cell necrosis. These cells are generally arranged in micropapillary and cribriform patterns.

A small proportion of cases of DCIS exhibit mixed features of differing nuclear grades.

Other rare, but morphologically distinct, subtypes of DCIS are recognized, but without firm evidence of distinction from more common DCIS forms with regard to their clinical presentation and/or behaviour, with the exception of encysted papillary carcinoma. These include apocrine, clear cell, signet ring, neuroendocrine, and cystic hypersecretory forms of DCIS and variants with a papillary structure, including papillary carcinoma in situ, solid papillary carcinoma in situ, and encysted papillary carcinoma.

(b) Molecular genetic changes of breast carcinoma in situ

Several molecular alterations have been characterized, some of which are related to survival. Molecular genetic studies of low-grade DCIS and ADH have provided evidence that these lesions are clonal and therefore fulfil the basic criterion of neoplastic transformation (Lakhani et al., 1995; Lopez-Garcia et al., 2010). Early molecular studies and particularly comparative genomic hybridization studies suggested that the genetic lesions of DCIS are associated with particular morphological subtypes (Buerger et al., 1999). Well-differentiated DCIS is associated with loss of 16q and 17p, whereas tumours of intermediate and high grades often have losses of significantly more allelic chromosomal arms, frequently including 1p, 1q, 6q, 9p, 11p, 11q, 13q, and 17q (Fujii et al., 1996). High-grade DCIS is associated with gains at 17q but also at 11q and 13q (Chuaqui et al., 1997). Intermediate-grade DCIS shows a combination of lesions, such as 16q loss and gains at other chromosomes, particularly 1q, or gain at 11q or 13q but not at 17q12, which is a feature of high-grade DCIS (Buerger et al., 1999). Similarly, ALH and LCIS show the same genetic mutations, with loss at 16p, 16q, 17p, and 22q and gain at 6q (Lu et al., 1998). Interestingly, low-grade DCIS and ADH share similar genetic alterations with LCIS and ALH but not with high-grade DCIS. These observations challenge the existing assumptions that lobular and ductal lesions are distinct and that DCIS is a homogeneous disease.

It has been shown that in situ and invasive elements of breast cancers have identical molecular alterations (Stratton et al., 1995; Hwang et al., 2004; Moelans et al., 2011) and similar morphological characteristics (Lampejo et al., 1994), thus supporting the hypothesis that low-grade carcinoma in situ gives rise to low-grade invasive carcinoma, and high-grade carcinoma in situ to high-grade invasive carcinoma.

In addition, complementary DNA (cDNA) expression studies have confirmed that the core intrinsic molecular subgroups, including the luminal, HER2-overexpressing, and basal-like subtypes, found in invasive breast cancer (Perou et al., 2000; Sørlie et al., 2001) are replicated in DCIS, although at different frequencies (Vincent-Salomon et al., 2008).

(c) Natural history of DCIS – association of DCIS with invasive carcinoma

Data on the natural history of untreated DCIS are limited, for ethical reasons. The available studies are historical and relate to symptomatic, extensive, high-grade comedo-type DCIS. In the past, DCIS was rare in clinical practice; patients typically presented with a mass lesion, nipple discharge, or Paget disease of the nipple, and were treated with mastectomy (Dean & Geshchicter, 1938).

More recent studies are virtually all examples of low-grade DCIS, with a progression rate of about 40% to invasive disease after 30 years (Page et al., 1995; Collins et al., 2005; Sanders et al., 2005), and invasive tumours occurring in the quadrant of the breast of the initial lesion (Page et al., 1995, Sanders et al., 2005). About 50% of DCIS recurrences are invasive carcinomas, and high-grade DCIS and DCIS with necrosis represent a biologically aggressive subset compared with low-grade DCIS lesions without necrosis (Solin et al., 1993; Silverstein et al., 1995, 1996; Fisher et al., 1999). One large randomized trial (Bijker et al., 2001a) showed that the margin status is the most important factor in the success of breast-conserving therapy for DCIS. The same trial suggested that local recurrence usually reflects outgrowth of residual DCIS, that progression of low-grade DCIS to high-grade DCIS or grade 3 invasive carcinoma is unusual, and that all forms of DCIS, even the lowest-grade flat/micropapillary type, have a risk of local recurrence, which is reduced by the use of adjuvant radiotherapy (Bijker et al., 2001b; Fisher et al., 2001; Donker et al., 2013).

Invasive lesions with an extensive intraductal component also show a predisposition to local recurrence after breast-conserving therapy (van Dongen et al., 1989). The grade of DCIS associated with invasive carcinoma has been shown to correlate with both disease-free interval and survival (Lampejo et al., 1994). It has been also reported that high-grade DCIS is associated with high-grade invasive carcinoma, and low-grade DCIS with low-grade invasive carcinoma (Lampejo et al., 1994; Douglas-Jones et al., 1996; Cadman et al., 1997). An association between grade 3 invasive carcinoma and poorly differentiated DCIS is seen whatever grading system is used (Douglas-Jones et al., 1996).

(d) LCIS in the context of DCIS

Particularly in some more extensive lesions, making a distinction between in situ lobular neoplasia and DCIS may be difficult, and this may lead to misclassification (Fisher et al., 2004), as in the case of a regular, evenly spaced monotonous population within both ducts and lobules. In such cases, E-cadherin membrane reactivity may be useful in distinguishing between the two pathologies. However, if both ducts and lobules contain epithelial proliferation of this type, particularly if E-cadherin is heterogeneous, categorization as both LCIS and DCIS is currently recommended, to imply the precursor risk of DCIS and the bilateral cancer risk of in situ lobular neoplasia.

There is evidence that some forms of LCIS that have similarities to DCIS will behave in a similar fashion to DCIS and should be managed as an established form of carcinoma in situ. Such types of LCIS are described below.

(i) Pleomorphic variant of LCIS

See Lakhani et al. (2012) for review.

This LCIS subtype has larger cells of pleomorphic type (cytonuclear grade 3), with more abundant cytoplasm than the classic type. Pleomorphic LCIS is less frequently estrogen receptor (ER)-positive and more often HER2-positive than the classic forms. Based on abundant evidence, pleomorphic LCIS is widely regarded as a more aggressive form of the disease, and it is currently recommended that it should be managed similarly to DCIS rather than to classic LCIS, based on its biological and molecular profile (Masannat et al., 2013; Pieri et al., 2014).

(ii) Extensive and mass-forming LCIS with necrosis

See Lakhani et al. (2012) for review.

This variant of LCIS has classic cytology with central necrosis in distended acini. The degree of atypia is not sufficient for a diagnosis of pleomorphic LCIS. This variant is uncommon, and its clinical behaviour is not well established, but it can behave like DCIS (Fisher et al., 2004). This entity is usually regarded as an established form of carcinoma in situ, requiring therapeutic excision, equivalent to DCIS.

1.2.3 Invasive breast carcinoma

Invasive carcinoma of the breast is a malignant tumour, commonly adenocarcinoma, part or all of which penetrates the basement membrane of the mammary epithelial site of origin, particularly from the terminal duct lobular unit (NHSBSP, 2005; Perry et al., 2006; Lakhani et al., 2012). The morphological appearance of these tumours varies widely, and they show different prognostic or clinical characteristics. More recently, specific genetic alterations have been identified in some types.

(a) Histopathological characteristics and classification

The prognosis of a patient with breast cancer relies on two distinct groups of variables. The first are time-dependant variables that influence tumour stage, such as the histological size of the tumour, the presence and extent of lymph-node metastatic disease, and the presence of systemic metastatic disease. The second group of variables, sometimes referred to as intrinsic characteristics, are related to the inherent biology of the individual tumour and include the histological grade, tumour type, growth fraction, hormone and growth factor receptor status, and molecular genetic characteristics.

(i) Histological type and prognosis

A wide range of morphological patterns can be seen in invasive carcinomas, usually with distinct prognostic characteristics (Table 1.3; NHSBSP, 2005; Perry et al., 2006; Lakhani et al., 2012). The favourable prognosis of certain histological types of invasive carcinoma of the breast is well established (Ellis et al., 1992; Pereira et al., 1995; NHSBSP, 2005; Perry et al., 2006; Lakhani et al., 2012). These "special" or "specific" forms of invasive carcinoma have also been found at higher frequency in the prevalence round of mammographic breast screening programmes (Anderson et al., 1991; Ellis et al., 1993) and have been found more frequently at screening than as interval cancers found between screening rounds (Porter et al., 1999). The recent revision of the WHO classification, after consideration of clinical relevance and diagnostic reproducibility issues, has revised the requirements for absolute purity of features and suggested the designation of "medullary-like carcinoma" for tumours that exhibit some or all medullary characteristics and have a moderate prognosis (Lakhani et al., 2012). This contrasts with tubular carcinoma, which has recently been shown to have an exceptionally favourable long-term prognosis (Rakha et al., 2010b). Overall, patients with infiltrating lobular carcinoma have a slightly better prognosis than those with invasive ductal carcinoma, not otherwise specified (Haagensen, 1986; Ellis et al., 1992), although recent longer-term follow-up studies have shown that patients with lobular carcinoma may experience very late recurrence.

Invasive tumours are classified based on the purity of special type characteristics, if present, and are broadly categorized as follows (NHSBSP, 2005; Perry et al., 2006; Lakhani et al., 2012).

Pure special type

For an invasive tumour to be characterized as pure special type, at least 90% of the tumour should have the characteristic features of that particular type (e.g. a tumour showing 90% mucinous features is classified as being of pure mucinous carcinoma type). In general, tumours of special type show favourable clinical prognostic characteristics.

Invasive carcinoma of no special type

This is the most common category of invasive breast carcinoma, showing none, or less than 50%, of the characteristic morphology of the special type tumour. It is often described as invasive ductal carcinoma, although the term "invasive carcinoma of no special type" or "invasive carcinoma of no specific type" is preferred.

Mixed invasive carcinoma

This is a relatively common pattern of invasive breast carcinoma. The tumour may be heterogeneous in morphology, with more than 50% but less than 90% of special type areas, showing areas of pure tubular differentiation within a tumour otherwise showing no special type features.

Other primary breast carcinomas

This category includes rare variants such as carcinoma with apocrine differentiation, carcinoma with neuroendocrine differentiation, and salivary gland-type tumours (e.g. adenoid cystic carcinoma and secretory carcinoma).

Other malignant carcinomas

Non-epithelial tumours and secondary malignancies are included in this category.

(ii) Histological characteristics

Histological grade is a powerful prognostic method for grading invasive breast carcinomas based on the assessment of multiple cellular and architectural variables or nuclear variables. The early systems, in addition to a subjective histological assessment, were lacking strictly defined written criteria (Patey & Scarff, 1928; Bloom & Richardson, 1957). The method of Elston & Ellis (1991) was found to be reproducible (Dalton et al., 1994; Frierson et al., 1995; Robbins et al., 1995) and has been adopted internationally as the standard method (NHSBSP, 2005; Perry et al., 2006; Lakhani et al., 2012). It evaluates three main tumour characteristics: tubule formation as an expression of glandular differentiation, nuclear pleomorphism, and mitotic counts. After each factor is assessed individually, a numerical scoring system assigns an overall grade as follows:

- Grade 1: well differentiated; 3–5 points
- Grade 2: moderately differentiated; 6–7 points
- Grade 3: poorly differentiated; 8–9 points.

(b) Biological and molecular genetic characteristics

Several molecular alterations characterize invasive breast carcinomas. Some are related to survival and also represent tumour-specific molecular signatures, suggesting the possibility of developing targeted therapy.

(i) Estrogen and progesterone receptors

Estrogen is an important mitogen, and its expression is associated with response to hormone therapy, such as adjuvant tamoxifen (Osborne, 1998; Bundred, 2001; Isaacs et al., 2001; Ali & Coombes, 2002; Davies et al., 2011); thus, ER-positive tumours have a more favourable initial prognosis than ER-negative tumours (Ali & Coombes, 2002). ER is expressed in approximately 80% of invasive breast tumours. Progesterone receptors (PRs) serve as an indicator of an intact ER pathway and have been shown to also predict which patients will respond to hormone therapy (Bardou et al., 2003; Andre & Pusztai, 2006).

(ii) HER2

The *ERBB2/HER2* oncogene, located on 17q21, is amplified in approximately 20% of invasive breast carcinomas, leading to overexpression of the coded HER2 protein, a transmembrane receptor with tyrosine kinase activity. HER2 overexpression, measured by immunohistochemistry (Wolff et al., 2013), is a weak to moderate independent predictor of survival (Slamon et al., 1987). HER2 is targeted by the humanized anti-HER2 monoclonal antibody, the anticancer drug trastuzumab (Cobleigh et al., 1999), in combination with chemotherapy for efficacy in both the metastatic and adjuvant settings (Slamon et al., 2001; Perez et al., 2011).

(iii) Proliferation

Several markers of proliferation have been extensively investigated for their prognostic value (Stuart-Harris et al., 2008), including mitotic count, DNA flow cytometric measurement of the S-phase fraction, and immunohistochemistry with antibodies to Ki-67, which is strongly expressed in proliferating cells (Cheang et al., 2009; Yerushalmi et al., 2010; Dowsett et al., 2011). However, the widespread use of such molecular changes has been limited by the lack of methodological standardization, the lack of consensus on appropriate cut-off points for clinical use, and interobserver variability in scoring.

(iv) Gene expression and sequencing

A tumour classification system based on gene expression profiles is more informative than the morphology-based one (NICE, 2013). Variations in gene expression classify breast cancers into the following types: basal epithelial-like, luminal epithelial/ER-positive, HER2-overexpressing, and normal breast-like (Perou et al., 2000; Sørlie et al., 2001; Sotiriou & Pusztai, 2009). The luminal/ER-positive group might be further subdivided (Sotiriou & Pusztai, 2009), although the characterization of these subgroups is still controversial (Ades et al., 2014). The basal intrinsic subclass includes a high proportion of cancers that are triple-negative (ER-, PR-, and HER2-negative) (Andre & Pusztai, 2006). However, gene expression profiling has some limitations (Norum et al., 2014), and no established clinical relevance, although several commercial assays have emerged (Sinn et al., 2013). The most widely adopted to date is the 21-gene assay, which is used as a prognostic factor of recurrence in patients with ER-positive breast cancer treated with hormone therapy, but its cost–effectiveness has not been demonstrated (Isola et al., 2013). Combined genomic and transcriptomic studies have enabled the identification of a broader range of molecular subtypes (Curtis et al., 2012), and next-generation sequencing (Cancer Genome Atlas Network, 2012; Stephens et al., 2012) is improving our understanding of the biology and molecular genetics of breast cancer. Although at present the translation of this knowledge into the clinical setting is limited, there is considerable evidence that the molecular genetic signatures of breast cancer will play an increasing role in its clinical management (Balko et al., 2013).

(c) *Natural history of invasive breast carcinoma*

A very low 15-year survival rate of 5% for untreated breast cancer has been reported historically (Baum, 2013). Survival rates are higher in a modern screening setting, in which disease is detected early.

Historically, radical mastectomy was the treatment of choice, based on the assumption that breast cancer spread exclusively to and from the regional lymph nodes (Halsted, 1894). This approach has been proven ineffective, with high rates of metastatic development (Brinkley & Haybrittle, 1975). It has been demonstrated that breast cancer could also spread via the bloodstream, early and before symptomatic presentation, and may thus require systemic adjuvant treatment (Fisher et al., 2002). A strong and highly significant correlation exists between the tumour size at initiation of distant metastasis and involvement of the first lymph node, since the capacity for lymph-node metastatic spread is, on average, acquired much earlier than the capacity for systemic metastatic spread (Tubiana & Koscielny, 1991; Tabár et al., 1992). Further observations have led to the understanding that breast cancer has a long natural history and a propensity for late recurrence, compared with most other types of cancer (Brewster et al., 2008).

It has been shown that some clinically undetectable, small breast tumours can shed malignant cells with similar characteristics to the primary tumour but also with a relatively normal karyotype and few chromosomal aberrations in common (Schmidt-Kittler et al., 2003), supporting the hypothesis of cancer heterogeneity and Darwinian biological evolution (Klein, 2009; Burrell et al., 2013). These observations may shed light on the observed interindividual variability of apparently similar forms of breast cancer, as well as on the mechanisms of acquired resistance to treatment. Events at the time of surgery may have an impact on long-term survival, and a bimodal distribution of early and late recurrence is seen, possibly due to dormancy (Retsky et al., 2008) or surgical dissemination/autonomy (Badwe et al., 1999). For example, patients with ER-positive tumours have an annual recurrence rate of 2% for at least 15 years, even after 5 years of adjuvant tamoxifen therapy (Saphner et al., 1996). Currently, women who have a history of invasive breast cancer and who have been treated for 5 years with aromatase inhibitors have a risk of recurrence in the following 5 years (Early Breast Cancer Trialists' Collaborative Group, 2001; Cuzick et al., 2010). For this reason, adjuvant treatment has been extended to 10 years for women at high risk of recurrence (Sledge et al., 2014).

Spontaneous regression of breast cancer is exceptionally rare (Larsen & Rose, 1999), and although some studies suggest this possibility (Kaplan & Porzsolt, 2008; Zahl et al., 2008), their conclusions are not widely accepted as valid, given multiple methodological issues. The issue of overdiagnosis, indolence, and/or regression appears more compelling for in situ lesions, particularly non-high-grade DCIS and ADH. Hospital-based and forensic autopsy series of women not known to have had breast cancer during their lifetime have shown a frequency of 9% of DCIS (Welch & Black, 1997; Erbas et al., 2006). However, lesions identified in these studies are usually very small, low-nuclear-grade lesions and possibly ADH rather than established forms of DCIS. Also, a high proportion of these occult lesions identified histologically during postmortem examinations are not diagnosable by mammography and have been interpreted as being of questionable clinical relevance.

Pathologists use the term "overdiagnosis" to mean the incorrect pathological diagnosis of cancer, i.e. misdiagnosis or diagnostic error (Ellis et al., 2006). Epidemiologists and radiologists define "overdiagnosis" as the diagnosis of a cancer as a result of screening that would not have been diagnosed in the patient's lifetime if screening had not taken place. Under certain circumstances, the rate of overdiagnosis can be estimated by the excess proportion of cancers detected in women undergoing screening, compared with women in the non-screened control arm of a clinical trial (Kopans et al., 2011; Puliti et al., 2012). This definition implies that a proportion of breast cancers remain static, have a very indolent long-term course, or regress (Berlin, 2014). As discussed above, the evidence for regression remains highly controversial. There is compelling evidence that some cancers, particularly in situ and invasive low-grade hormone receptor-positive lesions, may remain indolent and do not progress to clinically relevant disease in a woman's lifetime. With respect to screening, these cancers would more correctly be described as "overdetected". However, in most cases it is not currently possible, based on mammographic signs, pathological features, or biological features, to determine which lesions are likely to progress or regress. The question of progression versus regression for non-high-grade forms of DCIS was investigated in two randomized trials currently under way: the Low Risk DCIS (LORIS) trial (Soumian et al., 2013; ISRCTN registry, 2014) and the Low-Risk DCIS (LORD) trial (Elshof et al., 2015).

1.2.4 Breast cancer with hereditary and somatic mutations

Two high-penetrance genes have been identified (*BRCA1* and *BRCA2*) that greatly increase the risk of developing breast cancer. Among age-matched cases, *BRCA1* mutation-related tumours are significantly different from sporadic breast tumours in their histopathological appearance and molecular characteristics (Lakhani et al., 1998, 2002; Honrado et al., 2006; Palacios et al., 2008; van der Groep et al., 2011; Vargas et al., 2011), possibly due to the expression of the basal-like phenotype. Invasive ductal carcinoma, not otherwise specified, is the most common histological type in both hereditary and sporadic breast cancers, although certain subtypes do occur more frequently in hereditary breast tumours than in sporadic breast tumours. *BRCA1* mutation-related tumours are frequently of histological grade 3 and of medullary-like type, characterized by syncytial architecture, absence of tubular or glandular structures, pushing or circumscribed margins, high nuclear grade, and a marked lymphoplasmacytic stromal infiltrate. *BRCA1*-related breast cancers are typically triple-negative and of basal phenotype or basal molecular gene expression class (Lakhani et al., 1998, 2002; Vargas et al., 2011; Mavaddat et al., 2012). In premenopausal patients with tumours of medullary and triple-negative histology, *BRCA1* mutation analysis is frequently performed regardless of the family history of breast and/or ovarian cancer. The specific biological origin of mammary tumours in *BRCA1* mutation carriers has been revealed by messenger RNA (mRNA) expression analyses and next-generation sequencing of breast cancer tissues (Sørlie, 2004; Stephens et al., 2012).

No consistently defined phenotype has been described for patients with *BRCA2* familial breast cancer, although some reports indicate a more frequent occurrence of tubular, lobular, and pleomorphic lobular carcinomas (Lakhani et al., 1998, 2002; Honrado et al., 2006; Palacios et al., 2008; van der Groep et al., 2011; Vargas et al., 2011). *BRCA2* mutation-related tumours show a high frequency of ER positivity, similar to sporadic cases, and they are usually HER2-negative. *BRCA2*-related tumours are of higher grade (grades 2 and 3) than sporadic tumours and may show more prominent lymphocytic infiltration, foci of necrosis, and pushing margins than sporadic tumours do. However, these features are exhibited less consistently by *BRCA2*-related tumours than are the medullary-like features by *BRCA1*-related tumours.

Both BRCA1-deficient cells and BRCA2-deficient cells display genomic instability due to impaired DNA repair, but cancers arising in *BRCA1/2* mutation carriers differ in their characteristics. The pathology and behaviour of *BRCA1/2*-related cancers have been extensively studied, and comprehensive review articles are available (Lakhani et al., 1998, 2002; Honrado et al., 2006; Atchley et al., 2008; Palacios et al., 2008; van der Groep et al., 2011; Vargas et al., 2011; Goodwin et al., 2012).

Breast cancers caused by other breast cancer susceptibility genes do not seem to differ significantly from sporadic breast cancers, but the numbers studied so far are small (van der Groep et al., 2011).

Other reported somatic point mutations, such as indels (insertions or deletions of bases), may be the consequence of the intrinsic infidelity of the DNA replication machinery, of exogenous or endogenous mutagen exposures, of enzymatic DNA modification, or of defective DNA repair. Somatically acquired mutations in triple-negative cancers vary extensively among breast tumours (Stephens et al., 2012). Integrative pathway analyses, comparing basal-like and luminal tumours, have identified hyperactivated FOXM1 as a transcriptional driver of proliferation and have found increased MYC and HIF1α/ARNT as key regulators (Kristensen et al., 2012). Integrative pathway analysis has also confirmed that loss of RB1 and BRCA1 expression are basal-like features.

Combined copy number aberrations and gene expression analyses have been used to classify and categorize breast cancer, and 10 integrative cluster groups have been defined (Curtis et al., 2012). Most of the triple-negative cancers were classified in integrative cluster 10, representing the core basal subgroup in this new classification. The highest rate of *TP53* mutations was found in integrative cluster 10, combined with intermediate levels of genomic instability, loss of 5q, and gains at 8q, 10p, and 12p (Jain et al., 2001; Curtis et al., 2012). Loss of 5q has been associated with the presence of a *TP53* mutation (Jain et al., 2001), and a basal-specific gene expression pattern has been linked with cell-cycle checkpoint control, DNA damage repair, and apoptosis (Dawson et al., 2013). Also, triple-negative cancers are characterized by increased lymphocytic infiltration (Chappuis et al., 2000).

1.2.5 Summary

(a) Benign breast disease

The vast majority of benign breast lesions, which can present symptomatically or be detected using breast screening methods including BSE, do not appear to develop to breast cancers. They are therefore clinically innocent and merit treatment by excision only if causing symptoms, otherwise requiring no intervention. In contrast, various forms of breast epithelial proliferation have been associated with an increased average risk of subsequent breast cancer (1.5–2.0-fold for usual epithelial hyperplasia and 2.5–4.0-fold for atypical hyperplasia).

(b) DCIS

The two forms of non-invasive breast carcinoma in situ are DCIS and LCIS, each with distinctive morphological and behavioural characteristics. The neoplastic cell populations are confined within the parenchymal site of origin, and the cells do not infiltrate beyond the limiting basement membrane. Nuclear grading is the recommended method for subclassification of DCIS into the categories of high, intermediate, and low nuclear grade, but mixed and rare subtypes are also recognized.

Both DCIS and LCIS harbour molecular alterations and intrinsic molecular subtype characteristics that are similar to those of their related forms of invasive breast cancer; thus, no distinct biological or molecular hallmarks of invasive potential have been identified.

The available data on low-grade DCIS show that at least 40% of cases progress to invasive cancer on long-term follow-up. For ethical reasons, only historical data are available for high-grade DCIS, and high rates of progression to invasive breast cancer are reported. There are no methods available to reliably distinguish between cases that will progress and those that will not.

DCIS is identified more frequently by mammography screening than by clinical examination, as small radiodense deposits of microcalcification.

(c) Invasive breast carcinoma

Invasive carcinoma of the breast is a malignant tumour, part or all of which penetrates the basement membrane of the epithelial site of origin (i.e. the duct or lobule).

The vast majority of these tumours are adenocarcinomas derived from mammary epithelial cells. The morphological appearance of these tumours varies widely, and many of the recognized morphological types have specific behavioural, prognostic, and clinical characteristics.

The morphological diversity of invasive breast cancer is directly related to the underlying molecular genetics. Distinct molecular intrinsic subtypes have been identified, including the luminal, HER2-overexpressing, and basal-like (often triple-negative) classes. Continued developments in molecular biology techniques will provide greater insights into the molecular pathology of breast cancer.

Invasive breast cancer may spread via both the blood and the lymphatic systems, and may progress via regional lymph nodes and systemic metastatic spread. The probability that metastatic spread has occurred is highly correlated with tumour size, and the capacity for lymph-node metastatic spread is, on average, acquired earlier than the capacity for systemic metastatic spread.

Historical studies of untreated invasive breast cancer show poor survival, with progression through the development of metastatic disease. Reviews of the medical literature indicate that confirmed examples of spontaneous regression of breast cancer are exceptionally infrequent.

(d) Related issues

When assessed by external quality assurance systems, the misclassification of cancer cases by pathologists as a cause of overdiagnosis is very rare.

In breast screening, overdiagnosis is defined as the diagnosis of a cancer as a result of screening that would not have been diagnosed in the patient's lifetime if screening had not taken place. The biological explanation for this theoretical concept remains unclear, but it is widely believed to relate to potential indolence of a low proportion of breast cancers.

1.3 Risk factors

Although it would be ideal to identify a subset of the population from which most cases would arise on the basis of established breast cancer risk factors, simulations of risk-based screening have not confirmed the validity of this approach. Screening of 17 543 women led to the conclusion that more than 50% of the cases would not have been detected if only women with either a previous breast biopsy or a family history of breast cancer had been screened, and that more than 40% of the cases would have been missed if women had been selected for screening on the basis of other established breast cancer risk factors (Solin et al., 1984). An analysis of the Edinburgh randomized trial similarly reported that if women had been selected for screening based on a previous biopsy or on a history of breast cancer in a mother or sister, only 19.8% of the first-round cancers would have been detected (Alexander et al., 1987). When menopausal status and nulliparity or first birth after age 30 years were included as high-risk factors, the proportion of first-round cases that would have been detected increased to 55.6%. Consequently, restricting screening to women with the most established risk factors would fail to identify the majority of prevalent cancers in an asymptomatic population. Madigan et al. reported population attributable risk estimates for breast cancer derived using data from the United States National Health and Nutrition Examination Survey Epidemiologic Follow-Up Study (Madigan et al., 1995). Well-established risk factors, such as later age at first live birth, nulliparity, higher family income, and family history of breast cancer in first-degree relatives, were associated with approximately 41% of the breast cancer cases in the USA. In the Netherlands, retrospective evaluation of a breast cancer screening programme showed that only 63% of the breast cancer cases would have been identified if the programme had screened only women with at least one established risk factor, representing only 37% of the study group (De Waard et al., 1988). The authors concluded that the "relevance of the high-risk group concept in screening for breast cancer is small". Finally, data from a large multicentre case–control study in Italy indicated that it would be necessary to screen 87% of the population in order to detect 95% of the cases (Paci et al., 1988). The authors concluded that breast cancer risk factors discriminated poorly for selective screening.

In each of these studies, the overall conclusion was that breast screening on the basis of selected breast cancer risk factors, individually or in combination, fails to identify a subset of women from which the majority of cases of breast cancer are expected to arise. It should also be stressed that the greater the complexity of the risk-based strategy, the greater the need for a regular risk assessment programme to ensure that as risk profiles change, women are cycled in and out of the programme. This necessity not only adds complexity and costs but also adds the potential for misspecification. From a public health standpoint, it appears that the single best strategy for breast cancer screening is a simple one, based on age-related invitation.

Breast cancer in women, as is the case for most cancers, is a multifactorial disease. Its risk factors strongly reflect the hormonal etiology; among the relevant biological exposures are levels of sex steroids, other hormones, and growth factors, including estrogens, androgens, prolactin, and insulin-like growth factors. Life-course reproductive, anthropometric, and lifestyle factors, many of which are prevalent in high-incidence countries, are well-established risk factors: early menarche, late menopause, later age at first pregnancy, nulliparity and low parity, little or no breastfeeding, higher body mass index (BMI) at postmenopausal ages, and tall stature. Lifestyle factors associated with increased risk include low physical activity levels, alcohol consumption, certain exogenous hormone therapies, and exposure to ionizing radiation. Breast density, history of benign breast disease, and family history of cancer are also linked to an increased risk of breast cancer. Also, a small proportion of breast cancers are hereditary, and specific genetic mutations have been identified.

In the following sections, breast cancer risk factors are broadly grouped into: hormonal and reproductive factors (Section 1.3.1), lifestyle factors and environmental exposures (Section 1.3.2), and risk factors that are not modifiable (Section 1.3.3). Exposure to ionizing radiation is described in Section 1.3.4, and genetic factors are described in Section 1.3.5. Population attributable fractions to known risk factors in different settings are summarized in Section 1.3.6. Table 1.4 presents the magnitude of relative risks for breast cancer associated with these risk factors.

1.3.1 Hormonal and reproductive factors

(a) Age at menarche

Women who have had an early menarche have higher breast cancer incidence rates. This association has been consistently observed across ethnic groups and countries. A collaborative

Table 1.4 Magnitude of relative risk for breast cancer associated with established risk factors

Risk factor	Categories	RR (95% confidence interval)	Reference
Hormonal and reproductive factors			
Age at menarche (years)	11	1.0 (reference)	Colditz et al. (2000)
	15	0.69 (0.65–0.74)	
Parity	Nulliparous	1.0 (reference)	
	Parous	1.26 (1.10–1.44)	
Age at first full-term pregnancy (years)	20	0.73 (0.63–0.86)	
	30	1.16 (0.96–1.41)	
Breastfeeding	Per 12 months of total breastfeeding	0.96 (0.94–0.97)	Collaborative Group on Hormonal Factors in Breast Cancer (2002)
Age at menopause (years)	45	1.0 (reference)	Colditz et al. (2000)
	55	1.44 (1.26–1.64)	
Type of menopause	Natural	1.0 (reference)	
	Bilateral oophorectomy	0.89 (0.80–0.98)	
Postmenopausal hormone use	None	1.0 (reference)	IARC (2012a)
	Estrogen only[a]	1.18 (1.08–1.30)	
	Combined estrogen–progestogen[a] for > 5 years	1.63 (1.22–2.18)	
Lifestyle factors			
Alcohol consumption	Per 12 g/day	1.12 (1.09–1.14)	Allen et al. (2009), WCRF/AICR (2010), IARC (2012b)
	Premenopausal	1.09 (1.01–1.17)	
	Postmenopausal	1.08 (1.05–1.10)	
Tobacco smoking (pack–years)	≥ 20	1.28 (1.17–1.39)	IARC (2012b), Warren et al. (2014)
Weight increase (per 5 kg/m^2 increase in BMI)	Postmenopausal	1.12 (1.08–1.16)	WCRF/AICR (2010)
	Premenopausal	0.92 (0.88–0.97)	
Physical activity, high vs low (METs)	Premenopausal	0.87 (0.84–0.92)	WCRF/AICR (2010), Chlebowski (2013), Wu et al. (2013)
	Postmenopausal	0.77 (0.72–0.84)	
	Moderate physical activity (3–5.9 METs)	0.81 (0.72–0.92)	
Non-modifiable factors			
Height (per 5 cm increase)	Premenopausal	1.09 (1.05–1.14)	WCRF/AICR (2010)
	Postmenopausal	1.11 (1.09–1.13)	
	Any age	1.03 (1.01–1.04)	
Age (years)	< 50	1.0 (reference)	Anderson et al. (2006)
	50–59	6.6 (6.5–6.7)	
	60–69	9.2 (9.1–9.3)	
	70–79	11.1 (10.9–11.2)	
	≥ 80	10.1 (10.0–10.3)	
Benign breast disease	No	1.0 (reference)	Colditz et al. (2000), Lakhani et al. (2012)
	Non-epithelial proliferative hyperplasia	1.57 (1.43–1.73)	

Table 1.4 (continued)

Risk factor	Categories	RR (95% confidence interval)	Reference
	Common epithelial hyperplasia	1.5–2.0	
	Atypical epithelial hyperplasia	2.5–4.0	
Breast density	Dense area, mean: 59.92–201.49 cm^2	1.57 (1.18–1.67)	Chiu et al. (2010)
Ionizing radiation			
Radiation exposure			See Table 1.6
Family and personal history of breast cancer			See also Section 1.3.5
Mother's age (years) at breast cancer	< 50	2.69 (2.29–3.15)	Anderson et al. (2000)
	≥ 50	1.88 (1.73–2.03)	

[a] Used continuously from age 50–60 years.
BMI, body mass index; CI, confidence interval; METs, metabolic equivalents; RR, relative risk.

pooled analysis demonstrated that each 1-year delay in menarche is associated with a reduction of approximately 5.0% (95% confidence interval [CI], 4.4–5.7%) in risk of breast cancer (Collaborative Group on Hormonal Factors in Breast Cancer, 2012).

(b) Parity

In general, nulliparous women have a higher risk of breast cancer (up to 2-fold increase) compared with parous women. It has been observed that parous women have a temporarily increased risk of breast cancer up to 15 years after childbirth; thereafter, the risk declines to below that of nulliparous women (Lambe et al., 1994). Each birth is associated with an average long-term reduction of 7% in the relative risk of breast cancer (Collaborative Group on Hormonal Factors in Breast Cancer, 2002).

(c) Age at first full-term pregnancy

Women who have their first full-term pregnancy at a younger age have a lower risk of breast cancer. Women aged 30 years or older at their first full-term pregnancy have consistently been shown to have a short-term increased risk of breast cancer, with relative risks ranging between 1.2 and 2.3, compared with women younger than 20 years at their first full-term pregnancy (MacMahon et al., 1973; Trichopoulos et al., 1983; Bruzzi et al., 1985; Gail et al., 1989; Ewertz et al., 1990; Harris et al., 1992; Madigan et al., 1995; Nagata et al., 1995; Byrne & Harris, 1996; Colditz et al., 2000; Wohlfahrt & Melbye, 2001; Tamakoshi et al., 2005; Washbrook, 2006; Iwasaki et al., 2007; Pike et al., 2007; Iwasaki & Tsugane, 2011; Kobayashi et al., 2012).

(d) Breastfeeding

Women who have breastfed their children have a reduced risk of breast cancer at both premenopausal and postmenopausal ages. At an equal number of full-term pregnancies, breast cancer risk decreases by approximately 4.3% (95% CI, 2.9–5.8%) for every 12 months of breastfeeding, whether consecutive or not, compared with women who never breastfed (Collaborative Group on Hormonal Factors in Breast Cancer, 2012). This protective effect cumulates with the effect of parity. The meta-analysis performed by the World Cancer Research Fund estimated the decreased breast cancer risk per 5 months of total breastfeeding to be 2% (pooled odds ratio, 0.98; 95% CI, 0.97–0.98) (WCRF/AICR, 2010).

(e) Age at menopause

Later age at menopause (≥55 years vs ≤45 years) is associated with an increased risk of breast cancer (1.9-fold vs 1.1-fold increased risk). Among women with natural menopause at age 55 years, the incidence is twice that among women with natural menopause at age 45 years (typically, relative risk [RR], 1.5 vs 0.7) and 3 times that among women with bilateral oophorectomy and menopause at age 35 years (RR, 0.4) (Harris et al., 1992; Kelsey & Bernstein, 1996; Colditz & Rosner, 2000; Iwasaki et al., 2007; Pike et al., 2007; Iwasaki & Tsugane, 2011). Each 1-year delay in the onset of menopause corresponds to an increase of approximately 3% in risk of breast cancer (Collaborative Group on Hormonal Factors in Breast Cancer, 1997; Cuzick, 2003; Washbrook, 2006), and each 5-year delay corresponds to an increase of 17% (95% CI, 1.11–1.22) in risk of breast cancer (Hsieh et al., 1990).

(f) Endogenous hormones

Among postmenopausal women, those with high blood levels of both estrogens and androgens have almost double the risk of breast cancer compared with those with low blood levels (Key et al., 2002; Missmer et al., 2004; Kaaks et al., 2005). The major known determinant of endogenous estrogen levels in postmenopausal women is BMI (estrogen levels in obese postmenopausal women are more than twice those in slender postmenopausal women), and this appears to largely explain the observed association (Key et al., 2003). Among premenopausal women, it is more difficult to estimate the breast cancer risk related to the levels of endogenous sex hormones, mainly because of the large variations in hormone levels across the menstrual cycle. However, high blood estrogen levels in premenopausal women have been reported to be associated with an increase of approximately 40% in breast cancer risk (Key et al., 2013). High blood levels of insulin-like growth factor 1 (IGF-1) are associated with an increase of approximately 30% in breast cancer risk in both premenopausal and postmenopausal women (Key et al., 2010), and high blood levels of prolactin are associated with an increase of approximately 30% in breast cancer risk in postmenopausal women (Tworoger et al., 2013; Tikk et al., 2014).

(g) Use of oral contraceptives

The use of combined estrogen–progestogen oral contraceptives causes breast cancer (IARC, 2012a). After 10 years of use of oral contraceptives, the relative risk is 1.24 (95% CI, 1.15–1.33) among current users, and it decreases with time since stopping the use of oral contraceptives. No significant excess risk of breast cancer has been observed 10 years or more after stopping the use of oral contraceptives. In general, the duration of use, the age at first use, and the dose and type of hormone within the oral contraceptives have not shown any additional effect on breast cancer risk (Collaborative Group on Hormonal Factors in Breast Cancer, 1996). The risk is particularly increased among current users with benign breast disease, or among users younger than 20 years (RR, 1.63; 95% CI, 1.02–2.62) (IARC, 2012a).

(h) Use of hormonal menopausal therapy

The use of estrogen–progestogen hormone replacement therapy (HRT) increases the risk of developing breast cancer. The relative risk is less than 2 for long-term users (≥ 5 years) or high-dose users (IARC, 2012a; Chlebowski et al., 2013; de Villiers et al., 2013b), but is already significantly increased (odds ratio [OR], 1.35; 95% CI, 1.16–1.57) after less than 5 years of use (Shah et al., 2005). In long-term users (> 5 years), the risk is still increased several years after stopping the use of HRT (hazard ratio for 5–10 years after stopping, 1.34; 95% CI, 1.04–1.73) (Fournier et al., 2014). Overall, the increase in risk is estimated to be 2% for each additional year of use. The association is clearer in slender women than in obese women (Collaborative Group on Hormonal Factors in Breast Cancer, 1997; Beral et al., 2005; Pike et al., 2007). A decreased breast cancer risk with estrogen-only menopausal therapy was observed among women who had undergone a hysterectomy (Stefanick et al., 2006). The trend for decreased breast cancer incidence among women aged 50 years and older observed in some countries (see Section 1.1) may be related to a reduction in use of HRT (Antoine et al., 2014), although this remains a complex issue (de Villiers et al., 2013a).

It appears that the effects of HRT on a woman's risk of breast cancer depend greatly on her BMI. Treatment with estrogen (conjugated equine estrogen at 0.625 mg/day) for 5 years has an estimated effect of increasing breast cancer risk by 30% in women with a BMI of 20 kg/m^2 and by 8% in women with a BMI of 30 kg/m^2. In contrast, use of combined estrogen–progestin therapy (medroxyprogesterone acetate at 2.5 mg/day) for 5 years is estimated to increase risk of breast cancer by 50% in women with a BMI of 20 kg/m^2 and by 26% in women with a BMI of 30 kg/m^2. With use at a higher dose (medroxyprogesterone acetate at 10 mg/day) for 5 years, the estimated increase in breast cancer risk is 59% and 34%, respectively (Pike et al., 2007).

When comparing continuous versus sequential combined therapy, the risk estimates per 5-year use are of 1.20 (95% CI, 1.01–1.44) for continuous therapy and of 1.32 (95% CI, 1.11–1.56) for sequential therapy in women in the USA; for women in Europe, the breast cancer risk increases by 88% for continuous therapy (RR, 1.88; 95% CI, 1.61–2.21) and by 40% for sequential therapy (RR, 1.40; 95% CI, 1.19–1.64) (Lee et al., 2005). The observed differences in risk between women in the USA and Europe may be explained by different treatment regimens and differences in women's BMI (Pike et al., 2007).

Whereas using percutaneous estradiol with or without micronized progesterone did not seem to increase breast cancer risk, a combination of estrogens with synthetic progestogens seemed to increase it by 40–50% (RR, 1.4; 95% CI, 1.2–1.7) (Fournier et al., 2005), except with dydrogesterone (Fournier et al., 2009).

(i) Other hormonal treatment

Women exposed to diethylstilbestrol while pregnant have an increased risk of breast cancer (IARC, 2012a).

1.3.2 Lifestyle factors and environmental exposures

(a) Alcohol consumption

Alcohol consumption is carcinogenic to humans (Group 1) and causes cancer of the female breast (IARC, 2012b). There is convincing evidence that the consumption of alcoholic beverages increases the incidence of breast cancer in both premenopausal and postmenopausal women, irrespective of the type of alcoholic beverage. Compared with not consuming any alcohol, the consumption of three or more alcoholic drinks per day is associated with an increase of 40–50% in breast cancer risk (Seitz et al., 2012). A linear exposure–response relationship is apparent, and the risk increases by 10% (RR, 1.10; 95% CI, 1.06–1.14) for each 10 g/day (WCRF/AICR, 2007). Even at low levels of alcohol consumption (1 drink/day, ~12.5 g of ethanol/drink, ~0.8 g of ethanol/mL), a significant association with breast cancer risk is seen (RR, 1.05; 95% CI, 1.02–1.08) (Bagnardi et al., 2013; Scoccianti et al., 2014). No threshold of consumption has been identified, and there is robust evidence for mechanisms of alcohol-associated carcinogenesis in humans (WCRF/AICR, 2007).

(b) Tobacco smoking

Although the evidence that tobacco smoking increases breast cancer risk is limited, several subgroup analyses support that smoking at early ages (before the first full-term pregnancy) and smoking for several decades do increase the risk (Secretan et al., 2009; IARC, 2012b). The 2014 United States Surgeon General's report concluded that "the evidence is suggestive but not sufficient to infer a causal relationship between active smoking and breast cancer" (Warren et al., 2014). The report noted that several epidemiological issues may prevent the assessment of an association between active smoking and breast cancer risk, including: (i) timing of exposure at early ages and/or long duration of smoking, (ii) potential confounding or effect modification, and (iii) the exact definition of the outcome (e.g. ER-positive breast cancer).

(c) Overweight, obesity, and change in body weight

There are consistent epidemiological data that support an inverse exposure–response relationship (protective effect) between high body fat and risk of breast cancer in premenopausal women, with a clear exposure–response relationship (IARC, 2002; WCRF/AICR, 2007, 2010). In contrast, increased abdominal fat and weight gain in adulthood are associated with an increased risk of developing postmenopausal breast cancer (RR, 1.19; 95% CI, 1.10–1.28 per 0.1 increment in waist-to-hip ratio; RR, 1.05; 95% CI, 1.04–1.07 per 5 kg weight gain), whereas higher birth weight is associated with an increased risk of premenopausal breast cancer (RR, 1.08; 95% CI, 1.04–1.13) (WCRF/AICR, 2007). The global burden of postmenopausal breast and corpus uteri cancers attributed to excess BMI is estimated at 221 000 cases and is concentrated in countries with very high and high HDI compared with countries with medium and low HDI (Arnold et al., 2015).

(d) Physical activity

Overall, results from prospective studies suggest that increased physical activity has a protective effect for both premenopausal and postmenopausal breast cancer. The evidence for postmenopausal breast cancer appears to be stronger than that for premenopausal breast cancer, but there is some heterogeneity in the exposure–response relationship depending on the study design. There are few data regarding the effects of frequency, duration, or intensity of activity on breast cancer risk (WCRF/AICR, 2007, 2010; Chlebowski, 2013; Wu et al., 2013).

1.3.3 Non-modifiable risk factors

(a) Height

Overall, there is abundant and consistent evidence of a clear exposure–response relationship and of plausible mechanisms in humans of the association between height and breast cancer risk. The World Cancer Research Fund reported that factors leading to greater adult attained height are associated with an increased risk of breast cancer in both premenopausal and postmenopausal women (RR, 1.03; 95% CI, 1.01–1.04 per 5 cm increase in height) (WCRF/AICR, 2010).

(b) Age

In many populations, breast cancer incidence rates appear to increase rapidly before age 50 years and generally flatten in later years (see Section 1.1). Data from the Surveillance, Epidemiology, and End Results (SEER) Program of the United States National Cancer Institute show that at postmenopausal ages, incidence rates of ER-positive breast cancer continue to increase, whereas those for more-aggressive, earlier-onset ER-negative breast cancer reach a plateau or decline (Anderson et al., 2006). Breast cancer shows an age–incidence pattern for ER expression, and relative risks compared with women younger than 50 years increase 6-fold at ages 50–59 years and up to 10-fold at ages 70 years and older (Anderson et al., 2006).

Table 1.5 Distribution of breast density on first and last screening mammography, by age group, for women without and with breast cancer diagnosed after the most recent or last screening mammography

Age (years)	BI-RADS category	No breast cancer (%)		Breast cancer patients (%)	
		First screen	Last screen	First screen	Last screen
40–49	1	4.9	4.8	0.9	1.3
	2	36.1	35.6	27.2	24.7
	3	44.6	47.6	49.6	57.1
	4	14.5	12.1	22.3	16.8
50–59	1	10.5	10.4	4.3	3.6
	2	49.1	49.8	45.8	47.3
	3	34.5	35.3	44.0	43.4
	4	6.0	4.5	5.9	5.7
60–69	1	16.8	14.4	11.5	7.6
	2	57.2	56.4	58.2	56.8
	3	23.5	26.8	27.2	33.5
	4	2.5	2.4	3.2	2.1

BI-RADS, American College of Radiology Breast Imaging Reporting and Data System.
Adapted from Kerlikowske et al. (2007). Longitudinal measurement of clinical mammographic breast density to improve estimation of breast cancer risk, *Journal of the National Cancer Institute*, volume 99, issue 5, pages 386–395, by permission of Oxford University Press.

(c) Benign breast disease

The majority of benign breast conditions are non-proliferative lesions with no associated increased risk of subsequent development to breast cancer. However, usual epithelial hyperplasia is associated with a 1.5–2.0-fold increased risk, and atypical hyperplasia, both ductal and lobular, with a 2.5–4.0-fold increased risk (London et al., 1992; Dupont et al., 1993; Fitzgibbons et al., 1998; Colditz et al., 2000; Lakhani et al., 2012).

(d) Breast density

Breast density, commonly referred to as "mammographic density", is the relative composition of mammary collagen-rich stromal tissues in the breast, as opposed to the lower-density adipose tissue. The American College of Radiology Breast Imaging Reporting and Data System (BI-RADS) has visually estimated and classified breast density into the following categories of increasing area density: category 1, < 25% (almost entirely fatty); category 2, 25–50% (scattered fibroglandular densities); category 3, 51–75% (heterogeneously dense); category 4, > 75% (extremely dense) (see Table 1.5 for the distribution of breast density by age group and cancer status; Lazarus et al., 2006; Kerlikowske et al., 2007). These categories serve during the routine interpretation of mammography and are measured on a mammogram as the percentage of the projected breast area that is radiodense (radiopaque), known as "percent mammographic density" (Boyd et al., 2005; McCormack & dos Santos Silva, 2006; Boyd et al., 2007; Chiu et al., 2010; Pike & Pearce, 2013).

Mammographic density appears to be correlated with several other breast cancer risk factors, including genetic predisposition (Becker & Kaaks, 2009; Boyd et al., 2009) and genetic polymorphisms (Dumas & Diorio, 2010; Lindström et al., 2011; Peng et al., 2011). Although after adjusting for other risk factors, mammographic density appears to remain independently associated with breast cancer risk (Pettersson et al., 2014), at present it has not proven to be a valuable component for modelling and predicting breast cancer risk (Barlow et al., 2006; Tice et al., 2008).

An important effect of mammographic density is the risk of a false-negative mammography finding due to the masking effect of dense tissue (Boyd et al., 2007). The effect of density on the sensitivity of mammographic screening is discussed and quantified in Section 2.1.9.

1.3.4 Ionizing radiation

Exposure to ionizing radiation is a well-established risk factor for breast cancer, as concluded by several international committees (National Research Council, 2006; INSERM, 2008; UNSCEAR, 2010, 2013; IARC, 2012c). Knowledge about radiation-related risk of breast cancer in women is derived mainly from studies of atomic bomb survivors, women exposed to diagnostic radiation, and patients exposed during therapy for benign disease or for cancer, mainly during childhood. Other useful information about the radiation-related risk of the general population derives from studies of occupationally exposed workers, such as medical workers (Table 1.6). The huge amount of evidence of an exposure–risk relationship comes from epidemiological studies of various populations, age groups, and exposure conditions (Ronckers et al., 2005; Telle-Lamberton, 2008). In summary, the majority of studies indicate that breast cancer may be induced after radiation exposure of women younger than 40 years. Studies of atomic bomb survivors or of patients medically exposed show very low or no risk from exposure after that age.

(a) Atomic bomb survivors

Regularly updated analyses of incidence and mortality in the Life Span Study of Japanese atomic bomb survivors have enabled detailed studies of the consequences of exposure received at one time and at a high exposure rate over a population exposed at various ages (Land et al., 2003; Preston et al., 2007; Ozasa et al., 2012). The dose–response for breast cancer risk is significant, is among the highest compared with other cancer sites, and is consistent with a statistical model in which the excess risk of breast cancer is proportional to the radiation dose received (the so-called linear, no-threshold model). An important and significant effect of age at exposure is observed, with a higher risk for women exposed before age 20 years, a less-increased risk for women exposed after age 40 years, and a not measurably increased risk for women exposed after age 50 years. Although it is challenging to separate the role of age at exposure from the role of attained age (or age at observation for risk), it is necessary to calculate the radiation-associated breast cancer risk, and this has enabled the identification of an early-onset group of women at high risk (before age 35 years). The general conclusions are similar whether based on incidence or on mortality studies.

(b) Women exposed for medical monitoring

Other informative studies are from women exposed for diagnostic purposes, as during fluoroscopic examinations of pulmonary tuberculosis. An incidence study was conducted in the USA (Boice et al., 1991) and a mortality study was conducted in Canada (Howe & McLaughlin, 1996). The doses to the breast were moderate but fractionated at a high dose rate and received at a mean age of 25 years, resulting in significant dose–response relationships. The estimated excess risks observed in studies of women undergoing multiple radiological examinations for spine deformities were similarly high and suggested a higher carcinogenic effect of radiation among women with a family history of breast cancer (Doody et al., 2000; Ronckers et al., 2008, 2010). The modifying effect of stage of reproductive development at exposure was not found to be significant. Overall, the excess risk of fractionated exposure is similar to the excess risk of acute exposure, such as that received by atomic bomb survivors.

Table 1.6 Epidemiological studies on radiation exposure and risk of breast cancer in women

Reference	Exposed population (size; number of breast cancer cases/ deaths)	Country	Exposure type	Exposure rate	Average dose (Gy)	ERR/Gy (95% CI) Main conclusion
Atomic bomb survivors						
Land et al. (2003), Preston et al. (2007)	Female atomic bomb survivors (70 000; 1060)	Japan	Gamma, neutron	Acute exposure at low doses	0.28	0.87 (0.55–1.30) at age 30 years. Linear dose–response relationship; −19% (−33% to 4%) change by 10-year increment of age at exposure
Ozasa et al. (2012)	Atomic bomb survivors (51 000; 320)	Japan	Gamma, neutron	Acute exposure at low doses	0.28	1.50 (0.93–2.30) −45% (−67% to −17%) change by 10-year increment of age at exposure
Medical monitoring						
Boice et al. (1991)	Women monitored for tuberculosis (2500; 150)	USA	X-rays (radiography, fluoroscopy)	Fractionated moderate dose rate	0.79	0.61 (0.30–1.01) Included in Preston et al. (2002)
Howe & McLaughlin (1996)	Women monitored for tuberculosis (32 000; 680)	Canada	X-rays (radiography, fluoroscopy)	Fractionated moderate dose rate	0.89 Sv	0.90 (0.55–1.39) ERR/Sv at age 15 years Strong dose–response relationship Modification by age at exposure
Doody et al. (2000), Ronckers et al. (2010)	Children and adolescents monitored for scoliosis (5000; 110)	USA	Chest X-rays	Various low dose rates	0.26	3.90 (1.00–9.30)
Ronckers et al. (2008)	Children and adolescents monitored for scoliosis (3000; 80)	USA	Chest X-rays	Various low dose rates	0.13	2.86 (−0.07 to 8.62) Excess only in group with family history of breast cancer No modification by stage of reproductive development at exposure
Radiotherapy for benign disease						
Shore et al. (1986)	Women with postpartum mastitis (600; 50)	USA	X-rays	Fractionated high dose rate	3.8	3.20 (2.30–4.30)
Mattsson et al. (1993, 1995)	Women with breast disease (1200; 280)	Sweden	X-rays	Fractionated high dose rate	5.8	1.63 (0.77–2.89)
Hildreth et al. (1989), Adams et al. (2010)	Infants irradiated for treatment of thymus hypertrophy (1200; 100)	USA	X-rays	Fractionated moderate dose rate	0.71	1.10 (0.61–1.86)
Lundell et al. (1999), Eidemüller et al. (2009)	Children irradiated for treatment of skin haemangioma (17 000; 680)	Sweden	Gamma	Protracted low dose rate	0.29	0.25 (0.14–0.37)

Table 1.6 (continued)

Reference	Exposed population (size; number of breast cancer cases/ deaths)	Country	Exposure type	Exposure rate	Average dose (Gy)	ERR/Gy (95% CI) Main conclusion
Radiotherapy for breast cancer						
Storm et al. (1992)	Women treated by radiotherapy, mainly at or after menopause (56 500; 529)	Denmark	X-rays	High dose rate	2.51	1.04 (0.74–1.46)
Boice et al. (1992)	Women treated by radiotherapy, mainly at or after menopause (41 000; 650)	USA	X-rays	High dose rate	2.82	1.59 (1.07–2.36) at age < 45 years Significant exposure–response only for women treated at age < 45 years
Survivors of childhood cancer						
van Leeuwen et al. (2000, 2003)	Children treated for Hodgkin lymphoma (1200; 50)	Netherlands	Mantle chest radiotherapy	Several fractions of very high dose rate	38	0.06 (0.01–0.45) Further risk reduction for women treated after age 30 years, and for women also receiving chemotherapy
Travis et al. (2003), Hill et al. (2005)	Children treated for Hodgkin lymphoma (3800; 105)	Denmark, Finland, Netherlands, Sweden, USA	Mantle chest radiotherapy	Several fractions of very high dose rate	25	0.15 (0.04–0.73) Higher risk for higher doses No modifying effect of time since radiotherapy No strong conclusion on modifying factors
Guibout et al. (2005)	Children treated for cancer at different sites (1300; 16)	France, United Kingdom	External beam radiotherapy	Several fractions of high dose rate	5.1	0.13 (< 0–0.75) High risk for survivors of Hodgkin lymphoma No effect of age at first cancer
Reulen et al. (2011)	Children treated for cancer at different sites (18 000; 100)	United Kingdom	External beam radiotherapy	Several fractions of moderate to high dose rate	NA	SIR, 2.2 (1.8–2.7)
Kenney et al. (2004), Friedman et al. (2010)	Children treated for cancer at different sites (6000; 200)	USA	External beam radiotherapy	Several fractions of moderate to high dose rate	NA	SIR, 9.8 (8.4–11.5) Larger excess of breast cancer for survivors of Hodgkin lymphoma Increased risk when family history of breast cancer No modifying effect of reproductive and menstrual histories

Table 1.6 (continued)

Reference	Exposed population (size; number of breast cancer cases/deaths)	Country	Exposure type	Exposure rate	Average dose (Gy)	ERR/Gy (95% CI) Main conclusion
Moskowitz et al. (2014)	Children treated for cancer at different sites (1200; 170)	Canada, USA	External beam radiotherapy	Several fractions of high to very high dose rate	14	SIR, 30.6 (18.4–50.7) for radiation to chest Large excess risks of breast cancer whatever type of radiotherapy Higher risk for mantle field and whole-lung field therapies
Lange et al. (2014)	Children treated for Wilms tumour (2500, 28)	Canada, USA	Chest radiotherapy	Several fractions of high dose rate	12	14.8% (8.7–24.5%) at age 40 years Large excess of breast cancer
Pooled analysis						
Preston et al. (2002)	Atomic bomb survivors, women with tuberculosis, women with postpartum mastitis, women with benign breast disease, children with thymus hypertrophy, and children with skin haemangioma (77 500; 1500)	Japan, Sweden, USA	X-rays, gamma, neutron	Acute and fractionated low to high dose rate	0.2–5.8	0.86 (0.7–1.04) Linear dose–response relationship, flattening at high doses −45% change by 10-year increase of age at exposure Similar risks for acute and fractionated rate
Occupational exposure – medical and radiation workers						
Sigurdson et al. (2003), Doody et al. (2006)	Radiologists and radiological technologists (56 600; 1050)	USA	X-rays	Protracted very low dose rate	~100 mSv/yr before 1940	2.9 (1.3–6.2) for women exposed before 1935 2.6 (1.3–5.1) for women exposed before age 17 years
Mohan et al. (2002), Liu et al. (2014)	Radiologists and radiological technologists (69 500; 520)	USA	X-rays	Protracted low to moderate dose rate	NA	HR, 2.51 (1.24–5.05) for women exposed before the 1940s Decline in breast cancer mortality with increasing number of times technologists held patient for X-ray
Muirhead et al. (2009)	Radiation workers (17 500; 150 cases/60 deaths)	United Kingdom	X-rays, gamma	Protracted very low dose rate	0.02 Sv	ERR/Sv Mortality, 2.28 (< 0–38.2) Incidence, −0.23 (< 0–18.1)

Table 1.6 (continued)

Reference	Exposed population (size; number of breast cancer cases/ deaths)	Country	Exposure type	Exposure rate	Average dose (Gy)	ERR/Gy (95% CI) Main conclusion
Buitenhuis et al. (2013)	Workers occupationally exposed to radiation (3000; 1200)	Australia	Occupational external radiation	Protracted very low dose rate	NA	OR, 1.16 (0.86–1.57)
Hammer et al. (2014)	Airline flight crews (44 700; 200)	Denmark, Finland, Germany, Greece, Iceland, Italy, Norway, Sweden, United Kingdom, USA	Cosmic radiation	Protracted very low dose rate	~2–6 mSv/ yr	SMR, 1.06 (0.89–1.27)

CI, confidence interval; ERR/Gy (Sv), dose-specific excess relative risk per Gy (per Sv); Gy, gray; HR, hazard ratio; NA, not applicable; OR, odds ratio; SIR, standardized incidence ratio; SMR, standardized mortality ratio; Sv, Sievert; yr, year or years.

(c) Women irradiated for benign disease

The risk of breast cancer after radiotherapy for treatment of benign diseases has been estimated mainly among women treated for postpartum mastitis (Shore et al., 1986) or for benign breast disease (Mattsson et al., 1993, 1995), and among children treated for thymus hypertrophy (Hildreth et al., 1989; Adams et al., 2010) or for skin haemangioma (Lundell et al., 1999; Eidemüller et al., 2009). The doses were low to moderate but were received at a fractionated high dose rate, except for the skin haemangioma study. All these studies overall reported significant excess risks of breast cancer. The mean age at exposure of women treated for postpartum mastitis was 26 years and for benign breast disease was 40 years, but in these two studies no effect of age at exposure was observed. Infants treated for thymus hypertrophy were exposed mainly before age 1 year, and an excess risk of breast cancer was still observed after a mean follow-up of 57 years (Adams et al., 2010). In children treated for haemangioma, who were exposed at low doses and at a low dose rate, the estimated dose–response was lower but significant (Eidemüller et al., 2009).

(d) Women irradiated for breast cancer

Two studies were conducted on the risk of contralateral cancer associated with radiotherapy for breast cancer (Boice et al., 1992; Storm et al., 1992). The study in Denmark was mostly of perimenopausal or postmenopausal women and reported little evidence of radiation-induced contralateral breast cancer at low doses (Storm et al., 1992). The study in the USA reported an excess risk that was significant only for women treated before age 45 years (Boice et al., 1992). These two studies concluded that radiotherapy for breast cancer, at average radiation doses of 2.8 Gy and after age 45 years, contributes little, if at all, to the risk of a second cancer in the opposite breast.

(e) Survivors of childhood cancer

Cohorts of survivors of childhood cancer in the United Kingdom and the USA who were treated by X-ray radiotherapy with moderate to very high doses of chest radiation, targeted to mantle and modified mantle fields, mediastinum, lung, and chest (Henderson et al., 2010) exhibit a much higher risk of developing breast cancer compared with the general population (Kenney et al., 2004; Friedman et al., 2010; Reulen et al., 2011). The excess risk of breast cancer was consistently higher among survivors of Hodgkin lymphoma, mainly because they received higher exposure (Henderson et al., 2010). Two pooled studies (Guibout et al., 2005; Moskowitz et al., 2014) reported similar increased risks and gave detailed results either by radiation field or by radiation dose. A significant increase in risk of breast cancer was observed in the pooled cohort from France and the United Kingdom, with each Gray unit received by any breast increasing the excess relative risk by 0.13 (95% CI, < 0.0–0.75) (Guibout et al., 2005). Higher risks for mantle-field therapy (very high doses) and whole-lung-field therapy (large volume of radiation) were reported among women in Canada and the USA treated for cancer during childhood (Moskowitz et al., 2014). Female survivors of Wilms tumour who had been treated with chest radiotherapy had a high risk of developing early breast cancer (Lange et al., 2014). A study of women treated for Hodgkin lymphoma during childhood focused on a good reconstruction of radiation dosimetry and reported a significant dose–response relationship that still increased at very high doses and remained significant with increasing time since therapy (Travis et al., 2003). An analysis of modifying factors in that study was not conclusive (Hill et al., 2005). Similarly, in another study, in the Netherlands, the risk of breast cancer increased significantly with radiation dose, and the relationship was still observed at high doses (van Leeuwen et al., 2000, 2003). In that study,

Fig. 1.17 Population estimates (mean, minimum, maximum) of glandular tissue dose (mGy) from mammography, by time period and CBT

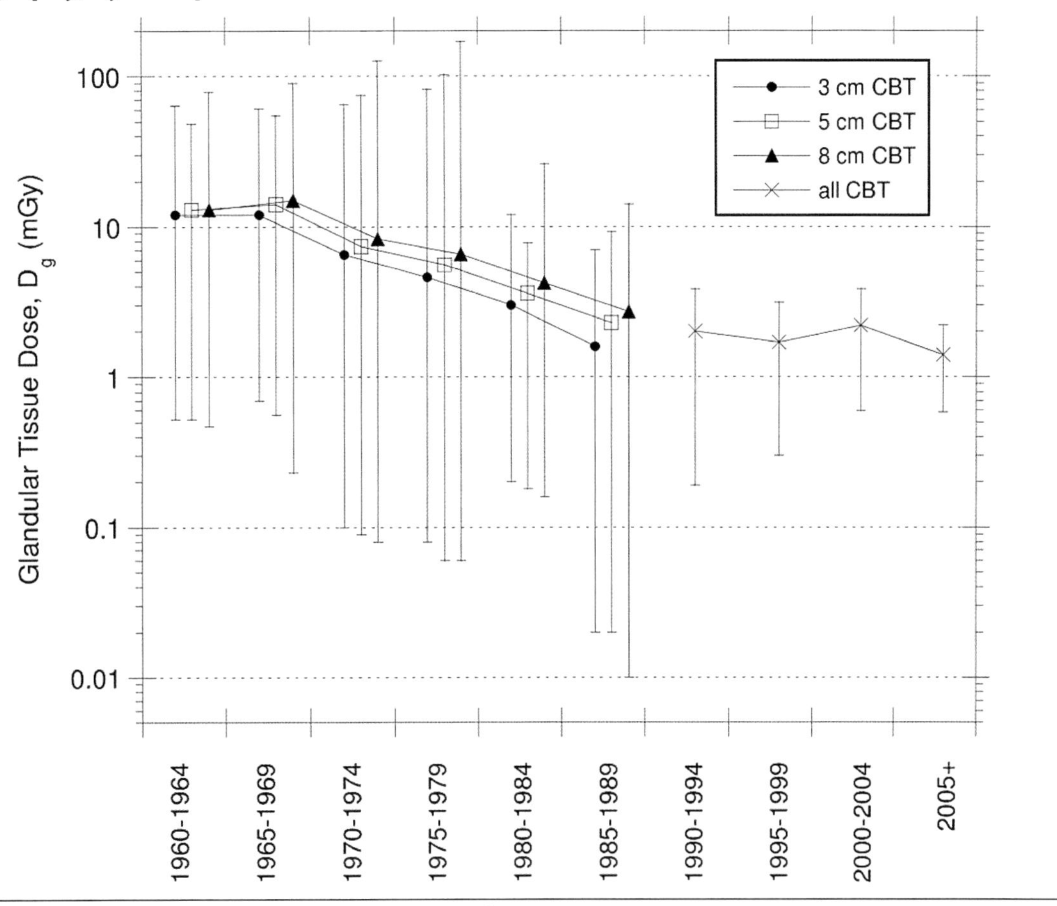

CBT, compressed breast thickness; D_g, glandular tissue dose; mGy, milligray.
From Thierry-Chef et al. (2012). Reconstruction of absorbed doses to fibroglandular tissue of the breast of women undergoing mammography (1960 to the present). *Radiat Res*, 177(1):92–108.

the risk seemed to decrease in women treated after age 30 years (compared with ≤ 20 years) and in women who received additional chemotherapy, partly due to the effect of chemotherapy on an earlier age at menopause.

(f) Women undergoing mammography

The risk of breast cancer induced by mammography is dependent on the dose received by the glandular tissue, as well as many other parameters, including age at exposure, dose rate, type of radiation, and dose–response relationship at low or high dose. Historical estimated doses to glandular breast tissue received from a single mammography view are presented in Fig. 1.17 (Thierry-Chef et al., 2012). Since the late 1990s, the dose received is about 2 mGy, about one sixth of the dose level in the 1960s and well below the dose level of most other exposures, apart from that received by radiation workers (see Table 1.6). Nevertheless, the detailed screening modalities (age range, frequency of screening, number of examinations at each screening, etc.) are necessary to accurately estimate the cumulative dose received by women during their entire participation in a screening programme. The risk of mammography-induced breast cancer is discussed in more detail in Section 5.3.4.

(g) Pooled analysis of non-occupational exposures

A very informative pooled analysis of eight cohort studies, of atomic bomb survivors, women with tuberculosis, women with post-partum mastitis, women with benign breast disease, infants treated for thymus hypertrophy, and children treated for skin hemangioma, included women from Japan, Sweden, and the USA exposed to a wide range of radiation doses at different ages (Preston et al., 2002). This study supports the linearity of the dose–response relationship for breast cancer, with evidence of a flattening at high doses. It highlights the independent modifying effect of age at exposure and attained age. Some heterogeneity of the dose–response relationship was observed across studies; this is partly explained by modifying factors such as family history of breast cancer. The study also suggests a similarity in dose–response for acute and fractionated high-dose-rate exposure.

(h) Women exposed occupationally

Incidence and mortality data on radiological technologists are available from large cohorts in Canada, the USA, Europe, and China (Mohan et al., 2002; Sigurdson et al., 2003; Doody et al., 2006). Doses received were elevated before 1940 and then decreased gradually; accordingly, current results show higher risks of breast cancer for women in their earlier years of employment. Other cohort studies of medical workers occupationally exposed to radiation are currently under way and may provide interesting results on breast cancer risk among women in the general population. Studies of nuclear workers are another important source of information on cancer risk at low doses and low-dose-rate exposure, but to date they have included too few women to be informative (Cardis et al., 2007). An incidence and mortality study from the United Kingdom National Registry for Radiation Workers showed no significant dose–response relationship for breast cancer (Muirhead et al., 2009). A case–control study in Australia found a low and non-significant excess risk of breast cancer among exposed women (Buitenhuis et al., 2013). Airline flight crews, composed mainly of women, are exposed to doses of cosmic radiation of up to 6 mSv per year. The most recent updated mortality study of an international joint analysis of cohorts of flight crews from 10 countries showed a breast cancer mortality rate similar to that of the general population, whereas a deficit was observed for almost all other cancer sites (Hammer et al., 2010).

(i) Increased radiosensitivity

Due to the involvement of *BRCA1/2* in the repair of DNA double-strand breaks, which can be caused by radiation, *BRCA1/2* mutation carriers show increased radiosensitivity (Nieuwenhuis et al., 2002; Venkitaraman, 2002; Powell & Kachnic, 2003; Yoshida & Miki, 2004; Boulton, 2006). In addition to the DNA repair mechanisms described in the above-mentioned studies, very recently a DNA damage-induced BRCA1 protein complex was described as part of the mRNA-splicing machinery. Mutations in BRCA1 and several proteins found within this complex lead to increased sensitivity to DNA damage (Savage et al., 2014).

It has been shown that female *BRCA1/2* mutation carriers have a higher risk of developing a radiation-induced breast cancer compared with non-carriers, and particularly before age 40 years (Broeks et al., 2007). A meta-analysis based on six case–control studies and one cohort study showed a non-significantly increased risk of breast cancer due to exposure to low-dose radiation (OR, 1.3; 95% CI, 0.9–1.8) among women with a familial or genetic predisposition (Jansen-van der Weide et al., 2010). The risk became significant at increasing cumulative doses compared with no or minimal radiation exposure (OR, 1.8; 95% CI, 1.1–3.0) and for exposure occurring before age 20 years (OR, 2.0; 95% CI, 1.3–3.1) (Jansen-van

Fig. 1.18 Schematic distribution of breast cancer incidence according to genetic risk

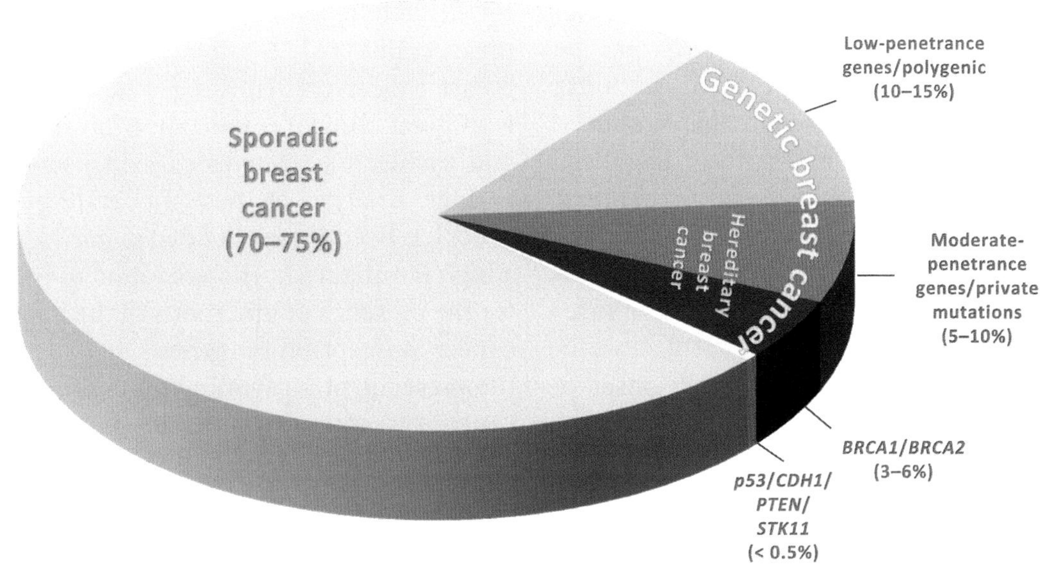

Created by the Working Group.

der Weide et al., 2010). Similarly, female *BRCA1/2* mutation carriers showed an increased risk of breast cancer before age 20–30 years associated with increasing cumulative doses of (low-dose) diagnostic radiation, and sensitivity analysis showed that this was not confounded by family history in this population (Pijpe et al., 2012).

1.3.5 Women at high genetic risk of breast cancer

Among the established risk factors for breast cancer (Mahoney et al., 2008), genetic factors are of particular importance. The current implementation of high-throughput technology has enabled the detection of hereditary alterations and related oncogenic pathways and of driver somatic mutations in mammary tumours, to characterize the phenotypic subtypes of pathologically heterogeneous breast tumours (Stephens et al., 2012).

As in other malignant tumours, the development of breast cancer is driven predominantly by the gradual and lifelong accumulation of acquired (somatic) mutations, but also by epigenetic changes in mammary cells and their progenitors (Polyak, 2007). Breast cancer is a highly pleomorphic disease, and numerous driver mutations (guiding the process of tumorigenesis) (Stratton et al., 2009) have been described by next-generation sequencing studies (Stephens et al., 2012). These mutations usually affect genes that code for key proteins regulating the maintenance of normal tissue homeostasis. A schematic distribution of breast cancer incidence according to genetic risk is given in Fig. 1.18. (See Section 5.6 for a discussion of the screening of women at an increased risk.)

(a) Hereditary breast cancer

Hereditary breast cancer is caused by germline mutations in highly penetrant breast cancer susceptibility genes, most commonly the *BRCA1/2* genes (Lichtenstein et al., 2000; Rahman, 2014a). Breast cancers attributable to heritable factors represent 5–10% of all breast cancer cases, which is a small but important proportion. Overall, the presence of breast cancer in any first-degree female relative nearly doubles the risk for a proband, and the inherited risk increases gradually with the number of affected relatives (Collaborative Group on Hormonal Factors in Breast Cancer, 2001). When risk is conferred through the mother, it increases gradually if the mother was diagnosed at a young age or had multiple diagnoses of breast or ovarian cancer (Anderson et al., 2000). For example, the presence of breast cancer in at least one first-degree relative accounts for 13% of cases (Collaborative Group on Hormonal Factors in Breast Cancer, 2001). Also, the early onset of breast cancer and other cancers in mutation carriers increases the probability of recurrence.

Other high- or moderate-penetrance breast cancer susceptibility genes that contribute to the hereditary breast cancer spectrum include *CHEK2*, *PTEN*, *TP53*, *ATM*, *STK11/LKB1*, *CDH1*, *NBS1*, *RAD50*, *BRIP1*, and *PALB2*, although none of them is comparable in frequency and clinical importance to *BRCA1/2* (Antoniou et al., 2014; Couch et al., 2014). Several common features of hereditary breast cancer, documented in both affected families and individuals, characterize this high-risk population.

(b) Penetrance of breast cancer susceptibility genes

Breast cancer susceptibility genes are usually categorized as high-penetrance, moderate-penetrance, or low-penetrance genes, reflecting the relative risk of breast cancer development in mutation carriers.

Mutations in high-penetrance genes (*BRCA1*, *BRCA2*, *PALB2*, *TP53*, *PTEN*, *STK11*, and *CDH1*) increase breast cancer risk more than 5-fold (Collaborative Group on Hormonal Factors in Breast Cancer, 2001). Within this group, the major breast cancer susceptibility genes *BRCA1* and *BRCA2* account for approximately 3–5% of all breast cancer cases and approximately 20–50% of all hereditary breast cancer cases (Rahman, 2014b).

Mutations in moderate- or intermediate-penetrance genes (such as *CHEK2*, *ATM*, *BRIP1*, *NBS1*, *RAD51C*, and *XRCC2*) increase breast cancer risk 2–5-fold. The identification of breast cancer-predisposing mutations in genes is of great clinical importance for both patients and unaffected relatives carrying a pathogenic variant. Analysis of these moderate-penetrance genes has been recommended in individuals with a high familial risk who are found to be negative for the presence of mutations in the major breast cancer susceptibility genes. Signs suggesting the presence of a germline mutation in a breast cancer susceptibility gene are: (i) unusual breast cancer appearance (early disease onset; tumour recurrence; bilateral tumour development; male breast cancer development; presence of rare or minor histopathological diagnoses [triple-negative, medullary, or atypical medullary type]; ER-negative); (ii) clustering of breast cancer in affected families; and (iii) cancer multiplicity (development of breast and other cancer types, including ovarian cancer, colorectal cancer, and melanoma).

Mutations in low-penetrance genes increase breast cancer risk less than 2-fold and have no clinical utility at present (Michailidou et al., 2013). However, the categorization of penetrance is not optimal and sometimes could be rather misleading, due to a limited understanding of the true phenotypic characteristics. Even the major breast cancer susceptibility genes exhibit polymorphisms that increase breast cancer risk only mildly (although with high statistical significance); examples are the *BRCA1* missense mutation R1699Q and the *BRCA2* truncating mutation c.K3326* (Michailidou et al., 2013). Deep sequencing analyses revealed that approximately 20% of triple-negative cancers have potentially druggable aberrations, which include *BRAF* V600E, *EGFR* amplifications, and *ERBB2/ERBB3* mutations (Shah et al., 2012). The incomplete knowledge of the disease characteristics and response to treatment in patients harbouring mutations in breast cancer susceptibility genes limits the clinical potential of dozens of recently characterized variants, making the assessment of cancer risk in this high-risk population uncertain (Kean, 2014).

The clinical utility of specific variants in the breast cancer susceptibility genes depends not only on their penetrance but also on the population-specific prevalence, which is inversely correlated with the risk of breast cancer development (John et al., 2007; Karami & Mehdipour, 2013). Mutations in breast cancer-predisposing genes other than *BRCA1/2* are usually not frequent and have large population variability. For example, the most common pathogenic variant in the *CHEK2* gene, c.1100delC (Bell et al., 1999), has a frequency of more than 1% in populations in northern Europe, whereas its frequency is lower in central Europe, extremely low in southern Europe, and practically null in Asian populations (Kleibl et al., 2005).

The large majority of breast cancer susceptibility genes code for tumour suppressor proteins that are involved in key DNA repair pathways (except for *PTEN*, *STK11*, and *CDH1*) and could thus represent a critical anticancer barrier; however, the molecular mechanisms through which hereditary alterations trigger the development of breast cancer remain to be elucidated (Bartek et al., 2007).

(c) BRCA1 *and* BRCA2 *mutation carriers*

The BRCA1 and BRCA2 proteins are coded by the most important breast cancer susceptibility genes responsible for the development of familial breast and ovarian cancer syndromes 1 and 2 (Online Mendelian Inheritance in Man [OMIM] #604370 and #612555; OMIM, 2015). The BRCA1 and BRCA2 proteins are structurally unrelated and form part of large multiprotein complexes involved in the repair of DNA double-strand breaks (Li & Greenberg, 2012). Currently, the Breast Cancer Information Core database (BIC, 2015) describes more than 1700 distinct variants in the *BRCA1* gene and more than 1900 in the *BRCA2* gene. The mutation frequency in both genes varies worldwide; it is highest in the Ashkenazi Jewish population, in which 2.5% of women are carriers (Warner et al., 1999; Karami & Mehdipour, 2013).

Among *BRCA1* and *BRCA2* mutation carriers, the cumulative risk to age 80 years was shown to reach 90% and 41%, respectively, for breast cancer and 24% and 8.4%, respectively, for ovarian cancer (Offit, 2006). Overall, the risk of mutations in either gene is comparable in patients from hereditary breast cancer-only families, is particularly increased in families with breast and/or ovarian cancer cases, and is inversely correlated with the age at onset (see above).

Carriers of mutations in either gene are also at increased risk of cancer at other anatomical sites. *BRCA1* mutations in women predispose to the development of fallopian tube and peritoneal cancers, and to a 5-fold increased risk of early-onset colorectal cancer in women younger than 50 years (Sopik et al., 2014).

It has been suggested that several lifestyle factors may modulate the risk of breast cancer in *BRCA1/2* mutation carriers, including breast-feeding, the use of oral contraceptives (associated with a reduced risk in *BRCA1/2* mutation carriers), and smoking (associated with an increased risk in *BRCA2* mutation carriers) (Friebel et al., 2014).

(d) *Putative* BRCA3 *candidate:* PALB2

The *PALB2* (partner and localizer of *BRCA2*) gene codes for a protein that serves as a scaffold for the BRCA1/2 proteins during the DNA double-strand break repair process. *PALB2* mutations have been associated with an increased risk of hereditary breast cancer and pancreatic cancer. A recent study estimated the cumulative risk to age 70 years of developing breast cancer to be 47.5% for carriers of *PALB2* loss-of-function mutations (Antoniou et al., 2014). Therefore, the risk is similar to that ascertained in *BRCA2* mutation carriers, although *PALB2* mutations are less frequent. The clinical management of *PALB2* mutation carriers should be similar to that of *BRCA2* mutation carriers.

(e) Other high-penetrance breast cancer susceptibility genes

Hereditary mutations in other high-penetrance genes conferring a high risk of breast cancer are very rare. Previously, they were usually analysed in cases with the clinical and histopathological characteristics of the associated genetic syndromes (Walsh et al., 2006). This practice has changed with the implementation of next-generation sequencing analyses in high-risk individuals (Couch et al., 2014; Tung et al., 2014). Interestingly, somatic mutations in these genes represent frequent driver mutations in sporadic breast cancer (Stephens et al., 2012).

Breast cancer is the most common cancer diagnosed in women affected by Li–Fraumeni syndrome (LFS; OMIM #151623; OMIM, 2015), mostly as ductal carcinoma or DCIS with ER and PR positivity and/or HER2/neu positivity (Masciari et al., 2012). LFS is a hereditary cancer predisposition syndrome caused by a *TP53* mutation (Gonzalez et al., 2009), which confers a cumulative risk of 49% of developing breast cancer by age 60 years. The probability of carrying a *TP53* mutation is increased in breast cancer patients younger than 30 years with a first- or second-degree relative with typical LFS-associated cancers at any age, and is almost null in patients diagnosed with breast cancer at age 30–49 years and with no family history of LFS-associated cancers (Gonzalez et al., 2009).

Female carriers of *CDH1* (human epithelial cadherin) mutations have a cumulative breast cancer risk to age 75 years of 52% (Kaurah et al., 2007), and the breast cancer is frequently of lobular type in patients older than 45 years (Schrader et al., 2011).

Hereditary heterozygous mutations in the *PTEN* (phosphatase and tensin homologue) gene, which codes for a phosphatase targeting phosphatidylinositol (3,4,5)-triphosphate, were characterized in individuals with Cowden syndrome (OMIM #158350; OMIM, 2015). Cowden syndrome is a rare, multisystem disease with an increased lifetime risk of developing breast cancer of 25–50% (Pilarski et al., 2013); higher lifetime risks of breast cancer (67%) and development of other cancer types (e.g. dysplastic cerebellar gangliocytoma) are also reported (Nieuwenhuis et al., 2014).

Mutations in the *STK11* (serine/threonine-protein kinase) gene have been associated with Peutz–Jeghers syndrome (OMIM #175200; OMIM, 2015), a rare disorder characterized by an increased risk of various neoplasms, including an increased risk of 45% of developing ductal breast cancer by age 70 years (Hearle et al., 2006).

(f) Moderate-penetrance breast cancer susceptibility genes

A representative of this group is the *CHEK2* (checkpoint kinase 2) gene, which codes for a regulatory serine/threonine kinase that phosphorylates various protein substrates (including p53 and BRCA1) in response to DNA damage. Mutations in *CHEK2* variants could be dispersed over the entire coding sequence, but only a few studies have analysed these in breast cancer patients (Desrichard et al., 2011). The most common variant, c.1100delC, increases breast cancer risk, with odds ratios of 2.7 for unselected breast cancer, 2.6 for early-onset breast cancer, and 4.8 for familial breast cancer (Weischer et al., 2008) and a hazard ratio of 3.5 and worsened survival for contralateral breast cancer (Weischer et al., 2012), in high-risk individuals not carrying *BRCA1/2* mutations (Meijers-Heijboer et al., 2002). The cumulative risk for patients with familial breast cancer and who are heterozygous carriers was estimated at 37% (Weischer et al., 2008). Breast tumours arising in c.1100delC mutation carriers are frequently of luminal type and express ER and/or PR (Nagel et al., 2012; Kriege et al., 2014), and do not occur at a particularly young age (Narod, 2010). *CHEK2* variants are highly population-specific, and four other variants were found to be associated with increased risk of multiple cancers, including cancers of the breast, colorectum, prostate, and thyroid (Cybulski et al., 2004). The p.I157T variant has been associated with a significantly increased breast cancer risk (OR, 4.2 for lobular breast cancer) (Liu et al., 2012a, b).

The upstream signalling activator of the CHEK2 protein is the large ATM (ataxia telangiectasia mutated) kinase. The frequency of hereditary variants of the *ATM* gene is estimated to be 0.3–1% in the general population (Prokopcova et al., 2007), and these variants have been associated with an increased relative risk of breast cancer of 2.4 (Renwick et al., 2006). Several studies led to the identification of only a limited number of mutation carriers in high-risk patients, characterized by a 2–3-fold increased breast cancer risk (Damiola et al., 2014).

Several other breast cancer susceptibility genes have been reported. *BRIP1* (also known as *BACH1*) is a BRCA1-binding helicase associated with breast cancer. Three genes – *MRE11*, *RAD50*, and *NBN* (*NBS1*) – that code for a protein complex (MRE11–RAD50–NBS1) required for DNA strand processing during the repair of DNA double-strand breaks have also been identified in breast cancer patients. Recent studies also indicate that mutations in non-canonical breast cancer susceptibility genes (e.g. mismatch repair genes, including *MLH1*, *MLH2*, and *PMS6*, which are associated with hereditary colorectal cancer) may contribute to the increased risk in patients with hereditary breast cancer (Castéra et al., 2014; Tung et al., 2014).

1.3.6 Attributable burden to known risk factors

Overall, established breast cancer risk factors are common across female populations worldwide and explain a large proportion of the 10-fold international variations in breast cancer incidence rates, as well as the increases seen in migrant studies. It has been estimated that the cumulative incidence of breast cancer to age 70 years in developed countries would drop from 6.3% to 2.7% if women had just two reproductive factors (parity and lifetime breastfeeding) similar to those of women in less-developed countries at the time (Collaborative Group on Hormonal Factors in Breast Cancer, 2002; see Table 1.7); in lower-incidence countries, such as those in Africa and Asia, the cumulative risks to age 70 years were 1–2%. International differences in age at first full-term pregnancy and age at menarche are likely to contribute further. Similarly, in the Million Women Study in the United Kingdom, lower breast cancer incidence rates in South Asian women (unadjusted RR, 0.82) and Black women (RR, 0.85) compared with White women were almost entirely attributed to eight reproductive and lifestyle risk factors (Gathani et al., 2014).

Within the same population, non-modifiable risk factors and family history appear to account for population attributable fractions of 40–50%, but most results are from higher-incidence countries. In terms of immediately modifiable risk factors, the 2005 Global Burden of Disease study estimated that 5% of deaths from breast cancer worldwide were attributable to alcohol consumption, 9% to overweight/obesity, and 10% to physical inactivity (with 21% attributable to their joint hazard) (Danaei et al., 2005). Joint population attributable fractions were considerably lower (18%) in low- and middle-income countries (LMICs) than in high-income countries (27%), largely due to lower alcohol consumption and lower prevalence of overweight/obesity in LMICs. [Note that this analysis did not include breastfeeding.]

Table 1.7 Population attributable fraction for breast cancer incidence associated with lifestyle factors in selected populations

Setting	Menopausal status	Risk factor	PAF (%)	References
High-income countries/countries with higher breast cancer incidence rates				
Worldwide		Alcohol consumption	9	Danaei et al. (2005), Arnold et al. (2015)
	Postmenopausal	Overweight/obesity	12.5	
Europe		Physical inactivity	9	
		Insufficiently active	20	Friedenreich et al. (2010)
		Sedentary lifestyle	10	
China		Number of children	4.7	Li et al. (2012)
		OC use	0.7	
		HRT use (1–5 years)	0.3	
Japan		Alcohol consumption, overweight/obesity, physical inactivity, and exogenous hormone use (including HRT and OC use)	10.5	Inoue et al. (2012)
Republic of Korea		Obesity (BMI ≥ 30 kg/m^2)	8.2	Park et al. (2014)
		Low leisure-time physical activity	8.8	
Brazil		Overweight/obesity	14	WCRF/AICR (2009)
Low- and middle-income countries/countries with lower breast cancer incidence rates				
Worldwide		Alcohol consumption	4	
	Postmenopausal	Overweight/obesity	4.4	Danaei et al. (2005), Arnold et al. (2015)
		Physical inactivity	10	
Islamic Republic of Iran	Postmenopausal	Parity < 7	52.6	Ghiasvand et al. (2012)
		BMI > 25 kg/m^2	24.8	
		Family history of breast cancer	15.7	
		OC use	13.7	
		Parity + BMI > 25 kg/m^3 + family history + OC use	71.3	

BMI, body mass index; HRT, hormone replacement therapy; OC, oral contraceptive; PAF, population attributable fraction.
The results collected may reflect some heterogeneity among the methods of the different source publications.

1.4 Stage at diagnosis, survival, and management

The diagnosis and management of breast cancer developed significantly during the late 1990s and early 2000s. Staging describes the size of a carcinoma and whether it has spread regionally to lymph nodes or metastasized to distant organs. Accurate staging provides key prognostic information, helps to tailor treatment protocols, and contributes to the planning and implementation of specific public health interventions, such as screening programmes, aiming to improve the detection of lesions at an early stage and to decrease overall cancer mortality rates.

The staging system routinely used for breast cancer is the tumour–node–metastasis (TNM) classification. It describes localized disease as stages I and II, regional disease as stage III, and distant disease as stage IV, mostly based on the anatomical extent of the primary tumour and the presence of spread to regional lymph nodes and of distant metastases (Table 1.8 and Table 1.9; UICC, 2010). This classification was first developed in 1940 and is periodically revised and updated by the Union for International Cancer Control (UICC) and the American Joint Committee on Cancer (AJCC) (Edge et al., 2010). Although the coding schema has evolved considerably over time, a good correlation has always been maintained between old and new classifications, especially for stages 0, I, II, and IV (Kwan et al., 2012; Walters et al., 2013b). The sixth edition of the TNM staging system was officially adopted by tumour registries in January 2003. The heterogeneity of small tumours was reflected in more subcategories in the lower levels of the staging system, and additional issues were assessed, including metastatic lesions detected by molecular biology techniques and/or immunohistochemical staining of sentinel node specimens and the clinical importance of the total number of positive axillary lymph nodes (Singletary & Greene, 2003). The most recent, seventh edition (Table 1.8 and Table 1.9) was published in 2010 and includes the use of specific imaging modalities and of circulating tumour cells detectable in blood or bone marrow to better estimate clinical tumour size (Edge et al., 2010; Murthy & Chamberlain, 2011). The eighth edition will be published in late 2016 and will incorporate further advances in cancer research, staging, diagnosis, and treatment (AJCC, 2014).

Although the TNM classification system is accepted worldwide, there is great variability in the process of stage recording, due to different technological advances in diagnostic procedures across the globe. Therefore, estimates of survival based on stage at diagnosis may be misleading, and survival by stagc at diagnosis may appear to have improved while overall survival does not change (Feinstein et al., 1985). International comparisons of survival by stage at diagnosis should take into consideration the variations in clinical classification and coding among cancer registries, which reflect the source of stage data, the time frame after the diagnosis within which the stage was recorded, whether the classification was defined clinically or pathologically, and whether tumour size was recorded before or after neo-adjuvant therapy (Walters et al., 2013a). The TNM system has become extremely complex and may be too complicated for use in developing countries. A much simpler system, such as the one used by the United States National Cancer Institute, could be a better option. The SEER staging, based on the widely accepted theory of cancer development, is the most basic staging system applicable to all anatomical sites (solid tumours). The five main categories of summary staging (in situ, localized, regional, distant, and unknown) are developed based on information available in the medical, clinical, and pathological records. However, although this system is frequently used by tumour registries, is not always properly understood by physicians (SEER, 2014b).

1.4.1 Stage at diagnosis and survival

Population-based cancer registries (PBCRs) provide information on the cancer burden in communities around the world, including incidence, mortality, stage at diagnosis, and survival. Currently, there are more than 700 PBCRs worldwide, although the quality and data coverage of registries differ substantially between developed and developing countries. PBCRs are especially valuable in LMICs, where the available population-based cancer data are few; poorly developed and inaccessible health services result in inconsistencies in early diagnosis, adequate treatment, and follow-up care, with a profound negative effect on cancer survival (Sankaranarayanan et al., 2010; Bray et al., 2014). A standardized minimum data set of variables with coding based on international systems like the TNM classification is required to facilitate the analysis of data

Table 1.8 Tumour–node–metastasis (TNM) clinical classification of breast cancer

T – Primary tumour
TX – Primary tumour cannot be assessed
T0 – No evidence of primary tumour
Tis – Carcinoma in situ
Tis (DCIS) – Ductal carcinoma in situ
Tis (LCIS) – Lobular carcinoma in situ
Tis (Paget) – Paget disease of the nipple not associated with invasive carcinoma and/or carcinoma in situ (DCIS and/or LCIS) in the underlying breast parenchyma
T1 – Tumour 2 cm or less in greatest dimension
T1mi – Microinvasion 0.1 cm or less in greatest dimension
T1a – More than 0.1 cm but not more than 0.5 cm in greatest dimension
T1b – More than 0.5 cm but not more than 1 cm in greatest dimension
T1c – More than 1 cm but not more than 2 cm in greatest dimension
T2 – Tumour more than 2 cm but not more than 5 cm in greatest dimension
T3 – Tumour more than 5 cm in greatest dimension
T4 – Tumour of any size with direct extension to chest wall and/or to skin (ulceration or skin nodules)
T4a – Extension to chest wall (does not include pectoralis muscle invasion only)
T4b – Ulceration, ipsilateral satellite skin nodules, or skin oedema (including peau d'orange)
T4c – Both 4a and 4b, above
T4d – Inflammatory carcinoma
N – Regional lymph nodes
NX – Regional lymph nodes cannot be assessed (e.g. previously removed)
N0 – No regional lymph-node metastasis
N1 – Metastasis in movable ipsilateral level I, II axillary lymph node(s)
N2 – Metastasis in ipsilateral level I, II axillary lymph node(s) that are clinically fixed or matted; or in clinically detected ipsilateral internal mammary lymph node(s) in the absence of clinically evident axillary lymph-node metastasis
N2a – Metastasis in axillary lymph node(s) fixed to one another (matted) or to other structures
N2b – Metastasis only in clinically detected internal mammary lymph node(s) and in the absence of clinically detected axillary lymph-node metastasis
N3 – Metastasis in ipsilateral infraclavicular (level III axillary) lymph node(s) with or without level I, II axillary lymph-node involvement; or in clinically detected ipsilateral internal mammary lymph node(s) with clinically evident level I, II axillary lymph-node metastasis; or metastasis in ipsilateral supraclavicular lymph node(s) with or without axillary or internal mammary lymph node involvement
N3a – Metastasis in infraclavicular lymph node(s)
N3b – Metastasis in internal mammary and axillary lymph nodes
N3c – Metastasis in supraclavicular lymph node(s)
M – Distant metastasis
M0 – No distant metastasis
M1 – Distant metastasis

Adapted from UICC (2010).

Table 1.9 Tumour–node–metastasis (TNM) stage grouping of breast cancer

Stage	T	N	M
Stage 0	Tis	N0	M0
Stage IA	T1[a]	N0	M0
Stage IB	T0, T1[a]	N1mi[b]	M0
Stage IIA	T0, T1[a]	N1	M0
	T2	N0	M0
Stage IIB	T2	N1	M0
	T3	N0	M0
Stage IIIA	T0,T1[a],T2	N2	M0
	T3	N1, N2	M0
Stage IIIB	T4	N0, N1, N2	M0
Stage IIIC	Any T	N3	M0
Stage IV	Any T	Any N	M1

[a] T1 includes T1mic.

[b] N1mi, micrometastases > 0.2 mm and ≤ 2 mm.

Used with the permission of the Union for International Cancer Control (UICC, 2010), Geneva, Switzerland. The original source for this material is TNM Classification of Malignant Tumours, 7th Edition, Sobin LH, Gospodarowicz MK, Wittekind C (editors), published by Wiley-Blackwell, 2009.

and to enable comparison of results among registries (Bray et al., 2014).

(a) *Stage at diagnosis*

In developing countries, an estimated 75% (range, 30–98%) of breast cancer cases are diagnosed at late clinical stages, such as stage III or IV (Sloan & Gelband, 2007; Coughlin & Ekwueme, 2009).

In African countries, retrospective studies have reported that 70–90% of breast cancers are diagnosed at stage III or IV (Fregene & Newman, 2005). A PBCR that covers the Gharbiah Governorate in Egypt reported an increase in the percentage of localized breast tumours from 14.8% in 1999 to 21.4% in 2008 (Hirko et al., 2013).

In India, more than 70% of patients are diagnosed with clinically advanced disease (stage III or IV) (Okonkwo et al., 2008).

In China, findings from a multicentre nationwide screening study showed a tendency towards higher cancer stages for disadvantaged women, with the majority of cases diagnosed at stage II (44.9% of cases) or stage III (18.7% of cases) (Li et al., 2011; Fan et al., 2014).

The proportion of breast cancer cases that are clinically advanced at diagnosis (stages III and IV) is reported as approximately 30–40% in Mexico and less than 20% in Uruguay, although in Uruguay the data come from a single institution. In Brazil, women are diagnosed earlier in the wealthier regions of the country; generally percentages of advanced disease (25–40%) are similar to those in Chile (30%) in 2003 (Justo et al., 2013).

Data from high-income countries for 2000–2007 reported the proportion of stage III or IV disease to be 8% in Sweden and 22% in Denmark and the proportion of localized disease to be 61–62% in Australia, Canada, Denmark, Norway, Sweden, and the United Kingdom (Walters et al., 2013a). For Norway in 2008–2012, the proportion was 0.7% for stage 0, 40.8% for stage I, 38.0% for stage II, 5.9% for stage III, and 3.5% for stage IV (Cancer Registry of Norway, 2014).

In British Columbia, Canada, a population-based cohort study of participants in the Screening Mammography Program reported that the majority of cases were detected at localized stages (38% at stage I and 32% at stage II)

Table 1.10 5-Year age-standardized breast cancer relative survival, by country/region

Country/region (type of registry)	5-Year relative survival (%)
The Gambia[b]	12
Uganda[b]	46
Philippines[b]	47 (40–55)
India[b]	52 (31–54)
Brazil (Brazilian registries)[a]	58.4 (52.7–64.6)
Thailand[b]	63
United Kingdom[a]	69.7 (69.4–70.1)
Europe (European registries)[a]	73.1 (72.9–73.4)
Singapore[b]	76
Costa Rica[b]	77
Turkey[b]	77
Republic of Korea[b]	79 (78–81)
Australia (national registry)[a]	80.7 (80.1–81.3)
Japan (Japanese registries)[a]	81.6 (79.7–83.5)
China[b]	82 (58–90)
Sweden[a]	82.0 (81.2–82.7)
Canada (Canadian registries)[a]	82.5 (81.9–83.0)
USA (North American registries)[a]	83.9 (83.7–84.1)

[a] International Cancer Survival Standard data (with 95% confidence interval) are for adults (aged 15–99 years) diagnosed during 1990–1994 and followed up until 1999. Adapted from Coleman et al. (2008).

[b] Data are the median percentage of an individual registry (and range, minimum–maximum, if more than one registry) for adults diagnosed during 1990–2001 and followed up until 2003. Adapted from Sankaranarayanan et al. (2010).

(Davidson et al., 2013). Similarly, in the USA in 1999–2005, 61% of cases were detected at localized stages (stages I and II), 32% at a regionally advanced stage (stage III), and only 5% at a distant-metastatic stage (stage IV) (Shulman et al., 2010). However, the proportion of cases diagnosed beyond the local stage and the 5-year cause-specific probability of death were higher among Black women than among White women (Harper et al., 2009). Data for 2003–2009 for all races showed that 61% of breast cancers were localized (among African-American women, only 52%), 32% were regional, and 5% were distant (Siegel et al., 2014).

(b) Survival

Worldwide, survival differences that persist after adjustment for tumour stage at diagnosis are likely to reflect differences in treatment, accuracy of staging, or tumour biology (Sant et al., 2003; Walters et al., 2013a). Overall, 5-year survival rates are consistently lower in LMICs compared with upper-middle- and high-income countries (Table 1.10; Anderson et al., 2011). Differences in 5-year survival between more- and less-developed health services for both localized and regional breast cancer are shown in Fig. 1.19.

A population-based study on breast cancer survival in countries in Africa, Asia, and Central America reported 5-year relative survival rates of 12% in The Gambia, 46% in Uganda, 52% in India, 82% in China, and 63% in Thailand. Rates in upper-middle- and high-income countries were 70% in Costa Rica, 77% in Turkey, 79% in the Republic of Korea, and 76% in Singapore (Sankaranarayanan et al., 2010). In Latin America, reported 5-year survival rates were 79% in Suriname, 72% in Chile, and 75% in Brazil (Mendonça et al., 2004; Navarrete Montalvo et al., 2008; van Leeuwaarde et al., 2011). In the

Fig. 1.19 Absolute survival for breast cancer, localized and regional extent of disease, by level of development of health services

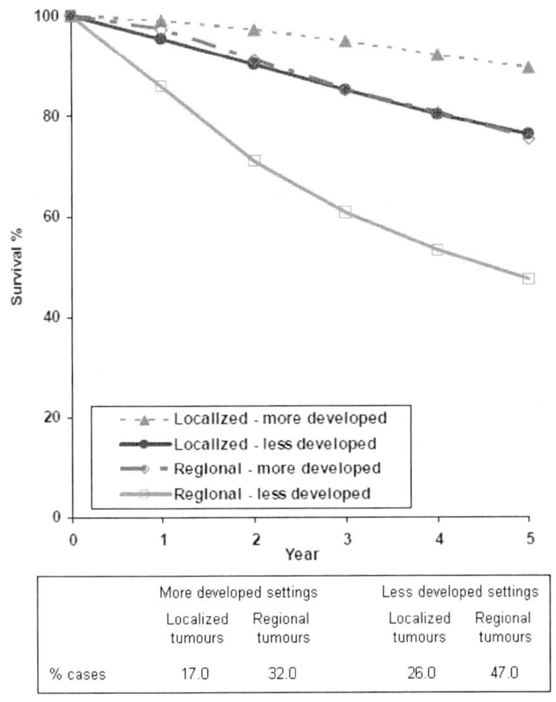

	More developed settings		Less developed settings	
	Localized tumours	Regional tumours	Localized tumours	Regional tumours
% cases	17.0	32.0	26.0	47.0

From Sankaranarayanan & Swaminathan (2011).

industrialized city of Shanghai, China, 5-year survival was 78% in 1992–1995, whereas in a rural neighbouring area, Qidong, it was only 58% in 1992–2000 (Fan et al., 2014).

Data from PBCRs in Canada (Alberta, British Columbia, Ontario, and Manitoba) showed a slight increase in 5-year survival rates over time, from 85.3% in 1995–2000 to 86.3% in 2005–2007 (Coleman et al., 2011) and to 88% in 2006–2008 (Canadian Cancer Society, 2014).

In the USA, the 5-year survival increased from 75% in 1975 to 89% in 2010, and was 98% for localized disease, 85% for regional disease, and 25% for distant disease (SEER, 2014a). A meta-analysis among African-American and White American breast cancer patients revealed that African-American ethnicity was associated with a 20% excess of mortality in 1980–2005 (Newman et al., 2006).

In Finland, the 5-year survival for breast cancer (all malignant neoplasms) of patients diagnosed in 2005–2010 and observed in 2010–2012 was 90% (Finnish Cancer Registry, 2015).

The largest cooperative study of population-based cancer survival in Europe (EUROCARE) shows a mean breast cancer survival rate of about 82% for breast cancer diagnosed in 2000–2007 (De Angelis et al., 2014). Geographical differences were reported, with higher survival in northern (84.7%), southern (83.6%), and central Europe (83.9%) and lower survival in the United Kingdom and Ireland (79.2%) and eastern Europe (73.7%). For most countries, the 5-year survival rate for breast cancer was fairly close to the European mean. Overall, survival rates in Europe increased over time, from 78.4% in 1999–2001 to 82.4% in 2005–2007. This increase was the most marked in eastern Europe and the United Kingdom and Ireland, so the survival gap between these countries and the rest of Europe decreased. Predictions of 10-year survival exceed 70% in most regions, with the highest value in northern Europe (74.9%) and the lowest in eastern Europe (54.2%), although 10-year survival is about 10% lower than 5-year survival in almost all European regions (Allemani et al., 2013). See Sections 1.5 and 1.6 and Section 4.1 for further details on the interpretation of survival findings with regard to mammographic screening.

1.4.2 Management

Breast cancer care has improved dramatically over the past 50 years, thanks to advances in multidisciplinary management, diagnosis, and treatment, including adjuvant treatments. Biological markers of prognosis have been identified, as well as biomarkers for targeted therapies, such as aromatase inhibitors for hormone receptor-positive breast cancers and anti-HER2 therapy for HER2/neu-overexpressing breast cancers.

The management of breast cancer often requires multimodality treatment involving surgery, radiotherapy, systemic treatment with chemotherapy, and/or hormone therapy and targeted therapy. Neo-adjuvant therapy may be given before surgery to shrink the tumour and after surgery to treat micrometastases.

(a) Surgery

Surgical treatment for breast cancer has been used for centuries. Radical mastectomy became the standard surgical approach towards the end of the 19th century and was popular until the 1980s, when randomized trials showed that it had a limited beneficial effect on survival. Modified radical mastectomy, simple mastectomy, and the evaluation of breast-conserving surgery were then introduced. Surgical interventions such as oophorectomies and adrenalectomies were relatively popular in the 20th century (Ahmed et al., 2011; American College of Surgeons, 2014). Nowadays, surgical treatment for the primary tumour may involve breast-conserving surgery plus radiotherapy, modified radical mastectomy, or simple mastectomy, depending on the size and location of the tumour, the suitability of breast-conserving surgery, and, in developing countries, the availability of radiotherapy.

Assessing the axillary lymph nodes is critical in staging and to determine prognosis and therapeutic options. Nowadays, axillary lymph node dissection as a staging procedure has largely been replaced by the less-invasive sentinel lymph node biopsy. Local surgical treatments have improved greatly without compromising locoregional control in breast cancer management (McWhirter, 1948; Lythgoe et al., 1978; Langlands et al., 1980; Fisher et al., 1981; Maddox et al., 1983).

(b) Radiotherapy

Radiotherapy is regularly indicated for locoregional treatment after breast-conserving surgery and in post-mastectomy patients to eradicate residual disease, thus reducing local recurrence. In women with axillary lymph node dissection and with up to three positive lymph nodes or with four or more positive nodes, radiotherapy reduced locoregional recurrence and overall recurrence (RR, 0.68; 95% CI, 0.57–0.82 versus RR, 0.79; 95% CI, 0.69–0.90) and reduced cancer mortality (RR, 0.80; 95% CI, 0.67–0.95 versus RR, 0.87; 95% CI, 0.77–0.99) (McGale et al., 2014). In women with no positive nodes, radiotherapy had no statistically significant effect on locoregional recurrence, overall recurrence, or cancer mortality, although it increased overall mortality (RR, 1.23; 95% CI, 1.02–1.49). Results were similar in the subset of trials in which women received systemic therapy (McGale et al., 2014). Women who receive breast-conserving surgery without radiotherapy have a risk of recurrence in the conserved breast of greater than 20% even when axillary lymph nodes are absent. It has been shown that radiotherapy to the conserved breast reduces the 10-year risk of any recurrence from 35.0% to 19.3% and the 15-year risk of mortality from 25.2% to 21.4%. The mortality reduction differed significantly between patients with node-positive and node-negative disease (Darby et al., 2011).

(c) Chemotherapy and adjuvant therapy

Chemotherapy was introduced into clinical cancer practice in the middle of the 20th century, and targeted therapy was introduced towards the end of the 20th century, whereas hormone therapy was already in use by the end of the 19th century (American College of Surgeons, 2014). The need for and the choice of adjuvant systemic treatment are determined by the stage and the molecular features of the disease. The side-effects must be considered before starting any treatment, as they can be immediate (appearing during treatment) or long-term (appearing weeks, months, or years after the treatment ends) and may be associated both with the patient's clinical conditions and stage at diagnosis and with the treatment (type and intensity).

Patients with ER-positive and/or PR-positive tumours, which account for 50–80% of breast cancers, usually receive hormone therapy, and patients with HER2-overexpressing tumours receive adjuvant anti-HER2 therapy in combination with chemotherapeutic agents, which may reduce mortality by one third and the risk of recurrence by 40% (Moja et al., 2012; Pinto et al., 2013). When neither HER2 overexpression nor hormone receptors are present, adjuvant therapy relies on chemotherapeutic regimens. It has been shown that 2 years of adjuvant anti-HER2 therapy is not more effective than 1 year of treatment for patients with HER2-positive early breast cancer, and thus 1 year of treatment remains the standard of care (Gianni et al., 2011; Goldhirsch et al., 2013), although cardiac toxicity is still a concern.

The classic adjuvant chemotherapy with cyclophosphamide, methotrexate, and 5-fluorouracil (CMF) (Bonadonna et al., 1976) was shown to improve survival in both node-positive and node-negative patients. Chemotherapy regimens such as 6 months of anthracycline as well as the addition of taxanes led to an additional decline in recurrence and mortality. A few years after its introduction in routine adjuvant practice, CMF was replaced by more-effective "third-generation" regimens containing anthracyclines and taxanes (Munzone et al., 2012). A meta-analysis showed that six cycles of anthracycline-based polychemotherapy, such as combination of 5-fluorouracil, doxorubicin, and cyclophosphamide or 5-fluorouracil, epirubicin, and cyclophosphamide, reduced the annual breast cancer death rate by about 38% in women younger than 50 years and by about 20% in women aged 50–69 years, irrespective of the use of tamoxifen and of ER status, nodal status, or other tumour characteristics (EBCTCG, 2005). The addition of four separate cycles of a taxane to such anthracycline-based regimens and the extension of treatment duration further reduced breast cancer mortality (RR, 0.86) (Peto et al., 2012).

It has been clearly demonstrated that neo-adjuvant chemotherapy such as tamoxifen reduces breast cancer mortality (RR, 0.71) and recurrence (RR, 0.68) in both node-positive and node-negative ER-positive breast cancers (Davies et al., 2011). Recent findings suggest that tamoxifen treatment is more beneficial for 10 years rather than for 5 years in women at high risk of recurrence (Davies et al., 2013). Studies have shown that the aromatase inhibitors offer an incremental improvement in survival and lower toxicity for postmenopausal women requiring hormone therapy. Pooled analyses of radiotherapy and systemic treatments reported a clinically significant improvement for both local and systemic therapy and provided evidence of modest but consistent effects of treatment.

As an example, the milestones of breast cancer treatment in the USA and their relationship with time trends in incidence, survival, and mortality are shown in Fig. 1.20.

(i) *Access to care and treatment in high-income countries*

In high-income countries and in populations where sufficient resources are available, access to optimal cancer treatment is promoted by well-developed infrastructures, due to the spending of 6–16% of gross domestic product (GDP) on health care (Coleman, 2010). The variations observed in survival trends mainly reflect later diagnosis or differences in treatment (Coleman et al., 2011), particularly among women in eastern European countries and non-Hispanic Black women in the USA (Kingsmore et al., 2004; Mikeljevic et al., 2004).

Expenditure on cancer therapy in Europe rose from €840 million in 1993 to €6.2 billion in 2004,

Fig. 1.20 Milestones of breast cancer therapy in the USA

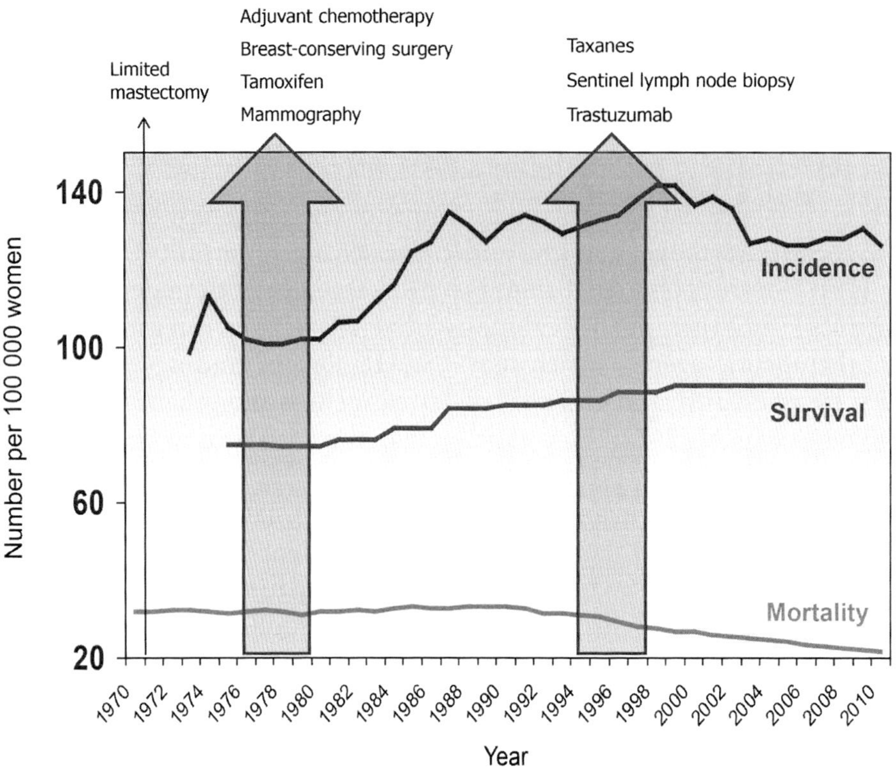

Courtesy of the IARC Screening Group, based on data from the American Society of Clinical Oncology (ASCO, 2014) and the SEER Program, USA (SEER, 2014a).

and is likely to increase further with the advent of targeted chemotherapy (Sullivan et al., 2011). Variations in breast cancer care across European countries are apparent (Allemani et al., 2010). Data from EUROCARE-3 show that 55% of women diagnosed with T1N0M0 breast cancers received breast-conserving surgery plus radiotherapy, ranging from 9% in Estonia to 78% in France. Of node-positive patients, chemotherapy was received by 52.1% of postmenopausal women and by 90.7% of premenopausal women, with marked variations among countries, particularly for postmenopausal women. For patients with ER-positive tumours, which constituted 45.3% of total cases, marked variations across countries in the availability of endocrine therapy were noted (Allemani et al., 2010).

Breast cancers are generally less advanced at diagnosis in the USA than in Europe, but the overall frequency of metastatic tumours is similar, at about 5–6% (Allemani et al., 2013). Currently, about 60% of cancer patients in the USA are treated with highly modern radiotherapy (Sullivan et al., 2011). Lymphadenectomy was reported in 86% of women in Europe and in 81% of women in the USA; surgical treatment was received by 91% of women in Europe and by 96% of women in the USA. Among women with early node-negative disease, 55% in Europe and 49% in the USA received breast-conserving surgery plus radiotherapy. Among women with node-positive tumours, 58% in Europe and 69% in the USA received chemotherapy. Compared with women aged 15–49 years, the proportion of women aged 50–99 years who received chemotherapy was higher in the USA (60%) than in Europe (46%), as was access to endocrine treatment for ER-positive tumours (62% in the USA and 55% in Europe) (Allemani et al., 2013).

(ii) Access to care and treatment in low- and middle-income countries

In many LMICs, major treatments (surgery, chemotherapy, and radiotherapy) are delivered within inadequate health services infrastructures. Rural areas, in particular, lack infusion equipment or other supplies, skilled oncology surgeons, and proper equipment; radiotherapy facilities are scarce (available to about 15% of patients) or non-existent, and access to chemotherapy and hormone therapy is limited (Anderson at al., 2011; Cesario, 2012).

In Latin America, the WHO Medical Devices Database reports inadequate cancer care due to limited physical and technological resources. The supply of radiotherapy units may vary, from 6 per 100 000 people in Bolivia and Paraguay to 57 per 100 000 people in Uruguay (Goss et al., 2013). In most Latin American countries, oncology services are concentrated in major cities, whereas rural regions often lack or have limited cancer care services. In Brazil, anti-HER2 targeted therapy for HER2-positive early breast cancer became available only in 2012. The situation is similar in other Latin American countries, such as Mexico, Argentina, and Colombia (Goss et al., 2013).

In sub-Saharan Africa, delayed presentation of breast cancer is common. Although mastectomy is not always culturally accepted in this region, it is the most widely used procedure for breast cancer treatment, due to the poor availability of adjuvant radiotherapy, chemotherapy, and resources for the assessment of sentinel lymph nodes. In a hospital in Uganda in 1996–2000, 75% of patients underwent surgery (58% of surgeries were modified radical mastectomy), 76% received radiotherapy, 60% received hormone therapy, and 29% received chemotherapy (Kingham et al., 2013). Locally advanced breast cancers are frequently treated with neo-adjuvant therapy; however, the frequencies of response and positive outcomes are not as high as those in high-income countries (Kingham et al., 2013).

In China, important disparities in access and timely care for breast cancer are reported. Although breast-conserving surgery has become the recommended surgical treatment since the 1990s, mastectomy still accounts for almost 89% of primary breast cancer surgery (Li et al., 2011; Fan et al., 2014). Even in developed urban areas, breast-conserving surgeries represented only 12.1% of surgeries in 2005 and 24.3% of surgeries in 2008. In Beijing in 2008, complete axillary lymph node dissection was performed for 84.1% of the patients. There is poor availability of radiotherapy as well as linear accelerator equipment, trained radiation oncologists, and technologists. Among patients who underwent breast-conserving surgery, 16.3% did not receive radiotherapy as per standard guidelines, and only 27% of patients nationwide received radiotherapy as part of their primary treatment. Access to systemic therapy is relatively frequent in China. About 81.4% of all patients with invasive breast cancer received adjuvant chemotherapy, and 80.2% of patients with HER2-positive tumours received adjuvant targeted therapy. Unfortunately, for many drugs the costs are not reimbursed by insurance, and the lack of access to new drugs also limits systemic treatment options for metastatic disease. For example, despite the approval of anti-HER2 therapy in 2002, in Beijing only 20.6% of patients with HER2-positive disease received targeted therapy (Fan et al., 2014).

Although cancer control programmes are becoming a higher priority and adequate multidisciplinary breast cancer treatment services generally exist, socioeconomic, geographical, or ethnic barriers are reflected in the inequity of cancer treatment. As the economies of middle-resource countries strengthen, higher breast cancer

Table 1.11 Recommended breast cancer treatment resources for low-resource countries

Resource level[a]	Local-regional treatment	Radiotherapy	Chemotherapy	Endocrine therapy	Supportive therapy
Basic	Modified radical mastectomy	[b]	Preoperative chemotherapy with AC, EC, FAC, or CMF[c]	Oophorectomy in premenopausal women Tamoxifen[d]	Non-opioid and opioid analgesics and symptom management
Limited	Breast-conserving surgery[e] Sentinel lymph node biopsy with blue dye[f]	Post-mastectomy irradiation of chest and regional nodes for high-risk cases[b]	See note	See note	See note

[a] Basic-level resources are defined as core resources or fundamental services that are absolutely necessary for any breast health care system to function. Limited-level resources or services are defined as those that produce major improvements in outcome but that are attainable with limited financial means and modest infrastructure.

[b] Chest wall and regional lymph node irradiation substantially decreases the risk of post-mastectomy local recurrence. If available, it should be used as a basic-level resource.

[c] Systemic chemotherapy requires blood chemistry profile and complete blood count testing for safety. When chemotherapy is available at the basic level, these tests should also be provided.

[d] Estrogen receptor (ER) testing by immunohistochemistry (IHC) is preferred for establishing hormone receptor status and is cost-effective when tamoxifen is available. When tamoxifen is available at the basic level, IHC testing of ER status should also be provided.

[e] Breast-conserving surgery can be provided as a limited-level resource but requires breast-conserving radiotherapy. If breast-conserving radiation is unavailable, patients should be transferred to a higher-level facility for post-lumpectomy radiation.

[f] Use of the sentinel lymph node (SLN) biopsy requires clinical and laboratory validation of SLN technique.

Note: The table stratification scheme implies incrementally increasing resource allocation at the basic and limited levels.

AC, doxorubicin and cyclophosphamide; CMF, cyclophosphamide, methotrexate, and 5-fluorouracil; EC, epirubicin and cyclophosphamide; FAC, 5-fluorouracil, doxorubicin, and cyclophosphamide.

Adapted from *Breast*, Volume 20, Supplement 2, El Saghir NS, Adebamowo CA, Anderson BO, Carlson RW, Bird PA, Corbex M et al., Breast cancer management in low resource countries (LRCs): consensus statement from the Breast Health Global Initiative, pages 3–11, Copyright (2011), with permission from Elsevier (El Saghir et al., 2011); and from *Cancer*, Volume 113, issue 8, Supplement 20, Anderson BO, Yip C-H, Smith RA, Shyyan R, Sener SF, Eniu A et al., Guideline implementation for breast healthcare in low-income and middle-income countries: overview of the Breast Health Global Initiative Global Summit 2007, pages 2221–2243, Copyright (2008), with permission from John Wiley & Sons, Inc. (Anderson et al., 2008).

survival rates are reported, due to earlier detection and better treatment options (Anderson at al., 2011). Identifying what can be done to diagnose and treat cancers more effectively at each level of the health system will require a global public health approach (Anderson et al., 2010). Recommended breast cancer treatment resources for low-resource countries from the Breast Health Global Initiative are shown in Table 1.11.

1.5 Breast awareness, early detection and diagnosis, and screening

Early detection of breast cancer aims to reduce mortality and other serious consequences of advanced disease through the early clinical diagnosis of symptomatic breast cancer or by screening asymptomatic women (Sankaranarayanan, 2000). When earlier treatments are available for detected cases, life expectancy, locoregional control of disease, and quality of life are much improved. In turn, early detection relies on access to prompt and effective diagnostic and treatment services (von Karsa et al., 2014a).

Early cancer detection is part of a cancer control strategy, which also should include: health education; breast cancer awareness; health-care providers with sufficient clinical skills, particularly at the primary care level; availability of accessible, affordable, and efficient health services with adequate infrastructure, human resources, and information systems; prompt diagnosis, staging, and treatment; and follow-up care (Richards et al., 1999; Norsa'adah et al., 2011; Ermiah et al., 2012; Caplan, 2014; Poum et al., 2014; Unger-Saldaña, 2014).

1.5.1 Breast awareness

Breast awareness is intended to encourage women to be conscious of how their breasts normally look and feel, so that they can recognize and report any abnormality. Breast awareness programmes also provide information about the efficacy of treatment when breast cancer is detected and treated early. Breast Cancer Awareness Month is observed worldwide every October.

Breast awareness is distinguished from breast self-examination (BSE). The purpose of BSE is to detect breast cancer by performing regular, systematic palpation and inspection of the breasts. The common goal of breast awareness and BSE is to improve breast cancer survival by detecting breast cancer at an early stage. The United Kingdom National Health Service (NHS) mammography screening programme historically emphasized breast awareness over BSE (Faulder, 1992) because BSE was thought to lead to an excessive preoccupation with cancer and to anxiety, while being theoretically equivalent to breast awareness. In 1991, the NHS emphasized a five-point plan for being breast aware: (i) knowing what is normal for you; (ii) looking at your breasts and feeling them; (iii) knowing what changes to look for; (iv) reporting any changes without delay; and (v) attending breast screening if you are aged 50 years or older (NHSBSP, 2006). Nowadays, it is pointed out that the distinction between breast awareness and BSE is not clear and that there is no evidence that morbidity or mortality are reduced by taking the recommended steps to become breast aware; in addition, it is not known whether the harms, such as anxiety and excess false-positive biopsies, are associated with both breast awareness and BSE (McCready et al., 2005; Thornton & Pillarisetti, 2008; Mac Bride et al., 2012; Mark et al., 2014). It has been suggested that breast awareness should be replaced with the concept of "sensible alertness" to the possibility of finding an abnormality, with women occasionally but regularly performing quick BSE (Thornton & Pillarisetti, 2008), because breast awareness may cause more harm than good unless it is followed up by prompt and effective diagnosis and treatment. At present, it is still not clear what breast awareness means to women, how it is acquired, and whether the balance of benefits and harms is favourable. Awareness about breast cancer is especially relevant for LMICs, compared with more developed countries, which rely heavily on mammographic screening to improve earlier detection and treatment of symptomatic cases (Yip et al., 2008).

1.5.2 Early diagnosis of symptomatic breast cancer

Given the fact that most breast cancers are first recognized by patients, an important aspect of early diagnosis is encouraging women to seek medical care without delay when they notice symptoms or signs. Referral occurs mostly in health centres, in dispensaries, and in the offices of general and family practitioners. It is critical that the doctors, nurses, and health workers at these primary care levels are knowledgeable and skilled about early symptoms and signs of breast cancer and about referral. A systematic review of 23 studies worldwide reported a 7% difference in pooled survival at 5 years between patients with a short delay (< 3 months) from onset of symptoms to initiation of treatment and those with a moderate delay (3–6 months) (Richards et al., 1999).

The common symptoms and clinical signs of breast cancer are: painless firm to hard lump in the breast; feeling of lumpiness in the breast; asymmetry of breasts; unilateral nipple retraction (as opposed to nipple inversion); unilateral bloody or serous nipple discharge; localized breast skin changes, such as tethering, oedema, puckering, or skin thickening; and eczematous changes in or around the nipple or areola. The clinical predictability of symptoms and signs should be considered together with family history of breast cancer (especially among first-degree relatives), past history of breast disease, and other risk factors, to avoid unnecessary referrals of women with normal breasts or benign lesions.

The single most important symptom of early breast cancer is the presence of a small palpable lump. The positive predictive value of a breast lump for breast cancer is reported to be about 1% or less in population-based studies (Mittra et al., 2010; Sankaranarayanan et al., 2011; Singh et al., 2015) and between 13% and 25% in hospital-based studies (Mahoney & Csima, 1982; Ohene-Yeboah & Amaning, 2008; Pradhan & Dhakal, 2008). The vast majority of breast lumps are fibroadenoma, fibroadenosis, fibrocystic mastopathy, mastitis, or solitary cysts, which are associated with benign breast disease (Mahoney & Csima, 1982; Ohene-Yeboah & Amaning, 2008; Pradhan & Dhakal, 2008; Sankaranarayanan et al., 2011). Discrete lumps with a hard consistency, lumps with skin or nipple changes, lumps associated with unilateral nipple discharge, and persistent breast lumps are associated with advanced breast cancer (Mahoney & Csima, 1982; Giess et al., 1998; Dolan et al., 2010; Chen et al., 2012). Breast pain and discomfort without a palpable breast lump is very common in menstrual and premenstrual women and is rarely, if ever, a sign of early breast cancer, whereas painless lumps should be brought to immediate medical attention (Ohene-Yeboah & Amaning, 2008).

Nipple changes are an important aspect of early detection and breast awareness. Inversion of one or both nipples is a common occurrence and is not typically associated with breast cancer. Unilateral bloody or serous nipple discharge, considered by many to be pathognomonic for breast cancer, is usually caused by benign conditions, most frequently papillomas and papillomatosis (Tabár et al., 1983). In contrast, extensive nipple retraction is associated with a tumour deep to the nipple causing retraction of the nipple towards the tumour. Serious nipple changes such as eczema and areola, with or without retraction, often accompanied by erythema and unpleasant or painful sensations, may be caused by Paget disease, which is associated with invasive or in situ breast cancer. As the disease advances, the surface of the skin breaks down, with a resulting oozing of fluid. A palpable tumour and nipple retraction are late symptoms of Paget disease. Any nipple rash or itchy, dry skin in or around the nipple should be brought to medical attention.

Early diagnosis of breast cancer can be facilitated by clinical breast examination or breast self-examination (see Sections 2.3 and 2.4, respectively).

Women referred with suspected breast cancer rarely require open surgery and usually undergo clinical assessment by a surgeon, oncologist, or radiologist, diagnostic imaging (magnetic resonance imaging or ultrasonography), and percutaneous tissue sampling (core needle biopsy provides greater sensitivity and specificity than fine-needle aspiration cytology) (Hukkinen et al., 2008). Triple assessment (comprising clinical examination, imaging, and tissue sampling) is an approach that is cost-effective, easy to perform, and time-saving but is achieved only in high-resource settings with excellent diagnostic imaging facilities and pathology services. In the lowest-resource settings, as in many countries in sub-Saharan Africa, clinical assessment is

Fig. 1.21 Early detection of breast cancer through screening asymptomatic women or early diagnosis of symptomatic women

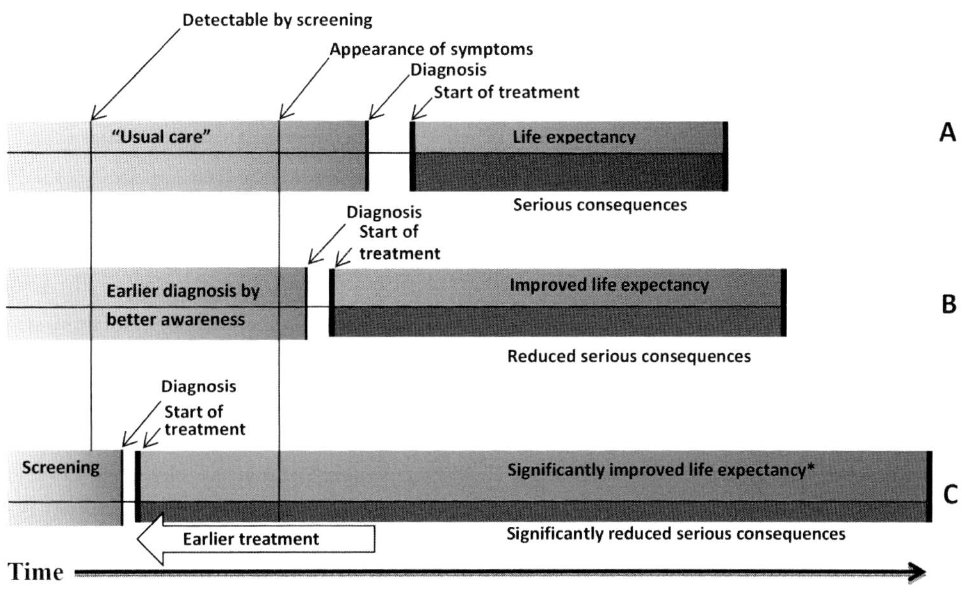

(A) Time intervals between the appearance of symptoms, the diagnosis, and the start of breast cancer treatment can be weeks to several months, depending on access to specialized care.
(B) Earlier diagnosis and good access to treatment may increase life expectancy and reduce serious consequences of the disease. Some overdiagnosis may also occur.
(C) Screening asymptomatic women leads to even earlier detection and treatment of breast cancer, albeit with some overdiagnosis but with a significantly increased life expectancy and less serious consequences of the cancer, provided screening services are adequate. The time intervals between positive screening results or the appearance of symptoms and the diagnosis and the start of treatment should be as short as possible. Well-organized screening programmes can shorten the interval between diagnosis and the start of treatment by prompt referral to qualified clinical units. They also provide an organizational framework for implementing the quality assurance.
Adapted with permission from de Koning (2009). The mysterious mass(es). [Inaugural address, Professor of Screening Evaluation.] Rotterdam, Netherlands: Erasmus MC. Available from: http://repub.eur.nl/res/pub/30689/oratie.pdf. (Figure 1, p. 7) and from Stewart BW, Wild CP, editors (2014). World Cancer Report 2014. Lyon, France: International Agency for Research on Cancer.

usually performed by biopsy. Improved breast cancer survival rates and reduced mortality were already observed in high-income countries before the introduction of widespread mammography screening (see Fig. 1.3; Sankaranarayanan et al., 2010; Tryggvadóttir et al., 2010). This has been attributed to increased breast awareness, improved medical assessment, early clinical diagnosis, the introduction of national universal medical insurance, and improved access to treatment (Taylor et al., 2003).

1.5.3 Screening asymptomatic women

Screening asymptomatic women, as part of early detection, includes both performing mammography screening at specified intervals and referring those women with positive screening findings for further diagnostic investigations and possibly treatment. Screening programmes may be either organized or unorganized (opportunistic) programmes (von Karsa et al., 2014a).

The main objective of screening asymptomatic women of appropriate age and average risk is to enable adequate treatment before the cancer poses a more serious threat to the individual woman (Fig. 1.21; Wilson & Jungner, 1968; Duffy et al., 2003; Perry et al., 2006, 2008; de Koning, 2009). As in any form of early detection, access to prompt and effective diagnosis and treatment is key to achieving the potential benefit of breast cancer screening (von Karsa et al., 2014a). In practice, less than one third of the breast cancers detected by mammography screening would also be detectable by clinical examination (Friedman et al., 2013). Also, some subtypes of breast cancer are more frequently detected at a more advanced stage, irrespectively of whether through screening or symptomatically (Tabár et al., 2014).

(a) Appropriate balance of benefits and harms

In recent decades, the principles of screening established by WHO in 1968 have been extended through experience gained from the implementation of population-based cancer screening programmes (WHO, 2007, 2013a, b). The careful consideration of the harm–benefit balance associated with the implementation of a cancer screening programme is particularly important in breast cancer screening, given the large number of women potentially involved.

The principal benefits of screening are the avoidance of death due to breast cancer (IARC, 2002; see Section 5.2), or of other serious consequences, such as advanced-stage breast cancer (Taplin et al., 2004; Norman et al., 2006; Malmgren et al., 2014; Fig. 1.21). The primary harms of screening include the morbidity and mortality from the procedures for detection and diagnosis, false-positive tests, overdiagnosis, and the side-effects of treatment (Sections 5.3.1–5.3.4). Another reported harm is anxiety, particularly when further investigation is required after a mammogram (see Section 5.3.5).

Exposure to these risks in the absence of any direct health benefit is of particular concern.

(b) Organized, population-based programmes

Organized programmes are characterized by centralized screening invitations to a well-defined target population, systematic call and recall for screening, delivery of test results, investigations, treatment and follow-up care, centralized quality assurance, and a programme database with linkages to other information systems, such as cancer registration systems and death registration systems, for monitoring and evaluation of the programme. Implementation of organized and opportunistic screening programmes is presented in Section 3.2, by WHO regions.

Most breast cancer screening programmes offer mammography to normal-risk women beginning at age 40–50 years and ending at age 69–74 years, typically at 2-year intervals (von Karsa et al., 2014b). The screening policy of an organized programme defines at least the screening protocol, the repeat interval, and the determinants of eligibility for screening. Effective communications should also be supported (Giordano et al., 2006; Webster & Austoker, 2006; Robb et al., 2010), enabling women to make an informed decision about whether to participate (Giordano et al., 2006, 2012; von Karsa et al., 2014a). In addition, organized programmes include an administrative structure, which is responsible for service delivery, including follow-up of detected lesions, quality assurance, and evaluation. Organized screening programmes generally include a national or regional implementation team, which is responsible for coordinating the delivery of the screening services, maintaining the requisite quality, reporting on performance and results, and defining standard operating procedures. In addition, information about all new cases and deaths from breast cancer occurring in the defined population served by the screening programme enables an estimate to be made of the impact of the programme on breast cancer mortality (IARC, 2002). Ideally, this can be

Fig. 1.22 The process of cancer screening

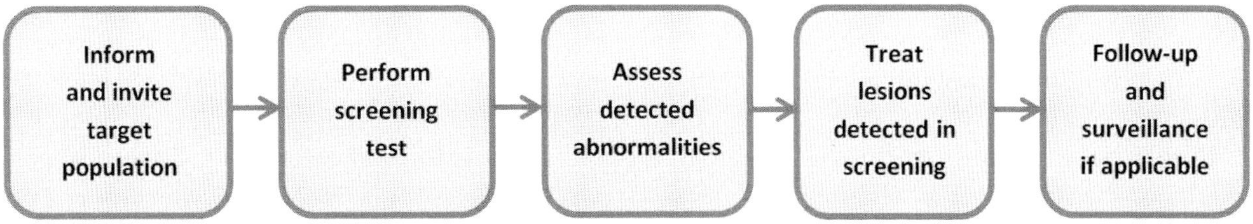

Inform and invite target population → Perform screening test → Assess detected abnormalities → Treat lesions detected in screening → Follow-up and surveillance if applicable

Adapted from von Karsa (1995) with permission from Deutscher Ärzte-Verlag.

achieved through linkage of individual data from a PBCR and a screening registry, if available (von Karsa & Arrossi, 2013; Anttila et al., 2014).

(c) *Opportunistic programmes*

Opportunistic programmes are not tailored to a predetermined eligible population and provide screening tests on request or at the time of routine health examinations. These programmes are less amenable to quality assurance than population-based screening, due, among other things, to the lack of administrative and organization infrastructure (de Gelder et al., 2009). They rely on the initiative of individual healthcare providers to offer screening or to encourage participation in a screening programme or outside the context of any programme (so-called wild screening). Organized breast screening programmes reach women who have not participated in opportunistic screening (Chamot et al., 2007; Gorini et al., 2014).

(d) *Quality assurance of screening programmes*

Quality assurance in breast cancer screening programmes goes beyond the need to ensure that any medical intervention is performed adequately, efficiently, and with minimum risk and maximum benefit. Screening involves a complex sequence of events and interrelated activities (see Fig. 1.22 for a summary of the process). To achieve maximum benefits with minimum risk, quality must be optimal at every step of the screening process (Perry et al., 2006, 2008; von Karsa & Arrossi, 2013). This can be achieved by a coordinated approach to programme planning and management, and by the availability of adequate human, financial, and technical resources. Overall, in Europe, the proportion of expenditure devoted to quality assurance should be no less than 10–20%, depending on the scale of the programme (Perry et al., 2013b; von Karsa et al., 2013, 2014a).

Numerous countries have adopted regulations, guidelines, and recommendations covering different aspects of quality assurance of mammography screening (Sibbering et al., 2009; Ellis, 2011; Gemeinsamen Bundesausschuss, 2011; Tonelli et al., 2011; Smith et al., 2012; BMV-Ä/EKV, 2014). The European Commission has published comprehensive multidisciplinary European guidelines for quality assurance in breast cancer screening and diagnosis (Perry et al., 2006, 2008, 2013a), and for establishing a population-based cancer screening programme (Lynge et al., 2012; Perry et al., 2013b; von Karsa & Arrossi, 2013; von Karsa et al., 2013) (see Section 3.2 for further information by country/region). In the USA, the Mammography Quality Standards Act (MQSA) made accreditation of mammography facilities mandatory (FDA, 2014). Professional and scientific societies provide additional guidance and standards, and training and technical support for the achievement of the standards, such as in preparation for accreditation, including comprehensive audits of professional and organizational performance (D'Orsi et al., 2013; American College of Surgeons, 2014; Canadian Association of Radiologists, 2014).

It may take several years to implement a population-based cancer screening programme, from the beginning of planning to completion of roll-out across an entire country or region. Sustainable institutional capacity is useful for programme management; computerized information systems, registration of breast cancer cases in the population, in screening registries and other data repositories and institutions are needed to collaborate in monitoring and evaluation, for regular audits of programme performance, and to assure the technical quality of equipment and services.

International collaboration can compensate for a local shortage of expertise in any given country, to facilitate process evaluation and avoid unnecessary delays in establishing fully functional screening programmes (von Karsa et al., 2014a).

(e) Denominators

As pointed out in the Working Procedures of this Handbook, the evaluation of the efficacy and effectiveness of breast cancer screening should measure the impact of a specific intervention, procedure, regimen, or service (Porta, 2008). The terms "breast cancer screening" and "mammography screening" are ambiguous; they may refer either to the invitation of women intended to be screened or to their actual participation by undergoing a screening mammogram. It is crucial to properly differentiate between the two concepts in order to evaluate breast cancer screening and to accurately interpret published reports.

The number of women, invited or participating, provides the denominator when the results of a screening programme are presented as rates or proportions. Results on women invited to screening are of particular interest to public health authorities when considering the potential benefits and harms to the population served by the programme. Participation in screening is fundamental to estimate the actual benefit of breast screening programmes and make informed decisions about whether to participate. In this Handbook, mammography screening programmes are examined using the number of women invited as the denominator, and the effects of participation in the screening programme are examined using the number of women participating as the denominator. Due consideration is given to the fact that the difference between the effect of invitation and the effect of attendance will depend on the proportion of women participating and so will not be generalizable from programme to programme.

References

Abdel-Fatah TM, Powe DG, Hodi Z, Reis-Filho JS, Lee AH, Ellis IO (2008). Morphologic and molecular evolutionary pathways of low nuclear grade invasive breast cancers and their putative precursor lesions: further evidence to support the concept of low nuclear grade breast neoplasia family. *Am J Surg Pathol*, 32(4):513–23. doi:10.1097/PAS.0b013e318161d1a5 PMID:18223478

Adams MJ, Dozier A, Shore RE, Lipshultz SE, Schwartz RG, Constine LS et al. (2010). Breast cancer risk 55+ years after irradiation for an enlarged thymus and its implications for early childhood medical irradiation today. *Cancer Epidemiol Biomarkers Prev*, 19(1):48–58. doi:10.1158/1055-9965.EPI-09-0520 PMID:20056622

Ades F, Zardavas D, Bozovic-Spasojevic I, Pugliano L, Fumagalli D, de Azambuja E et al. (2014). Luminal B breast cancer: molecular characterization, clinical management, and future perspectives. *J Clin Oncol*, 32(25):2794–803. doi:10.1200/JCO.2013.54.1870 PMID:25049332

Ahmed MI, Youssef M, Carr M (2011). Breast Cancer Care: A Historical Review. *Pak J Surg*, 27(2):135–9.

AJCC (2014). AJCC cancer staging manual, 8th edition updates. Chicago (IL), USA: American Joint Committee on Cancer. Available from: http://cancerstaging.org/About/Pages/8th-Edition.aspx.

Alexander FE, Roberts MM, Huggins A (1987). Risk factors for breast cancer with applications to selection for the prevalence screen. *J Epidemiol Community Health*, 41(2):101–6. doi:10.1136/jech.41.2.101 PMID:3498783

Ali S, Coombes RC (2002). Endocrine-responsive breast cancer and strategies for combating resistance. *Nat Rev Cancer*, 2(2):101–12. doi:10.1038/nrc721 PMID:12635173

Allemani C, Minicozzi P, Berrino F, Bastiaannet E, Gavin A, Galceran J et al.; EUROCARE Working Group (2013). Predictions of survival up to 10 years after diagnosis for European women with breast cancer in 2000–2002. *Int J Cancer*, 132(10):2404–12. doi:10.1002/ijc.27895 PMID:23047687

Allemani C, Storm H, Voogd AC, Holli K, Izarzugaza I, Torrella-Ramos A et al. (2010). Variation in 'standard care' for breast cancer across Europe: a EUROCARE-3 high resolution study. *Eur J Cancer*, 46(9):1528–36. doi:10.1016/j.ejca.2010.02.016 PMID:20299206

Allemani C, Weir HK, Carreira H, Harewood R, Spika D, Wang XS et al.; CONCORD Working Group (2014). Global surveillance of cancer survival 1995–2009: analysis of individual data for 25,676,887 patients from 279 population-based registries in 67 countries (CONCORD-2). *Lancet*, 385(9972):977–1010. doi:10.1016/S0140-6736(14)62038-9 PMID:25467588

Allen NE, Beral V, Casabonne D, Kan SW, Reeves GK, Brown A et al.; Million Women Study Collaborators (2009). Moderate alcohol intake and cancer incidence in women. *J Natl Cancer Inst*, 101(5):296–305. doi:10.1093/jnci/djn514 PMID:19244173

American College of Surgeons (2014). National Accreditation Program for Breast Centers. Available from: https://www.facs.org/quality%20programs/napbc.

Anderson B, Ballieu M, Bradley C, Elzawawy A, Cazap E, Enio A et al. (2010). Access to cancer treatment in low- and middle-income countries – an essential part of global cancer control. Working Paper. CanTreat International.

Anderson BO, Cazap E, El Saghir NS, Yip CH, Khaled HM, Otero IV et al. (2011). Optimisation of breast cancer management in low-resource and middle-resource countries: executive summary of the Breast Health Global Initiative consensus, 2010. *Lancet Oncol*, 12(4):387–98. doi:10.1016/S1470-2045(11)70031-6 PMID:21463833

Anderson H, Bladström A, Olsson H, Möller TR (2000). Familial breast and ovarian cancer: a Swedish population-based register study. *Am J Epidemiol*, 152(12):1154–63. doi:10.1093/aje/152.12.1154 PMID:11130621

Anderson TJ, Lamb J, Donnan P, Alexander FE, Huggins A, Muir BB et al. (1991). Comparative pathology of breast cancer in a randomised trial of screening. *Br J Cancer*, 64(1):108–13. doi:10.1038/bjc.1991.251 PMID:1854609

Anderson WF, Pfeiffer RM, Dores GM, Sherman ME (2006). Comparison of age distribution patterns for different histopathologic types of breast carcinoma. *Cancer Epidemiol Biomarkers Prev*, 15(10):1899–905. doi:10.1158/1055-9965.EPI-06-0191 PMID:17035397

Anderson BO, Yip CH, Smith RA, Shyyan R, Sener SF, Eniu A et al. (2008). Guideline implementation for breast healthcare in low-income and middle-income countries: overview of the Breast Health Global Initiative Global Summit 2007. *Cancer*, 113(8 Suppl):2221–43. doi:10.1002/cncr.23844 PMID:18816619

Andre F, Pusztai L (2006). Molecular classification of breast cancer: implications for selection of adjuvant chemotherapy. *Nat Clin Pract Oncol*, 3(11):621–32. doi:10.1038/ncponc0636 PMID:17080180

Antoine C, Ameye L, Paesmans M, Rozenberg S (2014). Systematic review about breast cancer incidence in relation to hormone replacement therapy use. *Climacteric*, 17(2):116–32. doi:10.3109/13697137.2013.829812 PMID:23909434

Antoniou AC, Casadei S, Heikkinen T, Barrowdale D, Pylkäs K, Roberts J et al. (2014). Breast-cancer risk in families with mutations in PALB2. *N Engl J Med*, 371(6):497–506. doi:10.1056/NEJMoa1400382 PMID:25099575

Anttila A, Lönnberg S, Ponti A, Suonio E, Villain P, Coebergh JW et al. (2014). Towards better implementation of cancer screening in Europe through improved monitoring and evaluation and greater engagement of cancer registries. *Eur J Cancer*, 51(2):241–51. doi:10.1016/j.ejca.2014.10.022 PMID:25483785

Arnold M, Pandeya N, Byrnes G, Renehan AG, Stevens GA, Ezzati M et al. (2015). Global burden of cancer attributable to high body-mass index in 2012: a population-based study. *Lancet Oncol*, 16(1):36–46. doi:10.1016/S1470-2045(14)71123-4 PMID:25467404

ASCO (2014). American Society of Clinical Oncology. Available from: http://cancerprogress.net/timeline/breast-cancer, accessed May 2011.

Atchley DP, Albarracin CT, Lopez A, Valero V, Amos CI, Gonzalez-Angulo AM et al. (2008). Clinical and pathologic characteristics of patients with BRCA-positive and BRCA-negative breast cancer. *J Clin Oncol*, 26(26):4282–8. doi:10.1200/JCO.2008.16.6231 PMID:18779615

Badwe RA, Dikshit R, Laversanne M, Bray F (2014). Cancer incidence trends in India. *Jpn J Clin Oncol*, 44(5):401–7. doi:10.1093/jjco/hyu040 PMID:24755545

Badwe RA, Mittra I, Havaldar R (1999). Timing of surgery with regard to the menstrual cycle in women with primary breast cancer. *Surg Clin North Am*, 79(5):1047–59. doi:10.1016/S0039-6109(05)70060-8 PMID:10572550

Bagnardi V, Rota M, Botteri E, Tramacere I, Islami F, Fedirko V et al. (2013). Light alcohol drinking and cancer: a meta-analysis. *Ann Oncol*, 24(2):301–8. doi:10.1093/annonc/mds337 PMID:22910838

Balko JM, Stricker TP, Arteaga CL (2013). The genomic map of breast cancer: which roads lead to better targeted therapies? *Breast Cancer Res*, 15(4):209. doi:10.1186/bcr3435 PMID:23905624

Bardou VJ, Arpino G, Elledge RM, Osborne CK, Clark GM (2003). Progesterone receptor status significantly improves outcome prediction over estrogen receptor status alone for adjuvant endocrine therapy in two large breast cancer databases. *J Clin Oncol*, 21(10):1973–9. doi:10.1200/JCO.2003.09.099 PMID:12743151

Barlow WE, White E, Ballard-Barbash R, Vacek PM, Titus-Ernstoff L, Carney PA et al. (2006). Prospective breast cancer risk prediction model for women undergoing screening mammography. *J Natl Cancer Inst*, 98(17):1204–14. doi:10.1093/jnci/djj331 PMID:16954473

Bartek J, Bartkova J, Lukas J (2007). DNA damage signalling guards against activated oncogenes and tumour progression. *Oncogene*, 26(56):7773–9. doi:10.1038/sj.onc.1210881 PMID:18066090

Baum M (2013). Modern concepts of the natural history of breast cancer: a guide to the design and publication of trials of the treatment of breast cancer. *Eur J Cancer*, 49(1):60–4. doi:10.1016/j.ejca.2012.07.005 PMID:22884336

Becker S, Kaaks R (2009). Exogenous and endogenous hormones, mammographic density and breast cancer risk: can mammographic density be considered an intermediate marker of risk? *Recent Results Cancer Res*, 181:135–57. doi:10.1007/978-3-540-69297-3_14 PMID:19213565

Bell DW, Varley JM, Szydlo TE, Kang DH, Wahrer DC, Shannon KE et al. (1999). Heterozygous germ line *hCHK2* mutations in Li-Fraumeni syndrome. *Science*, 286(5449):2528–31. doi:10.1126/science.286.5449.2528 PMID:10617473

Beral V, Reeves G, Banks E (2005). Current evidence about the effect of hormone replacement therapy on the incidence of major conditions in postmenopausal women. *BJOG*, 112(6):692–5. doi:10.1111/j.1471-0528.2005.00541.x PMID:15924521

Berlin L (2014). Point: Mammography, breast cancer, and overdiagnosis: the truth versus the whole truth versus nothing but the truth. *J Am Coll Radiol*, 11(7):642–7. doi:10.1016/j.jacr.2014.01.015 PMID:24794764

BIC (2015). Breast Cancer Information Core database. Bethesda (MD), USA: National Human Genome Research Institute. Available from: http://research.nhgri.nih.gov/bic/.

Bijker N, Peterse JL, Duchateau L, Julien JP, Fentiman IS, Duval C et al. (2001a). Risk factors for recurrence and metastasis after breast-conserving therapy for ductal carcinoma-in-situ: analysis of European Organization for Research and Treatment of Cancer Trial 10853. *J Clin Oncol*, 19(8):2263–71. PMID:11304780

Bijker N, Peterse JL, Duchateau L, Robanus-Maandag EC, Bosch CA, Duval C et al. (2001b). Histological type and marker expression of the primary tumour compared with its local recurrence after breast-conserving therapy for ductal carcinoma in situ. *Br J Cancer*, 84(4):539–44. doi:10.1054/bjoc.2000.1618 PMID:11207051

Bloom HJ, Richardson WW (1957). Histological grading and prognosis in breast cancer; a study of 1409 cases of which 359 have been followed for 15 years. *Br J Cancer*, 11(3):359–77. doi:10.1038/bjc.1957.43 PMID:13499785

BMV-Ä/EKV (2014). Provision of care in the Programme for Early Detection of Breast Cancer by Mammography Screening. Federal Collective Agreement – Physician fee schedule of the substitute funds, Annex 9.2, version 16 June 2014, valid from 1 July 2014 [in German]. Legal documents compendium of the German National Association of Statutory Health Insurance Physicians. Available from: http://www.kbv.de/media/sp/09.2_Mammographie.pdf.

Boice JD Jr, Harvey EB, Blettner M, Stovall M, Flannery JT (1992). Cancer in the contralateral breast after radiotherapy for breast cancer. *N Engl J Med*, 326(12):781–5. doi:10.1056/NEJM199203193261201 PMID:1538720

Boice JD Jr, Morin MM, Glass AG, Friedman GD, Stovall M, Hoover RN et al. (1991). Diagnostic x-ray procedures and risk of leukemia, lymphoma, and multiple myeloma. *JAMA*, 265(10):1290–4. doi:10.1001/jama.1991.03460100092031 PMID:2053936

Bombonati A, Sgroi DC (2011). The molecular pathology of breast cancer progression. *J Pathol*, 223(2):308–17. doi:10.1002/path.2808 PMID:21125683

Bonadonna G, Brusamolino E, Valagussa P, Rossi A, Brugnatelli L, Brambilla C et al. (1976). Combination chemotherapy as an adjuvant treatment in operable breast cancer. *N Engl J Med*, 294(8):405–10. doi:10.1056/NEJM197602192940801 PMID:1246307

Boulton SJ (2006). Cellular functions of the BRCA tumour-suppressor proteins. *Biochem Soc Trans*, 34(5):633–45. doi:10.1042/BST0340633 PMID:17052168

Boyd NF, Guo H, Martin LJ, Sun L, Stone J, Fishell E et al. (2007). Mammographic density and the risk and detection of breast cancer. *N Engl J Med*, 356(3):227–36. doi:10.1056/NEJMoa062790 PMID:17229950

Boyd NF, Martin LJ, Rommens JM, Paterson AD, Minkin S, Yaffe MJ et al. (2009). Mammographic density: a heritable risk factor for breast cancer. *Methods Mol Biol*, 472:343–60. doi:10.1007/978-1-60327-492-0_15 PMID:19107441

Boyd NF, Rommens JM, Vogt K, Lee V, Hopper JL, Yaffe MJ et al. (2005). Mammographic breast density as an intermediate phenotype for breast cancer. *Lancet Oncol*, 6(10):798–808. doi:10.1016/S1470-2045(05)70390-9 PMID:16198986

Bray F, Znaor A, Cueva P, Korir A, Swaminathan R, Ullrich A et al. (2014). Planning and developing population-based cancer registration in low- and middle-income settings. Lyon: International Agency for Research on Cancer (IARC Technical Publication Series, No. 43).

Available from: http://www.iarc.fr/en/publications/pdfs-online/treport-pub/treport-pub43/index.php.

Brewster AM, Hortobagyi GN, Broglio KR, Kau SW, Santa-Maria CA, Arun B et al. (2008). Residual risk of breast cancer recurrence 5 years after adjuvant therapy. *J Natl Cancer Inst*, 100(16):1179–83. doi:10.1093/jnci/djn233 PMID:18695137

Brinkley D, Haybrittle JL (1975). The curability of breast cancer. *Lancet*, 306(7925):95–7. doi:10.1016/S0140-6736(75)90003-3 PMID:49738

Broeks A, Braaf LM, Huseinovic A, Nooijen A, Urbanus J, Hogervorst FB et al. (2007). Identification of women with an increased risk of developing radiation-induced breast cancer: a case only study. *Breast Cancer Res*, 9(2):R26. doi:10.1186/bcr1668 PMID:17428320

Bruzzi P, Green SB, Byar DP, Brinton LA, Schairer C (1985). Estimating the population attributable risk for multiple risk factors using case-control data. *Am J Epidemiol*, 122(5):904–14. PMID:4050778

Buerger H, Otterbach F, Simon R, Poremba C, Diallo R, Decker T et al. (1999). Comparative genomic hybridization of ductal carcinoma in situ of the breast-evidence of multiple genetic pathways. *J Pathol*, 187(4):396–402. doi:10.1002/(SICI)1096-9896(199903)187:4<396::AID-PATH286>3.0.CO;2-L PMID:10398097

Buitenhuis W, Fritschi L, Thomson A, Glass D, Heyworth J, Peters S (2013). Occupational exposure to ionizing radiation and risk of breast cancer in Western Australia. *J Occup Environ Med*, 55(12):1431–5. doi:10.1097/JOM.0b013e3182a7e692 PMID:24270294

Bundred NJ (2001). Prognostic and predictive factors in breast cancer. *Cancer Treat Rev*, 27(3):137–42. doi:10.1053/ctrv.2000.0207 PMID:11417963

Burrell RA, McGranahan N, Bartek J, Swanton C (2013). The causes and consequences of genetic heterogeneity in cancer evolution. *Nature*, 501(7467):338–45. doi:10.1038/nature12625 PMID:24048066

Byrne C, Harris A (1996). Cancer rates and risks, 4th edition. Bethesda (MD), USA: US Department of Health and Human Services, National Institute of Health.

Cadman BA, Ostrowski JL, Quinn CM (1997). Invasive ductal carcinoma accompanied by ductal carcinoma in situ (DCIS): comparison of DCIS grade with grade of invasive component. *Breast*, 6(3):132–7. doi:10.1016/S0960-9776(97)90553-1

Canadian Association of Radiologists (2014). Mammography Accreditation Program (MAP). Available from: http://www.car.ca/en/accreditation/map.aspx.

Canadian Cancer Society (2014). Breast Cancer Statistics. Canadian Cancer Society's Advisory Committee on Cancer Statistics. Canadian Cancer Statistics 2014. Toronto: Canadian Cancer Society.

Cancer Genome Atlas Network (2012). Comprehensive molecular portraits of human breast tumours. *Nature*, 490(7418):61–70. doi:10.1038/nature11412 PMID:23000897

Cancer Registry of Norway (2014). Cancer in Norway 2012 – Cancer incidence, mortality, survival and prevalence in Norway. Oslo: Cancer Registry of Norway. Available from: http://www.kreftregisteret.no/global/cancer in norway/2012/cin_2012.pdf.

Caplan L (2014). Delay in breast cancer: implications for stage at diagnosis and survival. *Front Public Health*, 2:87. doi:10.3389/fpubh.2014.00087 PMID:25121080

Cardis E, Vrijheid M, Blettner M, Gilbert E, Hakama M, Hill C et al. (2007). The 15-country collaborative study of cancer risk among radiation workers in the nuclear industry: estimates of radiation-related cancer risks. *Radiat Res*, 167(4):396–416. doi:10.1667/RR0553.1 PMID:17388693

Castéra L, Krieger S, Rousselin A, Legros A, Baumann JJ, Bruet O et al. (2014). Next-generation sequencing for the diagnosis of hereditary breast and ovarian cancer using genomic capture targeting multiple candidate genes. *Eur J Hum Genet*, 22(11):1305–13. doi:10.1038/ejhg.2014.16 PMID:24549055

Cesario SK (2012). Global inequalities in the care of women with cancer. *Nurs Womens Health*, 16(5):372–85. doi:10.1111/j.1751-486X.2012.01761.x PMID:23067282

Chamot E, Charvet AI, Perneger TV (2007). Who gets screened, and where: a comparison of organised and opportunistic mammography screening in Geneva, Switzerland. *Eur J Cancer*, 43(3):576–84. doi:10.1016/j.ejca.2006.10.017 PMID:17223542

Chappuis PO, Nethercot V, Foulkes WD (2000). Clinico-pathological characteristics of *BRCA1*- and *BRCA2*-related breast cancer. *Semin Surg Oncol*, 18(4):287–95. doi:10.1002/(SICI)1098-2388(200006)18:4<287::AID-SSU3>3.0.CO;2-5 PMID:10805950

Cheang MC, Chia SK, Voduc D, Gao D, Leung S, Snider J et al. (2009). Ki67 index, HER2 status, and prognosis of patients with luminal B breast cancer. *J Natl Cancer Inst*, 101(10):736–50. doi:10.1093/jnci/djp082 PMID:19436038

Chen L, Zhou WB, Zhao Y, Liu XA, Ding Q, Zha XM et al. (2012). Bloody nipple discharge is a predictor of breast cancer risk: a meta-analysis. *Breast Cancer Res Treat*, 132(1):9–14. doi:10.1007/s10549-011-1787-5 PMID:21947751

Chiu SY, Duffy S, Yen AM, Tabár L, Smith RA, Chen HH (2010). Effect of baseline breast density on breast cancer incidence, stage, mortality, and screening parameters: 25-year follow-up of a Swedish mammographic screening. *Cancer Epidemiol Biomarkers Prev*, 19(5):1219–28. doi:10.1158/1055-9965.EPI-09-1028 PMID:20406961

Chlebowski RT (2013). Nutrition and physical activity influence on breast cancer incidence and outcome. *Breast*, 22(Suppl 2):S30–7. doi:10.1016/j.breast.2013.07.006 PMID:24074789

Chlebowski RT, Manson JE, Anderson GL, Cauley JA, Aragaki AK, Stefanick ML et al. (2013). Estrogen plus progestin and breast cancer incidence and mortality in the Women's Health Initiative Observational Study. *J Natl Cancer Inst*, 105(8):526–35. doi:10.1093/jnci/djt043 PMID:23543779

Chuaqui RF, Zhuang Z, Emmert-Buck MR, Liotta LA, Merino MJ (1997). Analysis of loss of heterozygosity on chromosome 11q13 in atypical ductal hyperplasia and in situ carcinoma of the breast. *Am J Pathol*, 150(1):297–303. PMID:9006344

Cobleigh MA, Vogel CL, Tripathy D, Robert NJ, Scholl S, Fehrenbacher L et al. (1999). Multinational study of the efficacy and safety of humanized anti-HER2 monoclonal antibody in women who have HER2-overexpressing metastatic breast cancer that has progressed after chemotherapy for metastatic disease. *J Clin Oncol*, 17(9):2639–48. PMID:10561337

Colditz GA, Atwood KA, Emmons K, Monson RR, Willett WC, Trichopoulos D et al. (2000). Harvard report on cancer prevention volume 4: Harvard Cancer Risk Index. Risk Index Working Group, Harvard Center for Cancer Prevention. *Cancer Causes Control*, 11(6):477–88. doi:10.1023/A:1008984432272 PMID:10880030

Colditz GA, Rosner B (2000). Cumulative risk of breast cancer to age 70 years according to risk factor status: data from the Nurses' Health Study. *Am J Epidemiol*, 152(10):950–64. doi:10.1093/aje/152.10.950 PMID:11092437

Coleman MP (2010). Cancer survival in the developing world. *Lancet Oncol*, 11(2):110–1. doi:10.1016/S1470-2045(09)70371-7 PMID:20005176

Coleman MP, Forman D, Bryant H, Butler J, Rachet B, Maringe C et al.; ICBP Module 1 Working Group (2011). Cancer survival in Australia, Canada, Denmark, Norway, Sweden, and the UK, 1995–2007 (the International Cancer Benchmarking Partnership): an analysis of population-based cancer registry data. *Lancet*, 377(9760):127–38. doi:10.1016/S0140-6736(10)62231-3 PMID:21183212

Coleman MP, Quaresma M, Berrino F, Lutz JM, De Angelis R, Capocaccia R et al.; CONCORD Working Group (2008). Cancer survival in five continents: a worldwide population-based study (CONCORD). *Lancet Oncol*, 9(8):730–56. doi:10.1016/S1470-2045(08)70179-7 PMID:18639491

Collaborative Group on Hormonal Factors in Breast Cancer (1996). Breast cancer and hormonal contraceptives: collaborative reanalysis of individual data on 53 297 women with breast cancer and 100 239 women without breast cancer from 54 epidemiological studies. *Lancet*, 347(9017):1713–27. doi:10.1016/S0140-6736(96)90806-5 PMID:8656904

Collaborative Group on Hormonal Factors in Breast Cancer (1997). Breast cancer and hormone replacement therapy: collaborative reanalysis of data from 51 epidemiological studies of 52,705 women with breast cancer and 108,411 women without breast cancer. *Lancet*, 350(9084):1047–59. doi:10.1016/S0140-6736(97)08233-0 PMID:10213546

Collaborative Group on Hormonal Factors in Breast Cancer (2001). Familial breast cancer: collaborative reanalysis of individual data from 52 epidemiological studies including 58,209 women with breast cancer and 101,986 women without the disease. *Lancet*, 358(9291):1389–99. doi:10.1016/S0140-6736(01)06524-2 PMID:11705483

Collaborative Group on Hormonal Factors in Breast Cancer (2002). Breast cancer and breastfeeding: collaborative reanalysis of individual data from 47 epidemiological studies in 30 countries, including 50302 women with breast cancer and 96973 women without the disease. *Lancet*, 360(9328):187–95. doi:10.1016/S0140-6736(02)09454-0 PMID:12133652

Collaborative Group on Hormonal Factors in Breast Cancer (2012). Menarche, menopause, and breast cancer risk: individual participant meta-analysis, including 118 964 women with breast cancer from 117 epidemiological studies. *Lancet Oncol*, 13(11):1141–51. doi:10.1016/S1470-2045(12)70425-4 PMID:23084519

Collins LC, Tamimi RM, Baer HJ, Connolly JL, Colditz GA, Schnitt SJ (2005). Outcome of patients with ductal carcinoma in situ untreated after diagnostic biopsy: results from the Nurses' Health Study. *Cancer*, 103(9):1778–84. doi:10.1002/cncr.20979 PMID:15770688

Corbex M, Burton R, Sancho-Garnier H (2012). Breast cancer early detection methods for low and middle income countries, a review of the evidence. *Breast*, 21(4):428–34. doi:10.1016/j.breast.2012.01.002 PMID:22289154

Couch FJ, Nathanson KL, Offit K (2014). Two decades after BRCA: setting paradigms in personalized cancer care and prevention. *Science*, 343(6178):1466–70. doi:10.1126/science.1251827 PMID:24675953

Coughlin SS, Ekwueme DU (2009). Breast cancer as a global health concern. *Cancer Epidemiol*, 33(5):315–8. doi:10.1016/j.canep.2009.10.003 PMID:19896917

Curtis C, Shah SP, Chin SF, Turashvili G, Rueda OM, Dunning MJ et al.; METABRIC Group (2012). The genomic and transcriptomic architecture of 2,000 breast tumours reveals novel subgroups. *Nature*, 486(7403):346–52. PMID:22522925

Cuzick J (2003). Epidemiology of breast cancer – selected highlights. *Breast*, 12(6):405–11. doi:10.1016/S0960-9776(03)00144-9 PMID:14659113

Cuzick J, Sestak I, Baum M, Buzdar A, Howell A, Dowsett M et al.; ATAC/LATTE investigators (2010). Effect of anastrozole and tamoxifen as adjuvant treatment for early-stage breast cancer: 10-year analysis of the ATAC trial. *Lancet Oncol*, 11(12):1135–41. doi:10.1016/S1470-2045(10)70257-6 PMID:21087898

Cybulski C, Górski B, Huzarski T, Masojć B, Mierzejewski M, Debniak T et al. (2004). *CHEK2* is a multiorgan cancer susceptibility gene. *Am J Hum Genet*, 75(6):1131–5. doi:10.1086/426403 PMID:15492928

D'Orsi CJ, Sickles EA, Mendelson EB, Morris EA et al. (2013). ACR BI-RADS® Atlas, Breast Imaging Reporting and Data System. Reston (VA), USA: American College of Radiology.

Dalton LW, Page DL, Dupont WD (1994). Histologic grading of breast carcinoma. A reproducibility study. *Cancer*, 73(11):2765–70. doi:10.1002/1097-0142(19940601)73:11<2765::AID-CNCR2820731119>3.0.CO;2-K PMID:8194018

Damiola F, Pertesi M, Oliver J, Le Calvez-Kelm F, Voegele C, Young EL et al. (2014). Rare key functional domain missense substitutions in *MRE11A*, *RAD50*, and *NBN* contribute to breast cancer susceptibility: results from a Breast Cancer Family Registry case-control mutation-screening study. *Breast Cancer Res*, 16(3):R58 doi:10.1186/bcr3669 PMID:24894818

Danaei G, Vander Hoorn S, Lopez AD, Murray CJ, Ezzati M; Comparative Risk Assessment collaborating group (Cancers) (2005). Causes of cancer in the world: comparative risk assessment of nine behavioural and environmental risk factors. *Lancet*, 366(9499):1784–93. doi:10.1016/S0140-6736(05)67725-2 PMID:16298215

Darby S, McGale P, Correa C, Taylor C, Arriagada R, Clarke M et al.; Early Breast Cancer Trialists' Collaborative Group (EBCTCG) (2011). Effect of radiotherapy after breast-conserving surgery on 10-year recurrence and 15-year breast cancer death: meta-analysis of individual patient data for 10,801 women in 17 randomised trials. *Lancet*, 378(9804):1707–16. doi:10.1016/S0140-6736(11)61629-2 PMID:22019144

Davidson A, Chia S, Olson R, Nichol A, Speers C, Coldman AJ et al. (2013). Stage, treatment and outcomes for patients with breast cancer in British Columbia in 2002: a population-based cohort study. *CMAJ Open*, 1(4):E134–41. doi:10.9778/cmajo.20130017 PMID:25077115

Davies C, Godwin J, Gray R, Clarke M, Cutter D, Darby S et al.; Early Breast Cancer Trialists' Collaborative Group (EBCTCG) (2011). Relevance of breast cancer hormone receptors and other factors to the efficacy of adjuvant tamoxifen: patient-level meta-analysis of randomised trials. *Lancet*, 378(9793):771–84. doi:10.1016/S0140-6736(11)60993-8 PMID:21802721

Davies C, Pan H, Godwin J, Gray R, Arriagada R, Raina V et al.; Adjuvant Tamoxifen: Longer Against Shorter (ATLAS) Collaborative Group (2013). Long-term effects of continuing adjuvant tamoxifen to 10 years versus stopping at 5 years after diagnosis of oestrogen receptor-positive breast cancer: ATLAS, a randomised trial. *Lancet*, 381(9869):805–16. doi:10.1016/S0140-6736(12)61963-1 PMID:23219286

Dawson SJ, Rueda OM, Aparicio S, Caldas C (2013). A new genome-driven integrated classification of breast cancer and its implications. *EMBO J*, 32(5):617–28. doi:10.1038/emboj.2013.19 PMID:23395906

De Angelis R, Sant M, Coleman MP, Francisci S, Baili P, Pierannunzio D et al.; EUROCARE-5 Working Group (2014). Cancer survival in Europe 1999–2007 by country and age: results of EUROCARE-5 – a population-based study. *Lancet Oncol*, 15(1):23–34. doi:10.1016/S1470-2045(13)70546-1 PMID:24314615

de Gelder R, Bulliard JL, de Wolf C, Fracheboud J, Draisma G, Schopper D et al. (2009). Cost-effectiveness of opportunistic versus organised mammography screening in Switzerland. *Eur J Cancer*, 45(1):127–38. doi:10.1016/j.ejca.2008.09.015 PMID:19038540

de Koning HJ (2009). The mysterious mass(es). [Inaugural address, Professor of Screening Evaluation.] Rotterdam, Netherlands: Erasmus MC. Available from: http://repub.eur.nl/res/pub/30689/oratie.pdf.

de Villiers TJ, Gass ML, Haines CJ, Hall JE, Lobo RA, Pierroz DD et al. (2013a). Global consensus statement on menopausal hormone therapy. *Climacteric*, 16(2):203–4. doi:10.3109/13697137.2013.771520 PMID:23488524

de Villiers TJ, Pines A, Panay N, Gambacciani M, Archer DF, Baber RJ et al.; International Menopause Society (2013b). Updated 2013 International Menopause Society recommendations on menopausal hormone therapy and preventive strategies for midlife health. *Climacteric*, 16(3):316–37. doi:10.3109/13697137.2013.795683 PMID:23672656

De Waard F, Collette HJ, Rombach JJ, Collette C (1988). Breast cancer screening, with particular reference to the concept of 'high risk' groups. *Breast Cancer Res Treat*, 11(2):125–32. doi:10.1007/BF01805836 PMID:3401604

Dean L, Geshchicter CF (1938). Comedo carcinoma of the breast. *Arch Surg*, 36(2):225–34. doi:10.1001/archsurg.1938.01190200057003

Desrichard A, Bidet Y, Uhrhammer N, Bignon YJ (2011). *CHEK2* contribution to hereditary breast cancer in non-*BRCA* families. *Breast Cancer Res*, 13(6):R119. doi:10.1186/bcr3062 PMID:22114986

Dixon JM, Sainsbury JRC (1998). Handbook of diseases of the breast, 2nd edition. Edinburgh, UK: Churchill Livingstone.

Dolan RT, Butler JS, Kell MR, Gorey TF, Stokes MA (2010). Nipple discharge and the efficacy of duct cytology in evaluating breast cancer risk. *Surgeon*, 8(5):252–8. doi:10.1016/j.surge.2010.03.005 PMID:20709281

Donker M, Litière S, Werutsky G, Julien JP, Fentiman IS, Agresti R et al. (2013). Breast-conserving treatment with or without radiotherapy in ductal carcinoma in situ: 15-year recurrence rates and outcome after a recurrence, from the EORTC 10853 randomized phase III trial. *J Clin Oncol*, 31(32):4054–9. doi:10.1200/JCO.2013.49.5077 PMID:24043739

Doody MM, Freedman DM, Alexander BH, Hauptmann M, Miller JS, Rao RS et al. (2006). Breast cancer incidence in U.S. radiologic technologists. *Cancer*, 106(12):2707–15. doi:10.1002/cncr.21876 PMID:16639729

Doody MM, Lonstein JE, Stovall M, Hacker DG, Luckyanov N, Land CE (2000). Breast cancer mortality after diagnostic radiography: findings from the U.S. Scoliosis Cohort Study. *Spine*, 25(16):2052–63. doi:10.1097/00007632-200008150-00009 PMID:10954636

Douglas-Jones AG, Gupta SK, Attanoos RL, Morgan JM, Mansel RE (1996). A critical appraisal of six modern classifications of ductal carcinoma in situ of the breast (DCIS): correlation with grade of associated invasive carcinoma. *Histopathology*, 29(5):397–409. doi:10.1046/j.1365-2559.1996.d01-513.x PMID:8951484

Dowsett M, Nielsen TO, A'Hern R, Bartlett J, Coombes RC, Cuzick J et al.; International Ki-67 in Breast Cancer Working Group (2011). Assessment of Ki67 in breast cancer: recommendations from the International Ki67 in Breast Cancer working group. *J Natl Cancer Inst*, 103(22):1656–64. doi:10.1093/jnci/djr393 PMID:21960707

Duffy SW, Tabár L, Vitak B, Day NE, Smith RA, Chen HH et al. (2003). The relative contributions of screen-detected in situ and invasive breast carcinomas in reducing mortality from the disease. *Eur J Cancer*, 39(12):1755–60. doi:10.1016/S0959-8049(03)00259-4 PMID:12888371

Dumas I, Diorio C (2010). Polymorphisms in genes involved in the estrogen pathway and mammographic density. *BMC Cancer*, 10(1):636. doi:10.1186/1471-2407-10-636 PMID:21092186

Dupont WD, Parl FF, Hartmann WH, Brinton LA, Winfield AC, Worrell JA et al. (1993). Breast cancer risk associated with proliferative breast disease and atypical hyperplasia. *Cancer*, 71(4):1258–65. doi:10.1002/1097-0142(19930215)71:4<1258::AID-CNCR2820710415>3.0.CO;2-I PMID:8435803

EBCTCG; Early Breast Cancer Trialists' Collaborative Group (2001). Tamoxifen for early breast cancer. *Cochrane Database Syst Rev*, (1):CD000486. PMID:11279694

EBCTCG; Early Breast Cancer Trialists' Collaborative Group (2005). Effects of chemotherapy and hormonal therapy for early breast cancer on recurrence and 15-year survival: an overview of the randomised trials. *Lancet*, 365(9472):1687–717. doi:10.1016/S0140-6736(05)66544-0 PMID:15894097

Edge S, Byrd DR, Compton CC, Fritz AG, Greene FL, Trotti A, editors (2010). AJCC cancer staging manuals. Preface, 7th edition. With CD-ROM.

Eidemüller M, Holmberg E, Jacob P, Lundell M, Karlsson P (2009). Breast cancer risk among Swedish hemangioma patients and possible consequences of radiation-induced genomic instability. *Mutat Res*, 669(1–2):48–55. doi:10.1016/j.mrfmmm.2009.04.009 PMID:19416732

El Saghir NS, Adebamowo CA, Anderson BO, Carlson RW, Bird PA, Corbex M et al. (2011). Breast cancer management in low resource countries (LRCs): consensus statement from the Breast Health Global Initiative. *Breast*, 20(Suppl 2):S3–11. doi:10.1016/j.breast.2011.02.006 PMID:21392996

Ellis I, editor (2011). Quality assurance guidelines for breast pathology services, 2nd edition. NHSBSP Publication No. 2. Sheffield, UK: NHS Cancer Screening Programmes.

Ellis IO, Coleman D, Wells C, Kodikara S, Paish EM, Moss S et al. (2006). Impact of a national external quality assessment scheme for breast pathology in the UK. *J Clin Pathol*, 59(2):138–45. doi:10.1136/jcp.2004.025551 PMID:16443727

Ellis IO, Galea M, Broughton N, Locker A, Blamey RW, Elston CW (1992). Pathological prognostic factors in breast cancer. II. Histological type. Relationship with survival in a large study with long-term follow-up. *Histopathology*, 20(6):479–89. doi:10.1111/j.1365-2559.1992.tb01032.x PMID:1607149

Ellis IO, Galea MH, Locker A, Roebuck EJ, Elston CW, Blamey RW et al. (1993). Early experience in breast cancer screening: emphasis on development of protocols for triple assessment. *Breast*, 2(3):148–53. doi:10.1016/0960-9776(93)90058-N

Elshof LE, Tryfonidis K, Slaets L, van Leeuwen-Stok AE, Skinner VP, Dif N et al. (2015). Feasibility of a prospective, randomised, open-label, international multicentre, phase III, non-inferiority trial to assess the safety of active surveillance for low risk ductal carcinoma in situ - The LORD study. *Eur J Cancer*, 51(12):1497–510. doi:10.1016/j.ejca.2015.05.008 PMID:26025767

Elston CW, Ellis IO (1991). Pathological prognostic factors in breast cancer. I. The value of histological grade in breast cancer: experience from a large study with long-term follow-up. *Histopathology*, 19(5):403–10. doi:10.1111/j.1365-2559.1991.tb00229.x PMID:1757079

Engholm G, Ferlay J, Christensen N, Kejs AMT, Johannesen TB, Khan S et al. (2014). NORDCAN: Cancer incidence, mortality, prevalence and survival in the Nordic countries, Version 7.0 (17.12.2014). Association of the Nordic Cancer Registries. Danish Cancer Society. Available from: http://www.ancr.nu, accessed 5 December 2014.

Erbas B, Provenzano E, Armes J, Gertig D (2006). The natural history of ductal carcinoma in situ of the breast: a review. *Breast Cancer Res Treat*, 97(2):135–44. doi:10.1007/s10549-005-9101-z PMID:16319971

Ermiah E, Abdalla F, Buhmeida A, Larbesh E, Pyrhönen S, Collan Y (2012). Diagnosis delay in Libyan female breast cancer. *BMC Res Notes*, 5(1):452. doi:10.1186/1756-0500-5-452 PMID:22909280

Ewertz M, Duffy SW, Adami HO, Kvåle G, Lund E, Meirik O et al. (1990). Age at first birth, parity and risk of breast cancer: a meta-analysis of 8 studies from the Nordic countries. *Int J Cancer,* 46(4):597–603. doi:10.1002/ijc.2910460408 PMID:2145231

Fan L, Strasser-Weippl K, Li JJ, St Louis J, Finkelstein DM, Yu KD et al. (2014). Breast cancer in China. *Lancet Oncol,* 15(7):e279–89. doi:10.1016/S1470-2045(13)70567-9 PMID:24872111

Faulder C (1992). Breast awareness: what do we really mean? *Eur J Cancer,* 28(10):1595–6. doi:10.1016/0959-8049(92)90048-7 PMID:1389471

FDA (2014). Mammography Quality Standards Act and Program. US Food and Drug Administration. Available from: http://www.fda.gov/Radiation-EmittingProducts/MammographyQualityStandardsActandProgram/default.htm.

Feinstein AR, Sosin DM, Wells CK (1985). The Will Rogers phenomenon. Stage migration and new diagnostic techniques as a source of misleading statistics for survival in cancer. *N Engl J Med,* 312(25):1604–8. doi:10.1056/NEJM198506203122504 PMID:4000199

Ferlay J, Bray F, Steliarova-Foucher E, Forman D (2014b). Cancer Incidence in Five Continents, CI5*plus*: IARC CancerBase No. 9 [Internet]. Lyon, France: International Agency for Research on Cancer. Available from: http://ci5.iarc.fr.

Ferlay J, Soerjomataram I, Dikshit R, Eser S, Mathers C, Rebelo M et al. (2014a). Cancer incidence and mortality worldwide: sources, methods and major patterns in GLOBOCAN 2012. *Int J Cancer,* 136(5):E359–86. doi:10.1002/ijc.29210 PMID:25220842

Ferlay J, Soerjomataram I, Ervik M, Dikshit R, Eser S, Mathers C et al. (2013). GLOBOCAN 2012 v1.0, Cancer Incidence and Mortality Worldwide: IARC CancerBase No. 11 [Internet]. Lyon, France: International Agency for Research on Cancer. Available from: http://globocan.iarc.fr, accessed 15 September 2014.

Finnish Cancer Registry (2015). Survival ratios of cancer patients in Finland. Institute for Statistical and Epidemiological Cancer Research. Available from: http://www.cancer.fi/syoparekisteri/en/statistics/survival-ratios-of-cancer-patien/.

Fisher B, Anderson S, Bryant J, Margolese RG, Deutsch M, Fisher ER et al. (2002). Twenty-year follow-up of a randomized trial comparing total mastectomy, lumpectomy, and lumpectomy plus irradiation for the treatment of invasive breast cancer. *N Engl J Med,* 347(16):1233–41. doi:10.1056/NEJMoa022152 PMID:12393820

Fisher B, Land S, Mamounas E, Dignam J, Fisher ER, Wolmark N (2001). Prevention of invasive breast cancer in women with ductal carcinoma in situ: an update of the National Surgical Adjuvant Breast and Bowel Project experience. *Semin Oncol,* 28(4):400–18. doi:10.1016/S0093-7754(01)90133-2 PMID:11498833

Fisher B, Wolmark N, Redmond C, Deutsch M, Fisher ER (1981). Findings from NSABP Protocol No. B-04: comparison of radical mastectomy with alternative treatments. II. The clinical and biologic significance of medial-central breast cancers. *Cancer,* 48(8):1863–72. doi:10.1002/1097-0142(19811015)48:8<1863::AID-CNCR2820480825>3.0.CO;2-U PMID:7284980

Fisher ER, Dignam J, Tan-Chiu E, Costantino J, Fisher B, Paik S et al. (1999). Pathologic findings from the National Surgical Adjuvant Breast Project (NSABP) eight-year update of Protocol B-17: intraductal carcinoma. *Cancer,* 86(3):429–38. doi:10.1002/(SICI)1097-0142(19990801)86:3<429::AID-CNCR11>3.0.CO;2-Y PMID:10430251

Fisher ER, Land SR, Fisher B, Mamounas E, Gilarski L, Wolmark N (2004). Pathologic findings from the National Surgical Adjuvant Breast and Bowel Project: twelve-year observations concerning lobular carcinoma in situ. *Cancer,* 100(2):238–44. doi:10.1002/cncr.11883 PMID:14716756

Fitzgibbons PL, Henson DE, Hutter RV; Cancer Committee of the College of American Pathologists (1998). Benign breast changes and the risk for subsequent breast cancer: an update of the 1985 consensus statement. *Arch Pathol Lab Med,* 122(12):1053–5. PMID:9870852

Forman D, Bray F, Brewster DH, Gombe Mbalawa C, Kohler B, Piñeros M et al. (2013). Cancer Incidence in Five Continents, Volume X (electronic version). Lyon, France: International Agency for Research on Cancer. Available from: http://ci5.iarc.fr.

Fournier A, Berrino F, Riboli E, Avenel V, Clavel-Chapelon F (2005). Breast cancer risk in relation to different types of hormone replacement therapy in the E3N-EPIC cohort. *Int J Cancer,* 114(3):448–54. doi:10.1002/ijc.20710 PMID:15551359

Fournier A, Mesrine S, Boutron-Ruault MC, Clavel-Chapelon F (2009). Estrogen-progestagen menopausal hormone therapy and breast cancer: does delay from menopause onset to treatment initiation influence risks? *J Clin Oncol,* 27(31):5138–43. doi:10.1200/JCO.2008.21.6432 PMID:19752341

Fournier A, Mesrine S, Dossus L, Boutron-Ruault MC, Clavel-Chapelon F, Chabbert-Buffet N (2014). Risk of breast cancer after stopping menopausal hormone therapy in the E3N cohort. *Breast Cancer Res Treat,* 145(2):535–43. doi:10.1007/s10549-014-2934-6 PMID:24781971

Fregene A, Newman LA (2005). Breast cancer in sub-Saharan Africa: how does it relate to breast cancer in African-American women? *Cancer,* 103(8):1540–50. doi:10.1002/cncr.20978 PMID:15768434

Friebel TM, Domchek SM, Rebbeck TR (2014). Modifiers of cancer risk in *BRCA1* and *BRCA2* mutation carriers: systematic review and meta-analysis. *J Natl Cancer Inst,* 106(6):dju091. doi:10.1093/jnci/dju091 PMID:24824314

Friedenreich CM, Neilson HK, Lynch BM (2010). State of the epidemiological evidence on physical activity and cancer prevention. *Eur J Cancer*, 46(14):2593–604. doi:10.1016/j.ejca.2010.07.028 PMID:20843488

Friedman DL, Whitton J, Leisenring W, Mertens AC, Hammond S, Stovall M et al. (2010). Subsequent neoplasms in 5-year survivors of childhood cancer: the Childhood Cancer Survivor Study. *J Natl Cancer Inst*, 102(14):1083–95. doi:10.1093/jnci/djq238 PMID:20634481

Friedman EB, Chun J, Schnabel F, Schwartz S, Law S, Billig J et al. (2013). Screening prior to breast cancer diagnosis: the more things change, the more they stay the same. *Int J Breast Cancer*, 2013:1. doi:10.1155/2013/327567 PMID:24159387

Frierson HF Jr, Wolber RA, Berean KW, Franquemont DW, Gaffey MJ, Boyd JC et al. (1995). Interobserver reproducibility of the Nottingham modification of the Bloom and Richardson histologic grading scheme for infiltrating ductal carcinoma. *Am J Clin Pathol*, 103(2):195–8. PMID:7856562

Fujii H, Szumel R, Marsh C, Zhou W, Gabrielson E (1996). Genetic progression, histological grade, and allelic loss in ductal carcinoma in situ of the breast. *Cancer Res*, 56(22):5260–5. PMID:8912866

Gail MH, Brinton LA, Byar DP, Corle DK, Green SB, Schairer C et al. (1989). Projecting individualized probabilities of developing breast cancer for white females who are being examined annually. *J Natl Cancer Inst*, 81(24):1879–86. doi:10.1093/jnci/81.24.1879 PMID:2593165

Gathani T, Ali R, Balkwill A, Green J, Reeves G, Beral V et al.; Million Women Study Collaborators (2014). Ethnic differences in breast cancer incidence in England are due to differences in known risk factors for the disease: prospective study. *Br J Cancer*, 110(1):224–9. doi:10.1038/bjc.2013.632 PMID:24169349

Gemeinsamen Bundesausschuss (2011). Regulation of the Joint Committee on Cancer Screening (cancer screening regulation/KFE-RL) [in German]. *Bundesanzeiger*, 34(S.864):1–5.

Ghiasvand R, Bahmanyar S, Zendehdel K, Tahmasebi S, Talei A, Adami HO et al. (2012). Postmenopausal breast cancer in Iran; risk factors and their population attributable fractions. *BMC Cancer*, 12(1):414. doi:10.1186/1471-2407-12-414 PMID:22992276

Gianni L, Dafni U, Gelber RD, Azambuja E, Muehlbauer S, Goldhirsch A et al.; Herceptin Adjuvant (HERA) Trial Study Team (2011). Treatment with trastuzumab for 1 year after adjuvant chemotherapy in patients with HER2-positive early breast cancer: a 4-year follow-up of a randomised controlled trial. *Lancet Oncol*, 12(3):236–44. doi:10.1016/S1470-2045(11)70033-X PMID:21354370

Giess CS, Keating DM, Osborne MP, Ng YY, Rosenblatt R (1998). Retroareolar breast carcinoma: clinical, imaging, and histopathologic features. *Radiology*, 207(3):669–73. doi:10.1148/radiology.207.3.9609889 PMID:9609889

Giordano L, Cogo C, Patnick J, Paci E; Euroscreen Working Group (2012). Communicating the balance sheet in breast cancer screening. *J Med Screen*, 19(Suppl 1): 67–71. doi:10.1258/jms.2012.012084 PMID:22972812

Giordano L, Webster P, Segnan N, Austoker J (2006). Guidance on breast screening communication. In: Perry N, Broeders M, de Wolf C, Törnberg S, Holland R, von Karsa L et al., editors. European guidelines for quality assurance in breast cancer screening and diagnosis. 4th ed. Luxembourg: European Commission, Office for Official Publications of the European Communities; pp. 379–94.

Go EM, Tsang JY, Ni YB, Yu AM, Mendoza P, Chan SK et al. (2012). Relationship between columnar cell changes and low-grade carcinoma in situ of the breast–a cytogenetic study. *Hum Pathol*, 43(11):1924–31. doi:10.1016/j.humpath.2012.02.001 PMID:22542249

Goldhirsch A, Gelber RD, Piccart-Gebhart MJ, de Azambuja E, Procter M, Suter TM et al.; Herceptin Adjuvant (HERA) Trial Study Team (2013). 2 years versus 1 year of adjuvant trastuzumab for HER2-positive breast cancer (HERA): an open-label, randomised controlled trial. *Lancet*, 382(9897):1021–8. doi:10.1016/S0140-6736(13)61094-6 PMID:23871490

Gonzalez KD, Noltner KA, Buzin CH, Gu D, Wen-Fong CY, Nguyen VQ et al. (2009). Beyond Li Fraumeni syndrome: clinical characteristics of families with *p53* germline mutations. *J Clin Oncol*, 27(8):1250–6. doi:10.1200/JCO.2008.16.6959 PMID:19204208

Goodwin PJ, Phillips KA, West DW, Ennis M, Hopper JL, John EM et al. (2012). Breast cancer prognosis in *BRCA1* and *BRCA2* mutation carriers: an International Prospective Breast Cancer Family Registry population-based cohort study. *J Clin Oncol*, 30(1):19–26. doi:10.1200/JCO.2010.33.0068 PMID:22147742

Gorini G, Zappa M, Cortini B, Martini A, Mantellini P, Ventura L et al. (2014). Breast cancer mortality trends in Italy by region and screening programme, 1980–2008. *J Med Screen*, 21(4):189–93. doi:10.1177/0969141314549368 PMID:25186117

Goss PE, Lee BL, Badovinac-Crnjevic T, Strasser-Weippl K, Chavarri-Guerra Y, St Louis J et al. (2013). Planning cancer control in Latin America and the Caribbean. *Lancet Oncol*, 14(5):391–436. doi:10.1016/S1470-2045(13)70048-2 PMID:23628188

Guibout C, Adjadj E, Rubino C, Shamsaldin A, Grimaud E, Hawkins M et al. (2005). Malignant breast tumors after radiotherapy for a first cancer during childhood. *J Clin Oncol*, 23(1):197–204. doi:10.1200/JCO.2005.06.225 PMID:15625374

Haagensen CD (1986). Diseases of the breast. Philadelphia (PA), USA: Saunders.

Halsted WS (1894). The results of operations for the cure of cancer of the breast performed at The Johns Hopkins Hospital from June 1889 to January 1894. *Ann Surg*, 20(5):497–555. doi:10.1097/00000658-189407000-00075 PMID:17860107

Hammer GP, Auvinen A, De Stavola BL, Grajewski B, Gundestrup M, Haldorsen T et al. (2014). Mortality from cancer and other causes in commercial airline crews: a joint analysis of cohorts from 10 countries. *Occup Environ Med*, 71(5):313–22. doi:10.1136/oemed-2013-101395 PMID:24389960

Hammer GP, Seidenbusch MC, Schneider K, Regulla D, Zeeb H, Spix C et al. (2010). Cancer incidence rate after diagnostic X-ray exposure in 1976–2003 among patients of a university children's hospital [in German]. *Rofo*, 182(5):404–14. doi:10.1055/s-0029-1245235 PMID:20234999

Harford JB (2011). Breast-cancer early detection in low-income and middle-income countries: do what you can versus one size fits all. *Lancet Oncol*, 12(3):306–12. doi:10.1016/S1470-2045(10)70273-4 PMID:21376292

Harper S, Lynch J, Meersman SC, Breen N, Davis WW, Reichman MC (2009). Trends in area-socioeconomic and race-ethnic disparities in breast cancer incidence, stage at diagnosis, screening, mortality, and survival among women ages 50 years and over (1987–2005). *Cancer Epidemiol Biomarkers Prev*, 18(1):121–31. doi:10.1158/1055-9965.EPI-08-0679 PMID:19124489

Harris JR, Lippman ME, Veronesi U, Willett W (1992). Breast cancer. *N Engl J Med*, 327(5):319–28. doi:10.1056/NEJM199207303270505 PMID:1620171

Hearle N, Schumacher V, Menko FH, Olschwang S, Boardman LA, Gille JJ et al. (2006). Frequency and spectrum of cancers in the Peutz-Jeghers syndrome. *Clin Cancer Res*, 12(10):3209–15. doi:10.1158/1078-0432.CCR-06-0083 PMID:16707622

Henderson TO, Amsterdam A, Bhatia S, Hudson MM, Meadows AT, Neglia JP et al. (2010). Systematic review: surveillance for breast cancer in women treated with chest radiation for childhood, adolescent, or young adult cancer. *Ann Intern Med*, 152(7):444–55, W144–54. doi:10.7326/0003-4819-152-7-201004060-00009 PMID:20368650

Hildreth NG, Shore RE, Dvoretsky PM (1989). The risk of breast cancer after irradiation of the thymus in infancy. *N Engl J Med*, 321(19):1281–4. doi:10.1056/NEJM198911093211901 PMID:2797100

Hill DA, Gilbert E, Dores GM, Gospodarowicz M, van Leeuwen FE, Holowaty E et al. (2005). Breast cancer risk following radiotherapy for Hodgkin lymphoma: modification by other risk factors. *Blood*, 106(10):3358–65. doi:10.1182/blood-2005-04-1535 PMID:16051739

Hirko KA, Soliman AS, Hablas A, Seifeldin IA, Ramadan M, Banerjee M et al. (2013). Trends in breast cancer incidence rates by age and stage at diagnosis in Gharbiah, Egypt, over 10 years (1999–2008). *J Cancer Epidemiol*, 2013:1. doi:10.1155/2013/916394 PMID:24282410

Honrado E, Benítez J, Palacios J (2006). Histopathology of *BRCA1*- and *BRCA2*-associated breast cancer. *Crit Rev Oncol Hematol*, 59(1):27–39. doi:10.1016/j.critrevonc.2006.01.006 PMID:16530420

Howe GR, McLaughlin J (1996). Breast cancer mortality between 1950 and 1987 after exposure to fractionated moderate-dose-rate ionizing radiation in the Canadian fluoroscopy cohort study and a comparison with breast cancer mortality in the atomic bomb survivors study. *Radiat Res*, 145(6):694–707. doi:10.2307/3579360 PMID:8643829

Hsieh CC, Trichopoulos D, Katsouyanni K, Yuasa S (1990). Age at menarche, age at menopause, height and obesity as risk factors for breast cancer: associations and interactions in an international case-control study. *Int J Cancer*, 46(5):796–800. doi:10.1002/ijc.2910460508 PMID:2228308

Hukkinen K, Kivisaari L, Heikkilä PS, Von Smitten K, Leidenius M (2008). Unsuccessful preoperative biopsies, fine needle aspiration cytology or core needle biopsy, lead to increased costs in the diagnostic workup in breast cancer. *Acta Oncol*, 47(6):1037–45. doi:10.1080/02841860802001442 PMID:18607862

Hwang ES, DeVries S, Chew KL, Moore DH 2nd, Kerlikowske K, Thor A et al. (2004). Patterns of chromosomal alterations in breast ductal carcinoma in situ. *Clin Cancer Res*, 10(15):5160–7. doi:10.1158/1078-0432.CCR-04-0165 PMID:15297420

IARC (2002). Breast cancer screening. *IARC Handb Cancer Prev*, 7:1–229. Available from: http://www.iarc.fr/en/publications/pdfs-online/prev/handbook7/Handbook7_Breast.pdf.

IARC (2012a). Pharmaceuticals. *IARC Monogr Eval Carcinog Risks Hum*. 100A:1–437. PMID:23189749 Available from: http://monographs.iarc.fr/ENG/Monographs/vol100A/index.php.

IARC (2012b). Personal habits and indoor combustions. *IARC Monogr Eval Carcinog Risks Hum*. 100E:1–575. PMID:23193840 Available from: http://monographs.iarc.fr/ENG/Monographs/vol100E/index.php.

IARC (2012c). Radiation. *IARC Monogr Eval Carcinog Risks Hum*. 100D:1–437. PMID:23189752 Available from: http://monographs.iarc.fr/ENG/Monographs/vol100D/index.php.

Inoue M, Sawada N, Matsuda T, Iwasaki M, Sasazuki S, Shimazu T et al. (2012). Attributable causes of cancer in Japan in 2005 – systematic assessment to estimate current burden of cancer attributable to known preventable risk factors in Japan. *Ann Oncol*, 23(5):1362–9. doi:10.1093/annonc/mdr437 PMID:22048150

INSERM (2008). Cancer et environnement. Rapport. Institut national de la santé et de la recherche médicale. Paris, France: Les éditions INSERM.

Isaacs C, Stearns V, Hayes DF (2001). New prognostic factors for breast cancer recurrence. *Semin Oncol*, 28(1):53–67. doi:10.1016/S0093-7754(01)90045-4 PMID:11254867

Isola J, Saijonkari M, Kataja V, Lundin J, Hytönen M, Isojärvi J et al. (2013). Gene profiling assays for planning breast cancer treatment [in Finnish]. *Suomen Lääkärilehti*, 68(50–52):3321–7ö. English summary available from: http://www.thl.fi/attachments/halo/summaries/SLL_2013_GeeniprofilointitestienMerkitysRintasyovanHoidonValinnassa_eng.pdf.

ISRCTN registry (2014). Surgery versus active monitoring for low risk ductal carcinoma in situ (DCIS). Available from: http://www.isrctn.com/ISRCTN27544579.

Iwasaki M, Otani T, Inoue M, Sasazuki S, Tsugane S; Japan Public Health Center-based Prospective Study Group (2007). Role and impact of menstrual and reproductive factors on breast cancer risk in Japan. *Eur J Cancer Prev*, 16(2):116–23. doi:10.1097/01.cej.0000228410.14095.2d PMID:17297387

Iwasaki M, Tsugane S (2011). Risk factors for breast cancer: epidemiological evidence from Japanese studies. *Cancer Sci*, 102(9):1607–14. doi:10.1111/j.1349-7006.2011.01996.x PMID:21624009

Jain AN, Chin K, Børresen-Dale AL, Erikstein BK, Eynstein Lonning P, Kaaresen R et al. (2001). Quantitative analysis of chromosomal CGH in human breast tumors associates copy number abnormalities with p53 status and patient survival. *Proc Natl Acad Sci USA*, 98(14):7952–7. doi:10.1073/pnas.151241198 PMID:11438741

Jansen-van der Weide MC, Greuter MJ, Jansen L, Oosterwijk JCW, Pijnappel RM, de Bock GH (2010). Exposure to low-dose radiation and the risk of breast cancer among women with a familial or genetic predisposition: a meta-analysis. *Eur Radiol*, 20(11):2547–56. doi:10.1007/s00330-010-1839-y PMID:20582702

John EM, Miron A, Gong G, Phipps AI, Felberg A, Li FP et al. (2007). Prevalence of pathogenic *BRCA1* mutation carriers in 5 US racial/ethnic groups. *JAMA*, 298(24):2869–76. doi:10.1001/jama.298.24.2869 PMID:18159056

Justo N, Wilking N, Jönsson B, Luciani S, Cazap E (2013). A review of breast cancer care and outcomes in Latin America. *Oncologist*, 18(3):248–56. doi:10.1634/theoncologist.2012-0373 PMID:23442305

Kaaks R, Rinaldi S, Key TJ, Berrino F, Peeters PH, Biessy C et al. (2005). Postmenopausal serum androgens, oestrogens and breast cancer risk: the European prospective investigation into cancer and nutrition. *Endocr Relat Cancer*, 12(4):1071–82. doi:10.1677/erc.1.01038 PMID:16322344

Kaplan RM, Porzsolt F (2008). The natural history of breast cancer. *Arch Intern Med*, 168(21):2302–3. doi:10.1001/archinte.168.21.2302 PMID:19029491

Karami F, Mehdipour P (2013). A comprehensive focus on global spectrum of *BRCA1* and *BRCA2* mutations in breast cancer. *BioMed Res Int*, 2013:1. doi:10.1155/2013/928562 PMID:24312913

Kaurah P, MacMillan A, Boyd N, Senz J, De Luca A, Chun N et al. (2007). Founder and recurrent *CDH1* mutations in families with hereditary diffuse gastric cancer. *JAMA*, 297(21):2360–72. doi:10.1001/jama.297.21.2360 PMID:17545690

Kean S (2014). Breast cancer. The 'other' breast cancer genes. *Science*, 343(6178):1457–9. doi:10.1126/science.343.6178.1457 PMID:24675950

Kelsey JL, Bernstein L (1996). Epidemiology and prevention of breast cancer. *Annu Rev Public Health*, 17(1):47–67. doi:10.1146/annurev.pu.17.050196.000403 PMID:8724215

Kenney LB, Yasui Y, Inskip PD, Hammond S, Neglia JP, Mertens AC et al. (2004). Breast cancer after childhood cancer: a report from the Childhood Cancer Survivor Study. *Ann Intern Med*, 141(8):590–7. doi:10.7326/0003-4819-141-8-200410190-00006 PMID:15492338

Kerlikowske K, Ichikawa L, Miglioretti DL, Buist DS, Vacek PM, Smith-Bindman R et al.; National Institutes of Health Breast Cancer Surveillance Consortium (2007). Longitudinal measurement of clinical mammographic breast density to improve estimation of breast cancer risk. *J Natl Cancer Inst*, 99(5):386–95. doi:10.1093/jnci/djk066 PMID:17341730

Key T, Appleby P, Barnes I, Reeves G; Endogenous Hormones and Breast Cancer Collaborative Group (2002). Endogenous sex hormones and breast cancer in postmenopausal women: reanalysis of nine prospective studies. *J Natl Cancer Inst*, 94(8):606–16. doi:10.1093/jnci/94.8.606 PMID:11959894

Key TJ, Appleby PN, Reeves GK, Roddam A, Dorgan JF, Longcope C et al.; Endogenous Hormones Breast Cancer Collaborative Group (2003). Body mass index, serum sex hormones, and breast cancer risk in postmenopausal women. *J Natl Cancer Inst*, 95(16):1218–26. doi:10.1093/jnci/djg022 PMID:12928347

Key TJ, Appleby PN, Reeves GK, Roddam AW; Endogenous Hormones and Breast Cancer Collaborative Group (2010). Insulin-like growth factor 1 (IGF1), IGF binding protein 3 (IGFBP3), and breast cancer risk: pooled individual data analysis of 17 prospective studies. *Lancet Oncol*, 11(6):530–42. doi:10.1016/S1470-2045(10)70095-4 PMID:20472501

Key TJ, Appleby PN, Reeves GK, Travis RC, Alberg AJ, Barricarte A et al.; Endogenous Hormones and Breast Cancer Collaborative Group (2013). Sex hormones and risk of breast cancer in premenopausal women: a collaborative reanalysis of individual participant data from seven prospective studies. *Lancet Oncol*, 14(10):1009–19. doi:10.1016/S1470-2045(13)70301-2 PMID:23890780

Kingham TP, Alatise OI, Vanderpuye V, Casper C, Abantanga FA, Kamara TB et al. (2013). Treatment of cancer in sub-Saharan Africa. *Lancet Oncol*, 14(4):e158–67. doi:10.1016/S1470-2045(12)70472-2 PMID:23561747

Kingsmore D, Hole D, Gillis C (2004). Why does specialist treatment of breast cancer improve survival? The role of surgical management. *Br J Cancer*, 90(10):1920–5. doi:10.1038/sj.bjc.6601846 PMID:15138472

Kleibl Z, Novotny J, Bezdickova D, Malik R, Kleiblova P, Foretova L et al. (2005). The *CHEK2* c.1100delC germline mutation rarely contributes to breast cancer development in the Czech Republic. *Breast Cancer Res Treat*, 90(2):165–7. doi:10.1007/s10549-004-4023-8 PMID:15803363

Klein CA (2009). Parallel progression of primary tumours and metastases. *Nat Rev Cancer*, 9(4):302–12. doi:10.1038/nrc2627 PMID:19308069

Kobayashi S, Sugiura H, Ando Y, Shiraki N, Yanagi T, Yamashita H et al. (2012). Reproductive history and breast cancer risk. *Breast Cancer*, 19(4):302–8. doi:10.1007/s12282-012-0384-8 PMID:22711317

Kopans DB, Smith RA, Duffy SW (2011). Mammographic screening and "overdiagnosis". *Radiology*, 260(3):616–20. doi:10.1148/radiol.11110716 PMID:21846757

Kriege M, Hollestelle A, Jager A, Huijts PE, Berns EM, Sieuwerts AM et al. (2014). Survival and contralateral breast cancer in *CHEK2* 1100delC breast cancer patients: impact of adjuvant chemotherapy. *Br J Cancer*, 111(5):1004–13. doi:10.1038/bjc.2014.306 PMID:24918820

Kristensen VN, Vaske CJ, Ursini-Siegel J, Van Loo P, Nordgard SH, Sachidanandam R et al. (2012). Integrated molecular profiles of invasive breast tumors and ductal carcinoma in situ (DCIS) reveal differential vascular and interleukin signaling. *Proc Natl Acad Sci USA*, 109(8):2802–7. doi:10.1073/pnas.1108781108 PMID:21908711

Kwan ML, Haque R, Lee VS, Joanie Chung WL, Avila CC, Clancy HA et al. (2012). Validation of AJCC TNM staging for breast tumors diagnosed before 2004 in cancer registries. *Cancer Causes Control*, 23(9):1587–91. doi:10.1007/s10552-012-0026-7 PMID:22798182

Lakhani SR, Collins N, Stratton MR, Sloane JP (1995). Atypical ductal hyperplasia of the breast: clonal proliferation with loss of heterozygosity on chromosomes 16q and 17p. *J Clin Pathol*, 48(7):611–5. doi:10.1136/jcp.48.7.611 PMID:7560165

Lakhani SR, Ellis IO, Schnitt SJ, Tan PH, van de Vijver MJ, editors (2012). WHO classification of tumours of the breast. 4th ed. Lyon, France: International Agency for Research on Cancer.

Lakhani SR, Jacquemier J, Sloane JP, Gusterson BA, Anderson TJ, van de Vijver MJ et al. (1998). Multifactorial analysis of differences between sporadic breast cancers and cancers involving *BRCA1* and *BRCA2* mutations. *J Natl Cancer Inst*, 90(15):1138–45. doi:10.1093/jnci/90.15.1138 PMID:9701363

Lakhani SR, Van De Vijver MJ, Jacquemier J, Anderson TJ, Osin PP, McGuffog L et al. (2002). The pathology of familial breast cancer: predictive value of immunohistochemical markers estrogen receptor, progesterone receptor, HER-2, and p53 in patients with mutations in *BRCA1* and *BRCA2*. *J Clin Oncol*, 20(9):2310–8. doi:10.1200/JCO.2002.09.023 PMID:11981002

Lambe M, Hsieh C, Trichopoulos D, Ekbom A, Pavia M, Adami HO (1994). Transient increase in the risk of breast cancer after giving birth. *N Engl J Med*, 331(1):5–9. doi:10.1056/NEJM199407073310102 PMID:8202106

Lampejo OT, Barnes DM, Smith P, Millis RR (1994). Evaluation of infiltrating ductal carcinomas with a DCIS component: correlation of the histologic type of the in situ component with grade of the infiltrating component. *Semin Diagn Pathol*, 11(3):215–22. PMID:7831533

Land CE, Tokunaga M, Koyama K, Soda M, Preston DL, Nishimori I et al. (2003). Incidence of female breast cancer among atomic bomb survivors, Hiroshima and Nagasaki, 1950–1990. *Radiat Res*, 160(6):707–17. doi:10.1667/RR3082 PMID:14640793

Lange JM, Takashima JR, Peterson SM, Kalapurakal JA, Green DM, Breslow NE (2014). Breast cancer in female survivors of Wilms tumor: a report from the national Wilms tumor late effects study. *Cancer*, 120(23):3722–30. doi:10.1002/cncr.28908 PMID:25348097

Langlands AO, Prescott RJ, Hamilton T (1980). A clinical trial in the management of operable cancer of the breast. *Br J Surg*, 67(3):170–4. doi:10.1002/bjs.1800670304 PMID:6988032

Larsen SU, Rose C (1999). Spontaneous remission of breast cancer. A literature review [in Danish]. *Ugeskr Laeger*, 161(26):4001–4. PMID:10402936

Lazarus E, Mainiero MB, Schepps B, Koelliker SL, Livingston LS (2006). BI-RADS lexicon for US and mammography: interobserver variability and positive predictive value. *Radiology*, 239(2):385–91. doi:10.1148/radiol.2392042127 PMID:16569780

Lee SA, Ross RK, Pike MC (2005). An overview of menopausal oestrogen-progestin hormone therapy and breast cancer risk. *Br J Cancer*, 92(11):2049–58. doi:10.1038/sj.bjc.6602617 PMID:15900297

Li J, Zhang BN, Fan JH, Pang Y, Zhang P, Wang SL et al. (2011). A nation-wide multicenter 10-year (1999–2008) retrospective clinical epidemiological study of female breast cancer in China. *BMC Cancer*, 11(1):364. doi:10.1186/1471-2407-11-364 PMID:21859480

Li L, Ji J, Wang JB, Niyazi M, Qiao YL, Boffetta P (2012). Attributable causes of breast cancer and ovarian cancer in China: reproductive factors, oral contraceptives and hormone replacement therapy. *Chin J Cancer Res*, 24(1):9–17. doi:10.1007/s11670-012-0009-y PMID:23359757

Li ML, Greenberg RA (2012). Links between genome integrity and *BRCA1* tumor suppression. *Trends Biochem Sci*, 37(10):418–24. doi:10.1016/j.tibs.2012.06.007 PMID:22836122

Lichtenstein P, Holm NV, Verkasalo PK, Iliadou A, Kaprio J, Koskenvuo M et al. (2000). Environmental and heritable factors in the causation of cancer – analyses of cohorts of twins from Sweden, Denmark, and Finland. *N Engl J Med*, 343(2):78–85. doi:10.1056/NEJM200007133430201 PMID:10891514

Lindström S, Vachon CM, Li J, Varghese J, Thompson D, Warren R et al. (2011). Common variants in *ZNF365* are associated with both mammographic density and breast cancer risk. *Nat Genet*, 43(3):185–7. doi:10.1038/ng.760 PMID:21278746

Liu C, Wang QS, Wang YJ (2012a). The *CHEK2* I157T variant and colorectal cancer susceptibility: a systematic review and meta-analysis. *Asian Pac J Cancer Prev*, 13(5):2051–5. doi:10.7314/APJCP.2012.13.5.2051 PMID:22901170

Liu C, Wang Y, Wang QS, Wang YJ (2012b). The *CHEK2* I157T variant and breast cancer susceptibility: a systematic review and meta-analysis. *Asian Pac J Cancer Prev*, 13(4):1355–60. doi:10.7314/APJCP.2012.13.4.1355 PMID:22799331

Liu JJ, Freedman DM, Little MP, Doody MM, Alexander BH, Kitahara CM et al. (2014). Work history and mortality risks in 90,268 US radiological technologists. *Occup Environ Med*, 71(12):819–35. doi:10.1136/oemed-2013-101859 PMID:24852760

London SJ, Connolly JL, Schnitt SJ, Colditz GA (1992). A prospective study of benign breast disease and the risk of breast cancer. *JAMA*, 267(7):941–4. doi:10.1001/jama.1992.03480070057030 PMID:1734106

Lopez-Garcia MA, Geyer FC, Lacroix-Triki M, Marchió C, Reis-Filho JS (2010). Breast cancer precursors revisited: molecular features and progression pathways. *Histopathology*, 57(2):171–92. doi:10.1111/j.1365-2559.2010.03568.x PMID:20500230

Lu YJ, Osin P, Lakhani SR, Di Palma S, Gusterson BA, Shipley JM (1998). Comparative genomic hybridization analysis of lobular carcinoma in situ and atypical lobular hyperplasia and potential roles for gains and losses of genetic material in breast neoplasia. *Cancer Res*, 58(20):4721–7. PMID:9788628

Lundell M, Mattsson A, Karlsson P, Holmberg E, Gustafsson A, Holm LE (1999). Breast cancer risk after radiotherapy in infancy: a pooled analysis of two Swedish cohorts of 17,202 infants. *Radiat Res*, 151(5):626–32. doi:10.2307/3580039 PMID:10319736

Ly D, Forman D, Ferlay J, Brinton LA, Cook MB (2013). An international comparison of male and female breast cancer incidence rates. *Int J Cancer*, 132(8):1918–26. doi:10.1002/ijc.27841 PMID:22987302

Lynge E, Törnberg S, von Karsa L, Segnan N, van Delden JJ (2012). Determinants of successful implementation of population-based cancer screening programmes. *Eur J Cancer*, 48(5):743–8. doi:10.1016/j.ejca.2011.06.051 PMID:21788130

Lythgoe JP, Leck I, Swindell R (1978). Manchester regional breast study. Preliminary results. *Lancet*, 1(8067):744–7. doi:10.1016/S0140-6736(78)90859-0 PMID:76750

Mac Bride MB, Pruthi S, Bevers T (2012). The evolution of breast self-examination to breast awareness. *Breast J*, 18(6):641–3. doi:10.1111/tbj.12023 PMID:23009674

MacMahon B, Cole P, Brown J (1973). Etiology of human breast cancer: a review. *J Natl Cancer Inst*, 50(1):21–42. PMID:4571238

Maddox WA, Carpenter JT Jr, Laws HL, Soong SJ, Cloud G, Urist MM et al. (1983). A randomized prospective trial of radical (Halsted) mastectomy versus modified radical mastectomy in 311 breast cancer patients. *Ann Surg*, 198(2):207–12. doi:10.1097/00000658-198308000-00016 PMID:6870379

Madigan MP, Ziegler RG, Benichou J, Byrne C, Hoover RN (1995). Proportion of breast cancer cases in the United States explained by well-established risk factors. *J Natl Cancer Inst*, 87(22):1681–5. doi:10.1093/jnci/87.22.1681 PMID:7473816

Mahoney L, Csima A (1982). Efficiency of palpation in clinical detection of breast cancer. *Can Med Assoc J*, 127(8):729–30. PMID:7139488

Mahoney MC, Bevers T, Linos E, Willett WC (2008). Opportunities and strategies for breast cancer prevention through risk reduction. *CA Cancer J Clin*, 58(6):347–71. doi:10.3322/CA.2008.0016 PMID:18981297

Malmgren JA, Parikh J, Atwood MK, Kaplan HG (2014). Improved prognosis of women aged 75 and older with mammography-detected breast cancer. *Radiology*, 273(3):686–94. doi:10.1148/radiol.14140209 PMID:25093690

Mark K, Temkin SM, Terplan M (2014). Breast self-awareness: the evidence behind the euphemism. *Obstet Gynecol*, 123(4):734–6. doi:10.1097/AOG.0000000000000139 PMID:24785598

Masannat YA, Bains SK, Pinder SE, Purushotham AD (2013). Challenges in the management of pleomorphic lobular carcinoma in situ of the breast. *Breast*, 22(2):194–6. doi:10.1016/j.breast.2013.01.003 PMID:23357705

Masciari S, Dillon DA, Rath M, Robson M, Weitzel JN, Balmana J et al. (2012). Breast cancer phenotype in women with *TP53* germline mutations: a Li-Fraumeni syndrome consortium effort. *Breast Cancer Res Treat*, 133(3):1125–30. doi:10.1007/s10549-012-1993-9 PMID:22392042

Mattsson A, Rudén BI, Hall P, Wilking N, Rutqvist LE (1993). Radiation-induced breast cancer: long-term follow-up of radiation therapy for benign breast disease. *J Natl Cancer Inst*, 85(20):1679–85. doi:10.1093/jnci/85.20.1679 PMID:8411245

Mattsson A, Rudén BI, Palmgren J, Rutqvist LE (1995). Dose- and time-response for breast cancer risk after radiation therapy for benign breast disease. *Br J Cancer*, 72(4):1054–61. doi:10.1038/bjc.1995.461 PMID:7547222

Mavaddat N, Barrowdale D, Andrulis IL, Domchek SM, Eccles D, Nevanlinna H et al.; HEBON; EMBRACE; GEMO Study Collaborators; kConFab Investigators; SWE-BRCA Collaborators; Consortium of Investigators of Modifiers of BRCA1/2 (2012). Pathology of breast and ovarian cancers among *BRCA1* and *BRCA2* mutation carriers: results from the Consortium of Investigators of Modifiers of BRCA1/2 (CIMBA). *Cancer Epidemiol Biomarkers Prev*, 21(1):134–47. doi:10.1158/1055-9965.EPI-11-0775 PMID:22144499

McCormack VA, dos Santos Silva I (2006). Breast density and parenchymal patterns as markers of breast cancer risk: a meta-analysis. *Cancer Epidemiol Biomarkers Prev*, 15(6):1159–69. doi:10.1158/1055-9965.EPI-06-0034 PMID:16775176

McCormack VA, Joffe M, van den Berg E, Broeze N, Silva IS, Romieu I et al. (2013). Breast cancer receptor status and stage at diagnosis in over 1,200 consecutive public hospital patients in Soweto, South Africa: a case series. *Breast Cancer Res*, 15(5):R84. doi:10.1186/bcr3478 PMID:24041225

McCready T, Littlewood D, Jenkinson J (2005). Breast self-examination and breast awareness: a literature review. *J Clin Nurs*, 14(5):570–8. doi:10.1111/j.1365-2702.2004.01108.x PMID:15840071

McGale P, Taylor C, Correa C, Cutter D, Duane F, Ewertz M et al.; Early Breast Cancer Trialists' Collaborative Group (EBCTCG) (2014). Effect of radiotherapy after mastectomy and axillary surgery on 10-year recurrence and 20-year breast cancer mortality: meta-analysis of individual patient data for 8135 women in 22 randomised trials. *Lancet*, 383(9935):2127–35. doi:10.1016/S0140-6736(14)60488-8 PMID:24656685

McWhirter R (1948). The value of simple mastectomy and radiotherapy in the treatment of cancer of the breast. *Br J Radiol*, 21(252):599–610. doi:10.1259/0007-1285-21-252-599 PMID:18099752

Meijers-Heijboer H, van den Ouweland A, Klijn J, Wasielewski M, de Snoo A, Oldenburg R et al.; CHEK2-Breast Cancer Consortium (2002). Low-penetrance susceptibility to breast cancer due to *CHEK2*(*)1100delC in noncarriers of *BRCA1* or *BRCA2* mutations. *Nat Genet*, 31(1):55–9. doi:10.1038/ng879 PMID:11967536

Mendonça GA, Silva AM, Caula WM (2004). Tumor characteristics and five-year survival in breast cancer patients at the National Cancer Institute, Rio de Janeiro, Brazil [in Portuguese]. *Cad Saude Publica*, 20(5):1232–9. PMID:15486666

Michailidou K, Hall P, Gonzalez-Neira A, Ghoussaini M, Dennis J, Milne RL et al.; Breast and Ovarian Cancer Susceptibility Collaboration; Hereditary Breast and Ovarian Cancer Research Group Netherlands (HEBON); kConFab Investigators; Australian Ovarian Cancer Study Group; GENICA (Gene Environment Interaction and Breast Cancer in Germany) Network (2013). Large-scale genotyping identifies 41 new loci associated with breast cancer risk. *Nat Genet*, 45(4):353–61, e1–2. doi:10.1038/ng.2563 PMID:23535729

Mikeljevic JS, Haward R, Johnston C, Crellin A, Dodwell D, Jones A et al. (2004). Trends in postoperative radiotherapy delay and the effect on survival in breast cancer patients treated with conservation surgery. *Br J Cancer*, 90(7):1343–8. doi:10.1038/sj.bjc.6601693 PMID:15054452

Missmer SA, Eliassen AH, Barbieri RL, Hankinson SE (2004). Endogenous estrogen, androgen, and progesterone concentrations and breast cancer risk among postmenopausal women. *J Natl Cancer Inst*, 96(24):1856–65. doi:10.1093/jnci/djh336 PMID:15601642

Mittra I, Mishra GA, Singh S, Aranke S, Notani P, Badwe R et al. (2010). A cluster randomized, controlled trial of breast and cervix cancer screening in Mumbai, India: methodology and interim results after three rounds of screening. *Int J Cancer*, 126(4):976–84. PMID:19697326

Moelans CB, de Wegers RA, Monsuurs HN, Maess AH, van Diest PJ (2011). Molecular differences between ductal carcinoma in situ and adjacent invasive breast carcinoma: a multiplex ligation-dependent probe amplification study. *Cell Oncol (Dordr)*, 34(5):475–82. doi:10.1007/s13402-011-0043-7 PMID:21547576

Mohan AK, Hauptmann M, Linet MS, Ron E, Lubin JH, Freedman DM et al. (2002). Breast cancer mortality among female radiologic technologists in the United States. *J Natl Cancer Inst*, 94(12):943–8. doi:10.1093/jnci/94.12.943 PMID:12072548

Moinfar F, Man YG, Bratthauer GL, Ratschek M, Tavassoli FA (2000). Genetic abnormalities in mammary ductal intraepithelial neoplasia-flat type ("clinging ductal carcinoma in situ"): a simulator of normal mammary epithelium. *Cancer*, 88(9):2072–81. doi:10.1002/(SICI)1097-0142(20000501)88:9<2072::AID-CNCR13>3.0.CO;2-H PMID:10813719

Moja L, Tagliabue L, Balduzzi S, Parmelli E, Pistotti V, Guarneri V et al. (2012). Trastuzumab containing regimens for early breast cancer. *Cochrane Database Syst Rev*, 4:CD006243. doi:10.1002/14651858.CD006243.pub2 PMID:22513938

Moolgavkar SH, Stevens RG, Lee JA (1979). Effect of age on incidence of breast cancer in females. *J Natl Cancer Inst*, 62(3):493–501. PMID:283278

Moskowitz CS, Chou JF, Wolden SL, Bernstein JL, Malhotra J, Novetsky Friedman D et al. (2014). Breast cancer after chest radiation therapy for childhood cancer. *J Clin Oncol*, 32(21):2217–23. doi:10.1200/JCO.2013.54.4601 PMID:24752044

Muirhead CR, O'Hagan JA, Haylock RG, Phillipson MA, Willcock T, Berridge GL et al. (2009). Mortality and cancer incidence following occupational radiation exposure: third analysis of the National Registry for Radiation Workers. *Br J Cancer*, 100(1):206–12. doi:10.1038/sj.bjc.6604825 PMID:19127272

Munzone E, Curigliano G, Burstein HJ, Winer EP, Goldhirsch A (2012). CMF revisited in the 21st century. *Ann Oncol*, 23(2):305–11. doi:10.1093/annonc/mdr309 PMID:21715566

Murthy V, Chamberlain RS (2011). Recommendation to revise the AJCC/UICC breast cancer staging system for inclusion of proven prognostic factors: ER/PR receptor status and HER2 neu. *Clin Breast Cancer*, 11(5):346–7. doi:10.1016/j.clbc.2011.05.003 PMID:21820971

Nagata C, Hu YH, Shimizu H (1995). Effects of menstrual and reproductive factors on the risk of breast cancer: meta-analysis of the case-control studies in Japan. *Jpn J Cancer Res*, 86(10):910–5. doi:10.1111/j.1349-7006.1995.tb03000.x PMID:7493908

Nagel JH, Peeters JK, Smid M, Sieuwerts AM, Wasielewski M, de Weerd V et al. (2012). Gene expression profiling assigns *CHEK2* 1100delC breast cancers to the luminal intrinsic subtypes. *Breast Cancer Res Treat*, 132(2):439–48. doi:10.1007/s10549-011-1588-x PMID:21614566

Narod SA (2010). Testing for *CHEK2* in the cancer genetics clinic: ready for prime time? *Clin Genet*, 78(1):1–7. doi:10.1111/j.1399-0004.2010.01402.x PMID:20597917

National Research Council (2006). Health risks from exposure to low levels of ionizing radiation: BEIR VII Phase 2. Washington (DC), USA: National Academies Press.

Navarrete Montalvo D, González M N, Montalvo V MT, Jiménez A A, Echiburú-Chau C, Calaf GM (2008). Patterns of recurrence and survival in breast cancer. *Oncol Rep*, 20(3):531–5. PMID:18695902

Newman LA, Griffith KA, Jatoi I, Simon MS, Crowe JP, Colditz GA (2006). Meta-analysis of survival in African American and white American patients with breast cancer: ethnicity compared with socioeconomic status. *J Clin Oncol*, 24(9):1342–9. doi:10.1200/JCO.2005.03.3472 PMID:16549828

NHSBSP (2005). Pathology reporting of breast disease: a joint document incorporating the third edition of the NHS Breast Screening Programme's Guidelines for Pathology Reporting in Breast Cancer Screening and the second edition of The Royal College of Pathologists' Minimum Dataset for Breast Cancer Histopathology. NHSBSP Publication No. 58. Sheffield, UK: NHS Cancer Screening Programmes and The Royal College of Pathologists.

NHSBSP (2006). Be breast aware. NHS Cancer Screening Programmes information leaflet. London, UK: Department of Health. Available from: https://www.gov.uk/government/publications/nhs-breast-screening-awareness-leaflet.

NICE (2013). Gene expression profiling and expanded immunohistochemistry tests for guiding adjuvant chemotherapy decisions in early breast cancer management: MammaPrint, Oncotype DX, IHC4 and Mammostrat. NICE diagnostics guidance [DG10]. London, UK: National Institute for Health and Care Excellence. Available from: http://www.nice.org.uk/guidance/dg10/.

Nieuwenhuis B, Van Assen-Bolt AJ, Van Waarde-Verhagen MA, Sijmons RH, Van der Hout AH, Bauch T et al. (2002). *BRCA1* and *BRCA2* heterozygosity and repair of X-ray-induced DNA damage. *Int J Radiat Biol*, 78(4):285–95. doi:10.1080/09553000110097974 PMID:12020440

Nieuwenhuis MH, Kets CM, Murphy-Ryan M, Yntema HG, Evans DG, Colas C et al. (2014). Cancer risk and genotype-phenotype correlations in *PTEN* hamartoma tumor syndrome. *Fam Cancer*, 13(1):57–63. doi:10.1007/s10689-013-9674-3 PMID:23934601

Norman SA, Localio AR, Zhou L, Weber AL, Coates RJ, Malone KE et al. (2006). Benefit of screening mammography in reducing the rate of late-stage breast cancer diagnoses (United States). *Cancer Causes Control*, 17(7):921–9. doi:10.1007/s10552-006-0029-3 PMID:16841259

Norsa'adah B, Rampal KG, Rahmah MA, Naing NN, Biswal BM (2011). Diagnosis delay of breast cancer and its associated factors in Malaysian women. *BMC Cancer*, 11(1):141. doi:10.1186/1471-2407-11-141 PMID:21496310

Norum JH, Andersen K, Sørlie T (2014). Lessons learned from the intrinsic subtypes of breast cancer in the quest for precision therapy. *Br J Surg*, 101(8):925–38. doi:10.1002/bjs.9562 PMID:24849143

Offit K (2006). BRCA mutation frequency and penetrance: new data, old debate. *J Natl Cancer Inst*, 98(23):1675–7. doi:10.1093/jnci/djj500 PMID:17148764

Ohene-Yeboah M, Amaning E (2008). Spectrum of complaints presented at a specialist breast clinic in Kumasi, Ghana. *Ghana Med J*, 42(3):110–3. PMID:19274109

Okonkwo QL, Draisma G, der Kinderen A, Brown ML, de Koning HJ (2008). Breast cancer screening policies in developing countries: a cost-effectiveness analysis for India. *J Natl Cancer Inst*, 100(18):1290–300. doi:10.1093/jnci/djn292 PMID:18780864

OMIM (2015). Online Mendelian Inheritance in Man database. Baltimore (MD), USA: McKusick-Nathans Institute of Genetic Medicine, Johns Hopkins University. Available from: www.omim.org.

Osborne CK (1998). Tamoxifen in the treatment of breast cancer. *N Engl J Med*, 339(22):1609–18. doi:10.1056/NEJM199811263392207 PMID:9828250

Ozasa K, Shimizu Y, Suyama A, Kasagi F, Soda M, Grant EJ et al. (2012). Studies of the mortality of atomic bomb survivors, Report 14, 1950–2003: an overview of cancer and noncancer diseases. *Radiat Res*, 177(3):229–43. doi:10.1667/RR2629.1 PMID:22171960

Paci E, Del Turco MR, Palli D, Buiatti E, Bruzzi P, Piffanelli A (1988). Selection of high-risk groups for breast cancer screening. Evidence from an Italian multicentric case control study. *Tumori*, 74(6):675–9. PMID:3068864

Page DL, Dupont WD, Rogers LW, Jensen RA, Schuyler PA (1995). Continued local recurrence of carcinoma 15–25 years after a diagnosis of low grade ductal carcinoma in situ of the breast treated only by biopsy. *Cancer*, 76(7):1197–200. doi:10.1002/1097-0142(19951001)76:7<1197::AID-CNCR2820760715>3.0.CO;2-0 PMID:8630897

Palacios J, Robles-Frías MJ, Castilla MA, López-García MA, Benítez J (2008). The molecular pathology of hereditary breast cancer. *Pathobiology*, 75(2):85–94. doi:10.1159/000123846 PMID:18544963

Park S, Kim Y, Shin HR, Lee B, Shin A, Jung KW et al. (2014). Population-attributable causes of cancer in Korea: obesity and physical inactivity. *PLoS ONE*, 9(4):e90871. doi:10.1371/journal.pone.0090871 PMID:24722008

Patey DH, Scarff RW (1928). The position of histology in the prognosis of carcinoma of the breast. *Lancet*, 211(5460):801–4. doi:10.1016/S0140-6736(00)76762-6

Peng S, Lü B, Ruan W, Zhu Y, Sheng H, Lai M (2011). Genetic polymorphisms and breast cancer risk: evidence from meta-analyses, pooled analyses, and genome-wide association studies. *Breast Cancer Res Treat*, 127(2):309–24. doi:10.1007/s10549-011-1459-5 PMID:21445572

Pereira H, Pinder SE, Sibbering DM, Galea MH, Elston CW, Blamey RW et al. (1995). Pathological prognostic factors in breast cancer. IV: Should you be a typer or a grader? A comparative study of two histological prognostic features in operable breast carcinoma. *Histopathology*, 27(3):219–26. doi:10.1111/j.1365-2559.1995.tb00213.x PMID:8522285

Perez EA, Romond EH, Suman VJ, Jeong JH, Davidson NE, Geyer CE Jr et al. (2011). Four-year follow-up of trastuzumab plus adjuvant chemotherapy for operable human epidermal growth factor receptor 2-positive breast cancer: joint analysis of data from NCCTG N9831 and NSABP B-31. *J Clin Oncol*, 29(25):3366–73. doi:10.1200/JCO.2011.35.0868 PMID:21768458

Perou CM, Sørlie T, Eisen MB, van de Rijn M, Jeffrey SS, Rees CA et al. (2000). Molecular portraits of human breast tumours. *Nature*, 406(6797):747–52. doi:10.1038/35021093 PMID:10963602

Perry N, Broeders M, de Wolf C, Törnberg S, Holland R, von Karsa L et al., editors (2006). European guidelines for quality assurance in breast cancer screening and diagnosis. Fourth edition. Luxembourg: European Commission, Office for Official Publications of the European Communities; pp. 15–56. Available from: http://ec.europa.eu/health/ph_projects/2002/cancer/cancer_2002_01_en.htm.

Perry N, Broeders M, de Wolf C, Törnberg S, Holland R, von Karsa L (2008). European guidelines for quality assurance in breast cancer screening and diagnosis. Fourth edition–summary document. *Ann Oncol*, 19(4):614–22. doi:10.1093/annonc/mdm481 PMID:18024988

Perry N, Broeders M, de Wolf C, Törnberg S, Holland R, von Karsa L (2013a). European guidelines for quality assurance in breast cancer screening and diagnosis. Fourth edition, Supplements. Luxembourg: European Commission, Office for Official Publications of the European Union.

Perry N, Broeders M, de Wolf C, Törnberg S, Holland R, von Karsa L (2013b). Executive summary. In: Perry N, Broeders M, de Wolf C, Törnberg S, Holland R, von Karsa L, editors. European guidelines for quality assurance in breast cancer screening and diagnosis. Fourth edition, Supplements. Luxembourg: European Commission, Office for Official Publications of the European Union; pp. XIV–XX.

Peto R, Davies C, Godwin J, Gray R, Pan HC, Clarke M et al.; Early Breast Cancer Trialists' Collaborative Group (EBCTCG) (2012). Comparisons between different polychemotherapy regimens for early breast cancer: meta-analyses of long-term outcome among 100,000 women in 123 randomised trials. *Lancet*, 379(9814):432–44. doi:10.1016/S0140-6736(11)61625-5 PMID:22152853

Pettersson A, Graff RE, Ursin G, Santos Silva ID, McCormack V, Baglietto L et al. (2014). Mammographic density phenotypes and risk of breast cancer: a meta-analysis. *J Natl Cancer Inst*, 106(5):dju078. doi:10.1093/jnci/dju078 PMID:24816206

Pieri A, Harvey J, Bundred N (2014). Pleomorphic lobular carcinoma in situ of the breast: can the evidence guide practice? *World J Clin Oncol*, 5(3):546–53. doi:10.5306/wjco.v5.i3.546 PMID:25114868

Pijpe A, Andrieu N, Easton DF, Kesminiene A, Cardis E, Noguès C et al.; GENEPSO; EMBRACE; HEBON (2012). Exposure to diagnostic radiation and risk of breast cancer among carriers of *BRCA1/2* mutations: retrospective cohort study (GENE-RAD-RISK). *BMJ*, 345:e5660. doi:10.1136/bmj.e5660 PMID:22956590

Pike MC, Pearce CL (2013). Mammographic density, MRI background parenchymal enhancement and breast cancer risk. *Ann Oncol*, 24(Suppl 8):viii37–41. doi:10.1093/annonc/mdt310 PMID:24131968

Pike MC, Wu AH, Spicer DV, Lee S, Pearce CL (2007). Estrogens, progestins, and risk of breast cancer. *Ernst Schering Found Symp Proc*, 2007(1):127–50. PMID:18540571

Pilarski R, Burt R, Kohlman W, Pho L, Shannon KM, Swisher E (2013). Cowden syndrome and the *PTEN* hamartoma tumor syndrome: systematic review and revised diagnostic criteria. *J Natl Cancer Inst*, 105(21):1607–16. doi:10.1093/jnci/djt277 PMID:24136893

Pinto AC, Ades F, de Azambuja E, Piccart-Gebhart M (2013). Trastuzumab for patients with HER2 positive breast cancer: delivery, duration and combination therapies. *Breast*, 22(Suppl 2):S152–5. doi:10.1016/j.breast.2013.07.029 PMID:24074778

Polyak K (2007). Breast cancer: origins and evolution. *J Clin Invest*, 117(11):3155–63. doi:10.1172/JCI33295 PMID:17975657

Porta M (2008). A dictionary of epidemiology, 5th edition. Oxford, UK: Oxford University Press.

Porter PL, El-Bastawissi AY, Mandelson MT, Lin MG, Khalid N, Watney EA et al. (1999). Breast tumor characteristics as predictors of mammographic detection: comparison of interval- and screen-detected cancers. *J Natl Cancer Inst*, 91(23):2020–8. doi:10.1093/jnci/91.23.2020 PMID:10580027

Poum A, Promthet S, Duffy SW, Parkin DM (2014). Factors associated with delayed diagnosis of breast cancer in northeast Thailand. *J Epidemiol*, 24(2):102–8. doi:10.2188/jea.JE20130090 PMID:24335087

Powell SN, Kachnic LA (2003). Roles of *BRCA1* and *BRCA2* in homologous recombination, DNA replication fidelity and the cellular response to ionizing radiation. *Oncogene*, 22(37):5784–91. doi:10.1038/sj.onc.1206678 PMID:12947386

Pradhan M, Dhakal HP (2008). Study of breast lump of 2246 cases by fine needle aspiration. *JNMA J Nepal Med Assoc*, 47(172):205–9. PMID:19079396

Preston DL, Mattsson A, Holmberg E, Shore R, Hildreth NG, Boice JD Jr (2002). Radiation effects on breast cancer risk: a pooled analysis of eight cohorts. *Radiat Res*, 158(2):220–35. doi:10.1667/0033-7587(2002)158[0220:REOBCR]2.0.CO;2 PMID:12105993

Preston DL, Ron E, Tokuoka S, Funamoto S, Nishi N, Soda M et al. (2007). Solid cancer incidence in atomic bomb survivors: 1958–1998. *Radiat Res*, 168(1):1–64. doi:10.1667/RR0763.1 PMID:17722996

Prokopcova J, Kleibl Z, Banwell CM, Pohlreich P (2007). The role of *ATM* in breast cancer development. *Breast Cancer Res Treat*, 104(2):121–8. doi:10.1007/s10549-006-9406-6 PMID:17061036

Puliti D, Duffy SW, Miccinesi G, de Koning H, Lynge E, Zappa M et al.; EUROSCREEN Working Group (2012). Overdiagnosis in mammographic screening for breast cancer in Europe: a literature review. *J Med Screen*, 19(Suppl 1):42–56. doi:10.1258/jms.2012.012082 PMID:22972810

Rahman N (2014a). Realizing the promise of cancer predisposition genes. *Nature*, 505(7483):302–8. doi:10.1038/nature12981 PMID:24429628

Rahman N (2014b). Mainstreaming genetic testing of cancer predisposition genes. *Clin Med*, 14(4):436–9. doi:10.7861/clinmedicine.14-4-436 PMID:25099850

Rakha EA, Lee AH, Evans AJ, Menon S, Assad NY, Hodi Z et al. (2010b). Tubular carcinoma of the breast: further evidence to support its excellent prognosis. *J Clin Oncol*, 28(1):99–104. doi:10.1200/JCO.2009.23.5051 PMID:19917872

Renwick A, Thompson D, Seal S, Kelly P, Chagtai T, Ahmed M et al.; Breast Cancer Susceptibility Collaboration (UK) (2006). *ATM* mutations that cause ataxia-telangiectasia are breast cancer susceptibility alleles. *Nat Genet*, 38(8):873–5. doi:10.1038/ng1837 PMID:16832357

Retsky MW, Demicheli R, Hrushesky WJ, Baum M, Gukas ID (2008). Dormancy and surgery-driven escape from dormancy help explain some clinical features of breast cancer. *APMIS*, 116(7–8):730–41. doi:10.1111/j.1600-0463.2008.00990.x PMID:18834415

Reulen RC, Frobisher C, Winter DL, Kelly J, Lancashire ER, Stiller CA et al.; British Childhood Cancer Survivor Study Steering Group (2011). Long-term risks of subsequent primary neoplasms among survivors of childhood cancer. *JAMA*, 305(22):2311–9. doi:10.1001/jama.2011.747 PMID:21642683

Richards MA, Westcombe AM, Love SB, Littlejohns P, Ramirez AJ (1999). Influence of delay on survival in patients with breast cancer: a systematic review. *Lancet*, 353(9159):1119–26. doi:10.1016/S0140-6736(99)02143-1 PMID:10209974

Robb K, Wardle J, Stubbings S, Ramirez A, Austoker J, Macleod U et al. (2010). Ethnic disparities in knowledge of cancer screening programmes in the UK. *J Med Screen*, 17(3):125–31. doi:10.1258/jms.2010.009112 PMID:20956722

Robbins P, Pinder S, de Klerk N, Dawkins H, Harvey J, Sterrett G et al. (1995). Histological grading of breast carcinomas: a study of interobserver agreement. *Hum Pathol*, 26(8):873–9. doi:10.1016/0046-8177(95)90010-1 PMID:7635449

Ronckers CM, Doody MM, Lonstein JE, Stovall M, Land CE (2008). Multiple diagnostic X-rays for spine deformities and risk of breast cancer. *Cancer Epidemiol Biomarkers Prev*, 17(3):605–13. doi:10.1158/1055-9965.EPI-07-2628 PMID:18349278

Ronckers CM, Erdmann CA, Land CE (2005). Radiation and breast cancer: a review of current evidence. *Breast Cancer Res*, 7(1):21–32. doi:10.1186/bcr970 PMID:15642178

Ronckers CM, Land CE, Miller JS, Stovall M, Lonstein JE, Doody MM (2010). Cancer mortality among women frequently exposed to radiographic examinations for spinal disorders. *Radiat Res*, 174(1):83–90. doi:10.1667/RR2022.1 PMID:20681802

Sanders ME, Schuyler PA, Dupont WD, Page DL (2005). The natural history of low-grade ductal carcinoma in situ of the breast in women treated by biopsy only revealed over 30 years of long-term follow-up. *Cancer*, 103(12):2481–4. doi:10.1002/cncr.21069 PMID:15884091

Sankaranarayanan R (2000). Integration of cost-effective early detection programs into the health services of developing countries. *Cancer*, 89(3):475–81. doi:10.1002/1097-0142(20000801)89:3<475::AID-CN-CR1>3.0.CO;2-8 PMID:10931445

Sankaranarayanan R, Ramadas K, Thara S, Muwonge R, Prabhakar J, Augustine P et al. (2011). Clinical breast examination: preliminary results from a cluster randomized controlled trial in India. *J Natl Cancer Inst*, 103(19):1476–80. doi:10.1093/jnci/djr304 PMID:21862730

Sankaranarayanan R, Swaminathan R (2011). Cancer survival in Africa, Asia, the Caribbean and Central America. Introduction. *IARC Sci Publ*, 162(162):1–5. PMID:21675400

Sankaranarayanan R, Swaminathan R, Brenner H, Chen K, Chia KS, Chen JG et al. (2010). Cancer survival in Africa, Asia, and Central America: a population-based study. *Lancet Oncol*, 11(2):165–73. doi:10.1016/S1470-2045(09)70335-3 PMID:20005175

Sant M, Allemani C, Capocaccia R, Hakulinen T, Aareleid T, Coebergh JW et al.; EUROCARE Working Group (2003). Stage at diagnosis is a key explanation of differences in breast cancer survival across Europe. *Int J Cancer*, 106(3):416–22. doi:10.1002/ijc.11226 PMID:12845683

Saphner T, Tormey DC, Gray R (1996). Annual hazard rates of recurrence for breast cancer after primary therapy. *J Clin Oncol*, 14(10):2738–46. PMID:8874335

Savage KI, Gorski JJ, Barros EM, Irwin GW, Manti L, Powell AJ et al. (2014). Identification of a BRCA1-mRNA splicing complex required for efficient DNA repair and maintenance of genomic stability. *Mol Cell*, 54(3):445–59. doi:10.1016/j.molcel.2014.03.021 PMID:24746700

Schmidt-Kittler O, Ragg T, Daskalakis A, Granzow M, Ahr A, Blankenstein TJ et al. (2003). From latent disseminated cells to overt metastasis: genetic analysis of systemic breast cancer progression. *Proc Natl Acad Sci USA*, 100(13):7737–42. doi:10.1073/pnas.1331931100 PMID:12808139

Schrader KA, Masciari S, Boyd N, Salamanca C, Senz J, Saunders DN et al.; kConFab (2011). Germline mutations in *CDH1* are infrequent in women with early-onset or familial lobular breast cancers. *J Med Genet*, 48(1):64–8. doi:10.1136/jmg.2010.079814 PMID:20921021

Scoccianti C, Lauby-Secretan B, Bello PY, Chajes V, Romieu I (2014). Female breast cancer and alcohol consumption: a review of the literature. *Am J Prev Med*, 46(3 Suppl 1):S16–25. doi:10.1016/j.amepre.2013.10.031 PMID:24512927

Secretan B, Straif K, Baan R, Grosse Y, El Ghissassi F, Bouvard V et al.; WHO International Agency for Research on Cancer Monograph Working Group (2009). A review of human carcinogens – Part E: tobacco, areca nut, alcohol, coal smoke, and salted fish. *Lancet Oncol*, 10(11):1033–4. doi:10.1016/S1470-2045(09)70326-2 PMID:19891056

SEER (2014a). Cancer statistics fact sheets: female breast cancer. Bethesda (MD), USA: Surveillance, Epidemiology, and End Results Program, US National Cancer Institute. Available from: http://seer.cancer.gov/statfacts/html/breast.html.

SEER (2014b). Staging a cancer case. Bethesda (MD), USA: Surveillance, Epidemiology, and End Results Program, US National Cancer Institute. Available from: http://training.seer.cancer.gov/staging/, accessed 24 September 2014.

Seitz HK, Pelucchi C, Bagnardi V, La Vecchia C (2012). Epidemiology and pathophysiology of alcohol and breast cancer: update 2012. *Alcohol Alcohol*, 47(3):204–12. doi:10.1093/alcalc/ags011 PMID:22459019

Shah NR, Borenstein J, Dubois RW (2005). Postmenopausal hormone therapy and breast cancer: a systematic review and meta-analysis. *Menopause*, 12(6):668–78. doi:10.1097/01.gme.0000184221.63459.e1 PMID:16278609

Shah SP, Roth A, Goya R, Oloumi A, Ha G, Zhao Y et al. (2012). The clonal and mutational evolution spectrum of primary triple-negative breast cancers. *Nature*, 486(7403):395–9. PMID:22495314

Shore RE, Hildreth N, Woodard E, Dvoretsky P, Hempelmann L, Pasternack B (1986). Breast cancer among women given X-ray therapy for acute post-partum mastitis. *J Natl Cancer Inst*, 77(3):689–96. PMID:3462410

Shulman LN, Willett W, Sievers A, Knaul FM (2010). Breast cancer in developing countries: opportunities for improved survival. *J Oncol*, 2010:1. doi:10.1155/2010/595167 PMID:21253541

Sibbering M, Watkins R, Winstanley J, Patnick J, editors (2009). Quality assurance guidelines for surgeons in breast cancer screening, 4th edition. NHSBSP Publication No. 20. Sheffield, UK: NHS Cancer Screening Programmes.

Siegel R, Ma J, Zou Z, Jemal A (2014). Cancer statistics, 2014. *CA Cancer J Clin*, 64(1):9–29. doi:10.3322/caac.21208 PMID:24399786

Sigurdson AJ, Doody MM, Rao RS, Freedman DM, Alexander BH, Hauptmann M et al. (2003). Cancer incidence in the US radiologic technologists health study, 1983–1998. *Cancer*, 97(12):3080–9. doi:10.1002/cncr.11444 PMID:12784345

Silverstein MJ, Lagios MD, Craig PH, Waisman JR, Lewinsky BS, Colburn WJ et al. (1996). A prognostic index for ductal carcinoma in situ of the breast. *Cancer*, 77(11):2267–74. doi:10.1002/(SICI)1097-0142(19960601)77:11<2267::AID-CNCR13>3.0.CO;2-V PMID:8635094

Silverstein MJ, Poller DN, Waisman JR, Colburn WJ, Barth A, Gierson ED et al. (1995). Prognostic classification of breast ductal carcinoma-in-situ. *Lancet*,

345(8958):1154–7. doi:10.1016/S0140-6736(95)90982-6 PMID:7723550

Simpson PT, Gale T, Fulford LG, Reis-Filho JS, Lakhani SR (2003). The diagnosis and management of pre-invasive breast disease: pathology of atypical lobular hyperplasia and lobular carcinoma in situ. *Breast Cancer Res*, 5(5):258–62. doi:10.1186/bcr624 PMID:12927036

Simpson PT, Gale T, Reis-Filho JS, Jones C, Parry S, Sloane JP et al. (2005). Columnar cell lesions of the breast: the missing link in breast cancer progression? A morphological and molecular analysis. *Am J Surg Pathol*, 29(6):734–46. doi:10.1097/01.pas.0000157295.93914.3b PMID:15897740

Singh D, Malila N, Pokhrel A, Anttila A (2015). Association of symptoms and breast cancer in population-based mammography screening in Finland. *Int J Cancer*, 136(6):E630–7. doi:10.1002/ijc.29170 PMID:25160029

Singletary SE, Greene FL; Breast Task Force (2003). Revision of breast cancer staging: the 6th edition of the TNM classification. *Semin Surg Oncol*, 21(1):53–9. doi:10.1002/ssu.10021 PMID:12923916

Sinn P, Aulmann S, Wirtz R, Schott S, Marmé F, Varga Z et al. (2013). Multigene assays for classification, prognosis, and prediction in breast cancer: a critical review on the background and clinical utility. *Geburtshilfe Frauenheilkd*, 73(9):932–40. doi:10.1055/s-0033-1350831 PMID:24771945

Slamon DJ, Clark GM, Wong SG, Levin WJ, Ullrich A, McGuire WL (1987). Human breast cancer: correlation of relapse and survival with amplification of the HER-2/neu oncogene. *Science*, 235(4785):177–82. doi:10.1126/science.3798106 PMID:3798106

Slamon DJ, Leyland-Jones B, Shak S, Fuchs H, Paton V, Bajamonde A et al. (2001). Use of chemotherapy plus a monoclonal antibody against HER2 for metastatic breast cancer that overexpresses HER2. *N Engl J Med*, 344(11):783–92. doi:10.1056/NEJM200103153441101 PMID:11248153

Sledge GW, Mamounas EP, Hortobagyi GN, Burstein HJ, Goodwin PJ, Wolff AC (2014). Past, present, and future challenges in breast cancer treatment. *J Clin Oncol*, 32(19):1979–86. doi:10.1200/JCO.2014.55.4139 PMID:24888802

Sloan FA, Gelband H, editors (2007). Cancer control opportunities in low- and middle-income countries. Washington (DC), USA: Institute of Medicine of the National Academies.

Smith E, Heaney E, Dooher P (2012). Interim quality assurance guidelines for clinical nurse specialists in breast cancer screening, 5th edition. NHSBSP Publication No. 29. Sheffield, UK: NHS Cancer Screening Programmes.

Solin L, Schwartz G, Feig S, Shaber G, Patchefsky A (1984). Risk factors as criteria for inclusion in breast cancer screening programs. In: Ames F, Blumenschein G, Montague E, editors. Current controversies in breast cancer. Austin (TX), USA: University of Texas Press; pp. 565–73.

Solin LJ, Yeh IT, Kurtz J, Fourquet A, Recht A, Kuske R et al. (1993). Ductal carcinoma in situ (intraductal carcinoma) of the breast treated with breast-conserving surgery and definitive irradiation. Correlation of pathologic parameters with outcome of treatment. *Cancer*, 71(8):2532–42. doi:10.1002/1097-0142(19930415)71:8<2532::AID-CNCR2820710817>3.0.CO;2-0 PMID:8384070

Sopik V, Phelan C, Cybulski C, Narod S (2014). *BRCA1* and *BRCA2* mutations and the risk for colorectal cancer. *Clin Genet*, 87(5):411–8. doi:10.1111/cge.12497 PMID:25195694

Sørlie T (2004). Molecular portraits of breast cancer: tumour subtypes as distinct disease entities. *Eur J Cancer*, 40(18):2667–75. doi:10.1016/j.ejca.2004.08.021 PMID:15571950

Sørlie T, Perou CM, Tibshirani R, Aas T, Geisler S, Johnsen H et al. (2001). Gene expression patterns of breast carcinomas distinguish tumor subclasses with clinical implications. *Proc Natl Acad Sci USA*, 98(19):10869–74. doi:10.1073/pnas.191367098 PMID:11553815

Sotiriou C, Pusztai L (2009). Gene-expression signatures in breast cancer. *N Engl J Med*, 360(8):790–800. doi:10.1056/NEJMra0801289 PMID:19228622

Soumian S, Verghese ET, Booth M, Sharma N, Chaudhri S, Bradley S et al. (2013). Concordance between vacuum assisted biopsy and postoperative histology: implications for the proposed Low Risk DCIS Trial (LORIS). *Eur J Surg Oncol*, 39(12):1337–40. doi:10.1016/j.ejso.2013.09.028 PMID:24209431

Stefanick ML, Anderson GL, Margolis KL, Hendrix SL, Rodabough RJ, Paskett ED et al.; WHI Investigators (2006). Effects of conjugated equine estrogens on breast cancer and mammography screening in postmenopausal women with hysterectomy. *JAMA*, 295(14):1647–57. doi:10.1001/jama.295.14.1647 PMID:16609086

Stephens PJ, Tarpey PS, Davies H, Van Loo P, Greenman C, Wedge DC et al.; Oslo Breast Cancer Consortium (OSBREAC) (2012). The landscape of cancer genes and mutational processes in breast cancer. *Nature*, 486(7403):400–4. PMID:22722201

Storm HH, Andersson M, Boice JD Jr, Blettner M, Stovall M, Mouridsen HT et al. (1992). Adjuvant radiotherapy and risk of contralateral breast cancer. *J Natl Cancer Inst*, 84(16):1245–50. doi:10.1093/jnci/84.16.1245 PMID:1640483

Stratton MR, Campbell PJ, Futreal PA (2009). The cancer genome. *Nature*, 458(7239):719–24. doi:10.1038/nature07943 PMID:19360079

Stratton MR, Collins N, Lakhani SR, Sloane JP (1995). Loss of heterozygosity in ductal carcinoma in situ of the breast. *J Pathol*, 175(2):195–201. doi:10.1002/path.1711750207 PMID:7738715

Stuart-Harris R, Caldas C, Pinder SE, Pharoah P (2008). Proliferation markers and survival in early breast cancer: a systematic review and meta-analysis of 85 studies in 32,825 patients. *Breast*, 17(4):323–34. doi:10.1016/j.breast.2008.02.002 PMID:18455396

Sullivan R, Peppercorn J, Sikora K, Zalcberg J, Meropol NJ, Amir E et al. (2011). Delivering affordable cancer care in high-income countries. *Lancet Oncol*, 12(10):933–80. doi:10.1016/S1470-2045(11)70141-3 PMID:21958503

Tabár L, Dean PB, Chen SL, Chen HH, Yen AM, Fann JC et al. (2014). Invasive lobular carcinoma of the breast: the use of radiological appearance to classify tumor subtypes for better prediction of long-term outcome. *J Clin Exp Pathol*, 4(4).

Tabár L, Dean PB, Péntek Z (1983). Galactography: the diagnostic procedure of choice for nipple discharge. *Radiology*, 149(1):31–8. doi:10.1148/radiology.149.1.6611939 PMID:6611939

Tabár L, Fagerberg G, Day NE, Duffy SW, Kitchin RM (1992). Breast cancer treatment and natural history: new insights from results of screening. *Lancet*, 339(8790):412–4. doi:10.1016/0140-6736(92)90090-P PMID:1346670

Tamakoshi K, Yatsuya H, Wakai K, Suzuki S, Nishio K, Lin Y et al.; JACC Study Group (2005). Impact of menstrual and reproductive factors on breast cancer risk in Japan: results of the JACC study. *Cancer Sci*, 96(1):57–62. doi:10.1111/j.1349-7006.2005.00010.x PMID:15649257

Taplin SH, Ichikawa L, Buist DS, Seger D, White E (2004). Evaluating organized breast cancer screening implementation: the prevention of late-stage disease? *Cancer Epidemiol Biomarkers Prev*, 13(2):225–34. doi:10.1158/1055-9965.EPI-03-0206 PMID:14973097

Taylor R, Davis P, Boyages J (2003). Long-term survival of women with breast cancer in New South Wales. *Eur J Cancer*, 39(2):215–22. doi:10.1016/S0959-8049(02)00486-0 PMID:12509954

Telle-Lamberton M (2008). Epidemiologic data on radiation-induced breast cancer [in French]. *Rev Epidemiol Sante Publique*, 56(4):235–43. doi:10.1016/j.respe.2008.05.024 PMID:18672338

Thierry-Chef I, Simon SL, Weinstock RM, Kwon D, Linet MS (2012). Reconstruction of absorbed doses to fibroglandular tissue of the breast of women undergoing mammography (1960 to the present). *Radiat Res*, 177(1):92–108. doi:10.1667/RR2241.1 PMID:21988547

Thornton H, Pillarisetti RR (2008). 'Breast awareness' and 'breast self-examination' are not the same. What do these terms mean? Why are they confused? What can we do? *Eur J Cancer*, 44(15):2118–21. doi:10.1016/j.ejca.2008.08.015 PMID:18805689

Tice JA, Cummings SR, Smith-Bindman R, Ichikawa L, Barlow WE, Kerlikowske K (2008). Using clinical factors and mammographic breast density to estimate breast cancer risk: development and validation of a new predictive model. *Ann Intern Med*, 148(5):337–47. doi:10.7326/0003-4819-148-5-200803040-00004 PMID:18316752

Tikk K, Sookthai D, Johnson T, Rinaldi S, Romieu I, Tjønneland A et al. (2014). Circulating prolactin and breast cancer risk among pre- and postmenopausal women in the EPIC cohort. *Ann Oncol*, 25(7):1422–8. doi:10.1093/annonc/mdu150 PMID:24718887

Tonelli M, Connor Gorber S, Joffres M, Dickinson J, Singh H, Lewin G et al.; Canadian Task Force on Preventive Health Care (2011). Recommendations on screening for breast cancer in average-risk women aged 40–74 years. *CMAJ*, 183(17):1991–2001. doi:10.1503/cmaj.110334 PMID:22106103

Travis LB, Hill DA, Dores GM, Gospodarowicz M, van Leeuwen FE, Holowaty E et al. (2003). Breast cancer following radiotherapy and chemotherapy among young women with Hodgkin disease. *JAMA*, 290(4):465–75. doi:10.1001/jama.290.4.465 PMID:12876089

Trichopoulos D, Hsieh CC, MacMahon B, Lin TM, Lowe CR, Mirra AP et al. (1983). Age at any birth and breast cancer risk. *Int J Cancer*, 31(6):701–4. doi:10.1002/ijc.2910310604 PMID:6862681

Tryggvadóttir L, Gislum M, Bray F, Klint A, Hakulinen T, Storm HH et al. (2010). Trends in the survival of patients diagnosed with breast cancer in the Nordic countries 1964–2003 followed up to the end of 2006. *Acta Oncol*, 49(5):624–31. doi:10.3109/02841860903575323 PMID:20429724

Tubiana M, Koscielny S (1991). Natural history of human breast cancer: recent data and clinical implications. *Breast Cancer Res Treat*, 18(3):125–40. doi:10.1007/BF01990028 PMID:1756255

Tung N, Battelli C, Allen B, Kaldate R, Bhatnagar S, Bowles K et al. (2014). Frequency of mutations in individuals with breast cancer referred for *BRCA1* and *BRCA2* testing using next-generation sequencing with a 25-gene panel. *Cancer*, 121(1):25–33. doi:10.1002/cncr.29010 PMID:25186627

Tworoger SS, Eliassen AH, Zhang X, Qian J, Sluss PM, Rosner BA et al. (2013). A 20-year prospective study of plasma prolactin as a risk marker of breast cancer development. *Cancer Res*, 73(15):4810–9. doi:10.1158/0008-5472.CAN-13-0665 PMID:23783576

UICC (2010). TNM classification of breast cancer [in French]. UICC stage, 7th edition. Geneva, Switzerland: Union for International Cancer Control. Available from: http://www.canceraquitaine.org/sites/default/files/documents/INFOS-PRO/surveillance-sein/kit/base-documentaire/TNM.pdf.

UNDP (2012). Human development reports. United Nations Development Programme. Available from: http://hdr.undp.org/en/content/table-1-human-development-index-and-its-components.

Unger-Saldaña K (2014). Challenges to the early diagnosis and treatment of breast cancer in developing countries. *World J Clin Oncol*, 5(3):465–77. doi:10.5306/wjco.v5.i3.465 PMID:25114860

United Nations (2012). World population prospects (demographic data). Available from: http://www.un.org/esa/population/unpop.htm.

UNSCEAR (2010). Sources and effects of ionizing radiation, UNSCEAR 2008 Report, Volume I: Sources - Report to the General Assembly Scientific Annexes A and B. New York (NY), USA: United Nations Scientific Committee on the Effects of Atomic Radiation. Available from: http://www.unscear.org/unscear/en/publications/2008_1.html.

UNSCEAR (2013). Sources, effects and risks of ionizing radiation, UNSCEAR 2013 Report, Volume II: Scientific Annex B: Effects of radiation exposure of children. New York (NY), USA: United Nations Scientific Committee on the Effects of Atomic Radiation. Available from: www.unscear.org/docs/reports/2013/UNSCEAR2013Report_AnnexB_Children_13-87320_Ebook_web.pdf.

van der Groep P, van der Wall E, van Diest PJ (2011). Pathology of hereditary breast cancer. *Cell Oncol (Dordr)*, 34(2):71–88. doi:10.1007/s13402-011-0010-3 PMID:21336636

van Dongen JA, Fentiman IS, Harris JR, Holland R, Peterse JL, Salvadori B et al. (1989). In-situ breast cancer: the EORTC consensus meeting. *Lancet*, 2(8653):25–7. doi:10.1016/S0140-6736(89)90263-8 PMID:2567800

van Leeuwaarde RS, Vrede MA, Henar F, Does R, Issa P, Burke E et al. (2011). A nationwide analysis of incidence and outcome of breast cancer in the country of Surinam, during 1994–2003. *Breast Cancer Res Treat*, 128(3):873–81. doi:10.1007/s10549-011-1404-7 PMID:21340478

van Leeuwen FE, Klokman WJ, Stovall M, Dahler EC, van't Veer MB, Noordijk EM et al. (2003). Roles of radiation dose, chemotherapy, and hormonal factors in breast cancer following Hodgkin's disease. *J Natl Cancer Inst*, 95(13):971–80. doi:10.1093/jnci/95.13.971 PMID:12837833

van Leeuwen FE, Klokman WJ, Veer MB, Hagenbeek A, Krol AD, Vetter UA et al. (2000). Long-term risk of second malignancy in survivors of Hodgkin's disease treated during adolescence or young adulthood. *J Clin Oncol*, 18(3):487–97. PMID:10653864

Vargas AC, Reis-Filho JS, Lakhani SR (2011). Phenotype-genotype correlation in familial breast cancer. *J Mammary Gland Biol Neoplasia*, 16(1):27–40. doi:10.1007/s10911-011-9204-6 PMID:21400086

Venkitaraman AR (2002). Cancer susceptibility and the functions of *BRCA1* and *BRCA2*. *Cell*, 108(2):171–82. doi:10.1016/S0092-8674(02)00615-3 PMID:11832208

Vincent-Salomon A, Lucchesi C, Gruel N, Raynal V, Pierron G, Goudefroye R et al.; Breast cancer study group of the Institut Curie (2008). Integrated genomic and transcriptomic analysis of ductal carcinoma in situ of the breast. *Clin Cancer Res*, 14(7):1956–65. doi:10.1158/1078-0432.CCR-07-1465 PMID:18381933

von Karsa L (1995). Mammography screening – comprehensive, population-based quality assurance is required! [in German]. *Z Allgemeinmed*, 71:1863–7.

von Karsa L, Anttila A, Primic Žakelj M, de Wolf C, Bielska-Lasota M, Törnberg S et al. (2013). Stockholm statement on successful implementation of population-based cancer screening programmes. Annex 1a. In: Perry N, Broeders M, de Wolf C, Törnberg S, Holland R, von Karsa L, editors. European guidelines for quality assurance in breast cancer screening and diagnosis. Fourth edition, Supplements. Luxembourg: European Commission, Office for Official Publications of the European Union; pp. 123–8.

von Karsa L, Arrossi S (2013). Development and implementation of guidelines for quality assurance in breast cancer screening: the European experience. *Salud Publica Mex*, 55(3):318–28. PMID:23912545

von Karsa L, Dean PB, Arrossi S, Sankaranarayanan R (2014a). Screening – principles. In: Stewart BW, Wild CP, editors. World cancer report 2014. Lyon, France: International Agency for Research on Cancer; pp. 322–9.

von Karsa L, Qiao Y-L, Ramadas K, Keita N, Arrossi S, Dean PB et al. (2014b). Screening – implementation. In: Stewart BW, Wild CP, editors. World cancer report 2014. Lyon, France: International Agency for Research on Cancer; pp. 330–6.

Walsh T, Casadei S, Coats KH, Swisher E, Stray SM, Higgins J et al. (2006). Spectrum of mutations in *BRCA1*, *BRCA2*, *CHEK2*, and *TP53* in families at high risk of breast cancer. *JAMA*, 295(12):1379–88. doi:10.1001/jama.295.12.1379 PMID:16551709

Walters S, Maringe C, Butler J, Brierley JD, Rachet B, Coleman MP (2013b). Comparability of stage data in cancer registries in six countries: lessons from the International Cancer Benchmarking Partnership. *Int J Cancer*, 132(3):676–85. doi:10.1002/ijc.27651 PMID:22623157

Walters S, Maringe C, Butler J, Rachet B, Barrett-Lee P, Bergh J et al.; ICBP Module 1 Working Group (2013a). Breast cancer survival and stage at diagnosis in Australia, Canada, Denmark, Norway, Sweden and the UK, 2000–2007: a population-based study. *Br J Cancer*, 108(5):1195–208. doi:10.1038/bjc.2013.6 PMID:23449362

Warner E, Foulkes W, Goodwin P, Meschino W, Blondal J, Paterson C et al. (1999). Prevalence and penetrance of *BRCA1* and *BRCA2* gene mutations in unselected Ashkenazi Jewish women with breast cancer. *J Natl Cancer Inst*, 91(14):1241–7. doi:10.1093/jnci/91.14.1241 PMID:10413426

Warren GW, Alberg AJ, Kraft AS, Cummings KM (2014). The 2014 Surgeon General's report: "The health consequences of smoking – 50 years of progress": a paradigm shift in cancer care. *Cancer*, 120(13):1914–6. doi:10.1002/cncr.28695 PMID:24687615

Washbrook E (2006). Risk factors and epidemiology of breast cancer. *Women's Health Med*, 3(1):8–14. doi:10.1383/wohm.2006.3.1.8

WCRF/AICR (2007). Food, nutrition, physical activity, and the prevention of cancer: a global perspective. Washington (DC), USA: World Cancer Research Fund and American Institute for Cancer Research.

WCRF/AICR (2009). Ministério da Saúde, Instituto Nacional de Câncer, Políticas e ações para prevenção do câncer no Brasil: alimentação, nutrição e atividade física. Rio de Janeiro, Brazil: World Cancer Research Fund and American Institute for Cancer Research.

WCRF/AICR (2010). Continuous Update Project Report. Food, nutrition, physical activity, and the prevention of breast cancer. World Cancer Research Fund and American Institute for Cancer Research. Available from: http://www.dietandcancerreport.org/cancer_resource_center/downloads/cu/Breast-Cancer-2010-Report.pdf.

Webster P, Austoker J (2006). Women's knowledge about breast cancer risk and their views of the purpose and implications of breast screening–a questionnaire survey. *J Public Health (Oxf)*, 28(3):197–202. doi:10.1093/pubmed/fdl030 PMID:16902075

Weischer M, Bojesen SE, Ellervik C, Tybjaerg-Hansen A, Nordestgaard BG (2008). *CHEK2**1100delC genotyping for clinical assessment of breast cancer risk: meta-analyses of 26,000 patient cases and 27,000 controls. *J Clin Oncol*, 26(4):542–8. doi:10.1200/JCO.2007.12.5922 PMID:18172190

Weischer M, Nordestgaard BG, Pharoah P, Bolla MK, Nevanlinna H, Van't Veer LJ et al. (2012). *CHEK2**1100delC heterozygosity in women with breast cancer associated with early death, breast cancer-specific death, and increased risk of a second breast cancer. *J Clin Oncol*, 30(35):4308–16. doi:10.1200/JCO.2012.42.7336 PMID:23109706

Welch HG, Black WC (1997). Using autopsy series to estimate the disease "reservoir" for ductal carcinoma in situ of the breast: how much more breast cancer can we find? *Ann Intern Med*, 127(11):1023–8. doi:10.7326/0003-4819-127-11-199712010-00014 PMID:9412284

WHO (2007). Cancer control: Knowledge into action. WHO guide for effective programmes. Module 3: Early detection. Geneva, Switzerland: World Health Organization. Available from: http://www.who.int/cancer/publications/cancer_control_detection/en/index.html.

WHO (2013a). WHO guidelines for screening and treatment of precancerous lesions for cervical cancer prevention. Geneva, Switzerland: World Health Organization. Available from: http://www.who.int/reproductivehealth/publications/cancers/screening_and_treatment_of_precancerous_lesions/en/.

WHO (2013b). Implementation tools: Package of Essential Noncommunicable (PEN) disease interventions for primary health care in low-resource settings. Geneva, Switzerland: World Health Organization. Available from: http://apps.who.int/iris/bitstream/10665/133525/1/9789241506557_eng.pdf?ua=1&ua=1.

WHO (2014). World Health Organization Cancer Mortality Database. Available from: http://www-dep.iarc.fr/WHOdb/WHOdb.htm.

Wilson JMG, Jungner G (1968). Principles and practice of screening for disease. Geneva, Switzerland: World Health Organization. Public Health Papers No. 34. Available from: http://whqlibdoc.who.int/php/WHO_PHP_34.pdf.

Wohlfahrt J, Melbye M (2001). Age at any birth is associated with breast cancer risk. *Epidemiology*, 12(1):68–73. doi:10.1097/00001648-200101000-00012 PMID:11138822

Wolff AC, Hammond ME, Hicks DG, Dowsett M, McShane LM, Allison KH et al.; American Society of Clinical Oncology; College of American Pathologists (2013). Recommendations for human epidermal growth factor receptor 2 testing in breast cancer: American Society of Clinical Oncology/College of American Pathologists clinical practice guideline update. *J Clin Oncol*, 31(31):3997–4013. doi:10.1200/JCO.2013.50.9984 PMID:24101045

Wu Y, Zhang D, Kang S (2013). Physical activity and risk of breast cancer: a meta-analysis of prospective studies. *Breast Cancer Res Treat*, 137(3):869–82. doi:10.1007/s10549-012-2396-7 PMID:23274845

Yerushalmi R, Woods R, Ravdin PM, Hayes MM, Gelmon KA (2010). Ki67 in breast cancer: prognostic and predictive potential. *Lancet Oncol*, 11(2):174–83. doi:10.1016/S1470-2045(09)70262-1 PMID:20152769

Yip CH, Smith RA, Anderson BO, Miller AB, Thomas DB Ang ES et al.; Breast Health Global Initiative Early Detection Panel (2008). Guideline implementation for breast healthcare in low- and middle-income countries: early detection resource allocation. *Cancer*, 113(8 Suppl):2244–56. doi:10.1002/cncr.23842 PMID:18837017

Yoshida K, Miki Y (2004). Role of *BRCA1* and *BRCA2* as regulators of DNA repair, transcription, and cell cycle in response to DNA damage. *Cancer Sci*, 95(11):866–71. doi:10.1111/j.1349-7006.2004.tb02195.x PMID:15546503

Zahl PH, Maehlen J, Welch HG (2008). The natural history of invasive breast cancers detected by screening mammography. *Arch Intern Med*, 168(21):2311–6. doi:10.1001/archinte.168.21.2311 PMID:19029493

2. SCREENING TECHNIQUES

2.1 X-ray techniques

The original technique for mammography was introduced by Salomon in Germany in 1913, 18 years after the discovery of X-rays by Roentgen (Salomon, 1913). A mammogram is formed by recording the two-dimensional (2D) pattern of X-rays transmitted through the volume of the breast onto an image receptor. Breast cancer is detected radiographically on the basis of four major signs: a mass density with specific shape and border characteristics, microcalcifications, architectural distortions, and asymmetries between the radiological appearance of the left and right breast (Kopans, 2006). These signs are often very subtle, and in order for them to be detected accurately and when the cancer is at the smallest detectable size, the technical image quality of the mammograms must be excellent (Young et al., 1994; Taplin et al., 2002). At the same time, because ionizing radiation is carcinogenic, it is desirable that the radiation dose received by the patient is as low as is reasonably achievable consistent with the required image quality (Young et al., 1997). The trade-off between imaging performance and radiation doses inevitably involves compromises, and optimization of imaging is inextricably linked to technical design elements in the imaging system. Fig. 2.1 shows examples of mammograms obtained during different periods and with different equipment. Fig. 2.1a shows a mammogram from one of the randomized controlled trials (RCTs) in the early 1980s; the image is poorly exposed, and both the contrast and the spatial resolution are poor, making detection of small lesions difficult. The mammogram in Fig. 2.1b, from the same era, is of much higher quality and illustrates a cancer seen on the basis of an irregularly shaped mass (black arrow). Fig. 2.1c shows a digital mammogram, illustrating the enormous improvement that has occurred in both technology and technique. Breast positioning, penetration of the tissue, and contrast are excellent, allowing visualization of a small area of ductal carcinoma in situ (DCIS) seen on the basis of microcalcifications, and, more importantly, providing the opportunity to detect an immediately adjacent high-grade invasive cancer 1.7 mm in diameter.

Excellent image quality is an essential component but not, on its own, a sufficient component to ensure a high level of accuracy in cancer detection. Of equal or perhaps greater importance are the skill of the radiographer who conducts the examination and sets the equipment operating factors and the skill, experience, and judgement of the radiologist who interprets the images. This emphasizes the need for thorough training and ongoing maintenance of skills of these individuals.

2.1.1 X-ray equipment

Mammography was originally carried out using general-purpose X-ray imaging systems. Although the principles remain the same, it was gradually recognized that the specific imaging requirements for effective detection of breast

Fig. 2.1 Examples of mammograms of different quality

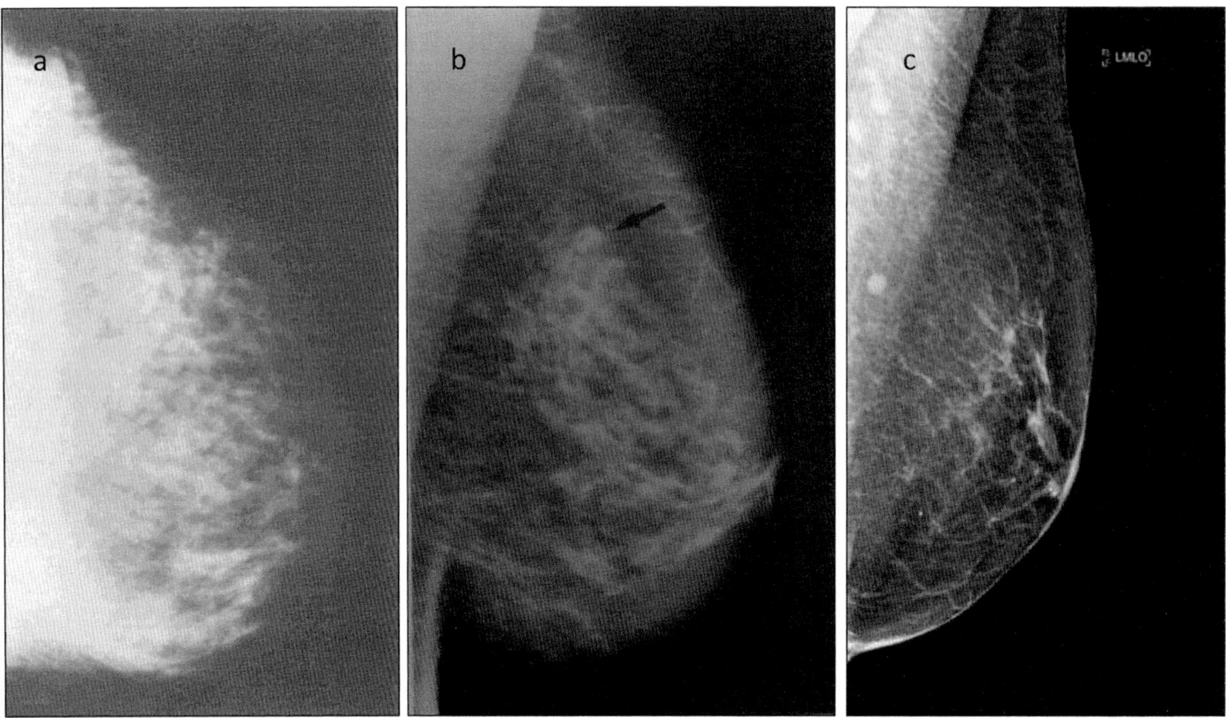

(a) Mammogram produced in the early 1980s. (b) Mammogram from the same era produced with better breast compression, exposure factors, and film processing, illustrating a tumour mass (arrow). (c) Mediolateral oblique digital screening mammogram of a woman aged 62 years, illustrating a cluster of microcalcifications near the nipple, later diagnosed as high-grade ductal carcinoma in situ (DCIS) 4 mm in diameter, and an adjacent area of invasive cancer 1.7 mm in diameter.
Unpublished clinical mammograms kindly provided by (a) Dr Roberta Jong, Toronto, Canada, (b) Dr László Tabár, Falun Central Hospital, Sweden, and (c) Dr Pavel Crystal, Mount Sinai Hospital, Toronto, Canada.

cancer would be better met if equipment were adapted specifically for the purpose of mammography (AAPM, 1990; NCRP, 2004). Between the mid-1960s and 1990, several important technical improvements were introduced, and these resulted in a highly specialized imaging system (Feig, 1987; Haus, 1987). A major technical change came about in 2000 when the first digital mammography systems became available.

Some of the specialized features of mammography systems are briefly described here.

Very high spatial resolution is required in mammography to allow discrimination of fine microcalcifications and morphological features of soft tissue structures such as masses. To support this resolution requirement, the effective size of the X-ray source for mammography (known as the focal spot or target) is much smaller than that used for most general radiography procedures. Modern mammography systems most frequently use a nominal focal spot size of 0.3 mm for regular mammography and of 0.1 mm for magnification procedures (IAEA, 2014).

The spectrum, or distribution of X-rays of different energies in the beam, is also specialized for mammography (Jennings et al., 1981; Beaman & Lillicrap, 1982). To maximize the contrast between soft tissues such as normal fibroglandular tissue and carcinoma, it is desirable to use an energy spectrum with much lower energies than are used for general radiography.

The X-ray spectrum is determined by three factors: the material used to form the X-ray target, the type and thickness of metallic filter placed in the X-ray beam, and the kilovoltage applied to the X-ray tube (IAEA, 2014). These factors affect both the spectral shape and the intensity of X-rays in the beam that is incident upon the breast for imaging. Two other variables directly influence the amount of X-rays incident on the breast, but not the contrast characteristics of the beam: the tube current, typically measured in milliamperes (referred to as "the mA") and the exposure time (the time during which this current flows from the cathode of the tube to the target to produce the exposure).

Decreasing the energy of the X-ray spectrum increases the differences in X-ray absorption between different tissue types, thereby increasing contrast. However, low-energy X-rays are more heavily absorbed in the breast, and therefore more need to be used to obtain an acceptable number of photons reaching the imaging system. This results in an increased radiation dose to the breast. As in any type of X-ray imaging, a compromise is required between maximizing contrast and controlling radiation dose.

In 1967, a specialized mammography tube was introduced by Gros in France (Gros, 1967). The tube was equipped with a molybdenum (Mo) target, rather than the tungsten used in general-purpose tubes. Mo emits characteristic X-rays at 17.5 keV and 19.5 keV in addition to a broader-energy bremsstrahlung spectrum (X-rays emitted when an electron suddenly slows down when impinging on a target material). Operated at a tube potential of 24–32 kV for imaging using a screen-film detector, the tube provides a more optimal compromise between low energy (with high contrast and the accompanying high dose) and a more-penetrating, high-energy spectrum that allows low-dose imaging but at the penalty of reduced image contrast.

The Mo target is typically used in conjunction with an external Mo beam filter. X-ray attenuation of the Mo filter increases sharply just above the characteristic energies emitted by the Mo target, creating a relatively transmissive energy "window" that allows the characteristic X-rays (emitted just below the K-edge energy of Mo) to pass through the filter and expose the image. The result is selective removal of both the low-energy and high-energy X-rays, leaving a fairly narrow spectrum (Fig. 2.2) with an effective energy suitable for imaging the breast.

In general radiography, it is customary to compensate for increased body-part thickness or attenuation properties by adjusting the kilovoltage applied to the tube (IAEA, 2014). However, when the spectrum is formed largely with characteristic X-rays, as is the case with many mammography systems, changing the kilovoltage has a limited effect on the energy spectrum, and this could make it difficult to adequately penetrate dense breast tissue to obtain the required image contrast in some parts of the breast. Inadequate contrast could result in cancers being missed. To alter the effective energy of the beam to a greater degree, most modern mammography systems provide a second, readily interchangeable filter, typically composed of rhodium (Rh). Together with a selection of increased kilovoltage, this Mo–Rh combination provides a more-penetrating spectrum than is possible with the Mo–Mo target–filter combination. A further increase in energy can be achieved by fitting the X-ray tube with dual target materials, for example with a Rh target in addition to the standard Mo target. The higher energy of the characteristic X-rays from Rh provides a more-penetrating beam, albeit with lower contrast. Depending on the breast thickness and fibroglandular content (often referred to as breast density), target–filter combinations of Mo–Mo, Mo–Rh, or Rh–Rh can today be selected and used in conjunction with a kilovoltage selection that optimizes imaging performance.

Fig. 2.2 Use of selected target materials and K-edge filters to define the energy spectrum for mammography

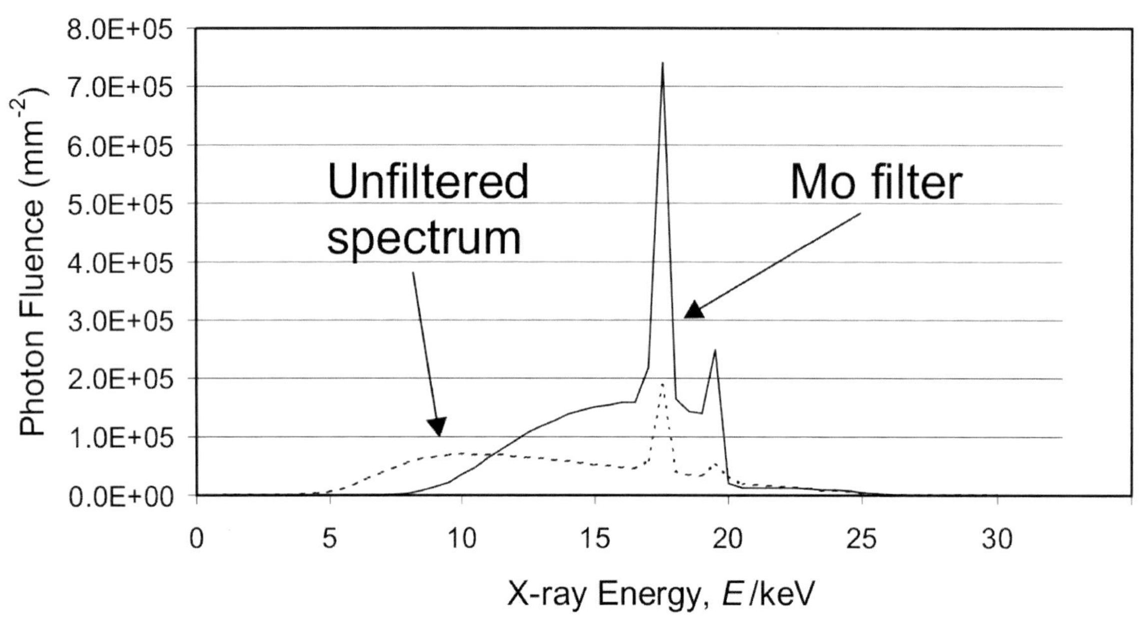

The filtered spectrum has been scaled upwards for clarity. Characteristic emission peaks from molybdenum (Mo) are seen at 17.5 keV and 19.5 keV.
Courtesy of Dr. M. Yaffe.

2.1.2 Screen-film mammography

To achieve high spatial resolution, the first mammograms were recorded on film exposed directly to X-rays (IAEA, 2014). The X-rays produce a latent image on the film, and this image is rendered visible by chemical processing of the film emulsion. This causes the silver bromide in the emulsion to be converted to metallic silver, which appears black upon trans-illumination of the processed film with white light. The degree of blackness, or optical density, increases with the amount of exposure of the film, which, in turn, is related to the transmission of X-rays through the breast. The optical density provides the visual signal, conveying information to the radiologist about the breast composition and the presence of suspicious lesions. Cancers and microcalcifications tend to be more absorbing of X-rays than fat or normal fibroglandular tissue; they therefore appear as areas of decreased optical density (white), whereas the fatty areas appear darker.

The characteristic curve of a mammography film is shown schematically in Fig. 2.3. The characteristic curve of the film transforms the X-ray fluence transmitted through the breast into the optical density of the processed film. Because the curve is sigmoidal in shape, the brightness of the image at each point will vary nonlinearly with X-ray exposure. The curve also transforms the contrast in the X-ray fluence transmitted through the breast into a difference in the optical density of the processed film (the displayed image contrast). Therefore, the displayed contrast is dependent on the gradient or slope of the characteristic curve at each point. Because the curve is nonlinear, the displayed contrast, which would ideally depend only on the tissue composition and the presence of lesions in the breast, also

Fig. 2.3 Characteristic curve of mammographic screen-film X-ray detector

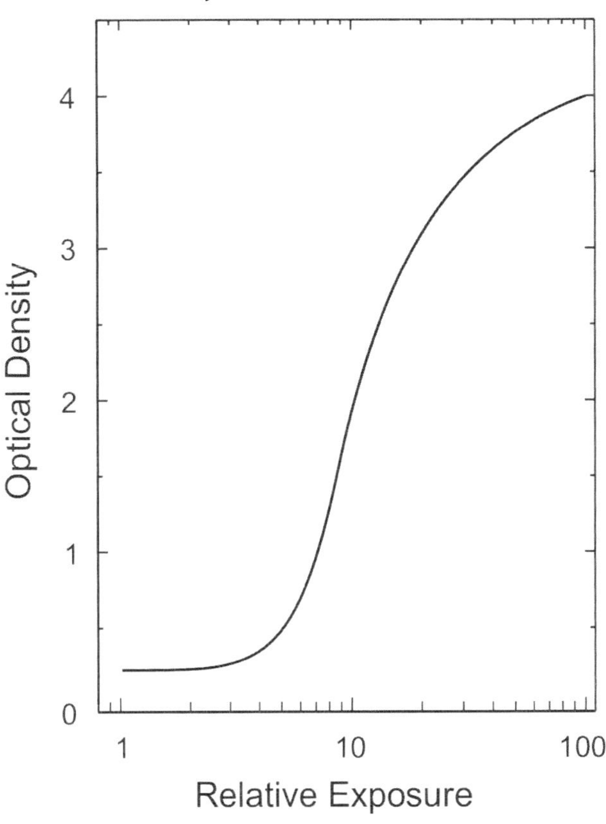

This creates a compromise between the range of exposure that can be recorded and the contrast in different parts of the image.
Courtesy of Dr. M. Yaffe.

depends on the degree of X-ray exposure to the film at each point.

In the earliest systems, the fraction of incident X-rays interacting with the film (referred to as the quantum efficiency) was very low, and so a relatively high exposure was required to achieve a useful working optical density, to provide adequate image brightness and contrast.

In the mid to late 1970s, non-screen film was largely replaced by dedicated mammographic screen-film image recording systems (Haus, 1987). Typically, these use a single thin screen to preserve spatial resolution and a film coated with emulsion on only one side. The system is used with a back screen, i.e. the X-rays pass through the film to strike and be absorbed by the phosphor of the screen, and the light emitted by the screen travels backwards towards the breast to be absorbed by the film emulsion. Intimate screen-film contact is essential for good resolution, and several different mechanisms have been used to maintain contact, including sealable plastic vacuum envelopes and cassettes containing a foam layer behind the screen to serve as a spring. These systems are considerably more sensitive to X-rays compared with non-screen film, and the peak gradient occurs at a much lower exposure. Further improvement in image quality came about, stimulated to a considerable extent by Logan-Young, a radiologist in Rochester, New York, USA, who brought together radiologists and scientists to promote scientific analysis of the performance of mammography systems and their technical advancement (Logan-Young & Muntz, 1979).

Rare-earth phosphor screens, which were introduced in the 1980s and improved progressively over the next decade (Brixner et al., 1985), provided a large increase in sensitivity. This occurred both through improved quantum efficiency of the screen compared with film alone and because of the amplification resulting when one X-ray, carrying say 20 keV, was absorbed and created thousands of light quanta, each carrying only 2–3 eV.

Logan-Young also advocated the use of firm compression of the breast during exposure. Compression serves several important purposes in improving image quality while reducing doses. It spreads out the tissues, reducing superposition, and thereby makes the boundaries of lesions easier to see. With a thinner breast, the transmission of primary radiation is higher, allowing a dose reduction while at the same time reducing the scatter-to-primary ratio of the X-ray beam exiting the breast and incident on the imaging system. More-uniform breasts represent less of a range of X-ray intensities and therefore require less exposure latitude or dynamic range from the film. This allows the use of higher-gradient films, thereby offering greater contrast. When the breast is immobilized, there is less image blurring due to anatomical motion, and therefore improvement in spatial resolution. Compression also reduces the degree of geometric magnification of tissues within the breast, since all parts of the breast are closer to the imaging system. This last factor reduces the amount of blurring caused by the X-ray focal spot, again improving spatial resolution. Inadequate compression can contribute to poor image quality and reduce the detectability of small or subtle lesions.

Even at the relatively low energies used for mammography, X-rays scattered in the breast and recorded by the image receptor are still a major problem, degrading image quality by producing a haze over the image, reducing the contrast produced by the directly transmitted primary X-rays, and also adding random quantum noise without providing useful information (IAEA, 2014). The scatter-to-primary ratio at the image receptor can be as high as 0.6–1.0. When film is used to record the image, part of its limited range is "used up" in recording scattered radiation. In the 1980s, specially designed anti-scatter moving grids were introduced for mammography. These grids reduced the scatter-to-primary ratio to about 0.1, thereby markedly improving image contrast. However, a grid does not transmit all of the useful primary radiation; some is blocked by the septa of the grid, and some is absorbed in the interspace material that separates the septa. In addition, because some of the film-darkening energy of scattered X-rays is removed from the beam, it is necessary to increase the patient's exposure to maintain the chosen film optical density. The resulting Bucky factor (the factor by which patient dose must be increased) when a grid is used is about 2.5–3. Nevertheless, the improvement is considered so important that grids are now routinely used in mammography. For medium to large breasts of medium to high density, the gridless technique is now considered inadequate for film mammography, due to insufficient contrast and significantly decreased visibility of cancers in such breasts.

A major improvement in mammography technology was the introduction of automatic exposure control (IAEA, 2014). One of the limitations of radiographic film is that the gradient of the characteristic curve varies with exposure level. It is very small at low and high exposures and has a maximum value within a limited range of intermediate exposures. It is difficult for the technologist to determine the appropriate exposure factors to ensure that the most important part of the breast parenchyma is imaged with the highest gradient. The automatic exposure control incorporates a sensor located beyond the image receptor (so that the shadow of the sensor is not seen on the mammogram) that discontinues the exposure when a predetermined amount of radiation has fallen onto the sensor. The location of the sensor can be moved around the image plane to select the area of anatomy of greatest interest. The automatic exposure control played a very important role in improving the consistency of film optical density, contrast, and radiation exposure in mammography.

Modern mammography systems have advanced further in terms of automatic selection of exposure parameters (IAEA, 2014). The X-ray attenuation of the breast depends on both compressed thickness and composition. Whereas the automatic exposure control controls only the exposure time according to the overall attenuation of the breast, it is valuable to tune the X-ray spectrum according to compressed breast thickness and composition. This can be done by measuring both the compressed breast thickness, by means of a sensor attached to the compression device, and the rate of X-ray transmission through the breast. The rate can be determined via a short test exposure (lasting only a few milliseconds) conducted at the beginning of the imaging sequence using standard exposure conditions appropriate for the breast thickness. Based on the measured transmitted X-ray exposure rate, the choice of X-ray target, filter, and kilovoltage can be adjusted automatically by the mammography equipment to optimize penetration and contrast in imaging, providing a better balance between image quality and radiation dose for each image produced.

2.1.3 Digital mammography

Despite the established value of film-based mammography for diagnosis and screening, screen-film mammography has several technological shortcomings that reduce its accuracy. Most of these stem from the fact that film is used both as part of the detector for image acquisition and as a display device. This necessitates certain compromises in performance for each of these roles. Because the gradient of the characteristic curve of the film depends on the exposure level (Fig. 2.3), the image contrast between tissues in the breast is reduced at both low and high exposures, corresponding to the most radiopaque and radiolucent parts of the breast. This loss of contrast can impair the visibility of structures within the breast in the image. Attempting to improve contrast by using a film emulsion with a higher gradient only reduces the exposure range over which the contrast is high (the exposure latitude or dynamic range), again causing parts of the breast to be imaged suboptimally.

Digital mammography attempts to overcome these limitations by decoupling image acquisition from display and archiving functions, and optimizing each separately. An electronic detector replaces the screen-film system for acquisition. Images are stored in digital form in computer memory and displayed on a high-resolution monitor. Additional advantages of digital mammography are the ability to make a detector that has increased quantum efficiency while maintaining spatial resolution, the elimination of the components of image noise due to film granularity and non-uniform sensitivity of the phosphor screen, the possibility of more-efficient approaches to reducing the effects of scattered radiation, and the ability to perform quantitative operations or analysis on the digital images.

Several different detector technologies have been developed and used for digital mammography. Further information on this topic is available (Pisano & Yaffe, 2005; Yaffe, 2010a).

Unlike screen-film technology, in which the elements of a phosphor X-ray absorber in contact with a film coated with photographic emulsion in a light-tight cassette are fairly common across all vendors, there is more diversity in the technology used for digital mammography, especially for the X-ray detectors used. This leads to differences in spatial resolution, signal-to-noise ratio, scatter-rejection characteristics, and radiation doses delivered to the breast. The photostimulable phosphor system, also often referred to as computed radiography, was introduced as a generic technology for use in digital mammography. In a series of physics measurements, computed radiography was found to have inferior performance characteristics, in terms of spatial resolution and signal-to-noise ratio at equivalent dose to the breast, to the other digital mammography technologies, which are typically collectively referred to as digital radiography systems (Young & Oduko, 2005; Yaffe et al., 2013).

These findings were later corroborated by observations of lower cancer detection rates and positive predictive values (PPVs) in screening programmes (Chiarelli et al., 2013) where computed radiography systems were used compared with those obtained with other types of digital mammography systems. Subsequently, the use of computed radiography systems was prohibited in the Ontario, Canada, screening programme. Similar observations were also made in the breast screening programme in France (INCa, 2010). Overall, among mammography systems, digital radiography systems appear to produce the highest and most consistent diagnostic image quality with a lower radiation dose.

Although digital mammography has considerably wider exposure latitude than screen-film mammography, it must still be optimized to provide excellent image quality at the lowest dose consistent with those quality requirements. The automatic exposure control need not be set to provide a target image optical density, as this can be adjusted on the computer monitor during image display, but instead a target image signal-to-noise ratio. There is also evidence that performance will be more optimal if digital systems are used with X-ray spectra of slightly higher beam quality than those used for screen-film mammography (Berns et al., 2003; Huda et al., 2003; Young et al., 2006).

(a) Image processing of digital mammograms

The digital mammogram is recorded on a numerical scale, where each pixel is given a value from 0 to 16 383 (where 16 383 represents the maximum transmitted X-ray intensity) (Yaffe, 2010b). This range exceeds the capability for optimal viewing by the human eye and also that of electronic display devices. Various types of image processing can be used to improve the conspicuity of relevant anatomical information before display by compressing or transforming this range and by correcting for certain imperfections in the imaging system. The first operation is commonly referred to as flat-fielding, gain correction, or uniformity correction. Detectors used to produce digital images frequently contain many (several million) elements, referred to as dels or pixels. These tend to vary slightly in sensitivity. In addition, the X-ray beam is not perfectly uniform in intensity. This causes variations across the image that would create fluctuations in the image unrelated to any features of the breast itself, a type of image granularity (referred to as structural or fixed-pattern noise). Fortunately, with digital technology these variations are generally temporally quite stable. The point-to-point fluctuations can be removed by recording an image of a uniform slab of X-ray absorbing material and using it to correct all subsequent images, thereby creating a very uniform image field.

It is also possible to improve the sharpness of display by various edge enhancement techniques, such as unsharp masking. Here, a blurred version of the original mammogram is made by filtering the image in the computer with a function that controls the degree of blurring. When this blurred mask is subtracted from the original image, the resulting difference image is composed mainly of the sharp features of the mammogram without the broad area structures. This edge map is then added to the original image to provide enhancement of the edges of microcalcifications, fine fibres, and blood vessels. The amount of edge enhancement is controlled by a weighting constant by which the edge image is multiplied before the addition takes place. Excessive enhancement also increases the intrinsic granularity of the image, and such noise can interfere with image interpretation. After flat-field correction and sharpening have been applied to the image, it is referred to as the "for processing" or "raw" digital mammogram.

A useful image processing feature applied to digital mammograms is referred to as peripheral equalization. The breast varies in thickness, and therefore in attenuation of X-rays, from the central region out towards its periphery. Such a variation in X-ray transmission is seldom relevant to the task of detecting suspicious compositional changes in the breast, and its recording would waste part of the limited display range of the viewing monitor. Therefore, it is common to implement a correction to the image that suppresses the overall change in image signal due to the changes in breast thickness, preserving the range to allow more-sensitive detection of lesions (Byng et al., 1997; Stefanoyiannis et al., 2000).

Another means of enhancing the display is through modification of the histogram of image display values. If the histogram is calculated, it is frequently found that certain display values are not used or are used infrequently. Histogram equalization is a technique to remap the image display values so that all grey levels in the display are used with approximately equal frequency. This can help to make better use of the capability of the display (Pizer et al., 1987; Pisano et al., 1998; Goldstraw et al., 2010). The correction is applied in small subregions of the image to optimize the local contrast. Again, care must be taken to control the amplification of display contrast to avoid excessive appearance of noise. After these operations have been applied to the original "for processing" image, it is referred to as the "for presentation" image.

(b) Display of digital mammograms

Digital mammograms can be printed; however, the advantage of being able to manipulate the brightness, contrast, and sharpness of the images interactively while viewing them is then lost. High-resolution, 5-megapixel monitors are available for "soft copy" display, and this is now the preferred means of viewing and interpreting digital mammograms (IAEA, 2014).

The final, and perhaps most useful, image processing operations are look-up table modifications. Most digital mammography systems are configured such that this is done by the radiologist interactively while viewing the "for presentation" image. The range of values of a digital mammogram exceeds the sensitivity capability of the eye for contrast perception and also the capability of most electronic display devices. Typically, on a monitor it is considered feasible to display the image in terms of 10 bits or 1024 shades of brightness at any one time. A look-up table is used by the digital mammography computer to map the original range of image data at 16 384 levels to the 1024 levels available for display (Pisano, 2004).

A simple use of look-up table modification, illustrated in Fig. 2.4, is called linear scaling and clipping. It is familiar to users of computed tomography systems, where a window level, L, is set, which describes the image value that will be displayed as the mid-value of display intensity, and a window, W, is chosen, which is the range of original image values to be displayed. Image values below L − W/2 are displayed as black, and those above L + W/2 are displayed at the maximum intensity of white. Intermediate values are displayed on a linear range of grey values between black and white, so that the entire range of display values is used. This allows the user to ensure that the anatomy of interest will be viewed in the optimal part of the display brightness as well as to adjust contrast as desired. By controlling WL, the display window can be used to inspect regions of the breast that vary greatly in density. The degree of contrast with which the image is displayed is increased (without the necessity to re-image the breast) by reducing W.

The value of W can be reduced until the appearance of noise in the displayed image becomes unacceptable. This is determined by the intrinsic noise of the image acquisition, which, in turn, can be controlled by the use of very-low-noise X-ray detection systems and by the dose to the breast. The dose can be chosen according to the required signal-to-noise ratio for a particular imaging situation, rather than by the need to produce an image of a given "brightness".

More generally, it may be found that other, nonlinear mappings from image intensity to display brightness may be more suitable. These may be found to better compensate for deficiencies in the display device or for the perceptual characteristics of the observer. An optimal look-up table modification remains to be determined.

One of the important advantages of digital imaging is that these image processing features can be turned on and off instantly to allow the radiologist to view the images under different enhancement conditions. This can facilitate decisions about whether suspicious structures are real or artefactual. Although very sophisticated image processing is possible, it is likely that the main benefit of image enhancement will derive from relatively simple operations that improve contrast in dense regions or sharpen subtle

Fig. 2.4 Interactive control of image brightness and contrast characteristics during viewing by look-up table adjustment

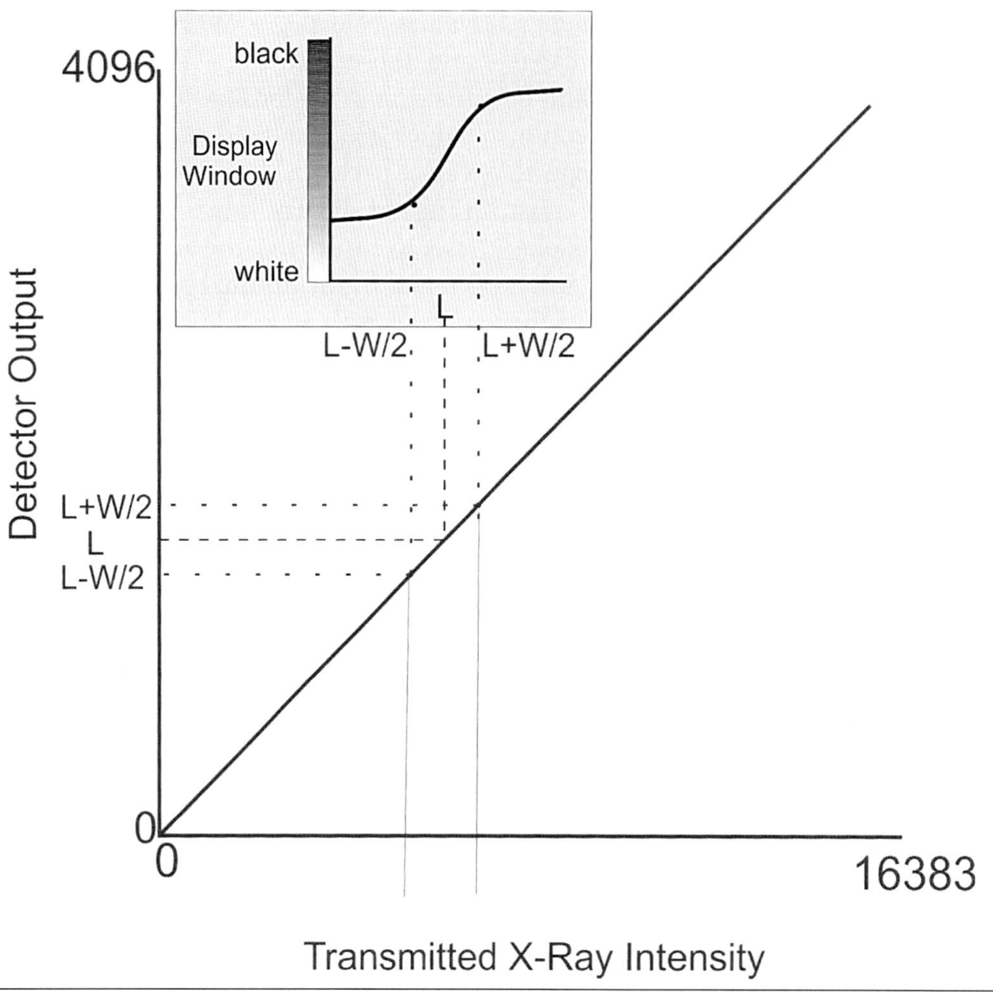

L, window level, digital pixel value set to mid-value of display intensity; W, window, range of original digital pixel values to be displayed between full black and full white.
Created by the Working Group.

structures. The optimal manner in which to display image contrast scales, the possible value of equalization, and the role of edge enhancement and other image sharpening techniques in digital mammography must be carefully investigated in terms of their efficacy.

Another important advantage of digital mammography is the immediate availability of current and previous examinations. Comparison with previous mammograms is extremely valuable for screening mammography, considering that each breast is individually different. Consideration of changes from a previous mammogram allows detection of subtle abnormalities, whereas a finding that is stable over time may not require a recall.

Digital mammography has been available since 2000. Due to the number of pixels available on high-resolution monitors (typically about 5 million), it is usually not possible to present even a single mammogram at full resolution on a monitor. In screening the radiologist is often required to work with eight images, four from the current examination and four from a previous examination. This implies that multiple monitors be used in a digital mammography workstation and, even so, that it would be necessary to present images at reduced spatial resolution when viewing the entire mammogram and then to apply zooming or scrolling operations to inspect areas of interest at full spatial resolution. This requires that the image manipulation tools provided with the digital mammography workstation are fast and user-friendly and that the radiologist undergoes a learning process to develop a regimen for efficiently and thoroughly inspecting the mammograms.

2.1.4 Digital breast tomosynthesis

An important limitation in mammography is that it is a projection imaging technique, where shadows from structures throughout the thickness of the breast superpose to form the image. The conspicuity of a lesion is frequently reduced by the obscuring effect of normal fibroglandular tissue of similar X-ray attenuation properties located along the path of the X-ray beam, above and below the lesion. This is most pronounced for women with dense breasts (those in which there is a high proportion of fibroglandular tissue; see Section 2.1.9). Overlap of tissues from different planes in the breast creates structural complexity in projection images that can mask the presence of a cancer in the dense breast, reducing sensitivity, or can mimic the presence of a lesion that does not exist, resulting in reduced specificity. Reducing the effect of tissue superposition in images should improve both sensitivity and specificity.

Digital breast tomosynthesis is a technique that produces quasi three-dimensional (3D) images of X-ray attenuation coefficients from a series of about 9–25 projection images (very-low-dose conventional mammograms) acquired over a limited range of angles around the breast (Fig. 2.5; Yaffe & Mainprize, 2014). The 3D image is created by mathematical reconstruction of the data in this set of 2D images. It is possible to make lesions more conspicuous by largely eliminating the effects of tissue superposition from the planar images that are presented. Furthermore, the morphology of lesions can be appreciated more easily, improving discrimination between malignant and benign lesions. This may simplify the diagnostic imaging algorithm by reducing the number of additional assessment procedures. Finally, using tomosynthesis, lesions can be localized in three dimensions, facilitating more accurate planning of surgery or radiation therapy.

Tomosynthesis can be performed on a modified digital mammography system that has a motorized gantry system (Niklason et al., 1997; Wu et al., 2003). This can be advantageous because conventional projection mammography could be performed on the same unit as the need arises (for screening, magnification viewing, characterization of microcalcification, etc.). Reconstruction is accomplished using algorithms similar to those used for computed tomography (Gordon et al., 1970; Mueller et al., 1998; Chidlow & Möller, 2003). Doses can be kept low while maintaining high-quality images; the dose for a tomosynthesis examination is of 3–5 mGy, comparable to that for a two-view digital mammography (Yaffe & Mainprize, 2014).

The reconstructed images are often viewed as a "movie loop" in which adjacent *x*–*y* planes (parallel to the X-ray detector) are displayed sequentially and resemble a series of 2D mammograms, each representing a "slice" of tissue in the breast (Yaffe & Mainprize, 2014). Within these 2D images, the spatial resolution (*x*–*y* plane) is the same as or similar to that of a conventional digital mammogram (0.05–0.14 mm), but the slice-to-slice resolution (*z* plane) is considerably coarser (0.5–1 mm). Also, because a complete range of angular data is not obtained, the data set is highly undersampled, giving rise to artefacts.

The quality of the reconstructed image and the dose to the breast are dependent on the

Fig. 2.5 Schematic of a digital breast tomosynthesis system

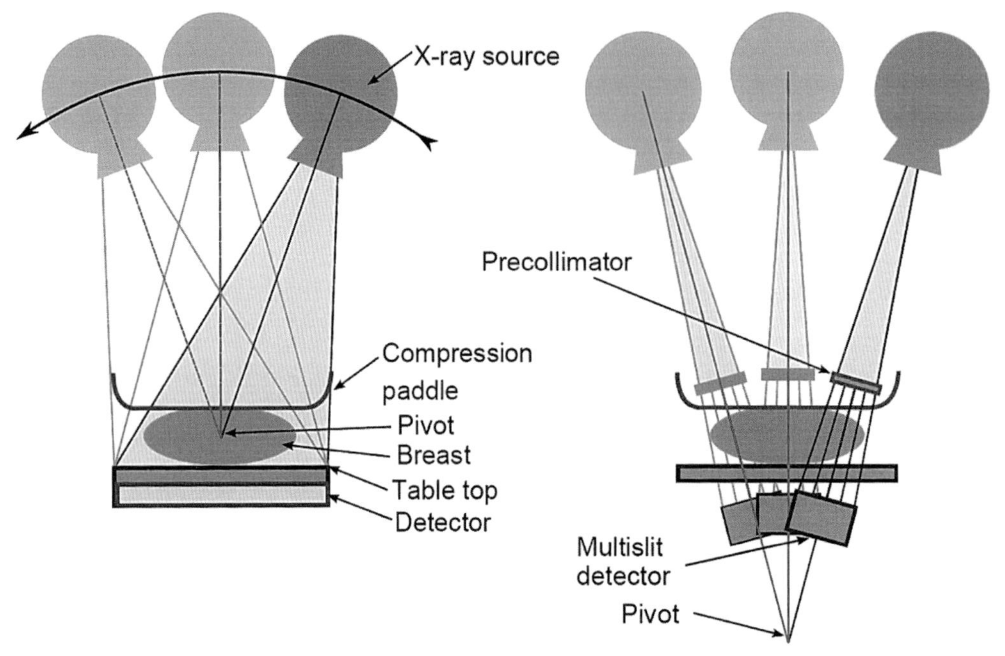

The X-ray source moves in an arc around a pivot axis, generally placed near the breast support.
Reprinted from Yaffe & Mainprize (2014). *Radiologic Clinics of North America*, Volume 52, issue 3, Digital tomosynthesis: technique, Pages 489–497, Copyright (2014), with permission from Elsevier.

angular range and number of projections, the dose used per projection, and the performance of the X-ray detector and electronics.

An examination that consists of the 3D mammogram plus the conventional 2D mammogram requires a higher total radiation dose to the breast than either mammogram alone. Once a 3D data set has been created, it is possible to synthesize 2D views by projecting through the data set onto traditional 2D planes, thereby simulating either the craniocaudal or mediolateral oblique views. This can be done without any additional radiation dose, and appears to provide acceptable image quality and adequate clinical performance (Skaane et al., 2014a; Zuley et al., 2014).

Studies on the performance of tomosynthesis are presented in Section 5.5. Radiation doses are discussed in Section 2.1.6.

2.1.5 Breast computed tomography

The availability of flat-panel digital radiography detectors has stimulated recent efforts to develop true 3D dedicated breast computed tomography systems. These consist of a table on which the patient lies in the prone position with the breast pendant into the centre of a digital X-ray system that rotates in a horizontal plane below the table (Boone et al., 2001). These systems produce tomographic images, with isotropic spatial resolution elements, although spatial resolution is generally designed to be coarser in the *x*–*y* plane compared with tomosynthesis to allow control of the required radiation doses to achieve adequate signal-to-noise ratio. Clinical evaluation of prototype breast computed tomography systems is currently under way (Chen & Ning, 2002, 2003; Lindfors et al., 2008).

2.1.6 Radiation dose

The majority of the X-ray dose received from mammography examinations is to the breast. With proper imaging technique, the thyroid is not exposed to direct radiation and receives only a very small dose scattered towards the thyroid from breast tissue. Similarly, if a woman is pregnant, the direct dose received by the embryo or fetus is close to zero. The small amount of radiation directed towards the pelvis is greatly reduced, first by attenuation by the breast and the breast support of the mammography unit, then by X-ray absorption by tissue overlying the conceptus, and finally due to the distance from the breast.

In the early use of mammography, the image was recorded on direct-exposure film without intensifying screens. It is estimated that the dose to each breast of average compressed thickness and composition from a two-view examination was on the order of 30 mGy (Conway et al., 1994). The xeroradiographic method, using a sheet of amorphous selenium as the X-ray detector, was introduced in the early 1970s and resulted in doses to the two breasts of about 8 mGy (Haus, 1983; Conway et al., 1994).

A series of technical developments introduced for mammography enabled a reduction of the radiation doses received by the breast (Feig, 1987; Haus, 1987; AAPM, 1990; Yaffe, 1990; NCRP, 2004). These included (i) the introduction in the late 1970s of intensifying screens, which provided improved quantum efficiency (absorption of the X-rays) compared with direct-exposure film, as well as a high degree of signal amplification; (ii) improved sensitivity of film emulsions to light; and (iii) technical advances in the chemistry and technique used to process the film. The original screen-film combinations for mammography were introduced in the late 1970s and were used without an X-ray anti-scatter grid. These required doses to the breast of about 1 mGy for the two views (Hammerstein et al., 1979; Haus, 1983).

Other technical developments or alterations in imaging technique had the effect of increasing radiation dose while improving image contrast or reducing noise. Factors that caused an increase in dose, accompanied by better image quality, included (i) use of a grid, which doubled or tripled doses but produced much better image contrast; (ii) the necessity to use thin phosphor screens, to preserve high spatial resolution; (iii) use of reduced kilovoltage, to improve contrast; (iv) use of increased optical density in images, to make use of the highest gradient available with the film; and (v) the choice of fine-grained films, to reduce the image-degrading effects of film granularity. More aggressive compression of the breast improved contrast while reducing dose.

The overall result of the many technical developments that occurred mainly in the 1980s and 1990s was a major decrease in dose from the levels used with non-screen film technology; doses to the breast for screen-film mammography in 2000 were considerably lower than those required with xeroradiography (8 mGy) but higher than those used with the earliest screen-film systems (1 mGy) (Suleiman et al., 1999).

Digital mammography with more-efficient X-ray detectors requires lower doses without loss of diagnostic accuracy. Digital radiography mammography systems operate at doses that are on average 22% lower than those used for screen-film mammography (Table 2.1). However, if a system uses an inefficient detector technology or is not operated optimally, the doses can be similar to or exceed those used for film (Young & Oduko, 2005).

The combined procedure of digital mammography plus tomosynthesis increases the total radiation dose. In their comparison of digital mammography versus combined digital breast tomosynthesis and digital mammography for screening, Skaane et al. (2013) estimated the dose as 3.2 mGy for two-view digital mammography

Table 2.1 Radiation dose to each breast (mGy) from a two-view examination with different mammographic techniques

Reference	Screen-film mammography	Digital mammography	Digital breast tomosynthesis	Digital breast tomosynthesis + digital mammography
Hendrick et al. (2010)	4.7	3.7		
Yaffe et al. (2013)	3.2	2.3		
Skaane et al. (2013)		3.2	3.9	~7

alone and approximately 7 mGy (3.2 mGy for digital mammography plus 3.9 mGy for digital breast tomosynthesis) for the combined procedure (Table 2.1). If the synthesized 2D projection image can be used to replace the standard digital mammography, then no further radiation is required than that needed for digital breast tomosynthesis alone.

The dose values discussed correspond to a standard screening examination with two views to each breast. Single-view protocols will result in doses that are about 50% lower but will increase the risk that some breast tissue will not be included in the examination. Those women who are recalled due to abnormal findings at screening will have additional imaging procedures performed. Ultrasonography and magnetic resonance imaging (MRI) are used for some purposes, but women may also receive additional X-ray views, for example magnification mammography. This will result in increased dose to those women. The actual increase will depend on the specifics of the procedure (e.g. whether the entire breast is imaged or only an area of concern), but is roughly one half of the two-view mammography dose (digital or screen-film, as appropriate) for each additional X-ray image acquired of the breast. Evaluation of the radiation risk is presented in Section 5.3.4.

2.1.7 Quality assurance and quality control in mammography

The ability of a breast cancer screening programme to achieve an impact is heavily dependent on two general categories of activities. Both fall under the overall umbrella of quality assurance (see also Section 1.5.3d).

The first aspect of quality is closely related to the operational standards of a screening facility or programme. This includes procedures for encouraging participation in screening and compliance with the recommended screening intervals, assessment of positive screening findings, and monitoring of performance and outcomes. There are many excellent references setting out these standards (BreastScreen Australia, 2001; Klabunde et al., 2001; NHSBSP, 2005; Perry et al., 2006a, 2013; CPAC, 2013).

The second category is more closely related to the activities of acquiring and interpreting the screening images. The ability to detect breast cancer with high sensitivity and specificity is closely linked to the technical quality of the mammograms and the skill of the radiologists. These aspects of quality begin with the establishment of appropriate standards for qualifications, the training requirements of personnel, the specifications for the purchase of equipment, and the definition of the exposure factors for imaging.

Once an initial high-quality environment is established for screening, quality control refers to the set of procedures and tests that will enable that high quality to be maintained over time.

Guidelines for quality control in mammography for both screening and diagnostic purposes have been developed by many countries and by several international organizations (see Hendrick et al., 2002), including by the International Atomic Energy Agency (IAEA, 2009, 2011) and the European Reference Organisation for Quality Assured Breast Screening and Diagnostic Services (EUREF) (Perry et al., 2006b), in Germany through mammography screening legislation (Kassenärztliche Bundesvereinigung, 2004), in the United Kingdom through the National Health Service (NHS) Breast Screening Programme (NHSBSP, 2013), in the USA through the United States Food and Drug Administration (FDA, 2013) Mammography Quality Standards Act (Fintor et al., 1995; Houn et al., 1995; Linver et al., 1995) and the American College of Radiology (ACR, 2013a), and in Canada (Health Canada, 2013) (see Section 3.2 for further information by country/region).

Many of the quality control programmes in different countries are quite similar in content, providing in-depth discussions of the necessary equipment for mammography imaging, the standards that the equipment must meet, the upkeep of that equipment, the duties and qualifications of the radiographers involved in performing the procedures, the standards for interpretation, recall rates, and the testing procedures performed by medical physicists necessary to confirm that mammography units are performing optimally and in accordance with applicable regulations. Frequently, ranges are defined for the results to define what is acceptable (if results fall outside the range, imaging should be discontinued until a problem is corrected) and achievable (a desirable range for facilities with modern equipment and experienced personnel to aim for).

The quality control testing programme recommended by the International Atomic Energy Agency for screen-film mammography is given in Table 2.2 and Table 2.3, which outline the responsibilities of the radiographers and medical physicists, respectively. The corresponding tests for digital mammography systems are given in Table 2.4 and Table 2.5, respectively.

In addition, several jurisdictions (economic regions, countries, states, and provinces) operate accreditation programmes for mammography. These include components to monitor that quality assurance and quality control practices and procedures are in place. For example, accreditation programmes have been implemented by the American College of Radiology in the USA (McLelland et al., 1991), the NHS Cancer Screening Programme in the United Kingdom (Wilson & Liston, 2011), and the Canadian Association of Radiologists (Canadian Association of Radiologists, 2012).

One critical point to be considered for quality assurance is the criterion for credentialing professionals involved in the mammography process. The team of health-care professionals involved in the mammography process includes radiologists, radiographers, and medical physicists. Also needed are equipment specifications, monitoring and maintenance schedules, standards for image quality, standardized image evaluation procedures, meticulous record-keeping, and periodic review of data for outcomes of mammography services. All of these requirements are of vital importance in ensuring the quality of the screening programme.

An opportunity provided by the introduction of digital mammography is the potential to perform automated quality control (Brooks et al., 1993; Karssemeijer et al., 1995; Jacobs et al., 2006). When specially designed phantoms and test objects are imaged, relevant information about the imaging system can be discerned, and quantitative, objective measurements can be produced either by manual measurement or by automated algorithms. This makes it possible to detect (and correct) problems before they become clinically significant. Several manufacturers provide test tools and algorithms that can be used to verify

Table 2.2 Radiographer's quality control tests for screen-film mammography

Test	Priority[a]	Suggested frequency	Tolerances
Visual inspection			
Visual inspection and evaluation of the mammography unit	E	Monthly	
Film storage			
Temperature Humidity	E	Monthly	15–21 °C 40–60%
Position of film boxes and cassettes	E	Monthly	
Film inventory	D	Monthly	Time period for inventory updating < 3 months
Darkroom and film processing			
Darkroom cleanliness	E	Daily	—
Temperature Humidity Ventilation conditions	E E D	Monthly Monthly Monthly	15–21 °C 30–70%
White light leakage	E	Annually	
Safe lights	E	Annually	Rating ≥ 15 W FSL < 0.05 OD in 2 minutes
Developer temperature	E	Daily	Achievable: ± 0.5 °C Acceptable: ± 1.0 °C of the manufacturer-recommended value
Sensitometry	E	Daily	
Development time, specific gravity, pH, and replenishment rate		Only when problems are detected	
Artefact detection during processing	E	Weekly	Acceptable: no clinically significant artefacts
Imaging system			
Screen cleanliness	E	Weekly	
Screen-film contact	E	Semi-annually	Acceptable: spots ≤ 5 mm
Light-tightness of cassettes	E	Semi-annually	Acceptable: blackening ≤ 2 mm chest wall edge, ≤ 5 mm other edges
Matching of cassette sensitivity[b]	E	Semi-annually	Achievable: maximum deviation ≤ 0.20 OD Acceptable: maximum deviation ≤ 0.30 OD
Cassettes uniformity	D	Semi-annually	Acceptable: maximum deviation ≤ 5% mAs
Artefacts from each cassette	E	Semi-annually	Acceptable: no clinically significant artefacts
AEC			
Test of system constancy	E	Daily	Achievable: $OD = OD_{target} \pm 0.15$ Acceptable: $OD = OD_{target} \pm 0.20$ Acceptable: mAs within ± 10% of mAs that produces OD_{target} Acceptable: no clinically significant artefacts
Compensation of the AEC for different thickness	E	Monthly	Achievable: $OD = OD_{target} \pm 0.15$ Acceptable: $OD = OD_{target} \pm 0.20$ Acceptable: ± 10% of baseline mAs
Image quality			
ACR phantom score	D	Weekly	Acceptable: fibres: ≥ 4; microcalcifications: ≥ 3; masses: ≥ 3
OD difference between disc and background	D	Weekly	Achievable: ≥ 0.55 OD Acceptable: ≥ 0.40 OD

Table 2.2 (continued)

Test	Priority[a]	Suggested frequency	Tolerances
Reject analysis			
Reject films analysis	E	Quarterly	Achievable: ≤ 3% Acceptable: ≤ 8%

ACR, American College of Radiology; AEC, automatic exposure control; FSL, fog due to the safety light; OD, optical density.

[a] D, desirable, recommended; E, essential, basic requirement.

[b] This includes speed of screens and cassette attenuation.

From IAEA (2009). Table reproduced with permission from IAEA. IAEA Human Health Series No. 2: Quality assurance programme for screen film mammography. IAEA, Vienna (2009).

optimal performance. Some vendors provide automated quality control and tracking.

2.1.8 Mammography screening performance

(a) Interpreter training, skills, and experience

The setting for screening mammography is different from that of diagnostic mammography, where the woman generally presents with symptoms and the probability of cancer may be 10% or higher. In screening, women are asymptomatic and the cancer detection rates are typically in the range of 2–8 per 1000 examinations (Breast Cancer Surveillance Consortium, 2009; CPAC, 2013). Detecting these cancers against a background that is overwhelmingly non-cancer, while avoiding an unacceptably high abnormal recall rate, is a challenging task for the radiologist and requires training and maintenance of skills in identifying subtle signs of small lesions with a reasonable likelihood of being cancer. This may present a challenge in screening facilities where examination volumes per interpreter are low, because a given individual may see only one or two screening cancers per year in their screening workload.

This challenge can be approached in several ways; which, if any, are practical will depend on the individual screening environment (availability of interpreters, population density, etc.). One study found that the annual volume of examinations interpreted did not predict accuracy but that recent training and working in a facility where diagnostic mammograms and breast intervention procedures were performed were predictive of accuracy (Beam et al., 2003). Another factor associated with high performance in that study was working in a comprehensive breast centre or specialized mammography facility. These may point to the value of being able to gain feedback from the downstream outcome of screening through assessment, follow-up results, and radiological–pathological correlation, and being able to share knowledge gained with colleagues. Other studies observed a correlation between examination volume and screening accuracy (Esserman et al., 2002, Moss et al., 2005; Smith-Bindman et al., 2005). In addition, Smith-Bindman et al. found that radiologists with more years of screening experience tended to have higher specificity compared with more junior radiologists.

Other measures that have been implemented in large organized screening programmes to support the quality of image interpretation are outcome audits (cancer detection rates, percentage of small invasive cancers, specificity or PPV for screening) and review of programme interval cancers. Feedback on performance is essential for radiologists to improve their skills. A well-annotated set of cases, including screen-detected cancers, benign findings, and normal breasts, that could be made available for self-education and testing, such as the one developed by the University of Washington, USA (Dee, 2002; UW Medicine, 2015), may also be valuable.

Table 2.3 Medical physicist's quality control tests for screen-film mammography

Test	Priority[a]	Suggested frequency	Tolerances
Unit assembly evaluation			
Unit assembly evaluation	E	Annually	
Sensitometry and darkroom			
Sensitometry and darkroom	E	At commissioning and annually	
Darkroom radiation level	D	As required	Acceptable: < 20 μGy/week
Radiological equipment			
Radiation leakage	D	At acceptance and after changes	Acceptable: ≤ 1 mGy/h at 1 m
Accuracy and repeatability of the tube kVp	E	Annually	Acceptable: accuracy: ± 5%; repeatability: COV ≤ 2%
Half-value layer	E	Annually	
Output: repeatability and linearity	E	Annually	Acceptable: repeatability: COV ≤ 5%; linearity: ± 10%
Normalized output value	D	Annually	Acceptable: > 30 μGy/mAs at 1 m, 28 kV, Mo/Mo
Compression			
Compression force and thickness	E	Annually	
AEC			
Repeatability of the AEC	E	Annually	Acceptable: COV in mAs: ≤ 5%
Constancy of OD with baseline value	E	Annually	Acceptable: $OD = OD_{target} \pm 0.20$
Exposure time for 45 mm slab	E	Annually	Contact mammography: Achievable: $t \leq 1.5$ s Acceptable: $t \leq 2$ s Magnification mammography: Achievable: $t \leq 2$ s Acceptable: $t \leq 3$ s
Compensation of the AEC for different thickness and beam quality	E	Annually	Achievable: $OD = OD_{target} \pm 0.15$ Acceptable: $OD = OD_{target} \pm 0.20$
Increase of OD for each step of the density control	E	Annually	Acceptable: ΔOD = 0.1–0.2
Collimation system			
Light field/radiation field coincidence	D	Annually	Achievable: ≤ 1% of FFD for all edges
Radiation field/image receptor coincidence	E	Annually	Achievable: completely irradiate the image receptor, but does not extend beyond the shielded breast support except at the chest wall, where it may extend by ≤ 5 mm Acceptable: as above for the chest wall and within the breast support by ≤ 2% of FFD for the other edges
Compression paddle/breast support alignment	E	Annually	Acceptable: paddle not visible in image and edge of paddle ≤ 1% of FFD beyond chest wall edge of image receptor
Image viewing conditions			
Luminance of the viewboxes	E	Annually	> 3000 cd/m^2 (nit)
Viewboxes homogeneity and colour	E	Annually	Acceptable: < 30% for each viewbox and < 15% between panels in a viewbox
Ambient interpretation room illumination	E	Annually	Achievable: ≤ 10 lux Acceptable: ≤ 50 lux

Table 2.3 (continued)

Test	Priority[a]	Suggested frequency	Tolerances
Image quality[b]			
Target background density	E	Annually	Acceptable: OD = OD_{target} ± 0.20
OD difference between disc and background	E	Annually	Achievable: ≥ 0.55 OD Acceptable: ≥ 0.40 OD
Phantom image quality evaluation (ACR)	E	Annually	Acceptable: fibre score: ≥ 4 ; speck score: ≥ 3; mass score: ≥ 3
System spatial resolution	E	Annually	Achievable: ≥ 15 lp/mm Acceptable: ≥ 11 lp/mm
Dosimetry[c]			
Mean glandular dose (D_G)	E	Annually	Achievable: $D_G \leq 2$ mGy Acceptable: $D_G \leq 2.5$ mGy

ACR, American College of Radiology; AEC, automatic exposure control; COV, coefficient of variation; Δ, change in parameter; FFD, focus film distance; Mo, molybdenum; OD, optical density.

[a] D, desirable, recommended; E, essential, basic requirement.

[b] The ACR phantom has been taken as an example because it is probably the one most commonly used.

[c] Values obtained with grid for a compressed breast of thickness 53 mm and composition of 71% fat and 29% fibroglandular tissue.

From IAEA (2009). Table reproduced with permission from IAEA. IAEA Human Health Series No. 2: Quality assurance programme for screen film mammography. IAEA, Vienna (2009).

(b) One versus two views

In mammography it is customary to acquire two views of each breast, typically the mediolateral oblique projection and the craniocaudal projection. This results in more complete imaging coverage of tissue than can usually be obtained from a single view, due to the curved shape of the chest (which makes it impossible to include all breast tissue on a single rectangular view) and varying individual anatomy. It also allows correlation between the views to estimate the 3D location of structures of interest and to rule out anomalous findings created by superposition of tissue shadows from different planes in the breast in the projection images. Some screening programmes used single-view mammography to reduce screening costs and the radiation dose received by the breast. However, in a study conducted in the United Kingdom, it was found that two-view mammography resulted in 24% higher breast cancer detection rate while simultaneously reducing the screening recall rate by 15%; i.e. increasing both sensitivity and specificity (Wald et al., 1995; Patnick, 2004).

Another study in the United Kingdom found that the rate of detection of invasive cancers less than 15 mm in diameter was 45% higher when two-view mammography was used (Blanks et al., 1997). A further study suggested that many of the cancers often missed on a single oblique view of the breast can be seen in retrospect when guided by information seen on the craniocaudal view (Hackshaw et al., 2000). These cancers tend to be smaller by about 4 mm and lack some of the more pathognomonic features of malignancies, suggesting that the availability of the second view provides supporting information and raises the confidence in the radiologist to assess the lesion as positive.

(c) Double reading

Human observers attain performance in mammography screening with sensitivities typically above 80% and specificities between 88% and 96% (Stout et al., 2014). As mentioned previously, both sensitivity and specificity tend to be reduced for the dense breast. The relationship between sensitivity and specificity is described

Table 2.4 Radiographer's quality control tests for digital mammography

Test	Priority[a]	Comments
Daily tests		
Monitor inspection, cleaning, and viewing conditions	D	Daily (D); weekly (E)
Digital mammography equipment daily checklist	E	
Daily flat-field phantom image	D	
Visual inspection for artefacts (CR systems only)	E	
Laser printer sensitometry	E	Wet processor: daily (D); on day of use (E) Dry processor: monthly
Image plate erasure (CR systems only)	E	Secondary erasure: daily Primary erasure: weekly or as per manufacturer's instructions
Weekly tests		
Monitor QC	E	
Viewbox cleanliness	E	
Weekly QC test object and full field artefacts	E	
Image quality with breast-mimicking phantom	D	
Monthly tests		
Safety and function checks of examination room and equipment	E	
Full field artefacts	E	
Laser printer artefacts	E	
Quarterly tests		
Printed image quality	E	
Repeat image analysis	E	
Spatial resolution test (CR and scanning systems only)	E	
Semi-annual tests		
CR plate sensitivity matching	E	
CR plate artefacts	E	

CR, computed radiography; QC, quality control.

[a] D, desirable; E, essential, basic requirement.

From IAEA (2011). Table reproduced with permission from IAEA. IAEA Human Health Series No. 17: Quality assurance programme for digital mammography. IAEA, Vienna (2011).

by the receiver operating characteristic curve (a graph that plots the sensitivity versus the false-positive fraction, which is also 1 – specificity), and unless the intrinsic performance of the observer or the imaging system is increased, any attempt to improve sensitivity in detecting cancer will be met by a corresponding decrease in specificity.

Double reading is practised in some screening programmes to increase screening performance. Double reading can be implemented in several possible ways: (i) two readers individually interpret the mammography examination, and the patient is referred for further assessment if either of them reports a suspicious finding; (ii) the readers interpret the examination independently and then create a consensus opinion, upon which assessment is based; or (iii) after independent interpretation, a third radiologist arbitrates only if the two findings are different.

In a population screening programme using screen-film mammography, Thurfjell et al. (1994) showed a 15% increase in cancer detection rate and Anderson et al. (1994) showed a 10% increase in cancer detection rate with double reading, but with a 1.8% decrease in specificity. In studying

Table 2.5 Medical physicist's quality control tests for digital mammography

Test	Priority[a]	Suggested frequency	Tolerances
Unit assembly			
Unit assembly evaluation	E	Annually (E) Semi-annually (D)	
Compression			
Compression force and thickness accuracy	E	Annually (E) Semi-annually (D)	Powered: 150 N to ≤ 200 N Manual: ≤ 300 N
AEC evaluation			
Technique chart and AEC evaluation	E	Annually or after changes to AEC software	
Site baseline settings for radiographer SDNR test	E	At commissioning and after changes to AEC software	Not applicable
Detector performance			
Baseline detector performance	E	At commissioning and after detector change	Not applicable
Detector response and noise	E	Annually and after detector service	
Spatial linearity and geometric distortion of detector	E	Annually and after detector change	
Detector ghosting	E	Annually and after detector change	Ghost image SDNR ≤ 2.0
Detector uniformity and artefact evaluation	E	Annually and after detector change	
Evaluation of system resolution			
Modulation transfer function	E	Annually and after detector change	
Limiting spatial resolution	E	Annually and after detector change	
X-ray equipment characteristics			
Half-value layer	E	Annually and after X-ray tube change	
Incident air kerma at the entrance surface of PMMA slabs	E	Annually and after X-ray tube change	Not applicable
Dosimetry			
Mean glandular dose (D_G)	E	Annually	
Collimation system			
Radiation field/image receptor coincidence	E	Annually and after X-ray tube service/replacement	
Compression paddle/breast support alignment	E	Annually and after X-ray tube service/replacement	Acceptable: paddle not visible in image and edge of paddle ≤ 5 mm beyond chest wall edge
Missing tissue at chest wall	E	Annually and after X-ray tube service/replacement	Achievable: ≤ 5 mm Acceptable: ≤ 7 mm
Image display quality			
Artefacts and uniformity (soft copy)	E D	Annually Semi-annually	
Monitor luminance response and viewing conditions	E	Annually and after monitor service	
Viewbox luminance and viewing conditions	E	Annually	
Laser printer (where applicable)			
Artefacts and uniformity	E D	Annually Semi-annually	

Table 2.5 (continued)

Test	Priority[a]	Suggested frequency	Tolerances
Film densities	E	Annually	
Image quality			
Phantom image quality	E	Annually	

AEC, automatic exposure control; PMMA, polymethylmethacrylate; SDNR, signal-difference-to-noise ratio.
[a] D, desirable; E, essential, basic requirement.
From IAEA (2011). Table reproduced with permission from IAEA. IAEA Human Health Series No. 17: Quality assurance programme for digital mammography. IAEA, Vienna (2011).

several different double reading programmes, Blanks et al. found that double reading, especially when practised with arbitration, was better than single reading for the detection of small (which they defined as < 15 mm) invasive cancers, and the increase in detection rate was 32% for prevalent screens (two-view mammograms) and 73% for incident screens (single-view mammograms) (Blanks et al., 1998). These improvements were not observed for larger cancers. Unfortunately, much of the work on double reading was confounded by factors such as the number of radiographic views used.

If performed by radiologists, double reading is labour-intensive and therefore expensive, and in some locations the availability of radiologists is limited. In the NHS Breast Screening Programme in England, highly trained radiographers are used as second readers (Bennett et al., 2012). In some cases, two radiographers may perform double reading together without a radiologist.

(d) Computer-aided detection

Another approach to improving the accuracy of interpretation is through computer-aided detection (Nishikawa, 2010). Computer-aided detection consists of a set of computer image analysis operations applied to a digital mammogram or to a digitized film mammogram. Typically, the algorithm uses a set of segmentation operations to identify the area of the breast on the mammogram and to select areas, generally corresponding to increased X-ray attenuation, as candidates for lesions. Further operations, which can include image texture analysis and morphological analysis, can then be applied to assign "features" to the image. The features are used collectively, often with different weighting factors, to classify an area of the mammogram as normal or suspicious for cancer. Typically, computer-aided detection algorithms produce marks on an overlay image of the mammogram to indicate the possible presence of microcalcifications, potentially malignant masses, asymmetry, or architectural distortion, and the accuracy of computer-aided detection algorithms generally decreases in that order.

In any detection task there will be a trade-off between sensitivity and specificity; for example, if all mammograms were interpreted as positive, the sensitivity would be 1.0 but the specificity would be 0. The operating point of a computer-aided detection algorithm, i.e. its aggressiveness in discriminating between suspicious and normal areas, can be set by the manufacturer.

Computer-aided detection is most frequently used as a prompt to the radiologist, indicating by marks areas that should be given special consideration in interpreting the image. This has been demonstrated to contribute to improving sensitivity of mammography, although generally the number of false-positive marks on the image is considered to be excessively high. This is an annoyance to experienced radiologists, and it may lead to an excessively high recall rate for inexperienced interpreters who rely heavily on the computer-aided detection marks (Fenton et al., 2007; Philpotts, 2009).

Another application of computer-aided detection is as a surrogate for the second reader in double reading. In the NHS Breast Screening Programme in England, it was found that, with such practice, a single reader with computer-aided detection was able to detect cancers with similar pathological characteristics, achieving almost identical sensitivity (87.2% vs 87.7%), with slightly reduced specificity (96.9% vs 97.4%), compared with double reading (Taylor et al., 2004; Gilbert et al., 2008). Another study showed a 9% increase in sensitivity for a single reader plus computer-aided detection compared with single reading only, and a 2.4% non-significant increase compared with double reading, with a small increase in recall rate (Gromet, 2008).

2.1.9 Host factors that affect performance

(a) Breast density

To detect breast cancer mammographically, there must be adequate contrast for the lesion to be distinguished from surrounding tissue, and the contrast must exceed the random fluctuation (noise) in the image by a sufficient factor (contrast-to-noise ratio) to ensure that statistically reliable information is conveyed to the viewer. There must also be adequate spatial resolution to delineate the characteristic features of a lesion. Finally, masking effects due to overlapping tissues or image artefacts must not be excessive.

Tumours tend to be somewhat more attenuating of X-rays than adipose tissue and slightly more attenuating than surrounding fibroglandular tissue, although there the difference may be extremely small (Hammerstein et al., 1979; Johns & Yaffe, 1987). Therefore, the challenge of accurately detecting a tumour is greatest in the dense (highly fibroglandular) breast, where the contrast and contrast-to-noise ratio for lesions are likely to be diminished and the potential for masking is elevated (see Section 1.3.3d). Both sensitivity and specificity tend to be lower in the dense breast compared with the fatty breast (Table 2.6 and Table 2.7). Digital mammography tends to provide improved lesion conspicuity in the dense breast compared with film mammography. The accuracy of digital mammography relative to screen-film mammography was evaluated in a large trial (Pisano et al., 2005) in which more than 40 000 women received both film and digital examinations. Digital mammography was found to have a better diagnostic accuracy (superior area under the receiver operating characteristic curve and superior relative sensitivity, without loss of specificity) in women with dense breasts, those younger than 50 years, and those who were premenopausal or perimenopausal (groups overlap). Similar results were reported in observational data from the Breast Cancer Surveillance Consortium in the USA (Stout et al., 2014).

(b) Size of lesion

Sensitivity also depends on the size of the lesion (generally it is much easier to detect large cancers because they provide greater contrast) and on whether microcalcifications are present.

Radiologists frequently consider changes between the current mammogram and previous examinations, especially densities that increase in size over time, suggestive of a cancer. Therefore, the presence of previous images for comparison is of great value. Table 2.6 and Table 2.7 provide data on sensitivity and specificity of mammography by age range, breast density, and whether the examination is an initial one or one of a sequence (where there is the possibility for comparisons to be made). In screening, sensitivity typically increases with the time since the previous screen because the cancer has had more time to grow. Conversely, to obtain optimal lead time in mammography, the system (equipment, technique, and radiologist) must achieve high sensitivity for small lesions.

Table 2.6 Sensitivity of mammography by age group, breast density, and screening interval

Screening interval	Breast density	Age at examination (years)							
		40–49		50–59		60–69		70–79	
		Film	Digital	Film	Digital	Film	Digital	Film	Digital
Initial screen	Extremely dense	0.75	0.81	0.79	0.89	0.82	0.91	0.86	0.92
	Heterogeneously dense	0.85	0.90	0.88	0.88	0.91	0.91	0.93	0.93
	Scattered density	0.89	0.92	0.91	0.93	0.93	0.95	0.94	0.96
	Mainly fatty	0.90	0.94	0.92	0.86	0.94	0.89	0.95	0.91
Recurring annual screen	Extremely dense	0.57	0.65	0.62	0.78	0.66	0.81	0.71	0.85
	Heterogeneously dense	0.73	0.79	0.77	0.78	0.80	0.81	0.84	0.85
	Scattered density	0.78	0.85	0.82	0.85	0.85	0.88	0.89	0.91
	Mainly fatty	0.80	0.85	0.83	0.73	0.86	0.77	0.89	0.81
Recurring biennial screen	Extremely dense	0.68	0.73	0.70	0.83	0.74	0.86	0.79	0.89
	Heterogeneously dense	0.79	0.84	0.82	0.83	0.85	0.86	0.88	0.89
	Scattered density	0.84	0.88	0.86	0.89	0.89	0.91	0.91	0.92
	Mainly fatty	0.85	0.89	0.87	0.80	0.90	0.83	0.92	0.87
Recurring triennial screen	Extremely dense	0.68	0.82	0.72	0.85	0.76	0.88	0.80	0.91
	Heterogeneously dense	0.81	0.81	0.84	0.84	0.87	0.87	0.90	0.90
	Scattered density	0.85	0.88	0.87	0.90	0.90	0.92	0.92	0.93
	Mainly fatty	0.86	0.78	0.88	0.81	0.91	0.84	0.93	0.87

Values interpolated by the Working Group using data from Stout et al. (2014) and British Columbia Cancer Agency (2011).

Table 2.7 Specificity of mammography by age group, breast density, and screening interval

Screening interval	Breast density	Age at examination (years)							
		40–49		50–59		60–69		70–79	
		Film	Digital	Film	Digital	Film	Digital	Film	Digital
Initial screen	Extremely dense	0.84	0.82	0.86	0.84	0.87	0.85	0.88	0.87
	Heterogeneously dense	0.82	0.78	0.84	0.80	0.85	0.82	0.87	0.83
	Scattered density	0.86	0.83	0.87	0.84	0.88	0.86	0.90	0.87
	Mainly fatty	0.92	0.90	0.93	0.91	0.94	0.92	0.94	0.93
Recurring annual screen	Extremely dense	0.91	0.90	0.92	0.91	0.93	0.92	0.94	0.93
	Heterogeneously dense	0.90	0.87	0.91	0.88	0.92	0.89	0.93	0.91
	Scattered density	0.92	0.90	0.93	0.91	0.94	0.92	0.94	0.93
	Mainly fatty	0.96	0.95	0.96	0.95	0.97	0.96	0.97	0.96
Recurring biennial screen	Extremely dense	0.90	0.88	0.91	0.90	0.92	0.91	0.93	0.92
	Heterogeneously dense	0.88	0.85	0.89	0.87	0.90	0.88	0.91	0.89
	Scattered density	0.91	0.89	0.92	0.90	0.93	0.91	0.93	0.92
	Mainly fatty	0.95	0.94	0.96	0.94	0.96	0.95	0.97	0.95
Recurring triennial screen	Extremely dense	0.89	0.88	0.90	0.89	0.91	0.90	0.92	0.91
	Heterogeneously dense	0.87	0.84	0.89	0.86	0.90	0.87	0.91	0.88
	Scattered density	0.90	0.88	0.91	0.89	0.92	0.90	0.93	0.91
	Mainly fatty	0.95	0.93	0.95	0.94	0.96	0.95	0.96	0.95

Values interpolated by the Working Group using data from Stout et al. (2014) and British Columbia Cancer Agency (2011).

2.2 Non-mammographic imaging techniques

Non-mammographic imaging methods might be considered as the only screening method or as adjunct (supplementary) to mammography. The evidence reviewed here, as far as available, includes (i) sensitivity and specificity in a defined consecutively examined screening population (at average, intermediate, or increased risk) and/or incremental detection rates when the technique is used as an adjunct, where specified; (ii) potential side-effects of the screening application that can be assessed immediately (e.g. false-positive recommendations of biopsy or of 6-month follow-up); (iii) potential side-effects inherent to the method (such as risks associated with radiation or the contrast agent); and (iv) any other data on test accuracy or biological background of the test. An overview of the results is presented in Table 2.8.

Proof of efficacy and effectiveness (reduction in mortality or more-aggressive treatment of late changes among screened vs non-screened women) and other outcomes (stage shifting, interval cancer rate) are discussed in Section 5.5 and Section 5.6. Information on potential overdiagnosis can only be expected after long-term follow-up and is not available for any of the non-mammographic imaging modalities.

2.2.1 Ultrasonography

(a) Equipment

Currently, breast ultrasonography can be performed using equipment for handheld ultrasonography (HHUS) or equipment for automated breast ultrasonography (ABUS), which has also been named 3D ultrasonography.

HHUS is performed manually, like ultrasonography of other organs. Adequately high resolution is needed. HHUS can also be used to screen the whole breast, but screening with HHUS is time-consuming and is known to be operator-dependent. So far, documentation has relied on imaging of representative slices, and the representative slices need to be selected by the operator.

Earlier ABUS systems, developed about 30 years ago, had low image quality and different types of artefacts. A new generation of ABUS equipment has now become commercially available, which allows all the breast tissue to be covered in a reproducible manner. Image acquisition is performed by trained health professionals and takes up to 10 minutes per breast. During ABUS, the transducer moves automatically over the breast; all images and their corresponding location in the breast are automatically recorded. Artefacts are significantly reduced compared with former systems. Reading requires adequate software and storage space (approximately 1 gigabyte per breast) and takes about 5–10 minutes per patient.

The anticipated advantage of ABUS systems is the decoupling of image acquisition and reading, which improves the possibilities for implementing breast ultrasonography in a screening setting and reduces the required time of an expert.

Sonoelastography is a new feature that is now offered by many manufacturers. Elastography calculates elasticity values based on the small shift of echoes, which occurs due to respiratory or cardiac motion, as a result of manual pressure or application of a shear wave. The type of elastography depends on the equipment and yields semiquantitative or quantitative measurements. The information from elastography is then provided by colour-coding of the B-mode image. Elastography provides additional diagnostic information to breast ultrasonography. It cannot be used as a stand-alone method but requires combination with B-mode ultrasound. So far, it has been used only for targeted analysis of lesions, not for screening of the whole breast (Wojcinski et al., 2010; Berg et al., 2012c;

Table 2.8 Non-mammographic imaging techniques – comparison of technologies

Technology	Diagnostic advantages for screening	Diagnostic drawbacks for screening	Reproducibility	Advantages inherent to technology	Disadvantages inherent to technology	Time needed for acquisition	Time needed for reading	Costs for screening[a]	Costs for assessment	Relevance to screening
HHUS ("2D")	Incremental detection of cancers in dense tissue	Low specificity, high biopsy rates, high rates of short-term follow-up	Depends strongly on diagnostic skills of operating health professional (crucial for teaching and for QA) Inter-reader variability (important for teaching and QA)	No radiation Absence of discomfort	None	20 min	10–20 min[b]	Equipment costs + Non-physician time ++ Physician/expert +++	Many assessments, low costs	Limited data
ABUS ("3D")	Incremental detection of cancers in dense tissue (limited data available to date)	Low specificity, high biopsy rates, high rates of short-term follow-up (limited data available to date)	Usual QA for adequate image acquisition required	No radiation Absence of discomfort	None	10 min	5–10 min (independent of acquisition)	Equipment costs ++ Storage space ++ Non-physician time ++ Physician/expert +++	Many assessments, low costs	Limited data
Non-contrast-enhanced MRI (including DWI and spectroscopy)	No data	No data	NA	No radiation No contrast agent	Side-effects of magnetic field Claustrophobia	> 20 min	Not tested	Equipment costs +++ Otherwise not tested	Very high	No data

Table 2.8 (continued)

Technology	Diagnostic advantages for screening	Diagnostic drawbacks for screening	Reproducibility	Advantages inherent to technology	Disadvantages inherent to technology	Time needed for acquisition	Time needed for reading	Costs for screening[a]	Costs for assessment	Relevance to screening
Contrast-enhanced MRI	High sensitivity	Low specificity, high biopsy rates, high rates of short-term follow-up	QA for image acquisition; see guidelines for contrast-enhanced breast MRI Inter-reader-variability No QA programme for screening available	No radiation	Side-effects of magnetic field Side-effects of contrast agent Claustrophobia	15 min	5–10 min (independent of acquisition)	Equipment costs +++ Cost for contrast agent ++ Non-physician time ++ Physician/ expert ++	Very high	Limited data
PET	No data	Low sensitivity for small cancers	No data		Very high radiation dose	20–40 min	5–10 min (independent of acquisition)	Equipment costs +++ Cost for tracer ++ Non-physician time ++ Physician/ expert ++	Not tested	No data for screening
PEM	No data for screening (high sensitivity in diagnostic studies)	No data for screening (specificity for diagnosis equal to that of MRI)	Not tested		Very high radiation dose	20–40 min	5–10 min (independent of acquisition)	Equipment costs +++ Cost for tracer ++ Non-physician time ++ Physician/ expert ++	Not tested	No data for screening
BSGI	One study with questionable applicability to screening (high sensitivity)	One study with questionable applicability to screening. (specificity similar to that of MRI)	Not tested		Very high radiation dose	20–30 min	5–10 min (independent of acquisition)	Equipment costs +++ Cost for tracer ++ Non-physician time ++ Physician/ expert ++	Not tested	Very limited data with questionable applicability to screening

Table 2.8 (continued)

Technology	Diagnostic advantages for screening	Diagnostic drawbacks for screening	Reproducibility	Advantages inherent to technology	Disadvantages inherent to technology	Time needed for acquisition	Time needed for reading	Costs for screening[a]	Costs for assessment	Relevance to screening
Electrical impedance imaging	NA	One study on screening; very low sensitivity	Not tested; high variation of results with equipment	No radiation	None	NA	NA	NA	NA	No data for screening
Thermography	NA	Low sensitivity and low accuracy for screening	Not tested; high variation of results with equipment	No radiation	None	NA	NA	NA	NA	Low accuracy
Near-infrared spectroscopy	NA	No data for screening; existing other data: low accuracy	Not tested; high variation of results with equipment	No radiation	None	NA	NA	NA	NA	No data for screening
Molecular imaging (other than MRI or BSGI)	NA	Not clinically applied	NA	Depend on vector	Depend on vector	NA	NA	NA	NA	Fundamental research

2D, two-dimensional 3D, three-dimensional; ABUS, automated breast ultrasonography; BSGI, breast-specific gamma imaging; DWI, diffusion-weighted imaging; HHUS, handheld ultrasonography; min., minute or minutes; MRI, magnetic resonance imaging; NA, not available; PEM, positron emission mammography; PET, positron emission tomography; QA, quality assurance.

[a] +, low; ++, moderate; +++, high.

[b] Depending on the physician performing the examination.

Compiled by the Working Group.

Schäfer et al., 2013; Zhi et al., 2013; reviewed in Vreugdenburg et al., 2013).

(b) Technique

The technique of HHUS is described in national and international guidelines (Mainiero et al., 2013). Scanning, reading, and image documentation of HHUS are observer-dependent.

The technique of ABUS scanning depends on the equipment and is taught by the manufacturers. There still appears to be significant interobserver variability for the interpretation of ABUS as well; however, this might be improved by adequate training and by reading of ABUS together with mammography (Shin et al., 2011; Golatta et al., 2013; Kim et al., 2013; Skaane et al., 2014b; Wojcinski et al., 2013).

There exist few studies comparing the diagnostic accuracy of ABUS and HHUS. The latest studies have reported approximately comparable performance (Lin et al., 2012; Wang et al., 2012; Zhang et al., 2012; Chen et al., 2013). Whereas an experienced ultrasonographer might obtain more information from evaluating the elasticity and mobility of tissues when applying the ultrasound probe manually (Chang et al., 2011), automated ultrasonography avoids missing any areas of the breast tissue, a known problem of ultrasonography due to the mobility of breast tissue.

The technique of sonoelastography varies with the equipment and the manufacturer.

(c) Quality control

Some quality control for diagnostic HHUS of the breast is established in most national health systems. Currently, no recommendations or guidelines exist to assure high quality of ultrasonography screening examinations.

If HHUS screening is performed by health professionals, whereas reading is performed by a breast physician, then excellent training of the health professional is crucial since the operator has to select which images will be recorded and thus read by the physician. Any error of recording risks a miss. Thus, the health professional must have a high level of diagnostic skills and quality assurance.

To date, quality assurance of ABUS has been taught by the manufacturer. Overall quality assurance of ABUS image acquisition is far less demanding than for HHUS since the health professional only needs to warrant complete coverage of the breast tissue and adequate coupling. Thus, ABUS may aid in reducing the operator-dependence of the image acquisition.

Currently, no recommendations or guidelines exist to assure high quality of ultrasonography screening examinations.

(d) Screening performance

Based on existing data, ultrasonography is not envisaged as a stand-alone screening modality in most countries where it is in use (Albert et al., 2009). Instead, with rare exceptions with limited data (Hou et al., 2002; Honjo et al., 2007), it has been investigated almost exclusively as a supplementary test for screening women with dense breast tissue. This selective application is based on the suggested increased breast cancer risk with increased mammographic density (McCormack & dos Santos Silva, 2006; Price et al., 2013; see Section 1.3.3d) and the decreased sensitivity of mammography in dense breasts caused by the masking effect of dense tissue (Blanch et al., 2014; Boyd et al., 2014; see Section 2.1.9). Furthermore, use of ultrasonography in large and fatty breasts has limitations.

Recently, prospective studies from China have become available, where ultrasonography was used consecutively in women at average risk, alone or together with other modalities.

A recent study in China (Kang et al., 2014) reported the exclusive prospective use of ultrasonography in 2471 asymptomatic women at average risk, and achieved a sensitivity, specificity, and PPV in this population of 78.6%, 99.7%, and 11.4%, respectively.

Another study in China (Xu et al., 2010) reported the prospective use of ultrasonography, mammography, and clinical breast examination in 118 273 women. Cancer was detected in 0.66% of the population, and 34.8% at an early stage. In women younger than 44 years, the detection rate of early disease was better with ultrasonography, and in women older than 44 years, it was better with mammography.

A large study in China (Xu et al., 2014) reported on the use of ultrasonography, mammography, and clinical breast examination in 23 910 consecutive women at increased risk. The overall detection rate was 1.3 per 1000 women. With respect to sensitivity, specificity, and area under the receiver operating characteristic curve, the combination of all methods performed best (90.3%, 94.6%, and 0.95, respectively). Mammography alone (74.2%, 91.7%, and 0.85, respectively) and ultrasonography alone (71.0%, 90.3%, and 0.81, respectively) were comparable but inferior to the combination of all methods. CBE proved inferior to the other methods (41.9%, 82.7%, and 0.68, respectively).

Further studies (Huang et al., 2012; Wang et al., 2013) comparing the sensitivities of different screening modalities in a Chinese population, including very young women (< 25 years), confirm the increased screening performance of ultrasonography in dense breasts and in younger women (< 55 years). [The authors pointed out an earlier onset of breast cancer and the generally higher tissue density in the Chinese population.]

Incremental cancer detection rates by adjunct ultrasonography reported in several prospective and retrospective studies range from about 2 per 1000 to about 5 per 1000 (reviewed in Nothacker et al., 2009).

This incremental detection is achieved at the cost of high biopsy rates (1.8–5.3%) and mostly high rates of incremental short-term follow-up recommendations, ranging from 1.2% to 7.5%.

For further details and implications concerning prognostic impact, see Section 5.5 for the screening of women at average risk and Section 5.6 for the screening of women at an increased risk.

Recent studies comparing the use of ABUS and HHUS in asymptomatic women with dense tissue and normal mammograms reported comparable results (Kelly et al., 2010; Giuliano & Giuliano, 2013; Brem et al., 2014).

Currently, elastography is used for diagnosis only. The first multicentre studies and a meta-analysis indicate that sonoelastography promises improved diagnostic accuracy of imaging assessment (Wojcinski et al., 2010; Barr et al., 2012; Berg et al., 2012c; Schäfer et al., 2013; Vreugdenburg et al., 2013; Zhi et al., 2013). With further technical development, elastographic information might become applicable to ABUS as well. However, so far no data exist on the use and the diagnostic accuracy that could be achieved if sonoelastography were used for screening.

(e) Host factors that affect performance

Decreased accuracy may be expected for large breasts. The reasons include limited penetration and the risk of missing part of the breast tissue (with HHUS). Since most breast cancers are hypoechoic, sensitivity may decrease in breasts with hypoechoic breast tissue (largely fatty breast tissue) and in breasts with heterogeneous echogenicity (due to hypoechoic mastopathic regions or many interposed fat lobules).

2.2.2 Magnetic resonance imaging

(a) Equipment

Breast MRI is performed on state-of-the-art MRI scanners. National and international updated guidelines recommend scanners of 1.5 T or more, special breast coils, and imaging protocols that allow dynamic contrast studies at high spatial and temporal resolution. Pulse sequences and evaluation software are provided by manufacturers.

Since contrast-enhanced MRI can detect small lesions not detected at mammography, MRI-guided biopsy and/or marking may be performed simultaneously. For such interventions, dedicated software, an MRI-compatible biopsy vacuum pump, and appropriate one-way MRI-compatible biopsy needles are indispensable. Solutions are expensive.

Diffusion-weighted imaging (DWI) is a new option on state-of-the-art MRI scanners of 1.5 T or 3 T. It is performed without contrast agent and allows calculation of the apparent diffusion coefficients of the imaged tissues. Apparent diffusion coefficient values provide a measure of the motion of water molecules in tissue, which appears restricted in many malignancies.

MRI spectroscopy also yields information on molecular binding of the imaged protons. It thus allows the identification of certain groups of molecules contained in the imaged voxel. The most promising results concern imaging of phosphocholines, which are also increased in many malignancies. This method is technologically demanding, is less promising on scanners of less than 3 T, and is not widely available.

Thus, both above-mentioned methods promise additional potentially valuable pathophysiological information. Their imaging resolution is restricted, and their accuracy is predicted to decrease with small lesion size and in cancers with a diffuse growth pattern (dispersed malignant cells). Their value for diagnosis is currently being investigated.

(b) Technique

When MRI is used (for diagnostic applications or for screening of women at an increased risk), dynamic contrast-enhanced breast MRI (CE-MRI) is currently considered state-of-the-art for reliable detection or exclusion of malignancy. With CE-MRI, the complete breast is imaged before and several times after intravenous administration of the MRI contrast agent (a gadolinium chelate). Standard procedures have been published in national and international guidelines (Sardanelli et al., 2010; Mainiero et al., 2013; Breast Imaging Working Group of the German Radiological Society, 2014).

To improve performance and feasibility, modified pulse sequences have been suggested, which might enable the specificity to be improved further (Mann et al., 2014) and/or the imaging time to be shortened (Kuhl et al., 2014). So far very limited experience concerning their diagnostic performance and reproducibility is available.

Even though gadolinium chelates are generally well tolerated and risks are much lower than for X-ray contrast agents, patients must be informed about potential side-effects. These include allergic reactions and nephrogenic fibrosing dermopathy/nephrogenic systemic fibrosis. Slight allergic reactions occur in up to 2.4% of applications; however, severe allergic reactions are rare (1–10 per 100 000 applications) (ACR, 2013b). Nephrogenic systemic fibrosis has been described in up to 3 per 100 000 applications (ACR, 2010). Among other risk factors, end-stage chronic kidney disease is associated with the highest risk of nephrogenic systemic fibrosis (up to 7%). Therefore, blood tests are officially recommended in patients who are older than 60 years or have pre-existing renal problems (Widmark, 2007; ACR, 2013b; Matsumura et al., 2013). Finally, the absence of cardiac pacemakers, certain metallic implants, or pumps must be ensured before MRI can be performed, to avoid severe injury to the patient (Expert Panel on MRI Safety, 2013).

Methods for MRI-guided marking and percutaneous breast biopsy have been developed and tested and are widely available (Perlet et al., 2006; Siegmann-Luz et al., 2014).

(c) Quality control

National and international guidelines concerning quality assurance of breast MRI have been published (Sardanelli et al., 2010; Mainiero et al., 2013; Breast Imaging Working Group of the German Radiological Society, 2014). No dedicated protocol for quality assurance of MRI screening has so far been developed or tested. Consensus recommendations for the use of MRI-guided vacuum-assisted breast biopsy have been issued, to assure adequate assessment of MRI-detected lesions (Heywang-Köbrunner et al., 2009).

(d) Screening performance

To date, no RCTs or observational prospective studies exist in which MRI has been applied consecutively for screening of **asymptomatic women at average risk**. Considering the high costs of MRI, the costs for further assessment of MRI-detected benign changes, the very large number of women at average risk, and the potential side-effects of the contrast agent or the magnetic field, MRI screening does not appear to be a sensible option for women at average risk.

"**Intermediate risk**" defines a broad range between average risk (< 15% lifetime risk) and increased risk (> 30% lifetime risk according to the definition in Europe, or > 20% lifetime risk according to the definition in the USA). This group of women at intermediate risk is heterogeneous and consists of different subgroups, such as women with a personal history of breast cancer or DCIS, women with a moderate family risk of breast cancer, or women with histologically proven high-risk lesions, such as atypical ductal hyperplasia (ADH) or lobular carcinoma in situ (LCIS).

Data for the use of MRI for screening of women at intermediate risk are limited. The largest body of data probably exists for MRI screening of the contralateral breast to the tumoural breast. A large prospective multicentre study (Lehman et al., 2007) in 969 women showed a significant incremental detection rate (compared with mammography) of 3.1%. The corresponding sensitivity was 91% and the specificity 88%. A meta-analysis (Brennan et al., 2009) that included this prospective study and a further 21 small and heterogeneous prospective and retrospective studies yielded an incremental detection rate of 4.1%. A retrospective single-centre study (Gweon et al., 2014) reported an incremental detection rate of only 1.8% in 607 patients. These incremental detections were at the cost of an increased rate of indicated percutaneous biopsies of 13.9% (Lehman et al., 2007), 9.3% (Brennan et al., 2009), and 9.4% (Gweon et al., 2014). PPVs varied from 21% (Lehman et al., 2007) to 43.5% (Gweon et al., 2014).

One recent study (Kuhl et al., 2014) assessed the use of MRI for "screening" women at "mildly to moderately increased risk". However, it included a mixture of variable indications (diagnostic problems, personal history of breast cancer) and thus cannot contribute significant evidence to this question.

In women with increased risk due to a history of LCIS, retrospective studies of MRI examinations on limited numbers of patients showed low incremental detection rates (of DCIS or invasive carcinoma), high rates of biopsy recommendations, and high rates of short-term follow-up (Friedlander et al., 2011; Sung et al., 2011). Similar results were also reported from studies of women with mixed intermediate risks (Kuhl et al., 2010; Berg et al., 2011, 2012b).

For **women at an increased risk** (with or without *BRCA1* or *BRCA2* mutation), there is ample evidence of significant incremental detection by MRI. It is based on at least 16 single-armed large cohort studies and three systematic reviews (Lord et al., 2007; Warner et al., 2008; Phi et al., 2015).

A recent meta-analysis showed an average sensitivity and specificity both of 84% for the diagnostic use of DWI (Chen et al., 2010). A first attempt at an MRI protocol that included plain MRI and DWI achieved a sensitivity of 76–78% and a specificity of 90% (Trimboli et al., 2014). Thus, to date DWI does not appear to be applicable for screening. The same is true for MRI spectroscopy, for which sensitivities and specificities of about 80% have been reported (Baltzer & Dietzel, 2013).

For further details and implications concerning prognostic impact, see Section 5.5.

(e) Host factors that affect performance

Contrast-enhanced MRI may not be possible for claustrophobic patients. It is not indicated in women with a known allergy to the MRI contrast agent or with a severe other disease that increases the risk of the contrast agent. It is contraindicated in women with pacemakers or other metallic devices (Expert Panel on MRI Safety, 2013).

Accuracy may be heavily degraded by motion artefacts. This must be considered in particular for women who – due to neurological disorders, lack of compliance, or other reasons – cannot lie still during the procedure.

Finally, high levels of progesterone may cause strong background enhancement and may interfere with the diagnostic accuracy. Therefore, whenever possible, MRI should be scheduled with respect to the menstrual cycle and progesterone treatment should be stopped for about 4 weeks before the MRI is performed (Sardanelli et al., 2010).

2.2.3 Positron emission tomography/ mammography

Positron emission tomography (PET) monitors the uptake of a radiotracer, and thus measures the activity of a metabolic pathway without interfering with it. Most PET studies have been performed using [^{18}F]-fluorodeoxyglucose (FDG), which represents glucose metabolism. Glucose metabolism is assumed to be increased in tumours. Other agents, such as [^{18}F]-fluorothymidine as a proliferation marker or [^{18}F]-labelled annexin V as an apoptosis marker, are under investigation (Surti, 2013).

(a) Equipment

Whole-body PET scanners allow imaging not only of the primary cancer but also of the lymph nodes and of distant metastases. However, due to insufficient resolution and signal-to-noise ratio, whole-body PET has low sensitivity for small tumours, and it is thus considered inappropriate for imaging of early breast cancer (Avril et al., 2000). Therefore, dedicated breast PET scanners have been developed. These dedicated scanners are called positron emission mammography (PEM) scanners. Their resolution, which is about 2–3 mm, is much higher than that of PET scanners.

(b) Technique

Most PEM scanners resemble mammography units. Imaging with these scanners is performed on the moderately compressed breast. Compression is applied to improve signal-to-noise ratio. Other PEM systems under development examine the breast in the prone position or may function as an add-on to whole-body PET scanners (Surti, 2013). The radiotracer (usually 370 MBq or 10 mCi FDG) is injected intravenously, and imaging can be performed after about 60 minutes. The time reported for a complete scan of both breasts is about 20–40 minutes. Toxic or allergic side-effects of the tracer are extremely rare and are negligible. However, the radiation dose, which is applied to the whole body, is high (~7 mSv). Due to the intravenous administration and its clearance time from the body, the lifetime attributable risk of one PEM scan has been calculated to be about 23 times that of a digital mammogram (~0.4 mSv) for a woman aged 40 years and more than 75 times that of a digital mammogram for a woman aged 60 years (Hendrick, 2010).

(c) Quality control

Standard doses of the tracer have been established. No protocol has yet been developed for PEM or for screening by PEM. Studies assessing interobserver variability and reproducibility of PEM diagnoses showed different results (Narayanan et al., 2011; Berg et al., 2012a). Thus, special training and quality assurance of PEM remain issues to be solved.

(d) Screening performance

No studies on the use of PEM (or PET) for screening asymptomatic women have been published. Data on accuracy are available from the use of PEM for diagnosis in patients with suspicious lesions or for preoperative staging (Berg et al., 2011; Schilling et al., 2011; Kalles et al., 2013). These studies show sensitivities of 85–90%, which are comparable to that of MRI.

(e) Host factors that affect performance

Limited sensitivity of PEM is expected in patients with uncontrolled diabetes mellitus since high blood levels of glucose interfere with FDG uptake in tumour tissue. In fertile women, physiological breast uptake of FDG may interfere with interpretation since FDG uptake is increased during all phases of the menstrual cycle except the proliferative phase (Rabkin et al., 2010; Park et al., 2013). Individual anatomical problems that prevent proper positioning are as crucial for PEM as they are for mammography.

2.2.4 Scintimammography

Breast-specific gamma imaging (BSGI), or scintimammography, is considered another method of molecular imaging. ^{99}Tc-sestamibi or ^{99}Tc-tetrofosmin binds to mitochondria (Sun et al., 2013). The density of mitochondria is assumed to be increased within cancer cells.

(a) Equipment

Dedicated scintimammography systems (BSGI systems) have been developed and are commercially available. The dedicated systems allow imaging of small breast lesions with sufficient reliability. Based on positive results in diagnostic examinations, the method has already been tested as a complementary tool for early detection and imaging of the mammographically dense breast. The initial BSGI systems required intravenous administration of a dose of 750–1100 MBq or 20–30 mCi ^{99}Tc-sestamibi. The most recent systems have improved detector technology (cadmium zinc telluride detectors and dual detector heads), leading to improved sensitivity and/or a reduction of the required applied radiation dose.

(b) Technique

Imaging with BSGI scanners is performed on the moderately compressed breast to increase signal-to-noise ratio. Individual anatomical problems that prevent proper positioning are as crucial for BSGI as they are for mammography.

The radiotracer (usually 750–1100 MBq or 20–30 mCi ^{99}Tc-sestamibi) is injected, and imaging can be performed after about 10 minutes. The time reported for a complete scan of both breasts is about 20–30 minutes. The radiation dose, which is applied by intravenous injection to the whole body with single-head systems, is even higher than that for PEM. Compared with a mean calculated radiation dose of mammography of 0.44 mSv to the breast, the dose for ^{99}Tc-sestamibi has been calculated to be about 9 mSv. The associated lifetime attributable cancer risk of one ^{99}Tc-sestamibi scan has been calculated to be about 20–30 times that of a digital mammogram for a woman aged 40 years (Hendrick, 2010). New technologies are expected to reduce the radiation dose to about 4 mSv.

(c) Quality control

So far, no official guidelines beyond the usual quality assurance of nuclear medicine exist for scintimammography. However, correct positioning is a prerequisite to allow imaging and thus detection of at least part of the lesion. Dose optimization studies for this technology are in progress. No quality assurance protocol exists for BSGI screening.

(d) Screening performance

No data exist on screening performance in women at average risk.

In one study (Rhodes et al., 2011), BSGI and mammography were performed in 936 women with mammographically dense tissue (ACR categories 3 and 4) and with additional risk factors (including family history, *BRCA* mutation, personal history, and other risks). The authors reported a sensitivity of 82% and a specificity of 93% for BSGI, and an astonishingly low sensitivity of 27% and a specificity of 91% for mammography. [The low sensitivity of mammography is explained by the diversity of patients. The study included women at an increased risk, who may develop tumour types that are particularly difficult to diagnose mammographically, and women with a personal history of breast cancer, where scarring impairs mammographic evaluation. The correct comparison would have been with MRI. Overall selection bias is probable (see Section 5.5 and BlueCross BlueShield Association, 2013).]

For the diagnostic use of BSGI, a sensitivity of 95% and a specificity of 80% were reported (Sun et al., 2013), which approximate those of MRI. No publications were available on BSGI-guided biopsy.

(e) Host factors that affect performance

Individual anatomical problems that prevent proper positioning are as crucial for PEM as they are for mammography.

2.2.5 Electrical impedance imaging

(a) Equipment

Electrical impedance, which derives from electrical conductivity and permittivity, is measured at different frequencies. Conductivity and permittivity vary with frequency in the different breast tissues (Hope & Iles, 2004). Electrical impedance imaging relies on the assumption that cancer cells have increased conductivity and thus decreased impedance (Vreugdenburg et al., 2013).

Different types of equipment have been developed for non-invasive measurement of the electrical properties of breast tissue (Ng et al., 2008). Electrical impedance tomography yields 2D and 3D tomographic images of the impedance (conductivity and permittivity). Electrical impedance mapping yields surface images of the distribution of conductivity and permittivity. One system did not yield images but solely allowed a classification as probably benign or malignant based on measurements from one selected location. (That system can, of course, not be used for screening.) The systems allow either areas of low impedance ("white spot") to be detected or a grading of suspicion or a classification as benign or malignant to be assigned based on selected algorithms (Zou & Guo, 2003; Ng et al., 2008).

The most commonly described devices in clinical studies were the electrical impedance scanner TransScan TS2000 system and the multiprobe resonance-frequency-based electrical impedance spectroscopy system (Malich et al., 2001; Martín et al., 2002; Wersebe et al., 2002; Diebold et al., 2005; Fuchsjaeger et al., 2005; Zheng et al., 2008, 2011; Wang et al., 2010; Lederman et al., 2011). Some of the electrical impedance technologies only detect asymmetry between breasts but do not localize the abnormality, and therefore may require another imaging technique, such as ultrasonography, to localize the abnormality (Zheng et al., 2008, 2011; Wang et al., 2010; Lederman et al., 2011).

(b) Technique

The technique varies with the equipment and is taught by the manufacturer (Ng et al., 2008).

(c) Quality control

Given the different types of equipment and techniques, no standard procedures exist that would be valid for all equipment types.

(d) Screening performance

Only one study applied electrical impedance scanning in asymptomatic women (Stojadinovic et al., 2008). It yielded a sensitivity of 26.4%.

A recent systematic review identified 10 studies that reported results concerning the diagnostic use of electrical impedance scanning. Most of these assessed initial testing with or without blinding to the standard. Due to significant heterogeneity between the studies, pooled estimates of the diagnostic accuracy could not be calculated. Most studies reported sensitivities that ranged from 62.0% to 97.5% (median, 83%) and specificities that ranged from 42.0% to 80.9% (median, 68%). The large range of sensitivities and specificities and their median values do not support the diagnostic use of this method (Vreugdenburg et al., 2013).

This technology has not been validated for screening women.

(e) Host factors that affect performance

Lesions close to the chest wall or close to the nipple may not show adequately (Ng et al., 2008). Also, the results appear to vary with hormone levels (Sardanelli et al., 2010).

2.2.6 Other techniques

Thermography measures temperature distribution on the breast surface, assuming a higher temperature in malignant tumours. The method has been tested in several studies. In two systematic reviews of diagnostic studies, sensitivities ranged from 25% to 97% and specificities from 12% to 85% (Gohagan et al., 1980; Fitzgerald & Berentson-Shaw, 2012; Vreugdenburg et al., 2013). Given these limitations, the available data cannot justify the application of thermography for screening.

Near-infrared spectroscopy evaluates spectral differences of the examined tissue. Without the use of contrast agent, mainly tissue concentrations of haemoglobin and deoxyhaemoglobin can be measured. Higher proportions of deoxyhaemoglobin than haemoglobin are assumed to be present in malignant tumours. Initial results have not been encouraging. However, such a technology might become useful in the future if fluorescent probes can be developed for molecular imaging that can be administered intravenously and that attach to malignant cells and thus allow the identification of malignant tumours by this fluorescent marking.

2.3 Clinical breast examination

Clinical breast examination (CBE), also called physical breast examination, is part of the clinical examination for early detection of breast cancer and is practised routinely by health-care providers, i.e. nurses, physicians, and surgeons, in high-income countries. CBE for primary breast screening takes on importance in low- and middle-income countries (LMICs) where mammography screening is not feasible and/or affordable.

2.3.1 Technique

Fig. 2.6 gives a description and illustrations of CBE.

The CBE screening technique involves visual inspection and palpation of both breasts by a health-care provider. During visual inspection, the provider looks for subtle changes in breast

Fig. 2.6 Clinical breast examination

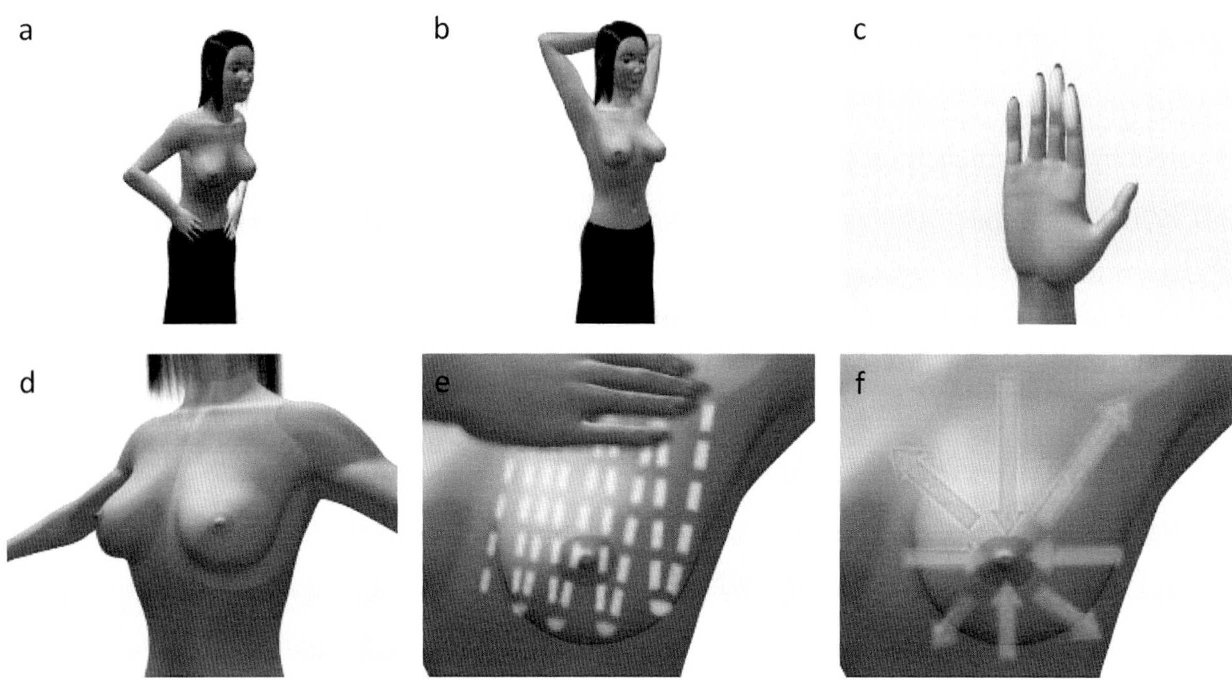

A visual examination should be performed with the woman in three different standing positions: with her arms relaxed at her sides, with her hands pressed firmly on her waist and leaning forward (a), and with her arms above her head (b). The examiner should seek subtle asymmetries in the appearance of the breasts. Three levels of pressure – superficial, medium, and deep – should be applied at each palpation site. Palpation is done with the finger pads of the middle three fingers (c), and pressure is applied with circular motions at each site. Palpation of the supraclavicular and axillary nodes is done with the woman seated, and re-palpation of the axillary nodes is done with the woman supine. Palpation of the breasts is performed over an area extending from the mid-axillary line to the mid-sternum and from above the subcostal margin (fifth rib) to the clavicle (d), including palpation of the nipple and areola. Palpation should be done systematically, either in vertical strips (e) or in circular motions from the centre to the periphery or vice versa (f). For the lateral half of the breast, the woman should be asked to rotate her body slightly in the opposite direction (right side for left breast, and left side for right breast); for the medial half of the breast, the body should be rotated laterally in order to spread out the breast tissue. When an abnormality in shape or contour is detected, the corresponding area of the other breast should be examined. If the finding is not bilateral, further investigation is required.

contour and skin and nipple changes that appear asymmetrically (i.e. not seen in both breasts), while the woman stands and clasps her waist tightly with both hands (Coleman & Heard, 2001). During palpation, the provider uses the soft pads of the middle three fingers to examine all areas of both breasts and axillae for the presence of lumps and thickening of breast tissue and lymph nodes. Palpation is performed with the woman in sitting and supine positions (Coleman & Heard, 2001). Several techniques for CBE have been described by researchers. Bassett (1985) described a "spoke and wheel" technique (f) for CBE as part of the Canadian National Breast Screening Study (CNBSS), whereas Saunders et al. (1986) described a vertical strip pattern (e). The most widely disseminated technique is probably that described by Pennypacker & Pilgrim (1993). Pennypacker et al. (1999) also suggested a minimum of 5 minutes of examination per breast. Fletcher et al. (1989) found that variations in CBE technique were responsible for 27–29% of variance in sensitivity and 14–33% of variance in specificity of lump detection. They also observed that increased duration of search time of the examination was correlated with higher sensitivity and lower specificity. However, there are no studies that have conclusively proven the superiority of any one technique over the others.

2.3.2 Training

Most training programmes use silicone models that simulate normal and abnormal human breast tissue (McDermott et al., 1996; Pennypacker et al., 1999). The effect of training on the improvement of providers' skills has been assessed (Costanza et al., 1995, 1999). Studies of medical students have shown low performance scores in many CBE components and also low sensitivity and specificity using silicone models (Sloan et al., 1994; Chalabian et al., 1996), whereas other studies have shown that CBE training on silicone breast models enhances the performance of examiners (Hall et al., 1980; Pilgrim et al., 1993).

Saslow et al. (2004) suggested that CBE training should be flexible and accommodate diverse settings and trainee needs. Miller et al. (1991) used the services of nurses who were trained by surgeons to provide CBE in the CNBSS. Pisani et al. (2006) trained nurses and midwives to perform CBE in an RCT in Manila, Philippines. Women in Mumbai, India, with a 10th grade education and good communication skills who were trained for 4 weeks to perform CBE per a modified version of the CNBSS protocol were able to perform CBE as well as trained surgeons ($\kappa = 0.849$) (Mittra et al., 2010). Sankaranarayanan et al. (2011) trained graduate female health workers for 3 weeks using silicone breast models to perform CBE in an RCT in Trivandrum, India (see Section 4.3).

2.3.3 Quality control

A general lack of quality control and standardization of technique is seen across CBE screening studies and programmes. Studies had reported that graduating primary care physicians were lacking adequate CBE skills and that healthcare providers expressed a need for CBE training (Chalabian & Dunnington, 1998; Pennypacker et al., 1999). In the CNBSS, the providers were trained per a designed CBE protocol, and the CBE skills of the providers were monitored (Baines et al., 1989; Baines, 1992a). The RCT in Mumbai, India, used a modified version of the CNBSS protocol and maintained quality control by comparing a 5% sample of the results of CBE examinations by the study providers with those of surgeons (Mittra et al., 2010). The RCTs in the Philippines and in Trivandrum, India, described structured CBE training of the providers, but there was no mention of quality monitoring of the process during the intervention (Pisani et al., 2006; Sankaranarayanan et al., 2011).

2.3.4 Screening performance

Morimoto et al. (1993) reported a sensitivity of 61% and a specificity of 94.5% for CBE in Zentsūji, Kagawa Prefecture, Japan. Ohuchi et al. (1995) reported a sensitivity of 85% and a specificity of 96% for CBE in Miyagi Prefecture, Japan. In these studies, sensitivity and specificity were calculated by observing all screening participants for a period of 2 years after screening. Barton et al. (1999) analysed the screening performance of CBE by pooling data from six studies: the Health Insurance Plan of Greater New York study, the United Kingdom Trial, the Breast Cancer Detection Demonstration Project of the United States National Cancer Institute, the West London Study, the CNBSS 1, and the CNBSS 2 (see Section 4.3 for descriptions of the studies). For the purpose of analysis, sensitivity was defined as the proportion of cancers detected by CBE, among all breast cancers detected/diagnosed within 12 months of screening; specificity was defined as the proportion of CBE-negative women who did not develop breast cancer within 12 months after screening, among all women who did not develop breast cancer within 12 months after screening. The authors reported a pooled sensitivity of 54.1% and a pooled specificity of 94.0%. Bobo et al. (2000) reported CBE sensitivity, specificity, and PPV of 58.8%, 93.4%, and

4%, respectively, from the United States Centers for Disease Control and Prevention's National Breast and Cervical Cancer Early Detection Program. Pisani et al. (2006) reported a sensitivity of 53.2% and a PPV of recall of 1.2%. Sankaranarayanan et al. (2011) reported CBE sensitivity, specificity, false-positive rate, and PPV of 51.7%, 94.3%, 5.7%, and 1.0%, respectively. Variances in screening performance by technique and duration of screening are discussed in Section 2.3.1.

2.3.5 Host factors that affect performance

Age, menopausal status, body weight, breast density, nodularity (lumpiness), ethnicity, and use of hormone replacement therapy are known to affect the performance of CBE. With respect to age and menopausal status, van Dam et al. (1988) observed that CBE sensitivity was significantly lower in premenopausal and perimenopausal women compared with postmenopausal women. Oestreicher et al. (2002) observed a bell-shaped pattern, with CBE sensitivity low in women aged 40–49 years, higher in women aged 50–59 years, and decreasing gradually in women aged 60 years and older. In contrast, Bobo & Lee (2000) found that CBE sensitivity was higher among women younger than 50 years than among those aged 50 years and older. Also, CBE sensitivity was reported to decrease with increasing body weight (Oestreicher et al., 2002). van Dam et al. (1988) observed that higher nodularity of breasts resulted in lower CBE specificity. The test characteristics of CBE reported from regions that are geographically separated and ethnically and demographically diverse are almost the same, although higher sensitivity values have been reported from one study in Japan (Ohuchi et al., 1995) and among Asian women in a study in the USA (Oestreicher et al., 2002).

2.4 Breast self-examination

Breast self-examination (BSE) is an examination of a woman's breasts by the woman herself, purportedly for early detection of breast cancer.

2.4.1 Technique

The essential components of BSE are visual inspection in front of a mirror and palpation of the breasts and nipples with the soft pads of the middle three fingers. Many techniques have been described for practising BSE (Mamon & Zapka, 1983; Carter et al., 1985; Baines, 1992b). Mamon & Zapka described a BSE technique with 34 systematic steps: 4 steps for visual inspection of both breasts in front of a mirror, 7 steps for each breast in an upright position, and 8 steps for each breast in a supine position. Carter et al. suggested a 21-step procedure, omitting the examinations in the supine position. It is unlikely that women would go through the rigours of such elaborate procedures. Therefore, Baines proposed a simpler technique. It is important to understand that a large proportion of women in LMICs cannot afford the privacy needed to perform BSE with such time-consuming procedures. Therefore, BSE has to be very simple for it to become a popular practice in LMICs.

2.4.2 Training

Clarke & Savage (1999) conducted a literature review of BSE training studies and found that BSE training improves compliance, confidence, and proficiency. Structured individual training in BSE improved the thoroughness of examination in terms of the depth of palpation and the duration of search time (Bragg Leight et al., 2000). Also, periodic reassessment and retraining are required to prevent deterioration of BSE skills (Pinto & Fuqua, 1991). In a study in Denmark, women showed a preference for individual instruction versus group instruction in BSE (Bech et al., 2005). Also, it has been reported

Fig. 2.7 Indicators appropriate for an evaluation of breast self-examination

- Is any visual examination done?
- Is most of the breast examined?
- Are the armpits examined?
- Is there a systematic search pattern?
- Are three fingers used?
- Are finger pads used?
- Is a rotary palpation applied?
- Is breast self-examination performed 12 times a year?

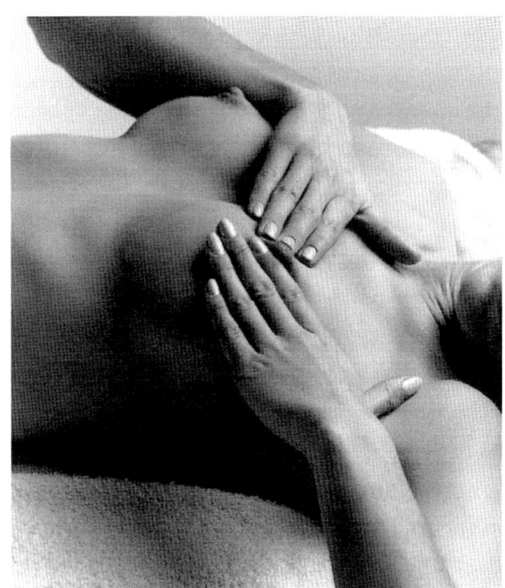

Photo from the United States National Cancer Institute Visuals Online, available from visualsonline.cancer.gov.

that individual instruction improved the proficiency and frequency of BSE performance compared with group instruction (Dorsay et al., 1988; Coleman & Pennypacker, 1991). Systematic training of women to perform BSE has been found to significantly increase the practice of BSE in several studies in Turkey (Hacihasanoğlu & Gözüm, 2008; Oezaras et al., 2010; Donmez et al., 2012).

2.4.3 Quality control

Very few studies have assessed quality control in BSE performance. Mamon & Zapka (1983) described a set of indicators for BSE quality (Fig. 2.7). The weakness is that they are equally weighted. Coleman & Pennypacker developed a weighted scoring system comprising: percentage of total breast area actually palpated, duration of examination, type of pressure, pattern and number of motions, and number and part of fingers used (Coleman & Pennypacker, 1991).

2.4.4 Screening performance

The sensitivity, specificity, and PPV of BSE to detect breast cancer have been reported as 58.3%, 87.4%, and 29.2%, respectively (Wilke et al., 2009). [The study was conducted in a single institution and among women at an increased risk.] In Shanghai, China, an RCT found that women in the BSE instruction group had greater specificity in lump finding in the silicone models compared with women in the control group (Thomas et al., 2002). A nested case–control study within the CNBSS compared the frequency and proficiency of BSE performance between the cases and controls at 1, 2, and 3 years before the diagnosis of the case (Harvey et al., 1997). No difference in BSE frequency was found between cases and controls. However, visual inspection, use of finger pads, and use of the middle three fingers were found to have a significant association with breast cancer diagnosis when performed 2 years before the diagnosis, with an odds ratio for death or distant metastases from breast cancer of 2.2 among women who omitted one, two, or three of these BSE components.

2.4.5 Host factors that affect performance

Because BSE might be of some value in the early detection of breast cancers in LMICs, it is most relevant to examine the host factors likely to affect BSE practice in such countries. A study among Iranian women identified lack of privacy as the principal barrier to BSE practice (Tavafian et al., 2009). In a study in Taiwan, China, personal and social factors were reported to affect the motivation of women attending BSE training (Yang et al., 2010). A study looking for predictors of BSE practice among Malaysian teachers found that higher level of knowledge about breast cancer, greater confidence in performing BSE, and regular visits to a physician were significant predictors for practising BSE (Parsa et al., 2011). Socioeconomic status, level of education, knowledge about breast cancer, and knowledge about BSE performance was found to affect BSE practice in Iranian women (Haji-Mahmoodi et al., 2002). Many studies in LMICs have identified the absence of breast symptoms, lack of breast cancer awareness, and lack of knowledge about BSE performance as the main host factors that affect BSE practice (Choi, 2005; Satitvipawee et al., 2009; Azage et al., 2013). A study in a mixed population of Caucasians and African-Americans in the USA found that high school education, employment status, and marital status were significant variables influencing BSE practice (Madan et al., 2000), whereas ethnicity did not affect compliance.

References

AAPM (1990). Equipment requirements and quality control for mammography. AAPM Report No. 29. American Association of Physicists in Medicine. Available from: https://www.aapm.org/pubs/reports/rpt_29.pdf.

ACR (2010). ACR manual on contrast media (version 7). American College of Radiology. Available from: http://www.acr.org/Quality-Safety/Resources/Contrast-Manual.

ACR (2013a). ACR practice guideline for the performance of screening and diagnostic mammography. American College of Radiology. Available from: http://www.acr.org/~/media/3484CA30845348359BAD4684779D492D.pdf, accessed 7 June 2013.

ACR (2013b). ACR manual on contrast media (version 9). American College of Radiology. Available from: http://www.acr.org/Quality-Safety/Resources/Contrast-Manual.

Albert US, Altland H, Duda V, Engel J, Geraedts M, Heywang-Köbrunner S et al. (2009). 2008 update of the guideline: early detection of breast cancer in Germany. *J Cancer Res Clin Oncol*, 135(3):339–54. doi:10.1007/s00432-008-0450-y PMID:18661152

Anderson EDC, Muir BB, Walsh JS, Kirkpatrick AE (1994). The efficacy of double reading mammograms in breast screening. *Clin Radiol*, 49(4):248–51. doi:10.1016/S0009-9260(05)81850-1 PMID:8162681

Avril N, Rosé CA, Schelling M, Dose J, Kuhn W, Bense S et al. (2000). Breast imaging with positron emission tomography and fluorine-18 fluorodeoxyglucose: use and limitations. *J Clin Oncol*, 18(20):3495–502. PMID:11032590

Azage M, Abeje G, Mekonnen A (2013). Assessment of factors associated with breast self-examination among health extension workers in West Gojjam Zone, Northwest Ethiopia. *Int J Breast Cancer*, 2013:814395. doi:10.1155/2013/814395 PMID:24298389

Baines CJ (1992a). Physical examination of the breasts in screening for breast cancer. *J Gerontol*, 47(Spec No):63–7. PMID:1430885

Baines CJ (1992b). Breast self-examination. *Cancer*, 69(Suppl 17):1942–6. doi:10.1002/1097-0142(19920401)69:7+<1942::AID-CNCR2820691712>3.0.CO;2-K PMID:1544096

Baines CJ, Miller AB, Bassett AA (1989). Physical examination. Its role as a single screening modality in the Canadian National Breast Screening Study. *Cancer*, 63(9):1816–22. doi:10.1002/1097-0142(19900501)63:9<1816::AID-CNCR2820630926>3.0.CO;2-W PMID:2702588

Baltzer PA, Dietzel M (2013). Breast lesions: diagnosis by using proton MR spectroscopy at 1.5 and 3.0 T – systematic review and meta-analysis. *Radiology*, 267(3):735–46. doi:10.1148/radiol.13121856 PMID:23468577

Barr RG, Destounis S, Lackey LB 2nd, Svensson WE, Balleyguier C, Smith C (2012). Evaluation of breast lesions using sonographic elasticity imaging: a multicenter trial. *J Ultrasound Med*, 31(2):281–7. PMID:22298872

Barton MB, Harris R, Fletcher SW (1999). The rational clinical examination. Does this patient have breast cancer? The screening clinical breast examination: should it be done? How? *JAMA*, 282(13):1270–80. doi:10.1001/jama.282.13.1270 PMID:10517431

Bassett AA (1985). Physical examination of the breast and breast self-examination. In: Miller AB, editor. Screening for cancer. Orlando (FL), USA: Academic Press; pp. 271–91.

Beam CA, Conant EF, Sickles EA (2003). Association of volume and volume-independent factors with accuracy in screening mammogram interpretation. *J Natl Cancer Inst*, 95(4):282–90. doi:10.1093/jnci/95.4.282 PMID:12591984

Beaman SA, Lillicrap SC (1982). Optimum X-ray spectra for mammography. *Phys Med Biol*, 27(10):1209–20. doi:10.1088/0031-9155/27/10/001 PMID:7146094

Bech M, Sorensen J, Lauridsen J (2005). Eliciting women's preferences for a training program in breast self-examination: a conjoint ranking experiment. *Value Health*, 8(4):479–87.

Bennett RL, Sellars SJ, Blanks RG, Moss SM (2012). An observational study to evaluate the performance of units using two radiographers to read screening mammograms. *Clin Radiol*, 67(2):114–21. doi:10.1016/j.crad.2011.06.015 PMID:22070944

Berg WA, Cosgrove DO, Doré CJ, Schäfer FKW, Svensson WE, Hooley RJ et al.; BE1 Investigators (2012c). Shear-wave elastography improves the specificity of breast US: the BE1 multinational study of 939 masses. *Radiology*, 262(2):435–49. doi:10.1148/radiol.11110640 PMID:22282182

Berg WA, Madsen KS, Schilling K, Tartar M, Pisano ED, Larsen LH et al. (2011). Breast cancer: comparative effectiveness of positron emission mammography and MR imaging in presurgical planning for the ipsilateral breast. *Radiology*, 258(1):59–72. doi:10.1148/radiol.10100454 PMID:21076089

Berg WA, Madsen KS, Schilling K, Tartar M, Pisano ED, Larsen LH et al. (2012a). Comparative effectiveness of positron emission mammography and MRI in the contralateral breast of women with newly diagnosed breast cancer. *AJR Am J Roentgenol*, 198(1):219–32. doi:10.2214/AJR.10.6342 PMID:22194501

Berg WA, Zhang Z, Lehrer D, Jong RA, Pisano ED, Barr RG et al.; ACRIN 6666 Investigators (2012b). Detection of breast cancer with addition of annual screening ultrasound or a single screening MRI to mammography in women with elevated breast cancer risk. *JAMA*, 307(13):1394–404. doi:10.1001/jama.2012.388 PMID:22474203

Berns EA, Hendrick RE, Cutter GR (2003). Optimization of technique factors for a silicon diode array full-field digital mammography system and comparison to screen-film mammography with matched average glandular dose. *Med Phys*, 30(3):334–40. doi:10.1118/1.1544674 PMID:12674233

Blanch J, Sala M, Ibáñez J, Domingo L, Fernandez B, Otegi A et al.; INCA Study Group (2014). Impact of risk factors on different interval cancer subtypes in a population-based breast cancer screening programme. *PLoS One*, 9(10):e110207. doi:10.1371/journal.pone.0110207 PMID:25333936

Blanks RG, Moss SM, Wallis MG (1997). Use of two view mammography compared with one view in the detection of small invasive cancers: further results from the National Health Service breast screening programme. *J Med Screen*, 4(2):98–101. PMID:9275268

Blanks RG, Wallis MG, Moss SM (1998). A comparison of cancer detection rates achieved by breast cancer screening programmes by number of readers, for one and two view mammography: results from the UK National Health Service breast screening programme. *J Med Screen*, 5(4):195–201. doi:10.1136/jms.5.4.195 PMID:9934650

BlueCross BlueShield Association (2013). Breast-specific gamma imaging (BSGI), molecular breast imaging (MBI), or scintimammography with breast-specific gamma camera. *Technol Eval Cent Assess Program Exec Summ*, 28(2):1–4. PMID:23865107

Bobo J, Lee N (2000). Factors associated with accurate cancer detection during a clinical breast examination. *Ann Epidemiol*, 10(7):463.

Bobo JK, Lee NC, Thames SF (2000). Findings from 752,081 clinical breast examinations reported to a national screening program from 1995 through 1998. *J Natl Cancer Inst*, 92(12):971–6. doi:10.1093/jnci/92.12.971 PMID:10861308

Boone JM, Nelson TR, Lindfors KK, Seibert JA (2001). Dedicated breast CT: radiation dose and image quality evaluation. *Radiology*, 221(3):657–67. doi:10.1148/radiol.2213010334 PMID:11719660

Boyd NF, Huszti E, Melnichouk O, Martin LJ, Hislop G, Chiarelli A et al. (2014). Mammographic features associated with interval breast cancers in screening programs. *Breast Cancer Res*, 16(4):417. doi:10.1186/s13058-014-0417-7 PMID:25346388

Bragg Leight S, Deiriggi P, Hursh D, Miller D, Leight V (2000). The effect of structured training on breast self-examination search behaviors as measured using biomedical instrumentation. *Nurs Res*, 49(5):283–9. doi:10.1097/00006199-200009000-00007 PMID:11009123

Breast Cancer Surveillance Consortium (2009). Screening performance. Available from: http://breastscreening.cancer.gov/statistics/performance/screening/2009/rate_age.html.

Breast Imaging Working Group of the German Radiological Society (2014). Updated recommendations for MRI of the breast. *Rofo*, 186(5):482–3. doi:10.1055/s-0034-1366404 PMID:24756386

BreastScreen Australia (2001). National Accreditation Standards. Quality Improvement Program. Available from: http://www.cancerscreening.gov.au/internet/screening/publishing.nsf/Content/br-accreditation/$File/standards.pdf.

Brem RF, Tabar L, Duffy SW, Inciardi MF, Guingrich JA, Hashimoto BE et al. (2014). Assessing improvement in detection of breast cancer with three-dimensional automated breast US in women with dense breast tissue: the SomoInsight Study. *Radiology*, 274(3):663–73. doi:10.1148/radiol.14132832 PMID:25329763

Brennan ME, Houssami N, Lord S, Macaskill P, Irwig L, Dixon JM et al. (2009). Magnetic resonance imaging screening of the contralateral breast in women with newly diagnosed breast cancer: systematic review and meta-analysis of incremental cancer detection and impact on surgical management. *J Clin Oncol*, 27(33):5640–9. doi:10.1200/JCO.2008.21.5756 PMID:19805685

British Columbia Cancer Agency (2011). Screening mammography programme, annual report. Available from: http://www.screeningbc.ca/NR/rdonlyres/D302DDFE-474D-48F2-912D-F5612AA8B204/61384/SMP_2012AR_WEB2.pdf.

Brixner L, Holland RS, Kellogg RE, Mickish D, Patten SH, Zegarski W (1985). Low print-through technology with rare earth tantalate phosphors. *Proc SPIE* 0555 Medical Imaging and Instrumentation, 85:84–90. doi:10.1117/12.949479

Brooks KW, Trueblood JH, Kearfott KJ (1993). Automated analysis of mammography quality control images. *Med Phys*, 20(3):881.

Byng JW, Critten JP, Yaffe MJ (1997). Thickness-equalization processing for mammographic images. *Radiology*, 203(2):564–8. doi:10.1148/radiology.203.2.9114122 PMID:9114122

Canadian Association of Radiologists (2012). Practice guidelines and technical standards for breast imaging and intervention. Available from: http://www.car.ca/uploads/standards%20guidelines/20131024_en_breast_imaging_practice_guidelines.pdf, accessed 25 April 2015.

Carter AC, Feldman JG, Tiefer L, Hausdorff JK (1985). Methods of motivating the practice of breast self-examination: a randomized trial. *Prev Med*, 14(5):555–72. doi:10.1016/0091-7435(85)90077-5 PMID:4070189

Chalabian J, Dunnington G (1998). Do our current assessments assure competency in clinical breast evaluation skills? *Am J Surg*, 175(6):497–502. doi:10.1016/S0002-9610(98)00075-0 PMID:9645781

Chalabian J, Garman K, Wallace P, Dunnington G (1996). Clinical breast evaluation skills of house officers and students. *Am Surg*, 62(10):840–5. PMID:8813167

Chang JM, Moon WK, Cho N, Park JS, Kim SJ (2011). Breast cancers initially detected by hand-held ultrasound: detection performance of radiologists using automated breast ultrasound data. *Acta Radiol*, 52(1):8–14. doi:10.1258/ar.2010.100179 PMID:21498319

Chen B, Ning R (2002). Cone-beam volume CT breast imaging: feasibility study. *Med Phys*, 29(5):755–70. doi:10.1118/1.1461843 PMID:12033572

Chen L, Chen Y, Diao XH, Fang L, Pang Y, Cheng AQ et al. (2013). Comparative study of automated breast 3-D ultrasound and handheld B-mode ultrasound for differentiation of benign and malignant breast masses. *Ultrasound Med Biol*, 39(10):1735–42. doi:10.1016/j.ultrasmedbio.2013.04.003 PMID:23849390

Chen X, Li WL, Zhang YL, Wu Q, Guo YM, Bai ZL (2010). Meta-analysis of quantitative diffusion-weighted MR imaging in the differential diagnosis of breast lesions. *BMC Cancer*, 10(1):693. doi:10.1186/1471-2407-10-693 PMID:21189150

Chen Z, Ning R (2003). Why should breast tumour detection go three dimensional? *Phys Med Biol*, 48(14):2217–28. doi:10.1088/0031-9155/48/14/312 PMID:12894980

Chiarelli AM, Edwards SA, Prummel MV, Muradali D, Majpruz V, Done SJ et al. (2013). Digital compared with screen-film mammography: performance measures in concurrent cohorts within an organized breast screening program. *Radiology*, 268(3):684–93. doi:10.1148/radiol.13122567 PMID:23674784

Chidlow K, Möller T (2003). Rapid emission tomography reconstruction. In: Fujishiro I, Mueller K, Kaufman A, editors. Volume graphics. The Eurographics Association.

Choi YH (2005). The factors influencing the compliance of breast self-examination of middle-aged women. *Taehan Kanho Hakhoe Chi*, 35(4):721–7. PMID:16037727

Clarke VA, Savage SA (1999). Breast self-examination training: a brief review. *Cancer Nurs*, 22(4):320–6. doi:10.1097/00002820-199908000-00010 PMID:10452210

Coleman EA, Heard JK (2001). Clinical breast examination: an illustrated educational review and update. *Clin Excell Nurse Pract*, 5(4):197–204. doi:10.1054/xc.2001.24219 PMID:11458314

Coleman EA, Pennypacker H (1991). Measuring breast self-examination proficiency. A scoring system developed from a paired comparison study. *Cancer Nurs*, 14(4):211–7. doi:10.1097/00002820-199114040-00007 PMID:1913636

Conway BJ, Suleiman OH, Rueter FG, Antonsen RG, Slayton RJ (1994). National survey of mammographic facilities in 1985, 1988, and 1992. *Radiology*, 191(2):323–30. doi:10.1148/radiology.191.2.8153301 PMID:8153301

Costanza ME, Greene HL, McManus D, Hoople NE, Barth R (1995). Can practicing physicians improve their counseling and physical examination skills in breast cancer screening? A feasibility study. *J Cancer Educ*, 10(1):14–21. PMID:7772460

Costanza ME, Luckmann R, Quirk ME, Clemow L, White MJ, Stoddard AM (1999). The effectiveness of using standardized patients to improve community physician skills in mammography counseling and clinical breast exam. *Prev Med*, 29(4):241–8. doi:10.1006/pmed.1999.0544 PMID:10547049

CPAC (2013). Quality determinants of breast cancer screening with mammography in Canada. Toronto: Canadian Partnership Against Cancer. Available from: http://www.cancerview.ca/idc/groups/public/documents/webcontent/manmmography_in_canada.pdf.

Dee KE (2002). MammoEd: digital interactive breast imaging education. *Med Educ*, 36(11):1103–4. doi:10.1046/j.1365-2923.2002.134723.x PMID:12406293

Diebold T, Jacobi V, Scholz B, Hensel C, Solbach C, Kaufmann M et al. (2005). Value of electrical impedance scanning (EIS) in the evaluation of BI-RADS III/IV/V-lesions. *Technol Cancer Res Treat*, 4(1):93–7. PMID:15649092

Donmez YC, Dolgun E, Yavuz M (2012). Breast self-examination practices and the effect of a planned training program in Western Turkey. *Asian Pac J Cancer Prev*, 13(12):6159–61. doi:10.7314/APJCP.2012.13.12.6159 PMID:23464423

Dorsay RH, Cuneo WD, Somkin CP, Tekawa IS (1988). Breast self-examination: improving competence and frequency in a classroom setting. *Am J Public Health*, 78(5):520–2. doi:10.2105/AJPH.78.5.520 PMID:3354734

Esserman L, Cowley H, Eberle C, Kirkpatrick A, Chang S, Berbaum K et al. (2002). Improving the accuracy of mammography: volume and outcome relationships. *J Natl Cancer Inst*, 94(5):369–75. doi:10.1093/jnci/94.5.369 PMID:11880475

Expert Panel on MRI Safety (2013). ACR guidance document on MR safe practices: 2013. *J Magn Reson Imaging*, 37(3):501–30. doi:10.1002/jmri.24011 PMID:23345200

FDA (2013). Mammography Quality Standards Act. US Food and Drug Administration. Available from: http://www.fda.gov/Radiation-EmittingProducts/MammographyQualityStandardsActandProgram/default.htm, accessed 6 June 2013.

Feig SA (1987). Mammography equipment: principles, features, selection. *Radiol Clin North Am*, 25(5):897–911. PMID:3306772

Fenton JJ, Taplin SH, Carney PA, Abraham L, Sickles EA, D'Orsi C et al. (2007). Influence of computer-aided detection on performance of screening mammography. *N Engl J Med*, 356(14):1399–409. doi:10.1056/NEJMoa066099 PMID:17409321

Fintor L, Alciati MH, Fischer R (1995). Legislative and regulatory mandates for mammography quality assurance. *J Public Health Policy*, 16(1):81–107. doi:10.2307/3342978 PMID:7738160

Fitzgerald A, Berentson-Shaw J (2012). Thermography as a screening and diagnostic tool: a systematic review. *N Z Med J*, 125(1351):80–91. PMID:22426613

Fletcher SW, O'Malley MS, Pilgrim CA, Gonzalez JJ (1989). How do women compare with internal medicine residents in breast lump detection? A study with silicone models. *J Gen Intern Med*, 4(4):277–83. doi:10.1007/BF02597396 PMID:2788213

Friedlander LC, Roth SO, Gavenonis SC (2011). Results of MR imaging screening for breast cancer in high-risk patients with lobular carcinoma in situ. *Radiology*, 261(2):421–7. doi:10.1148/radiol.11103516 PMID:21900618

Fuchsjaeger MH, Flöry D, Reiner CS, Rudas M, Riedl CC, Helbich TH (2005). The negative predictive value of electrical impedance scanning in BI-RADS category IV breast lesions. *Invest Radiol*, 40(7):478–85. doi:10.1097/01.rli.0000167425.34577.d1 PMID:15973141

Gilbert FJ, Astley SM, Gillan MG, Agbaje OF, Wallis MG, James J et al.; CADET II Group (2008). Single reading with computer-aided detection for screening mammography. *N Engl J Med*, 359(16):1675–84. doi:10.1056/NEJMoa0803545 PMID:18832239

Giuliano V, Giuliano C (2013). Improved breast cancer detection in asymptomatic women using 3D-automated breast ultrasound in mammographically dense breasts. *Clin Imaging*, 37(3):480–6. doi:10.1016/j.clinimag.2012.09.018 PMID:23116728

Gohagan JK, Rodes ND, Blackwell CW, Darby WP, Farrell C, Herder T et al. (1980). Individual and combined effectiveness of palpation, thermography, and mammography in breast cancer screening. *Prev Med*, 9(6):713–21. doi:10.1016/0091-7435(80)90016-X PMID:7454696

Golatta M, Franz D, Harcos A, Junkermann H, Rauch G, Scharf A et al. (2013). Interobserver reliability of automated breast volume scanner (ABVS) interpretation and agreement of ABVS findings with hand held breast ultrasound (HHUS), mammography and pathology results. *Eur J Radiol*, 82(8):e332–6. doi:10.1016/j.ejrad.2013.03.005 PMID:23540947

Goldstraw EJ, Castellano I, Ashley S, Allen S (2010). The effect of Premium View post-processing software on digital mammographic reporting. *Br J Radiol*, 83(986):122–8. doi:10.1259/bjr/96554696 PMID:19546175

Gordon R, Bender R, Herman GT (1970). Algebraic reconstruction techniques (ART) for three-dimensional electron microscopy and X-ray photography. *J Theor Biol*, 29(3):471–81. doi:10.1016/0022-5193(70)90109-8 PMID:5492997

Gromet M (2008). Comparison of computer-aided detection to double reading of screening mammograms: review of 231,221 mammograms. *AJR Am J Roentgenol*, 190(4):854–9. doi:10.2214/AJR.07.2812 PMID:18356428

Gros CM (1967). Methodology [in French]. *J Radiol Electrol Med Nucl*, 48(11):638–55. PMID:5591639

Gweon HM, Cho N, Han W, Yi A, Moon HG, Noh DY et al. (2014). Breast MR imaging screening in women with a history of breast conservation therapy. *Radiology*, 272(2):366–73. doi:10.1148/radiol.14131893 PMID:24635678 mammographic imaging screening trial. *AJR Am J Roentgenol*, 194(2):362–9. doi:10.2214/AJR.08.2114 PMID:20093597

Hacihasanoğlu R, Gözüm S (2008). The effect of training on the knowledge levels and beliefs regarding breast self-examination on women attending a public education centre. *Eur J Oncol Nurs*, 12(1):58–64. doi:10.1016/j.ejon.2007.06.005 PMID:17950665

Hackshaw AK, Wald NJ, Michell MJ, Field S, Wilson ARM (2000). An investigation into why two-view mammography is better than one-view in breast cancer screening. *Clin Radiol*, 55(6):454–8. doi:10.1053/crad.2000.0448 PMID:10873691

Haji-Mahmoodi M, Montazeri A, Jarvandi S, Ebrahimi M, Haghighat S, Harirchi I (2002). Breast self-examination: knowledge, attitudes, and practices among female health care workers in Tehran, Iran. *Breast J*, 8(4):222–5. doi:10.1046/j.1524-4741.2002.08406.x PMID:12100114

Hall DC, Adams CK, Stein GH, Stephenson HS, Goldstein MK, Pennypacker HS (1980). Improved detection of human breast lesions following experimental training. *Cancer*, 46(2):408–14. doi:10.1002/1097-0142(19800715)46:2<408::AID-CNCR2820460233>3.0.CO;2-P PMID:7388779

Hammerstein GR, Miller DW, White DR, Masterson ME, Woodard HQ, Laughlin JS (1979). Absorbed radiation dose in mammography. *Radiology*, 130(2):485–91. doi:10.1148/130.2.485 PMID:760167

Harvey BJ, Miller AB, Baines CJ, Corey PN (1997). Effect of breast self-examination techniques on the risk of death from breast cancer. *CMAJ*, 157(9):1205–12. PMID:9361639

Haus AG (1983). Physical principles and radiation dose in mammography. In: Feig SA, McClelland R, editors. Breast carcinoma: current diagnosis and treatment. New York (NY), USA: Masson; pp. 111–2.

Haus AG (1987). Recent advances in screen-film mammography. *Radiol Clin North Am*, 25(5):913–28. PMID:3306773

Health Canada (2013). Radiation protection and quality standards in mammography – safety procedures for the installation, use and control of mammographic X-ray equipment: safety code 36. Available from: http://www.hc-sc.gc.ca/ewh-semt/pubs/radiation/safety-code_36-securite/index-eng.php.

Hendrick RE (2010). Radiation doses and cancer risks from breast imaging studies. *Radiology*, 257(1):246–53. doi:10.1148/radiol.10100570 PMID:20736332

Hendrick RE, Klabunde C, Grivegnee A, Pou G, Ballard-Barbash R (2002). Technical quality control practices in mammography screening programs in 22 countries. *Int J Qual Health Care*, 14(3):219–26. doi:10.1093/oxfordjournals.intqhc.a002613 PMID:12108532

Hendrick RE, Pisano ED, Averbukh A, Moran C, Berns EA, Yaffe MJ et al. (2010). Comparison of acquisition parameters and breast dose in digital mammography and screen-film mammography in the American College of Radiology Imaging Network digital

Heywang-Köbrunner SH, Sinnatamby R, Lebeau A, Lebrecht A, Britton PD, Schreer I; Consensus Group (2009). Interdisciplinary consensus on the uses and technique of MR-guided vacuum-assisted breast biopsy (VAB): results of a European consensus meeting. *Eur J Radiol*, 72(2):289–94. doi:10.1016/j.ejrad.2008.07.010 PMID:18723305

Honjo S, Ando J, Tsukioka T, Morikubo H, Ichimura M, Sunagawa M et al. (2007). Relative and combined performance of mammography and ultrasonography for breast cancer screening in the general population: a pilot study in Tochigi Prefecture, Japan. *Jpn J Clin Oncol*, 37(9):715–20. doi:10.1093/jjco/hym090 PMID:17766996

Hope TA, Iles SE (2004). Technology review: the use of electrical impedance scanning in the detection of breast cancer. *Breast Cancer Res*, 6(2):69–74. doi:10.1186/bcr744 PMID:14979909

Hou MF, Chuang HY, Ou-Yang F, Wang CY, Huang CL, Fan HM et al. (2002). Comparison of breast mammography, sonography and physical examination for screening women at high risk of breast cancer in Taiwan. *Ultrasound Med Biol*, 28(4):415–20. doi:10.1016/S0301-5629(02)00483-0 PMID:12049952

Houn F, Elliott ML, McCrohan JL (1995). The Mammography Quality Standards Act of 1992. History and philosophy. *Radiol Clin North Am*, 33(6):1059–65. PMID:7480655

Huang Y, Kang M, Li H, Li JY, Zhang JY, Liu LH et al. (2012). Combined performance of physical examination, mammography, and ultrasonography for breast cancer screening among Chinese women: a follow-up study. *Curr Oncol*, 19(Suppl 2):eS22–30. doi:10.3747/co.19.1137 PMID:22876165

Huda W, Sajewicz AM, Ogden KM, Dance DR (2003). Experimental investigation of the dose and image quality characteristics of a digital mammography imaging system. *Med Phys*, 30(3):442–8. doi:10.1118/1.1543572 PMID:12674245

IAEA (2009). IAEA Human Health Series No. 2: Quality assurance programme for screen film mammography. Vienna, Austria: International Atomic Energy Agency. Available from: http://www-pub.iaea.org/MTCD/Publications/PDF/Pub1381_web.pdf, accessed 6 June 2013.

IAEA (2011). IAEA Human Health Series No. 17: Quality assurance programme for digital mammography. Vienna, Austria: International Atomic Energy Agency. Available from: http://www-pub.iaea.org/MTCD/Publications/PDF/Pub1482_web.pdf, accessed 6 June 2013.

IAEA (2014). Diagnostic radiology physics: a handbook for teachers and students. Vienna, Austria:

International Atomic Energy Agency. Available from: http://www-pub.iaea.org/books/IAEABooks/8841/Diagnostic-Radiology-Physics-A-Handbook-for-Teachers-and-Students.

INCa (2010). Enquête menée par l'INCa auprès des structures de gestion sur la mammographie numérique [in French]. Available from: http://www.sante.gouv.fr/IMG/pdf/Conf_presse_08_07_10_Enquete_menee_par_l_INCa_aupres_des_structures_de_gestion_sur_la_mammographie_numerique.pdf.

Jacobs J, Deprez T, Marchal G, Bosmans H (2006). MoniQA: a general approach to monitor quality assurance. *Proc SPIE*, 6145:614502. doi:10.1117/12.652093

Jennings RJ, Eastgate RJ, Siedband MP, Ergun DL (1981). Optimal X-ray spectra for screen-film mammography. *Med Phys*, 8(5):629–39. doi:10.1118/1.595021 PMID:7290015

Johns PC, Yaffe MJ (1987). X-ray characterisation of normal and neoplastic breast tissues. *Phys Med Biol*, 32(6):675–95. doi:10.1088/0031-9155/32/6/002 PMID:3039542

Kalles V, Zografos GC, Provatopoulou X, Koulocheri D, Gounaris A (2013). The current status of positron emission mammography in breast cancer diagnosis. *Breast Cancer*, 20(2):123–30. doi:10.1007/s12282-012-0433-3 PMID:23239242

Kang M, Zhao Y, Huang Y, Li J, Liu L, Li H (2014). Accuracy and direct medical cost of different screening modalities for breast cancer among Chinese women [in Chinese]. *Zhonghua Zhong Liu Za Zhi*, 36(3):236–40. PMID:24785288

Karssemeijer N, Trienekens DPC, Thijssen MAO (1995). Automated computation of contrast detail curves of mammographic imaging equipment. *Eur Radiol*, 5(Suppl):S6.

Kassenärztliche Bundesvereinigung (2004). Einführung eines bundesweiten Mammographie-Screening-Programms [in German]. Available from: https://www.mammascreen-bw.de/programmrichtlinien.pdf.

Kelly KM, Dean J, Comulada WS, Lee SJ (2010). Breast cancer detection using automated whole breast ultrasound and mammography in radiographically dense breasts. *Eur Radiol*, 20(3):734–42. doi:10.1007/s00330-009-1588-y PMID:19727744

Kim SH, Kang BJ, Choi BG, Choi JJ, Lee JH, Song BJ et al. (2013). Radiologists' performance for detecting lesions and the interobserver variability of automated whole breast ultrasound. *Korean J Radiol*, 14(2):154–63. doi:10.3348/kjr.2013.14.2.154 PMID:23482698

Klabunde C, Bouchard F, Taplin S, Scharpantgen A, Ballard-Barbash R; International Breast Cancer Screening Network (IBSN) (2001). Quality assurance for screening mammography: an international comparison. *J Epidemiol Community Health*, 55(3):204–12. doi:10.1136/jech.55.3.204 PMID:11160176

Kopans DB (2006). Breast imaging, Third edition. Philadelphia (PA), USA: Lippincott Williams & Wilkins.

Kuhl C, Weigel S, Schrading S, Arand B, Bieling H, König R et al. (2010). Prospective multicenter cohort study to refine management recommendations for women at elevated familial risk of breast cancer: the EVA trial. *J Clin Oncol*, 28(9):1450–7. doi:10.1200/JCO.2009.23.0839 PMID:20177029

Kuhl CK, Schrading S, Strobel K, Schild HH, Hilgers RD, Bieling HB (2014). Abbreviated breast magnetic resonance imaging (MRI): first postcontrast subtracted images and maximum-intensity projection – a novel approach to breast cancer screening with MRI. *J Clin Oncol*, 32(22):2304–10. doi:10.1200/JCO.2013.52.5386 PMID:24958821

Lederman D, Zheng B, Wang X, Sumkin JH, Gur D (2011). A GMM-based breast cancer risk stratification using a resonance-frequency electrical impedance spectroscopy. *Med Phys*, 38(3):1649–59. doi:10.1118/1.3555300 PMID:21520878

Lehman CD, Gatsonis C, Kuhl CK, Hendrick RE, Pisano ED, Hanna L et al.; ACRIN Trial 6667 Investigators Group (2007). MRI evaluation of the contralateral breast in women with recently diagnosed breast cancer. *N Engl J Med*, 356(13):1295–303. doi:10.1056/NEJMoa065447 PMID:17392300

Lin X, Wang J, Han F, Fu J, Li A (2012). Analysis of eighty-one cases with breast lesions using automated breast volume scanner and comparison with handheld ultrasound. *Eur J Radiol*, 81(5):873–8. doi:10.1016/j.ejrad.2011.02.038 PMID:21420814

Lindfors KK, Boone JM, Nelson TR, Yang K, Kwan ALC, Miller DF (2008). Dedicated breast CT: initial clinical experience. *Radiology*, 246(3):725–33. doi:10.1148/radiol.2463070410 PMID:18195383

Linver MN, Osuch JR, Brenner RJ, Smith RA (1995). The mammography audit: a primer for the mammography quality standards act (MQSA). *AJR Am J Roentgenol*, 165(1):19–25. doi:10.2214/ajr.165.1.7785586 PMID:7785586

Logan-Young WW, Muntz EP, editors (1979). Proceedings of the 2nd Reduced Dose Mammography Meeting, Roswell Park Institute, Buffalo, New York, October 4–6, 1978. New York (NY), USA: Masson.

Lord SJ, Lei W, Craft P, Cawson JN, Morris I, Walleser S et al. (2007). A systematic review of the effectiveness of magnetic resonance imaging (MRI) as an addition to mammography and ultrasound in screening young women at high risk of breast cancer. *Eur J Cancer*, 43(13):1905–17. doi:10.1016/j.ejca.2007.06.007 PMID:17681781

Madan AK, Barden CB, Beech B, Fay K, Sintich M, Beech DJ (2000). Socioeconomic factors, not ethnicity, predict breast self-examination. *Breast J*, 6(4):263–6. doi:10.1046/j.1524-4741.2000.99016.x PMID:11348376

Mainiero MB, Lourenco A, Mahoney MC, Newell MS, Bailey L, Barke LD et al. (2013). ACR appropriateness criteria breast cancer screening. *J Am Coll Radiol*, 10(1):11–4. doi:10.1016/j.jacr.2012.09.036 PMID:23290667

Malich A, Boehm T, Facius M, Freesmeyer MG, Fleck M, Anderson R et al. (2001). Differentiation of mammographically suspicious lesions: evaluation of breast ultrasound, MRI mammography and electrical impedance scanning as adjunctive technologies in breast cancer detection. *Clin Radiol*, 56(4):278–83. doi:10.1053/crad.2000.0621 PMID:11286578

Mamon J, Zapka J (1983). Determining the quality of breast self-examination and its relationship to other BSE measures. *Prog Clin Biol Res*, 130:313–22. PMID:6622465

Mann RM, Mus RD, van Zelst J, Geppert C, Karssemeijer N, Platel B (2014). A novel approach to contrast-enhanced breast magnetic resonance imaging for screening: high-resolution ultrafast dynamic imaging. *Invest Radiol*, 49(9):579–85. doi:10.1097/RLI.0000000000000057 PMID:24691143

Martín G, Martín R, Brieva MJ, Santamaría L (2002). Electrical impedance scanning in breast cancer imaging: correlation with mammographic and histologic diagnosis. *Eur Radiol*, 12(6):1471–8. doi:10.1007/s00330-001-1275-0 PMID:12042956

Matsumura T, Hayakawa M, Shimada F, Yabuki M, Dohanish S, Palkowitsch P et al. (2013). Safety of gadopentetate dimeglumine after 120 million administrations over 25 years of clinical use. *Magn Reson Med Sci*, 12(4):297–304. doi:10.2463/mrms.2013-0020 PMID:24172794

McCormack VA, dos Santos Silva I (2006). Breast density and parenchymal patterns as markers of breast cancer risk: a meta-analysis. *Cancer Epidemiol Biomarkers Prev*, 15(6):1159–69. doi:10.1158/1055-9965.EPI-06-0034 PMID:16775176

McDermott MM, Dolan NC, Huang J, Reifler D, Rademaker AW (1996). Lump detection is enhanced in silicone breast models simulating postmenopausal breast tissue. *J Gen Intern Med*, 11(2):112–4. doi:10.1007/BF02599588 PMID:8833020

McLelland R, Hendrick RE, Zinninger MD, Wilcox PA (1991). The American College of Radiology Mammography Accreditation Program. *AJR Am J Roentgenol*, 157(3):473–9. doi:10.2214/ajr.157.3.1872231 PMID:1872231

Medicine UW (2015). Breast imaging teaching files. Seattle (WA), USA: Department of Radiology, University of Washington. Available from: http://rad.washington.edu/teaching-files/.

Miller AB, Baines CJ, Turnbull C (1991). The role of the nurse-examiner in the National Breast Screening Study. *Can J Public Health*, 82(3):162–7. PMID:1884309

Mittra I, Mishra GA, Singh S, Aranke S, Notani P, Badwe R et al. (2010). A cluster randomized, controlled trial of breast and cervix cancer screening in Mumbai, India: methodology and interim results after three rounds of screening. *Int J Cancer*, 126(4):976–84. PMID:19697326

Morimoto T, Komaki K, Mori T, Sasa M, Ooshimo K, Miki H et al. (1993). The quality of mass screening for breast cancer by physical examination. *Surg Today*, 23(3):200–4. doi:10.1007/BF00309228 PMID:8467170

Moss SM, Blanks RG, Bennett RL (2005). Is radiologists' volume of mammography reading related to accuracy? A critical review of the literature. *Clin Radiol*, 60(6):623–6. doi:10.1016/j.crad.2005.01.011 PMID:16038688

Mueller K, Yagel R, Wheller JJ (1998). Fast and accurate projection algorithm for 3D cone-beam reconstruction with the Algebraic Reconstruction Technique (ART). *Proc SPIE*, 3336:724–32. doi:10.1117/12.317078

Narayanan D, Madsen KS, Kalinyak JE, Berg WA (2011). Interpretation of positron emission mammography and MRI by experienced breast imaging radiologists: performance and observer reproducibility. *AJR Am J Roentgenol*, 196(4):971–81. doi:10.2214/AJR.10.5081 PMID:21427351

NCRP (2004). A guide to mammography and other breast imaging procedures. NCRP Report No. 149. Bethesda (MD), USA: National Council on Radiation Protection and Measurements.

Ng EY, Sree SV, Ng KH, Kaw G (2008). The use of tissue electrical characteristics for breast cancer detection: a perspective review. *Technol Cancer Res Treat*, 7(4):295–308. doi:10.1177/153303460800700404 PMID:18642968

NHSBSP (2005). Monitoring NHSBSP standards – a guide for quality assurance reference centres, Version 3. Sheffield, UK: NHS Cancer Screening Programmes. Available from: http://www.cancerscreening.nhs.uk/breastscreen/publications/monitoring-standards.html.

NHSBSP (2013). Routine quality control tests for full-field digital mammography systems. Equipment Report NHSBSP 1303, 4th edition. Sheffield, UK: NHS Cancer Screening Programmes. Available from: http://www.cancerscreening.nhs.uk/breastscreen/publications/nhsbsp-equipment-report-1303.pdf.

Niklason LT, Christian BT, Niklason LE, Kopans DB, Castleberry DE, Opsahl-Ong BH et al. (1997). Digital tomosynthesis in breast imaging. *Radiology*, 205(2):399–406. doi:10.1148/radiology.205.2.9356620 PMID:9356620

Nishikawa RM (2010). Computer-aided detection and diagnosis. In: Bick U, Diekmann F, editors. Digital mammography. Berlin, Germany: Springer-Verlag; pp. 85–106. doi:10.1007/978-3-540-78450-0_6

Nothacker M, Duda V, Hahn M, Warm M, Degenhardt F, Madjar H et al. (2009). Early detection of breast cancer: benefits and risks of supplemental breast ultrasound in asymptomatic women with mammographically dense breast tissue. A systematic review. *BMC Cancer*, 9(1):335. doi:10.1186/1471-2407-9-335 PMID:19765317

Oestreicher N, White E, Lehman CD, Mandelson MT, Porter PL, Taplin SH (2002). Predictors of sensitivity of clinical breast examination (CBE). *Breast Cancer Res Treat*, 76(1):73–81. doi:10.1023/A:1020280623807 PMID:12408378

Oezaras G, Durualp E, Civelek FE, Gül B, Uensal M (2010). Analysis of breast self-examination training efficiency in women between 20–60 years of age in Turkey. *Asian Pac J Cancer Prev*, 11(3):799–802. PMID:21039057

Ohuchi N, Yoshida K, Kimura M, Ouchi A, Shiiba K, Ohnuki K et al. (1995). Comparison of false negative rates among breast cancer screening modalities with or without mammography: Miyagi trial. *Jpn J Cancer Res*, 86(5):501–6. doi:10.1111/j.1349-7006.1995.tb03084.x PMID:7790323

Park HH, Shin JY, Lee JY, Jin GH, Kim HS, Lyu KY et al. (2013). Discussion on the alteration of ^{18}F-FDG uptake by the breast according to the menstrual cycle in PET imaging. *Conf Proc IEEE Eng Med Biol Soc*, 2013:2469–72. PMID:24110227

Parsa P, Kandiah M, Parsa N (2011). Factors associated with breast self-examination among Malaysian women teachers. *East Mediterr Health J*, 17(6):509–16. PMID:21796969

Patnick J (2004). NHS breast screening: the progression from one to two views. *J Med Screen*, 11(2):55–6. doi:10.1258/096914104774061001 PMID:15153317

Pennypacker HS, Naylor L, Sander AA, Goldstein MK (1999). Why can't we do better breast examinations? *Nurse Pract Forum*, 10(3):122–8. PMID:10614356

Pennypacker HS, Pilgrim CA (1993). Achieving competence in clinical breast examination. *Nurse Pract Forum*, 4(2):85–90. PMID:8513268

Perlet C, Heywang-Kobrunner SH, Heinig A, Sittek H, Casselman J, Anderson I et al. (2006). Magnetic resonance-guided, vacuum-assisted breast biopsy: results from a European multicenter study of 538 lesions. *Cancer*, 106(5):982–90. doi:10.1002/cncr.21720 PMID:16456807

Perry N, Broeders M, de Wolf C, Törnberg S, Holland R, von Karsa L (2013). European guidelines for quality assurance in breast cancer screening and diagnosis. Fourth edition, Supplements. Luxembourg: European Commission, Office for Official Publications of the European Union.

Perry N, Broeders M, de Wolf C, Törnberg S, Holland R, von Karsa L et al., editors (2006a). European guidelines for quality assurance in breast cancer screening and diagnosis. 4th ed. Luxembourg: European Commission, Office for Official Publications of the European Communities. Available from: http://ec.europa.eu/health/ph_projects/2002/cancer/cancer_2002_01_en.htm.

Perry N, Holland R, Broeders M, Rijken H, Rosselli del Turco M, de Wolf C (2006b). Certification protocol for breast screening and breast diagnostic services. In: Perry N, Broeders M, de Wolf C, Törnberg S, Holland R, von Karsa L et al., editors. European guidelines for quality assurance in breast cancer screening and diagnosis. 4th ed. Luxembourg: European Commission, Office for Official Publications of the European Communities; pp. 369–78. Available from: http://ec.europa.eu/health/ph_projects/2002/cancer/cancer_2002_01_en.htm.

Phi XA, Houssami N, Obdeijn IM, Warner E, Sardanelli F, Leach MO et al. (2015). Magnetic resonance imaging improves breast screening sensitivity in *BRCA* mutation carriers age ≥ 50 years: evidence from an individual patient data meta-analysis. *J Clin Oncol*, 33(4):349–56. doi:10.1200/JCO.2014.56.6232 PMID:25534390

Philpotts LE (2009). Can computer-aided detection be detrimental to mammographic interpretation? *Radiology*, 253(1):17–22. doi:10.1148/radiol.2531090689 PMID:19789251

Pilgrim C, Lannon C, Harris RP, Cogburn W, Fletcher SW (1993). Improving clinical breast examination training in a medical school: a randomized controlled trial. *J Gen Intern Med*, 8(12):685–8. doi:10.1007/BF02598289 PMID:8120686

Pinto B, Fuqua RW (1991). Training breast self-examination: a research review and critique. *Health Educ Q*, 18(4):495–516. doi:10.1177/109019819101800407 PMID:1757270

Pisani P, Parkin DM, Ngelangel C, Esteban D, Gibson L, Munson M et al. (2006). Outcome of screening by clinical examination of the breast in a trial in the Philippines. *Int J Cancer*, 118(1):149–54. doi:10.1002/ijc.21343 PMID:16049976

Pisano ED (2004). Image display: softcopy and printed film basics of digital mammography display. In: Pisano ED, Yaffe MJ, Kuzmiak CM, editors. Digital mammography. Philadelphia (PA), USA: Lippincott Williams and Wilkins; pp. 58–66.

Pisano ED, Gatsonis C, Hendrick E, Yaffe M, Baum JK, Acharyya S et al.; Digital Mammographic Imaging Screening Trial (DMIST) Investigators Group (2005). Diagnostic performance of digital versus film mammography for breast-cancer screening. *N Engl J Med*, 353(17):1773–83. doi:10.1056/NEJMoa052911 PMID:16169887

Pisano ED, Yaffe MJ (2005). Digital mammography. *Radiology*, 234(2):353–62. doi:10.1148/radiol.2342030897 PMID:15670993

Pisano ED, Zong S, Hemminger BM, DeLuca M, Johnston RE, Muller K et al. (1998). Contrast limited adaptive histogram equalization image processing to improve the detection of simulated spiculations in dense mammograms. *J Digit Imaging*, 11(4):193–200. doi:10.1007/BF03178082 PMID:9848052

Pizer SM, Amburn EP, Austin JD, Cromartie R, Geselowitz A, Greer T et al. (1987). Adaptive Histogram Equalization and its variations. *Comput Vis Graph Image Process*, 39(3):355–68. doi:10.1016/S0734-189X(87)80186-X

Price ER, Hargreaves J, Lipson JA, Sickles EA, Brenner RJ, Lindfors KK et al. (2013). The California breast density information group: a collaborative response to the issues of breast density, breast cancer risk, and breast density notification legislation. *Radiology*, 269(3):887–92. doi:10.1148/radiol.13131217 PMID:24023072

Rabkin Z, Israel O, Keidar Z (2010). Do hyperglycemia and diabetes affect the incidence of false-negative ^{18}F-FDG PET/CT studies in patients evaluated for infection or inflammation and cancer? A comparative analysis. *J Nucl Med*, 51(7):1015–20. doi:10.2967/jnumed.109.074294 PMID:20554733

Rhodes DJ, Hruska CB, Phillips SW, Whaley DH, O'Connor MK (2011). Dedicated dual-head gamma imaging for breast cancer screening in women with mammographically dense breasts. *Radiology*, 258(1):106–18. doi:10.1148/radiol.10100625 PMID:21045179

Salomon A (1913). Beitrage zur Pathologie und Klinic der Mammacarzinome [in German]. *Arch Klin Chir*, 101:573–668.

Sankaranarayanan R, Ramadas K, Thara S, Muwonge R, Prabhakar J, Augustine P et al. (2011). Clinical breast examination: preliminary results from a cluster randomized controlled trial in India. *J Natl Cancer Inst*, 103(19):1476–80. doi:10.1093/jnci/djr304 PMID:21862730

Sardanelli F, Boetes C, Borisch B, Decker T, Federico M, Gilbert FJ et al. (2010). Magnetic resonance imaging of the breast: recommendations from the EUSOMA working group. *Eur J Cancer*, 46(8):1296–316. doi:10.1016/j.ejca.2010.02.015 PMID:20304629

Saslow D, Hannan J, Osuch J, Alciati MH, Baines C, Barton M et al. (2004). Clinical breast examination: practical recommendations for optimizing performance and reporting. *CA Cancer J Clin*, 54(6):327–44. doi:10.3322/canjclin.54.6.327 PMID:15537576

Satitvipawee P, Promthet SS, Pitiphat W, Kalampakorn S, Parkin DM (2009). Factors associated with breast self-examination among Thai women living in rural areas in Northeastern Thailand. *J Med Assoc Thai*, 92(Suppl 7):S29–35. PMID:20235356

Saunders KJ, Pilgrim CA, Pennypacker HS (1986). Increased proficiency of search in breast self-examination. *Cancer*, 58(11):2531–7. doi:10.1002/1097-0142(19861201)58:11<2531::AID-CNCR2820581128>3.0.CO;2-J PMID:3768844

Schäfer FK, Hooley RJ, Ohlinger R, Hahne U, Madjar H, Svensson WE et al. (2013). ShearWave™ Elastography BE1 multinational breast study: additional SWE™ features support potential to downgrade BI-RADS®-3 lesions. *Ultraschall Med*, 34(3):254–9. doi:10.1055/s-0033-1335523 PMID:23709241

Schilling K, Narayanan D, Kalinyak JE, The J, Velasquez MV, Kahn S et al. (2011). Positron emission mammography in breast cancer presurgical planning: comparisons with magnetic resonance imaging. *Eur J Nucl Med Mol Imaging*, 38(1):23–36. doi:10.1007/s00259-010-1588-9 PMID:20871992

Shin HJ, Kim HH, Cha JH, Park JH, Lee KE, Kim JH (2011). Automated ultrasound of the breast for diagnosis: interobserver agreement on lesion detection and characterization. *AJR Am J Roentgenol*, 197(3):747–54. doi:10.2214/AJR.10.5841 PMID:21862820

Siegmann-Luz KC, Bahrs SD, Preibsch H, Hattermann V, Claussen CD (2014). Management of breast lesions detectable only on MRI. *Rofo*, 186(1):30–6. PMID:23897532

Skaane P, Bandos AI, Eben EB, Jebsen IN, Krager M, Haakenaasen U et al. (2014a). Two-view digital breast tomosynthesis screening with synthetically reconstructed projection images: comparison with digital breast tomosynthesis with full-field digital mammographic images. *Radiology*, 271(3):655–63. doi:10.1148/radiol.13131391 PMID:24484063

Skaane P, Bandos AI, Gullien R, Eben EB, Ekseth U, Haakenaasen U et al. (2013). Comparison of digital mammography alone and digital mammography plus tomosynthesis in a population-based screening program. *Radiology*, 267(1):47–56. doi:10.1148/radiol.12121373 PMID:23297332

Skaane P, Gullien R, Eben EB, Sandhaug M, Schulz-Wendtland R, Stoeblen F (2014b). Interpretation of automated breast ultrasound (ABUS) with and without knowledge of mammography: a reader performance study. *Acta Radiol*, 56(4):404–12. doi:10.1177/0284185114528835 PMID:24682405

Sloan DA, Donnelly MB, Schwartz RW, Munch LC, Wells MD, Johnson SB et al. (1994). Assessing medical students' and surgery residents' clinical competence in problem solving in surgical oncology. *Ann Surg Oncol*, 1(3):204–12. doi:10.1007/BF02303525 PMID:7842290

Smith-Bindman R, Chu P, Miglioretti DL, Quale C, Rosenberg RD, Cutter G et al. (2005). Physician predictors of mammographic accuracy. *J Natl Cancer Inst*, 97(5):358–67. doi:10.1093/jnci/dji060 PMID:15741572

Stefanoyiannis AP, Costaridou L, Sakellaropoulos P, Panayiotakis G (2000). A digital density equalization technique to improve visualization of breast periphery in mammography. *Br J Radiol*, 73(868):410–20.

Stojadinovic A, Nissan A, Shriver CD, Mittendorf EA, Akin MD, Dickerson V et al. (2008). Electrical impedance scanning as a new breast cancer risk stratification tool for young women. *J Surg Oncol*, 97(2):112–20. doi:10.1002/jso.20931 PMID:18050282

Stout NK, Lee SJ, Schechter CB, Kerlikowske K, Alagoz O, Berry D et al. (2014). Benefits, harms, and costs for breast cancer screening after US implementation of digital mammography. *J Natl Cancer Inst*, 106(6):dju092. doi:10.1093/jnci/dju092 PMID:24872543

Suleiman OH, Spelic DC, McCrohan JL, Symonds GR, Houn F (1999). Mammography in the 1990s: the United States and Canada. *Radiology*, 210(2):345–51. doi:10.1148/radiology.210.2.r99fe45345 PMID:10207413

Sun Y, Wei W, Yang HW, Liu JL (2013). Clinical usefulness of breast-specific gamma imaging as an adjunct modality to mammography for diagnosis of breast cancer: a systemic review and meta-analysis. *Eur J Nucl Med Mol Imaging*, 40(3):450–63. doi:10.1007/s00259-012-2279-5 PMID:23151912

Sung JS, Malak SF, Bajaj P, Alis R, Dershaw DD, Morris EA (2011). Screening breast MR imaging in women with a history of lobular carcinoma in situ. *Radiology*, 261(2):414–20. doi:10.1148/radiol.11110091 PMID:21900617

Surti S (2013). Radionuclide methods and instrumentation for breast cancer detection and diagnosis. *Semin Nucl Med*, 43(4):271–80. doi:10.1053/j.semnuclmed.2013.03.003 PMID:23725989

Taplin SH, Rutter CM, Finder C, Mandelson MT, Houn F, White E (2002). Screening mammography: clinical image quality and the risk of interval breast cancer. *AJR Am J Roentgenol*, 178(4):797–803. doi:10.2214/ajr.178.4.1780797 PMID:11906848

Tavafian SS, Hasani L, Aghamolaei T, Zare S, Gregory D (2009). Prediction of breast self-examination in a sample of Iranian women: an application of the Health Belief Model. *BMC Womens Health*, 9(1):37. doi:10.1186/1472-6874-9-37 PMID:20040093

Taylor PM, Champness J, Given-Wilson RM, Potts HW, Johnston K (2004). An evaluation of the impact of computer-based prompts on screen readers' interpretation of mammograms. *Br J Radiol*, 77(913):21–7. doi:10.1259/bjr/34203805 PMID:14988134

Thomas DB, Gao DL, Ray RM, Wang WW, Allison CJ, Chen FL et al. (2002). Randomized trial of breast self-examination in Shanghai: final results. *J Natl Cancer Inst*, 94(19):1445–57. doi:10.1093/jnci/94.19.1445 PMID:12359854

Thurfjell EL, Lernevall KA, Taube AA (1994). Benefit of independent double reading in a population-based mammography screening program. *Radiology*, 191(1):241–4. doi:10.1148/radiology.191.1.8134580 PMID:8134580

Trimboli RM, Verardi N, Cartia F, Carbonaro LA, Sardanelli F (2014). Breast cancer detection using double reading of unenhanced MRI including T1-weighted, T2-weighted STIR, and diffusion-weighted imaging: a proof of concept study. *AJR Am J Roentgenol*, 203(3):674–81. doi:10.2214/AJR.13.11816 PMID:25148175

van Dam PA, Van Goethem ML, Kersschot E, Vervliet J, Van den Veyver IB, De Schepper A et al. (1988). Palpable solid breast masses: retrospective single- and multimodality evaluation of 201 lesions. *Radiology*, 166(2):435–9. doi:10.1148/radiology.166.2.3275983 PMID:3275983

Vreugdenburg TD, Willis CD, Mundy L, Hiller JE (2013). A systematic review of elastography, electrical impedance scanning, and digital infrared thermography for breast cancer screening and diagnosis. *Breast Cancer Res Treat*, 137(3):665–76. doi:10.1007/s10549-012-2393-x PMID:23288346

Wald NJ, Murphy P, Major P, Parkes C, Townsend J, Frost C (1995). UKCCCR multicentre randomised controlled trial of one and two view mammography in breast cancer screening. *BMJ*, 311(7014):1189–93. doi:10.1136/bmj.311.7014.1189 PMID:7488893

Wang F-L, Chen F, Yin H, Xu N, Wu XX, Ma JJ et al. (2013). Effects of age, breast density and volume on breast cancer diagnosis: a retrospective comparison of sensitivity of mammography and ultrasonography in China's rural areas. *Asian Pac J Cancer Prev*, 14(4):2277–82. doi:10.7314/APJCP.2013.14.4.2277 PMID:23725127

Wang T, Wang K, Yao Q, Chen JH, Ling R, Zhang JL et al. (2010). Prospective study on combination of electrical impedance scanning and ultrasound in estimating risk of development of breast cancer in young women. *Cancer Invest*, 28(3):295–303. doi:10.3109/07357900802203658 PMID:19857040

Wang ZL, Xu JH, Li JL, Huang Y, Tang J (2012). Comparison of automated breast volume scanning to hand-held ultrasound and mammography. Erratum in: Radiol Med. 2012; 117(8):1443. Xw, Jian Hong [corrected to Xu, Jian Hong]. *Radiol Med*, 117(8):1287–93. doi:10.1007/s11547-012-0836-4 PMID:22744341

Warner E, Messersmith H, Causer P, Eisen A, Shumak R, Plewes D (2008). Systematic review: using magnetic resonance imaging to screen women at high risk for breast cancer. *Ann Intern Med*, 148(9):671–9. doi:10.7326/0003-4819-148-9-200805060-00007 PMID:18458280

Wersebe A, Siegmann K, Krainick U, Fersis N, Vogel U, Claussen CD et al. (2002). Diagnostic potential of targeted electrical impedance scanning in classifying suspicious breast lesions. *Invest Radiol*, 37(2):65–72. doi:10.1097/00004424-200202000-00003 PMID:11799329

Widmark JM (2007). Imaging-related medications: a class overview. *Proc (Bayl Univ Med Cent)*, 20(4):408–17. PMID:17948119

Wilke LG, Broadwater G, Rabiner S, Owens E, Yoon S, Ghate S et al. (2009). Breast self-examination: defining a cohort still in need. *Am J Surg*, 198(4):575–9. doi:10.1016/j.amjsurg.2009.06.012 PMID:19800471

Wilson R, Liston J, editors (2011). Quality assurance guidelines for breast cancer screening radiology, 2nd edition. NHSBSP Publication No. 59. Sheffield, UK: NHS Cancer Screening Programmes. Available from:

http://www.cancerscreening.nhs.uk/breastscreen/publications/nhsbsp59.pdf.

Wojcinski S, Farrokh A, Weber S, Thomas A, Fischer T, Slowinski T et al. (2010). Multicenter study of ultrasound real-time tissue elastography in 779 cases for the assessment of breast lesions: improved diagnostic performance by combining the BI-RADS®-US classification system with sonoelastography. *Ultraschall Med*, 31(5):484–91. doi:10.1055/s-0029-1245282 PMID:20408116

Wojcinski S, Gyapong S, Farrokh A, Soergel P, Hillemanns P, Degenhardt F (2013). Diagnostic performance and inter-observer concordance in lesion detection with the automated breast volume scanner (ABVS). *BMC Med Imaging*, 13(1):36. doi:10.1186/1471-2342-13-36 PMID:24219312

Wu T, Stewart A, Stanton M, McCauley T, Phillips W, Kopans DB et al. (2003). Tomographic mammography using a limited number of low-dose cone-beam projection images. *Med Phys*, 30(3):365–80. doi:10.1118/1.1543934 PMID:12674237

Xu G, Hu Y, Kan X (2010). The preliminary report of breast cancer screening for 100000 women in China. *China Cancer*, 19(9):565–8. Available from: http://en.cnki.com.cn/Article_en/CJFDTOTAL-ZHLU201009004.htm.

Xu X, Wu Y, Li L (2014). An application evaluation on different screening methods of breast cancer. *Zhejiang J Prev Med*, 26(5):454–8.

Yaffe MJ (1990). AAPM tutorial. Physics of mammography: image recording process. *Radiographics*, 10(2):341–63. doi:10.1148/radiographics.10.2.2183301 PMID:2183301

Yaffe MJ (2010a). Detectors for digital mammography. In: Bick U, Diekmann F, editors. Digital mammography. Berlin, Germany: Springer-Verlag; pp. 13–31.

Yaffe MJ (2010b). Basic physics of digital mammography. In: Bick U, Diekmann F, editors. Digital mammography. Berlin, Germany: Springer-Verlag; pp. 1–11.

Yaffe MJ, Bloomquist AK, Hunter DM, Mawdsley GE, Chiarelli AM, Muradali D et al. (2013). Comparative performance of modern digital mammography systems in a large breast screening program. *Med Phys*, 40(12):121915. doi:10.1118/1.4829516 PMID:24320526

Yaffe MJ, Mainprize JG (2014). Digital tomosynthesis: technique. *Radiol Clin North Am*, 52(3):489–97. doi:10.1016/j.rcl.2014.01.003 PMID:24792651

Yang RJ, Huang LH, Hsieh YS, Chung UL, Huang CS, Bih HD (2010). Motivations and reasons for women attending a breast self-examination training program: A qualitative study. *BMC Womens Health*, 10(1):23. doi:10.1186/1472-6874-10-23 PMID:20618986

Young KC, Oduko JM (2005). Evaluation of Kodak DirectView mammography computerised radiography system. NHSBSP Equipment Report 0504. Sheffield, UK: NHS Cancer Screening Programmes. Available from: http://www.cancerscreening.nhs.uk.

Young KC, Oduko JM, Bosmans H, Nijs K, Martinez L (2006). Optimal beam quality selection in digital mammography. *Br J Radiol*, 79(948):981–90. doi:10.1259/bjr/55334425 PMID:17213303

Young KC, Ramsdale ML, Rust A, Cooke J (1997). Effect of automatic kV selection on dose and contrast for a mammographic X-ray system. *Br J Radiol*, 70(838):1036–42. doi:10.1259/bjr.70.838.9404208 PMID:9404208

Young KC, Wallis MG, Ramsdale ML (1994). Mammographic film density and detection of small breast cancers. *Clin Radiol*, 49(7):461–5. doi:10.1016/S0009-9260(05)81741-6 PMID:8088038

Zhang Q, Hu B, Hu B, Li WB (2012). Detection of breast lesions using an automated breast volume scanner system. *J Int Med Res*, 40(1):300–6. doi:10.1177/147323001204000130 PMID:22429369

Zheng B, Lederman D, Sumkin JH, Zuley ML, Gruss MZ, Lovy LS et al. (2011). A preliminary evaluation of multi-probe resonance-frequency electrical impedance based measurements of the breast. *Acad Radiol*, 18(2):220–9. doi:10.1016/j.acra.2010.09.017 PMID:21126888

Zheng B, Zuley ML, Sumkin JH, Catullo VJ, Abrams GS, Rathfon GY et al. (2008). Detection of breast abnormalities using a prototype resonance electrical impedance spectroscopy system: a preliminary study. *Med Phys*, 35(7):3041–8. doi:10.1118/1.2936221 PMID:18697526

Zhi H, Ou B, Xiao XY, Peng YL, Wang Y, Liu LS et al. (2013). Ultrasound elastography of breast lesions in Chinese women: a multicenter study in China. *Clin Breast Cancer*, 13(5):392–400. doi:10.1016/j.clbc.2013.02.015 PMID:23830799

Zou Y, Guo Z (2003). A review of electrical impedance techniques for breast cancer detection. *Med Eng Phys*, 25(2):79–90. doi:10.1016/S1350-4533(02)00194-7 PMID:12538062

Zuley ML, Guo B, Catullo VJ, Chough DM, Kelly AE, Lu AH et al. (2014). Comparison of two-dimensional synthesized mammograms versus original digital mammograms alone and in combination with tomosynthesis images. *Radiology*, 271(3):664–71. doi:10.1148/radiol.13131530 PMID:24475859

3. SCREENING PROGRAMMES

3.1 Determinants of participation in screening

Participation in breast cancer screening is not distributed equally. In this section, the personal, socioeconomic, and cultural factors that influence participation are presented, and the issues related to information and informed choice are described and discussed. Finally, the psychological consequences of mammography screening are addressed. This information may be more or less relevant for organized screening or opportunistic screening, depending on the context of the screening programme or practice.

3.1.1 *Personal and socioeconomic factors*

There are numerous known socioeconomic factors that influence participation in breast cancer screening (Edgar et al., 2013). Lower income, lower educational status, lack of health insurance, and unemployment are all factors associated with lower levels of participation. These factors may also be associated with less knowledge of breast cancer screening, in terms of both benefits and adverse effects. Socioeconomic differences in screening practices tend to decrease when participation is promoted, cultural and economic barriers are reduced, and social support is offered (Segnan, 1997).

(a) Income, education level, and socioeconomic status

Income and education level are significant factors that influence participation in breast cancer screening (George, 2000). Higher income and education level are associated with higher participation in mammography screening (Katz et al., 2000; Chamot et al., 2001; Samah & Ahmadian, 2012). Fear of costs has been reported as a barrier to participation among women with low incomes, and having health insurance is associated with not perceiving cost as a barrier (Fayanju et al., 2014). In Japan, providing screening free of charge does not influence participation rates (Sano et al., 2014). Having an organized screening programme also appeared to attract women of lower socioeconomic status who would not usually undergo mammography screening (Chamot et al., 2007). In a study in Sweden, education level did not predict participation, but women in the highest income quartile were less likely to be non-attenders compared with those in the lowest income quartile (Zackrisson et al., 2007). In contrast, a study in Denmark found that education level was associated with a bell-shaped pattern in participation, where women in the middle range of the educational scale were the most faithful participants (von Euler Chelpin et al., 2008). In Colombia, education level, income, and having health insurance have been shown to increase the probability of undergoing mammography screening (Charry et al., 2008; Avila et al., 2014). These tendencies were also found in a randomized controlled trial in India that explored determinants of participation (Dinshaw et al., 2007). Moreover, in Colombia, illiteracy was associated with a lower probability of undergoing mammography screening (Charry et al., 2008).

(b) Rural and urban residence

A meta-analysis of 28 studies found that the proportion of women who had ever had a mammogram was higher in the urban population than in the rural population in Australia, Canada, and the USA; there were contrasting findings in Northern Ireland and the Republic of Korea (Leung et al., 2014). Even in countries with screening programmes, their availability is not equally distributed among geographical districts, which may influence participation rates. Studies from both the Republic of Korea and the USA found that among rural women, recommendation by health professionals plays a key role in having a mammogram (Hur et al., 2005; Davis et al., 2012). In a study in Sweden, area-level factors, such as rates of employment and of immigration, were important determinants of neighbourhood rates of non-attendance in an urban mammography screening programme (Zackrisson et al., 2007).

Distance between the residence and the screening unit may also influence participation. A British study found a small decrease in participation with increasing distance to the screening unit (Maheswaran et al., 2006). In a study in Quebec, distance from the screening unit affected participation, but the distance at which the decrease started varied according to a rural–urban classification: for women living in small cities, reductions in participation were observed for distances of 12.5 km or more, whereas for women in rural areas, a clear reduction in participation was first seen for distances of 50 km or more (St-Jacques et al., 2013). In low- and middle-income countries, limited access to screening is a major challenge.

(c) Age

The influence of age on participation in screening has to be understood in the context of the screening system, or the lack thereof. Findings on whether age is a predictor of attendance in mammography screening are controversial. Several studies were conducted in women in different age ranges attending opportunistic screening. The younger women were more likely to have a mammogram, in a group of women older than 60 years in the USA (Michielutte et al., 1999), in women within the age range 50–75 years in Canada (Black et al., 2001), or in a group of women older than 65 years in the United Kingdom (Edwards & Jones, 2000). A review about Latinas in the USA found that in general women aged 50–64 years, and particularly in the age range 55–59 years, were more likely to have a mammogram than women aged 40–49 years (Wells & Roetzheim, 2007). Another study in the USA showed that women aged 51–64 years were more likely to have a mammogram than either younger or older women (Rutledge et al., 2001). A further study in the USA suggested that participation in mammography screening is higher in older women; for instance, African-American women aged 70 years and older were less likely to miss their mammography appointments compared with women in their forties (Crump et al., 2000). Other studies concluded that age is not indicative of non-attendance (Banks et al., 2002; Bulliard et al., 2004). [The cut-off age of screening programmes could potentially also explain why some age groups have higher participation rates in specific countries.]

(d) Health and disability

Poor health may inhibit women from participating in breast cancer screening, and lead to lower participation rates compared with women who have fewer health problems (Lostao & Joiner, 2001). However, women with diabetes have been found to have similar screening rates to women without diabetes (Giroux et al., 2000). Barriers such as sociability limitations and physical disabilities (Graham et al., 1998; Ahmed et al., 2009; Andresen et al., 2013) or intellectual disabilities (Taggart et al., 2011; Wilkinson et al., 2011) have been shown to decrease participation in screening. Also, obese women may face barriers to participation (Wee et al., 2000).

Mental health issues may also be a barrier to participation. One study found that non-attenders were significantly more depressed on the Hospital Anxiety and Depression Scale (Burton et al., 1998), and another showed that psychological distress was one of the strongest negative predictors of participation in breast cancer screening (O'Donnell et al., 2010) (see below).

(e) Social support and networks

Social networks may influence women's decision-making about mammography screening, among all socioeconomic groups (Stamler et al., 2000; Fowler, 2006). Different social settings may influence different groups of women. In a study in the USA, African-American women aged 65 years and older who had had a mammogram in the previous year, compared with those who had not, were more likely to have living children and grandchildren and to participate in social activities more frequently (Zhu et al., 2000).

In one study, co-workers were identified as having a strong influence for women older than 50 years, whereas friends and family were identified as being more influential for women in the younger age groups (Stamler et al., 2000). Data from a survey of 260 Samoan women aged 50 years and older in Los Angeles County, USA, over a 20-year period suggested that interpersonal networks may have accounted for the dramatic increase in the rate of adoption of screening within the 5 years preceding the survey (Levy-Storms & Wallace, 2003). Being part of a church-based health communication network appeared to increase the likelihood of having had a recent mammogram (Fox et al., 1998; Levy-Storms & Wallace, 2003). Also, among working Muslim Iranian women, there were suggestions of a link between religious involvement and increased participation in mammography screening (Hatefnia et al., 2010).

(f) Health-care services

Several factors within the health-care service system may influence participation in breast cancer screening. In a study in Canada among three age groups (< 30 years, 30–49 years, and ≥ 50 years), the physician was the most important influence for the different modalities of breast cancer screening in all age groups (Stamler et al., 2000).

In a study in the USA, women who had had a mammogram in the previous year, compared with those who had not, were 3 times as likely to have a regular doctor and about 6 times as likely to have a doctor's recommendation for a mammogram (Zhu et al., 2000).

Satisfaction with services could influence participation in screening. A study in the USA among 397 women undergoing a screening mammogram at three university-affiliated radiology clinics showed the importance of four major components: satisfaction with clinical services, physical experience, psychological experience, and communication with clinical personnel (Tang et al., 2009).

(g) Other barriers

Practical problems, such as being busy at work or at home, forgetting the appointment, or having other more pertinent tasks, may influence participation (Crump et al., 2000; Aro et al., 2001; Tsunematsu et al., 2013). This could affect women in either organized screening or opportunistic screening.

Experiencing or fearing pain during the mammography examination is a barrier to participation for some women (Aro et al., 2001; Papas & Klassen, 2005; Fayanju et al., 2014).

3.1.2 Cultural factors

Cultural understanding of breast cancer and breast cancer screening has been shown to influence women's decisions about participation in screening (Garbers & Chiasson, 2004; Pfeffer, 2004; Yu et al., 2005). Some women's cultural understanding of screening may be contrary to that of health professionals, and may be given priority over medical advice (Rajaram & Rashidi, 1998). In the USA, among 321 inner-city African-Americans, women who were more knowledgeable about cancer and its prevention were more likely to have been appropriately screened (Sung et al., 1997). Lack of knowledge about breast cancer could be related to socioeconomic group and could be a barrier to screening (McDonald et al., 1999; Farmer et al., 2007). However, studies from different cultural contexts as diverse as Nigeria, Turkey, and Chinese immigrants in the USA indicate that more knowledge about breast cancer does not automatically increase screening rates (Yu et al., 2005; Canbulat & Uzun, 2008; Bello et al., 2011). A study among 58 Latinas participating in focus-group interviews showed that women generally perceived breast cancer screening as a risky behaviour because of the many personal and interpersonal consequences associated with the detection of breast cancer (Borrayo et al., 2005).

Strong cultural beliefs of fatalism have been identified as a barrier to screening for Latinas (in Mexico and in the USA). In a literature review of 11 studies, most of them (64%) reported a statistically significant association between fatalism and non-use of cancer screening services among Latinas (Espinosa de Los Monteros & Gallo, 2011). Studies from Israel, Kenya, and the USA have all found that fatalism could be a barrier to screening (Mayo et al., 2001; Peek et al., 2008; Baron-Epel, 2010; Muthoni & Miller, 2010). If cancer is seen as a disease that is curable when detected early, screening can be perceived as worthwhile, but if cancer is seen as always fatal, early diagnosis might be seen as having no value (Straughan & Seow, 2000; Pfeffer, 2004). Moreover, women may experience fear of mastectomy as a barrier to screening participation because loss of a breast might have social consequences (Peek et al., 2008; Bodapati & Babu, 2013).

In late modern societies, discourses on women's participation in mammography screening have been characterized by morality, responsibility, and obligation to participate in available medical examinations (Kaufert, 1996; Klawiter, 2008; Willis, 2008; Solbjør et al., 2012a).

(a) Minority groups and acculturation

Ethnic background itself is not an independent predictor of attendance in mammography screening, but differences in participation have been found between ethnic groups (Consedine, 2012; Edgar et al., 2013). Results about the effect of ethnicity on breast cancer screening are ambiguous. A study from the USA suggested that even when controlling for education and income, some differences exist with ethnicity (Rawl et al., 2000). However, ethnicity is connected to culture, and cultural values and beliefs partially explain differences between ethnic groups. Moreover, the social situation in which women live is often also associated with ethnicity (Lindén-Boström et al., 2010; Flores et al., 2013).

Among immigrant women, the degree of acculturation to the culture into which they have moved could predict health status. Language acculturation has been found to be of specific importance for participation in mammography screening, among immigrant women to the USA from the former Soviet Union (Ivanov et al., 2010) and among Mexican-American women (Suarez & Pulley, 1995). Acculturation was associated with a higher likelihood of having had a recent mammogram, but this effect was not significant when controlling for sociodemographic factors (Abraído-Lanza et al., 2005). Period of residence in the country of immigration influences rates of screening (Ivanov et al., 2010). For Iraqi refugee women, psychosocial aspects, culturally mediated beliefs, and health consequences of war were identified as major barriers to their ability and motivation to obtain breast cancer screening (Saadi et al., 2012).

(b) Worry and perceived risk

There is an association between worry about breast cancer or perceived risk of breast cancer and participation in mammography screening. A meta-analysis of 12 prospective studies that measured worry about breast cancer and screening behaviour among 3342 women concluded that there is a positive relationship between worry about cancer and screening behaviour (Hay et al., 2006). A meta-analysis of 42 studies found an association between perceived risk and mammography screening (Katapodi et al., 2004). Another study found that worry about breast cancer risk appears to be associated with mammography use in a bell-shaped pattern, where women reporting moderate levels of worry were more likely to participate in mammography annually than those who were either mildly or severely worried (Andersen et al., 2003).

3.1.3 Information and understanding

This section addresses the issue of information provided by screening providers to women who are potential participants in screening, and how it may influence screening participation. In many countries, the mass media covers issues related to breast cancer screening and potentially contributes to communicating information on screening to the general public, but it is not included in this section (see Section 3.2 for region-specific data).

(a) Informed decision-making

Breast cancer screening programmes invite women who are presumably free of symptoms to a medical examination. Participation in screening may have both positive and negative effects for individuals, and ethical and legal considerations suggest that women should be fully informed about the benefits, limitations, and harms of a screening process and its aftermath. While some women trust the health authorities with the decision (Østerlie et al., 2008), many women want to make their own informed decision about mammography screening (Hersch et al., 2011). One study in the USA showed that most adults perceive mammography as valuable, probably due partly to decades of screening promotion campaigns (Schwartz et al., 2004). It is important to note that literature and debates on informed decision-making come primarily from high-income countries and that issues in low- and middle-income countries may be different.

The dominant approach to information about cancer screening has emphasized benefits, to improve participation in screening programmes. Many studies have examined how tailored information may increase screening participation (e.g. Champion et al., 1997; Rakowski et al., 1998; Latimer et al., 2005; Williams-Piehota et al., 2005). Albada et al. (2009) reviewed 18 studies of tailored information on mammography screening, and 6 of them reported that educational interventions increased adherence to mammography. [The authors did not assess whether these interventions increased women's informed decision-making.] In a more recent review (Biesecker et al., 2013), 5 of 8 interventions on screening for different diseases were reported to facilitate informed choice. [The Working Group noted that it remained unclear whether this was due to better understanding of information, and the review fell short of explaining the effective components of interventions that facilitate informed choice.]

If autonomy of choice is the leading ethical principle, women should be provided with balanced evidence-based information to enable them to make informed decisions about health care (Barratt, 2008). Several terms, such as "informed decision-making" and "informed choice", have been used to describe this process. Informed choice includes knowledge, attitudes, and test choice, and at least two different scales of measure have been developed to measure informed decision-making (the Multidimensional Measure of Informed Choice and the Decisional Conflict Scale) (Biesecker et al., 2013).

The issue of what constitutes balanced information on screening is subject to debate. Based on 12 articles, "balance" can be defined as "the complete and unbiased presentation of the relevant options and the information about those options – in content and in format – in a way that enables individuals to process this information without bias" (Abhyankar et al., 2013). Presenting information in a side-by-side display form was associated with more users/respondents judging the information as balanced (Abhyankar et al., 2013). However, sometimes patient decision aids may deviate from neutrality to counter pre-existing biases, such as pre-existing values and beliefs (Blumenthal-Barby et al., 2013). An example of pre-existing bias was found about the different recommendations for mammography for women younger than and older than 50 years (Schulz & Meuffels, 2012). The bias was the reluctance to accept that mammography is not usually recommended for women younger than 50 years, which was in contrast to the overwhelming acceptance of breast cancer screening for women older than 50 years. This points towards the difficulty of acceptance of "doing nothing". Balancing information means including the "doing nothing" option (Abhyankar et al., 2013). Others have argued that decisions about mammography screening should be individualized based on patients' risk profiles, preferences, and values (Pace & Keating, 2014). Yet others have argued that designing patient decision aids that lead patients to make a particular choice may be "more ethical" than balanced, nondirective content (Blumenthal-Barby et al., 2013). This controversial standpoint raises questions about who should decide what is the most ethical option, and which information should be provided to women.

Many studies have assessed women's knowledge of the benefits and risks of mammography screening. Text analyses of information material show that women are often not being informed about the likelihood of having a false-positive result, about overdiagnosis and overtreatment (Jørgensen & Gøtzsche, 2004, 2006; Giordano et al., 2005), or about the possibility and implications of a diagnosis of carcinoma in situ (Jørgensen & Gøtzsche, 2004). More recently, in a study in the Netherlands that measured 13 items of knowledge about breast cancer screening, 95% of the 229 respondents were deemed to have sufficient knowledge to make an informed choice about mammography screening; 68% of the women responded correctly on the item of overdiagnosis, and there was 90% consistency between intention to participate (or not) and attitude (van Agt et al., 2012). Other studies have found women to overestimate the benefit of mammography screening and their own risk of breast cancer (Chamot et al., 2001; Domenighetti et al., 2003). Many women who intend to participate in mammography screening believe that breast cancer can be prevented or cured through screening (Vahabi & Gastaldo, 2003). In addition, women of screening age may overestimate the mortality reduction due to mammography screening (Edgar et al., 2013). Women with strong "utility beliefs" in screening were more inclined to participate (Lauver et al., 2003), whereas belief that mammography screening is recommended every 4 years or not at all may lead to deciding not to participate (Chamot et al., 2001). Also, women might believe that mammography will detect all breast cancers, as the visualization technology convinces them of its potential (Solbjør 2008; Griffiths et al., 2010). Beliefs about breast cancer and screening can be seen as a hindrance to making an informed decision (Denberg et al.,

2005). Knowledge about the benefits and negative consequences of mammography screening must be present for women to make an informed choice about participation.

In a literature search in Germany, six studies on screening mammography showed that the majority of women were uninformed about the benefits of screening and the incidence of false-positive and false-negative test results in mammography (Dreier et al., 2012). In a cross-sectional study in south-western Nigeria, where a self-administered questionnaire was used to assess the knowledge, attitudes, and practice of breast cancer screening programmes among nurses in a university teaching hospital and among women in non-health professions, the authors concluded that good knowledge did not imply higher screening rates (Bello et al., 2011). Moreover, in a study in Switzerland, many women were not interested in detailed information about mammography screening that is deemed relevant by public health authorities (Chamot et al., 2005). Women may say "no" to professional recommendations about mammography screening because they see themselves as being at low risk of breast cancer, being their own health experts, and claiming responsibility for their own health, rather than conforming to professional perspectives on health care (Michaels et al., 2008).

Laypeople may conceptualize informed choice differently from policy-makers, and information about the disease could be as important as information about the risks and the limitations of screening (Jepson et al., 2007). Studies in Scandinavia have found that women may trust health authorities to offer relevant screening programmes and thus participate in screening on the basis of receiving an invitation (Forss et al., 2001; Østerlie et al., 2008; Willis, 2008). Moreover, women may see participation as a responsible action, as the morally right thing to do (Crossley, 2002; Pfeffer, 2004). For some women, very strong feelings lead to a reluctance to accept contrary information. For example, women with breast cancer participating in online breast cancer discussion boards were in opposition to the 2009 United States Preventive Services Task Force (USPSTF) recommendation against routine screening mammography for women in their forties (Barker & Galardi, 2011).

Several articles have argued that women must be informed about all possible outcomes of screening mammography, such as having a recall/false-positive result, having breast cancer or ductal carcinoma in situ (DCIS), or overdiagnosis on the population level. Some women express surprise at the possible extent of overdiagnosis (Hersch et al., 2013; Waller et al., 2013). About half of the women in a British study had ever heard of overdiagnosis before being confronted with the term during a survey (Waller et al., 2014). The concept of overdiagnosis was difficult to understand, and the study suggested that brief printed information on overdiagnosis is unlikely to have a major impact on participation in breast screening. Women who received information about the ratio of lives saved to overdiagnoses had a greater decrease in intention to participate than women who received information about the total number of overdiagnoses compared with lives saved in the United Kingdom (Waller et al., 2014). A randomized controlled trial is currently being conducted in Australia to investigate the consequences of providing information about overdetection of breast cancer to women approaching the age of invitation to mammography screening (Hersch et al., 2014). Not knowing about the uncertainties of mammography screening could change women's trust in mammography when they experience a false-negative/interval cancer (Solbjør et al., 2012a). A qualitative study with semi-structured interviews in 10 women diagnosed with DCIS as a result of mammography screening highlighted that the diagnosis had changed the women's information needs and that most of them would have liked to have had more information about DCIS when they were invited to routine screening (Prinjha et al., 2006).

(b) Ways of presenting information

Methods of communicating information are important to ensure that women's information needs are met. Which kind of information should be given to women is the subject of ongoing debate. However, information material has been criticized to be pro-screening and biased (Jørgensen & Gøtzsche, 2004, 2006; Gummersbach et al., 2010). Analyses of online health information have suggested that it is inadequate to support informed decision-making on screening (Burkell & Campbell, 2005). More information about breast cancer is included in brochures from programmes established earlier compared with newer programmes (Zapka et al., 2006).

The manner in which information is provided could also influence whether women will make an informed choice. Whether women prefer numerical or verbal information varies. In a study in Canada, two thirds of participants preferred numerical information, but comprehension was higher among women who received probabilistic information in verbal format (Vahabi, 2010). Numbers for screening effects can be presented as either relative risk reduction or absolute risk reduction. One study analysed how four different scenarios for presentation of data on screening affected women's decision-making and found that respondents indicated a significantly greater willingness to have a test when the benefit of a "new" screening test for breast cancer was expressed as relative risk reduction (88%) rather than either absolute risk reduction (78%) or all-cause mortality (53%) (Davey et al., 2005). Significantly more respondents considered information about absolute risk reduction to be "new" to them (65%) compared with information about relative risk reduction (30%). The results demonstrate that women's willingness as individuals to participate in mammography screening is influenced by how information is framed, and indicate that the quantitative content of information aids must be comprehensive and balanced to promote informed choice (Davey et al., 2005).

For women with low literacy, video material may be a way to communicate information, as has been tried among Latinas (Borrayo, 2004) and Chinese immigrants in the USA (Maxwell et al., 2011). Coleman et al. developed and tested a particular motivational book at a maximum third-grade literacy level, which led to increased knowledge and intent to follow guidelines among pilot participants (Coleman et al., 2003a). In the USA, several pilot studies that used health advisors to reach minority women with information about breast cancer screening have increased knowledge, uptake, and follow-up among Hispanic women (Koval et al., 2006; Fernández et al., 2009), Vietnamese-American women (Bird et al., 1998; Nguyen et al., 2009), Korean-American women (Han et al., 2009), African-American women (Coleman et al., 2003b; Crump et al., 2008), and Chinese-American women (Yu et al., 2007). In a study in Brazil, the mass media was found to be a source of information about breast self-examination (BSE) (Brito et al., 2010).

3.1.4 Psychological consequences of mammography screening

Participation in breast cancer screening could have psychological or psychosocial consequences for women, which are largely dependent on the result of the screening process. This section summarizes the psychological impacts of an invitation to screening, of a negative result, of a diagnosis of breast cancer, and of interval cancer, as well as the impact of a false-positive result on further participation. The psychological consequences of a false-positive result and of DCIS are evaluated in Section 5.3.5.

(a) Psychological consequences of an invitation to screening

Invitation to routine breast screening by itself may affect some women negatively, making them nervous, anxious, or depressed (Johnston et al., 1998). The invitation may also increase women's concern about breast cancer (Scaf-Klomp et al., 1997). However, such impacts of the invitation are not homogeneous. In a sample of 1253 women, the letter of invitation reduced anxiety about breast problems in 39.7%, increased anxiety in 24.6%, and had no appreciable effect in 35.7% (Swanson et al., 1996). A woman's perception of the impact of receiving the letter of invitation and undergoing the screening examination procedure is likely to be related to her previous levels of concern about breast problems.

(b) Psychological consequences of a normal screening result

Women who receive a clear negative result after participation in mammography screening generally have few negative psychological consequences from screening (Sutton et al., 1995; Scaf-Klomp et al., 1997; Lowe et al., 1999; Aro et al., 2000; Meystre-Agustoni et al., 2001) (reviewed by Brett et al., 2005; Hafslund & Nortvedt, 2009).

Some women may feel reassured by a clear negative result, perceiving mammography screening to be a reassuring preventive initiative (Brodersen et al., 2011). A few studies have even suggested improved psychological well-being and reduced anxiety after screening (Dean et al., 1986; Baines et al., 1990; Walker et al., 1994; Bakker et al., 1998), which lasted up to 2 months after screening (Scaf-Klomp et al., 1997) (reviewed by Hafslund & Nortvedt, 2009).

Although most articles report few psychological consequences of screening participation among women who receive a clear negative result, there have been discussions on how to measure anxiety due to participation in breast cancer screening. Questionnaires developed for measuring general psychiatric morbidity may not be able to measure changes among otherwise healthy individuals, and Cockburn et al. (1992) developed and validated a questionnaire (the psychological consequences questionnaire) to measure the psychological consequences of screening mammography. This questionnaire has been used both among the general population undergoing screening and among women who are recalled after mammography (Cockburn et al., 1994; Swanson et al., 1996; Olsson et al., 1999; Meystre-Agustoni et al., 2001; Brodersen et al., 2004). These studies point to small psychological consequences of mammography screening. Swanson et al. (1996) found that the psychological consequences questionnaire was sensitive in measuring changes in anxiety about breast problems, and concluded that screening procedures can either increase or decrease anxiety about breast problems or have no appreciable effect. Therefore, participants in breast screening programmes cannot be considered a homogeneous entity (Swanson et al., 1996).

(c) Psychological consequences of a breast cancer diagnosis

Having a breast cancer diagnosis will likely have psychological and psychosocial consequences. Psychological distress is strongly associated with the diagnostic phase for suspected breast cancer (Montgomery & McCrone, 2010). Being diagnosed with breast cancer after participating in mammography screening for women without symptoms may potentially have specific psychological consequences, but no studies were found comparing the mode of detection and its influence on the psychological aspects of having a breast cancer diagnosis. A qualitative interview study in Denmark found that women who are diagnosed with breast cancer through screening may feel optimistic about the future due to the internalization of arguments about how early detection of breast cancer may save lives (Ryle, 2009).

(d) Psychological consequences of interval cancer

No reviews or other articles were found about psychological consequences of having a false-negative result. However, it was shown that women's experiences with interval breast cancer may affect their trust in mammography screening (Solbjør et al., 2012a). A study in the Netherlands found that breast cancer patients with interval cancers attended the screening programme less often than breast cancer patients with screen-detected tumours, within 5 years as well as more than 5 years after treatment (de Munck et al., 2013). [One possible explanation is that the patients may have been disappointed and therefore reluctant to re-enter the programme.] One qualitative study showed that participation in a mammography screening programme may contribute to a delayed reaction when symptoms are detected between screening rounds (Solbjør et al., 2012b).

(e) Impact of a false-positive result on further participation

Negative psychological consequences of participation in screening may have an impact on further participation in mammography screening. Long-term psychological consequences of having a recall may negatively affect women's experiences at future screening rounds (Lampic et al., 2001) or affect future attendance in mammography screening (Marshall, 1994; Brett & Austoker, 2001; Brett et al., 2005). In their review on long-term effects of false-positive mammography results, Brewer et al. (2007) found that the effect of having a recall influenced women in different countries and within different screening regimes differently. Women in the USA were more likely than women in Europe to return for routine screening mammography after false-positive results. This may be explained by the opt-in system in the USA and the opt-out system in Europe (Brewer et al., 2007). If women opt in for mammography screening, they may already have considered eventualities such as a recall, whereas women who participate in an opt-out screening programme may be more surprised at having a false-positive result. Defrank & Brewer (2010) even suggested that having a false-positive mammography screening result increases women's perceived likelihood of having breast cancer and decreases their belief in test results, and that this will affect further participation in screening mammography. Experiences of false-positive results could lead to non-participation in the future, especially if coupled with a lack of advice on regular screening from the women's physicians (DeFrank et al., 2012). However, a study in Denmark found no significant difference in participation in the subsequent round between women with a false-positive test result and women with a negative test result (Andersen et al., 2008).

3.2 Availability and use of screening programmes

3.2.1 Europe

Breast cancer screening programmes are well established in many European countries. Most have organized programmes, several of which are now more than 25 years old, such as those in Finland, the Netherlands, and the United Kingdom. These programmes shared many aspects of their development from the outset and still have much the same form of delivery. For many years the European Union (EU) funded the European Breast Screening Network (EBSN), which encouraged the establishment of organized programmes and also the dissemination of knowledge from the more established programmes to pilot programmes. In 1993, the EBSN produced the first European guidelines for quality assurance in mammography screening (Kirkpatrick et al., 1993). These guidelines are now in their fourth edition (Perry et al., 2006).

The long-term support from the EBSN, when the screening service was new and needed to be developed in many countries, was a major influence on the common approach that developed across much of Europe. The EBSN included several pilot programmes and an annual meeting. It first focused on the delivery of high-quality screening and then moved on to publish quality standards and guidance for those establishing new programmes. The EBSN facilitated mutual cooperation and understanding, and enabled sharing of experiences about advances in technology and also about understanding of the science and epidemiology of breast screening. This international cooperation was also extended to countries that were not members of the EU, such as Norway and Switzerland, and in recent years was extended to include the countries in central and eastern Europe that had joined the EU.

The Council of the EU agreed on a recommendation on cancer screening in December 2003 (Council of Europe, 2003). This followed on the success of the EBSN, which had been emulated by the cervical cancer screening community and the burgeoning interest in colorectal cancer screening. The Council recommendation included the need to offer evidence-based cancer screening through a systematic population-based approach with quality assurance at all appropriate levels. The recommendation also included the requirement to ensure that the people participating in a screening programme were fully informed about the benefits, limitations, and adverse effects. Mammography screening for breast cancer in women aged 50–69 years in accordance with the European guidelines for quality assurance in mammography screening was then listed as one of the approved tests.

Health is not one of the areas in which the EU determines policy across all Member States. Therefore, the European guidelines for quality assurance in mammography screening are not mandatory, but they are a recognized authoritative view on best practice, with much practical advice for those countries operating, or beginning to operate, breast screening programmes. Member States are free to decide for themselves how to design and deliver the breast screening programmes in each country, and variations in protocols generally reflect societal pressures on the screening programme, the resources available, and the health-care system in which they operate. Thus, where health care is locally led, such as in Belgium, Portugal, and Sweden, the screening programme is run by the county or similar local authority. In the United Kingdom, there are effectively four screening programmes, reflecting the four constituent countries of the United Kingdom. Thus, initiatives to compare data across European countries face difficulties in obtaining comparative data.

(a) Systems, policies, and guidelines

Two Europe-wide surveys were recently carried out under different EU auspices, and Table 3.1 summarizes the key findings reported. The first European survey, published in 2012, described the organization of mammography screening in Europe and presented some basic quality indicators (Giordano et al., 2012a). Data were provided by only 18 of the 29 countries asked to participate; 10 countries provided national data, and the other 8 countries provided only regional data, although some (Portugal, Spain, and Sweden) from more than one regional programme. In 2014, the European Commission Joint Research Centre (JRC) carried out a further survey to prepare for consideration of a Europe-wide quality assurance system for breast cancer care, including screening (Lerda et al., 2014). This included a slightly different group of countries, and 25 of the 30 countries asked to participate provided a response. Whereas the first survey was peer-reviewed and aimed to provide comparative data, the JRC report came with the caveat that the figures were described as indicative only and not for comparison. The JRC report drew

Table 3.1 Policies and practice for breast cancer screening with mammography in Europe

Country, region	Start year	Target age (years)	Interval (years)	No. of mammography views[a]	Double reading?	No. of screening tests per year	Invitation coverage[b] (%)	Examination coverage[c] (%)	Participation rate[d] (%)	References[e]
Austria, Burgenland, Tyrol	Pilot	40–69	1–2	—	—	—	—	—	—	Lerda et al. (2014)
Austria, Vienna-Vorarlberg-Salzburg	Pilot	50–69	1–2	—	—	—	—	—	—	Lerda et al. (2014)
Belgium, Flanders	2001	50–69	2	2	Yes	134 356	82.2	37.4	37.9	Giordano et al. (2012a)
Cyprus	2003	50–69	2	—	—	—	100	65.0	—	Lerda et al. (2014)
Czech Republic	2002	45–69	2	2	Yes	374 157	—	41.0	—	Giordano et al. (2012a)
Denmark, Copenhagen	1992	50–69	2	2/1	Yes	16 987	64.6	46.7	—	Giordano et al. (2012a)
Estonia	2002	50–59	2	2	Yes	20 534	78.3	39.1	50.0	Giordano et al. (2012a)
Finland	1987	50–69	2	—	Yes	211 183	68.4	84.0	87.0	Giordano et al. (2012a), Finnish Cancer Registry (2014)
France	2004	50–74	2	2	Yes	2 361 548	—	52.4	—	Lastier et al. (2013)
Germany, pilot projects	2001	50–70	2	2	Yes	20 097	65.8	34.7	52.8	Giordano et al. (2012a)
Hungary	2002	45–65	2	2	Yes	219 406	75.9	29.0	38.2	Giordano et al. (2012a)
Ireland, east	2000	50–64	2	—	Yes	59 960	87.3	68.4	78.3	Giordano et al. (2012a)
Italy	1990	50–69	2	2/1	Yes	1 072 357	50.9	28.4	56.7	Giordano et al. (2012a)
Latvia	2009	50–69	2	—	—	—	99.0	34.0	—	Lerda et al. (2014)
Lithuania	2005	50–69	2	2	—	—	—	51.4	—	Lerda et al. (2014)
Luxembourg	1992	50–69	2	—	Yes	14 009	93.9	58.5	62.3	Giordano et al. (2012a)
Malta	2009	50–60	3	2	—	—	100	60.0	—	Lerda et al. (2014)
Netherlands	1988	50–75	2	2	Yes	890 837	94.8	78.5	82.6	Giordano et al. (2012a)
Norway	1996	50–69	2	2	Yes	185 389	94.2	72.1	76.6	Giordano et al. (2012a)
Poland	2007	50–69	2	2	No	935 416	115.2	39.4	19.4	Giordano et al. (2012a)
Portugal, centre	1990	45–69	2	2	Yes	73 182	97.4	60.4	62.1	Giordano et al. (2012a)
Portugal, north	1999	45–69	2	2	Yes	32 122	80.2	54.0	67.3	Giordano et al. (2012a)
Slovenia	2008	50–69	2	2/1	—	—	28.0	78.6	—	Lerda et al. (2014)
Spain, Asturias	1991	50–69	2	2	No	40 136	81.8	59.8	73.1	Giordano et al. (2012a)
Spain, Balearic Islands	1990	50–64	2	2	Yes	13 018	54.4	36.9	67.8	Giordano et al. (2012a)

Table 3.1 (continued)

Country, region	Start year	Target age (years)	Interval (years)	No. of mammography views[a]	Double reading?	No. of screening tests per year	Invitation coverage[b] (%)	Examination coverage[c] (%)	Participation rate[d] (%)	References[e]
Spain, Basque Country	1990	50–64	2	2/1	No	76 229	95.0	72.3	76.1	Giordano et al. (2012a)
Spain, Galicia	1992	50–66	2	2	Yes	86 170	84.6	66.7	78.9	Giordano et al. (2012a)
Spain, Navarra	1990	45–69	2	2	No	37 044	103.6	92.1	88.9	Giordano et al. (2012a)
Spain, Valencia	1992	45–69	2	2/1	Yes	209 271	101.9	73.9	72.5	Giordano et al. (2012a)
Sweden, Södermanland	1990	40–74	2	2/1	Yes	21 222	84.6	71.0	84.0	Giordano et al. (2012a)
Sweden, Stockholm	1989	40–69	2	2/1	Yes	76 371	95.5	66.8	70.0	Giordano et al. (2012a)
Sweden, Västmanland	1986	40–69	2	2/1	Yes	19 617	93.7	82.5	88.1	Giordano et al. (2012a)
Switzerland, Fribourg	2004	50–70	2	2/1	Yes	6886	88.7	46.7	44.3	Giordano et al. (2012a)
United Kingdom, England	1988	50–70	3	—	Yes	1 634 688	102.4	78.0	74.2	Giordano et al. (2012a)

[a] 2/1 indicates two views at first screening and one view at subsequent screening.

[b] Annual invitations as percentage of annual target population. Data from Lerda et al. (2014) should be considered mainly as indicative trends, as it was not possible for the authors to ensure that the data were consistently reported by country.

[c] Annual examinations as percentage of annual target population. Data from Lerda et al. (2014) should be considered mainly as indicative trends, as it was not possible for the authors to ensure that the data were consistently reported by country.

[d] Annual examinations as percentage of annual invitations.

[e] Data from Lerda et al. (2014) were provided by national authorities and are generally presented at a national level without the regional details. Data from Giordano et al. (2012a) were provided as part of the European Network for Information on Cancer (EUNICE) project, funded by the European Commission. Contributors were those involved with detailed operations of the screening programmes in their regions and countries. Most countries are represented in both surveys, but data from the Giordano et al. (2012a) survey are preferentially shown where available, as the data are more detailed and have been peer-reviewed. There are some differences between the two data sources, and more information is available on individual countries in the full survey reports.

on the previous work (Giordano et al., 2012a) and provided supplementary information. These surveys reflect the different ways in which breast screening is run in the different countries in Europe, although all aspire to the same quality standard defined in the European guidelines for quality assurance in mammography screening.

In 2007, 26 of the 27 Member States of the EU had breast screening programmes operating, and in 22 of those countries the programme was organized on a population basis (von Karsa et al., 2008). Overall, it has been estimated that screening programmes in those 26 countries offered breast screening by mammography regularly to more than 79% of their eligible populations, with some countries yet to achieve screening over their entire territory. The size of the populations served by a breast screening programme varies from the very large populations of England and France to the much smaller populations of Luxembourg or a Swiss canton. In some of the smallest programmes, fewer than 20 000 women are screened per year. Austria is piloting an organized programme, and Switzerland has local provision of screening, some of which is organized and some of which is opportunistic (Giordano et al., 2012a). Most countries report having a system that is mainly or totally public and that is provided at little or no cost to women, although in 20 countries at least some private sector provision of screening is involved (Lerda et al., 2014). Of the 20 countries with organized screening programmes included in the JRC survey, all reported a degree of national coordination, except for Belgium and Spain (Lerda et al., 2014).

Countries with regional programmes may have health-care decisions that differ between regions. For example, in Spain the different provinces make their own health policy decisions, and the age range for screening depends on where a woman lives (Giordano et al., 2012a).

All breast screening programmes in Europe use mammography, and two views and double reading are standard in most areas. The type of double reading (consensus, arbitration, etc.) varies among the programmes, and there are a few exceptions where a single view and/or single reading are used. France also includes clinical breast examination (CBE) (Lerda et al., 2014), but this is not usual. All countries screen women in the age group 50–59 years, although some start at age 40 or 45 years and most also invite women up to age 69 or 70 years (Giordano et al., 2012a). However, among the services reported, France, the Netherlands, and one county in Sweden (Södermanland) also invite women up to age 74 or 75 years. England, alone in the United Kingdom, is conducting a trial of also offering screening appointments to women aged 47–49 years or 71–73 years (Moser et al., 2011). All countries in Europe screen at 2-year intervals, with the exception of Malta and the United Kingdom, which use a 3-year interval, and there is some scope for annual screening in the pilot in Austria.

Screening for women at high risk of breast cancer at a more intensive level is generally available across Europe. Several European countries (Austria, Germany, Italy, the Netherlands, Norway, and the United Kingdom) have carried out cohort studies on high-risk women using magnetic resonance imaging (MRI) as well as mammography as the screening technique. The European Society of Breast Cancer Specialists has reviewed the evidence and produced consensus guidelines (Sardanelli et al., 2010) taking into account the recommendations from North America (Saslow et al., 2007). High-risk protocols focus on genetic risk (*BRCA1/2* and *TP53* mutation carriers) and family history. Provision of more intense breast screening for survivors of cancers in childhood and young adulthood is generally a local clinical decision. High-risk surveillance protocols have recently been formally incorporated into the screening programme in England (Department of Health, 2013). Recent legislation in some states in the

USA about breast density may influence practice in Europe in the future (see Section 3.2.2).

Across Europe, the switch to digital mammography is well established, but some analogue screen-film mammography sets are still in use. There has been extensive use of computed radiography in some countries, particularly in the early years of digital mammography, when this made the conversion cheaper and potentially quicker to achieve. There have been problems with computed radiography technology in some jurisdictions, and at the same time digital mammography has become more established. Computer-aided detection has not come into general use.

Discussion and research have now moved on to the use of digital breast tomosynthesis. Research trials are under way in some screening programmes to evaluate and assess this technology for routine use. There are some early adopters, but so far no single screening programme has moved to routine use of digital breast tomosynthesis.

The European quality assurance guidelines emphasize that the invitation to screening and initial imaging are only the start of the process. Women with abnormalities will need to have those abnormalities assessed, and any woman with cancer will require treatment. No screening programme encompasses treatment; several, such as the programmes in the United Kingdom, include the diagnostic workup in the programme, but others, such as the programme in the Netherlands, make a referral at that point. In France, the radiologist may undertake ultrasonography and clinical examination at the time of the initial imaging if this is thought to be warranted at that time (Lerda et al., 2014).

Across Europe, the need to deliver breast screening to the requisite quality has been accepted as the appropriate standard of care. Four editions of the European guidelines for quality assurance (Perry et al., 2006) have developed the concept, starting from the quality of the original image, to cover the diagnostic process, including histopathology and the underpinning epidemiology for the programmes. The basic importance of a high-quality image has remained over the years, and there are now guidelines to cover digital mammography, MRI, and the appropriate use of ultrasonography, including input about physics where necessary. Given the difference in population sizes across the different countries in Europe, the quality assurance operation can be regionally or nationally based, but often there is national coordination of data to enable evaluation of the overall activity. This has enabled the Europe-wide surveys to have an overview of the services that are delivered (Giordano et al., 2012a; Lerda et al., 2014).

The European guidelines for quality assurance specify that personnel should hold appropriate professional qualifications, but these vary from one state to another and there are complex EU rules governing recognition of medical and allied qualifications between states. However, universally after initial training, personnel are required to undergo specialist training for work in breast cancer screening, to participate in continuing education and update training, and to participate in any recognized quality assurance schemes. Also, who actually reports the mammogram can vary from one country to another. For example, in the United Kingdom, radiographers have evolved "advanced practice" and can not only report the images but also perform several diagnostic procedures, such as needle biopsies. In contrast, in the United Kingdom there is no role in breast cancer for the gynaecologist, which is standard practice in several other countries in Europe.

(b) Participation

Participation rates in organized programmes are reported to vary from just under 20% in Poland to nearly 90% in the Navarra region of Spain, with an average across Europe of just less than 50% (Giordano et al., 2012a). It is not known how many women are screened outside of the organized programmes (von Karsa et al., 2008). Estimates of opportunistic screening rates were sought in the JRC survey, but of the 22 countries that responded, no information was available for 5 and the rates were regarded as very low in 8 (Lerda et al., 2014). However, the contribution of opportunistic screening was regarded as significant in Austria, Belgium, Cyprus, Finland, France, Italy, Malta, Slovenia, and Switzerland.

Participation in breast cancer screening is influenced by personal, socioeconomic, cultural, and other factors (see Section 3.1). Generally, in Europe, the more affluent a woman, the more likely she is to participate in breast cancer screening (Maheswaran et al., 2006; Moser et al., 2009), whereas ethnic minority status and, particularly, being an immigrant are likely to decrease screening participation (Vermeer & Van den Muijsenbergh, 2010). These factors can be influenced by how the screening offer is made and how access to screening is organized (Palència et al., 2010). A randomized controlled trial in Italy that invited women to screening by different means of communication concluded that invitation letters with a fixed appointment to screening correlated with a higher attendance rate but did not overcome the social gradient in participation (Giordano et al., 2012c). However, a study from 22 European countries found socioeconomic inequalities in screening in countries with opportunistic screening but not in countries with nationwide population-based programmes (Palència et al., 2010). A study in France found that the existence of a screening programme decreased socioeconomic differences in participation, especially in women aged 60 years and older (Duport & Ancelle-Park, 2006). As part of the European initiative on screening participation funded by the European Commission, Molina et al. (2013) reported on social inequalities in participation in cancer screening programmes in Spain.

(c) Information and breast cancer awareness

The information provided to women who are invited to screening has developed a great deal since the early years, when the emphasis was on encouraging or even persuading women to participate. In 1999, Austoker wrote about the need to respect patients' autonomy and not to gloss over the uncertainties and harms, as well as describing the benefits (Austoker, 1999). The United Kingdom moved to an explicit policy of informed choice in 2003, and the fourth edition of the European quality assurance guidelines included, for the first time, a section on communication to support informed decision-making and described four ethical principles: autonomy, non-maleficence, beneficence, and justice (Perry et al., 2006). In reviewing the current state of knowledge on breast screening in Europe, the Euroscreen Working Group discussed how to communicate the issue of balancing benefits and harms in breast screening (Giordano et al., 2012b). One of the points made was that women did not make decisions about whether to participate in screening based solely on the quantitative and evidence-based information provided but also took into account cultural factors and other issues.

In the past 20 years, October has become Breast Cancer Awareness Month in many countries around the world, including most of Europe. Since 2008, 15 October has been designated as Breast Health Day to focus activity even further. Europa Donna, the European Breast Cancer Coalition, has promoted Breast Health Day in all the countries of the EU (Fricker, 2009). In 2014, the National Health Service in England ran a specific campaign to improve awareness about breast cancer in older women because of concern that older women were delaying presentation to their doctor after finding symptoms in their breasts (Grunfeld et al., 2002; NHS Choices, 2014).

3.2.2 North America

This discussion focuses on Canada and the USA.

Breast cancer screening is available and is well established in North America. In both Canada and the USA, some level of organized and opportunistic screening exists, but in Canada breast cancer screening is delivered mostly through organized programmes, whereas in the USA screening is mostly opportunistic. These two countries have unique health systems, and therefore they will be described separately.

(a) Canada

In 1992, the Canadian federal government launched the Canadian Breast Cancer Screening Initiative (CBCSI), which has since been integrated into the Canadian Partnership Against Cancer (CPAC, 2013). Currently, federal funding for the CBCSI is through the Public Health Agency of Canada.

(i) Systems, policies, and guidelines

Among the 13 provinces and territories in Canada, organized breast cancer screening programmes have been initiated in all except Nunavut; British Columbia started its programme in 1988, and the Northwest Territories started its in 2003 (see Table 3.2). Opportunistic screening, typically performed in facilities not participating in the organized programme, is also available in all provinces and territories, and some women who qualify for the organized programme, as well as women in age groups that are not invited to screening, can receive screening mammograms outside of the programme. For example, of the 60% of women aged 50–74 years in Ontario who were screened in 2011–2012, approximately 16% were screened outside of the organized programme (Cancer Quality Council of Ontario, 2014). The Public Health Agency of Canada promotes to the target population the advantages of organized screening compared with opportunistic screening, based on the reliability and quality of a programme that includes population-based recruitment, automatic recall/reminders for subsequent screening, coordinated follow-up for abnormal screening results, systematic quality assurance, and the ability to provide monitoring and evaluation of programme performance (CPAC, 2013). In Canada, there is no cost to women for screening mammography, regardless of whether they are screened in the organized programme or opportunistically.

The Canadian Task Force on Preventive Health Care recommends mammography screening every 2–3 years for women aged 50–74 years (Tonelli et al., 2011), but the provinces and territories set their own screening policies with respect to age, high-risk status, and invitation versus physician referral (Table 3.2). All provinces and territories invite women aged 50–69 years to biennial mammography screening; however, they differ in terms of whether mammography screening is available by invitation or by physician referral for women younger than 50 years and older than 70 years, and also in the type of mammography that is available. Screening mammograms are provided at fixed sites in the larger urban areas, and through mobile mammography for rural and distant communities. Digital mammography is available in Canada, both with digital radiography and with computed radiography, although computed radiography is no longer available in Ontario after evidence demonstrating lower sensitivity led Health Ontario to ban the use of computed radiography for breast cancer screening (Chiarelli et al., 2013; Montgomery, 2013). However, the penetration of digital radiography is highly variable both in the organized programmes and in settings that provide only opportunistic screening. For example, in Newfoundland, all 14 units in the screening centres are digital radiography units, and in Ontario, which accounts for 38% of the population of Canada, digital radiography units account for 95% of the screening

Table 3.2 Policies and practice for breast cancer screening with mammography in North America

Country	Start year	Target age (years)	Interval (years)	Examination coverage[a] (%)
Canada	All provinces invite women aged 50–69 years to biennial screening with 2-view mammography. Policies for other age groups vary by province; see below			47.3
Alberta	1990	40–49	1	7.5[b]
		70–74	2	
		≥ 75	NR	
British Columbia	1988	30–39	PR, NR	56.5
		40–49	1	
		70–79	2	
		≥ 80	PR, NR	
Manitoba	1995	40–49	PR, 2	58.4
		≥ 70	PR, NR	
Nunavut	No programme, but opportunistic screening is available			
New Brunswick	1995	40–49	PR, NR	59.2
		≥ 70	PR, NR	
Newfoundland and Labrador	1996	≥ 70	IPE, NR	40.1
Northwest Territories	2003	40–49	1	28.9
		≥ 70	2	
Nova Scotia	1991	40–49	1	59.9
		≥ 70	NR	
Ontario	1990	30–49	HR, PR, 1	42.5
		70–74	2	
		≥ 75	NR	
Prince Edward Island	1998	30–39	HR, PR, 1	—
		40–49	1	
		70–74	2	
Quebec	1998	35–49	PR, NR	60.1
		≥ 70	PR, NR	
Saskatchewan	1990	70–74	IPE, 2	50.0
		≥ 75	NR	
Yukon	1990	40–49	NR	—
		≥ 70	2	
USA	Mid-1980s	40–49	1	51.3
		50–74	2	

HR, high-risk; IPE, accept if previously enrolled in the screening programme; PR, physician referral; NR, no recall (indicates that women in this age group will be accepted for screening but will not be recalled for subsequent screening).

[a] Canada: women who had a screening mammogram within a 30-month period as percentage of target population, in 2009. USA: women who had a screening mammogram in the previous year as percentage of target population, in 2013.

Data for Canada from CPAC (2013); data for USA from USPSTF (2009) and Smith et al. (2015).

[b] Data for Alberta were collected from the Screen Test programme only, which conducts approximately 10–12% of screening mammograms in the province.

units. In contrast, all screening units in Manitoba are screen-film units. Some of the provinces and territories, such as British Columbia, are transitioning to digital radiography units (Dr Martin J. Yaffe, University of Toronto, Canada, personal communication, 2014).

In the organized screening programmes, the coordination of invitations and recall for screening is managed through a centralized programme or agency (Alberta, British Columbia, Manitoba, Northwest Territories, Nova Scotia, and Saskatchewan), through screening centres (New Brunswick, Newfoundland and Labrador, Ontario, Prince Edward Island, and Yukon), or through regional coordination centres (Quebec) (CPAC, 2014). Women are invited every 2 years, but some women are invited after 1 year, based on age, breast density, family history, and results of previous screening examinations. Five provinces or territories invite women on an annual basis if they have a mammographic density of more than 75% (Newfoundland and Labrador, Northwest Territories, Nova Scotia, Ontario, and Saskatchewan). If the screening mammogram is abnormal, either the screening programme or the woman's primary care provider coordinates follow-up testing (CPAC, 2013, 2014).

Six provinces or territories also have incorporated criteria for referral to MRI for women at high risk (Alberta, British Columbia, Newfoundland and Labrador, Nova Scotia, Ontario, and Prince Edward Island), principally for women who have undergone genetic testing and tested positive for a *BRCA1/2* mutation or other high-risk mutation of known penetrance, or women who had chest irradiation at age 10–30 years (CPAC, 2014).

All provinces have quality assurance programmes that focus on image quality. Most provinces and territories also have requirements for minimum numbers of screening examinations that radiologists should evaluate each year, and most evaluate radiologists' level of performance annually (Prince Edward Island and Yukon are exceptions) (CPAC, 2014). In Alberta, Northwest Territories, and Quebec, the minimum annual volume of mammography examinations is 480–500, which is similar to the minimum volume (480) in the USA under the Mammography Quality Standards Act (MQSA) (FDA, 1992); higher minimum annual volumes are required in Manitoba, Ontario, and Saskatchewan (1000), New Brunswick (1200), Newfoundland and Labrador and Nova Scotia (2000), and British Columbia (2500). In some provinces or territories, both screening and diagnostic examinations are acceptable for minimum volume requirements (Alberta, New Brunswick, and Ontario), whereas in the others, only screening examinations qualify. National targets also exist for screening outcomes on initial and subsequent screening examinations, including abnormal recall rate, invasive cancer detection rate, positive predictive value, proportion of screen-detected invasive cancers of 15 mm or smaller, and interval cancer rates (CPAC, 2013). Six provinces or territories solicit feedback from women undergoing screening about their satisfaction with the process (Alberta, British Columbia, Manitoba, Newfoundland and Labrador, Northwest Territories, and Nova Scotia) (CPAC, 2014).

(ii) Participation

The target participation rate for the breast cancer screening programmes in Canada is 70% attendance of women aged 50–69 years within a 30-month period. The programmes also have target retention rates of 75% for women aged 50–69 years who return for screening within 30 months after an initial screen and of 90% for a subsequent screen (CPAC, 2013). In 2009, 47.3% of women aged 50–69 years had been screened within the previous 30 months, with a range of 7.5% to 60.1% among the organized programmes (Table 3.2). Based on a review of 52 studies of mammography use among Canadian women, Hanson et al. concluded that the most common barriers to screening were ethnic minority status, older age, and concerns about radiation, pain, and embarrassment (Hanson et al., 2009). Lower income, low awareness about breast cancer and breast cancer screening, language and communication difficulties, and living in a rural area were also common barriers. While some studies identified lower educational status as a barrier to screening, others did not, leading to speculation that the expected influence of lower educational status on uptake of screening had been mitigated by programmes targeted at women with lower education levels. The reason reported most frequently by women for having had a recent mammogram was a provider's recommendation.

(iii) Information and breast cancer awareness

Strategies to increase screening uptake in Canada include letters of invitation, mass media campaigns, population-based invitations, and educating physicians to increase referrals to screening. Advocacy groups also provide educational information. On the website of the Canadian Breast Cancer Foundation, there is clear information about the benefits and limitations of mammography, including a discussion about overdiagnosis and advice to be informed about breast cancer screening and to make an informed decision about screening (Canadian Breast Cancer Foundation, 2014).

(b) USA

(i) Systems, policies, and guidelines

In the USA, mammography screening began to become available opportunistically during and after the initiation of the Breast Cancer Detection Demonstration Project by the American Cancer Society (ACS) and the National Cancer Institute (Baker, 1982), after the publication of favourable results from the Health Insurance Plan of Greater New York randomized trial of breast cancer screening (Shapiro et al., 1971). The increase in mammography screening was significantly influenced by advocacy groups and federal and state agencies' promotion of mammography to women and primary care providers during the late 1980s and early 1990s (CDC, 1989), as well as by advocacy groups' efforts to compel state and federal regulations to require mandated coverage of mammography by health insurance plans (CDC, 2000). In 1981, only one state in the USA (Illinois) mandated that health plans cover mammography, but by 2000 the District of Columbia and all but one state (Utah) mandated health insurance reimbursement for mammography screening. Despite state legislation, many women either had no health insurance or had a health plan that was not covered by state law, and thus still faced financial barriers to screening (Trivedi et al., 2008).

Many, but not all, of these shortcomings in coverage were resolved in 2010 by the passage of the Affordable Care Act, which requires that new or altered private health plans fully cover (i.e. no cost sharing) preventive health services, including mammography (Blumenthal & Collins, 2014). Thus, for all women with private health plans, screening mammography in the USA is fully covered. Some low-income women and all adults aged 65 years and older are covered by two federal programmes, Medicaid and Medicare. By statute or agency policy, Medicaid or public assistance programmes in all 50 states and the District of Columbia cover mammography screening for breast cancer either routinely or upon a physician's recommendation. Medicare covers annual mammography for women aged 65 years and older. Under the Affordable Care Act, women living in states that enter into an agreement with the federal government to expand Medicaid will have the same coverage for mammography screening as women with private health plans. However, in 2014 only about half of the states had chosen to expand Medicaid. Under Medicare, coverage for screening mammography every 2 years began in 1991, and coverage for screening mammography annually began in 1998 (NCI, 2013).

Recommendations for breast cancer screening for women at average risk are issued by numerous organizations in the USA, although the dominant guideline development organizations are the ACS and the USPSTF (Smith et al., 2003; USPSTF, 2009). ACS guidelines recommend that women undergo CBE at least every 3 years between age 20 years and age 40 years, and annually afterwards, and that they begin annual mammography at age 40 years and continuing screening until a woman likely will no longer benefit from screening due to poor health conditions. [Note added after the Meeting: These guidelines have recently been updated.] The USPSTF does not recommend CBE, and recommends biennial screening between age 50 years and age 74 years. However, under the Affordable Care Act, the United States Congress requires health plans to cover mammography screening beginning at age 40 years, according to previous USPSTF guidelines (NBCCEDP, 2002). Although neither the ACS nor USPSTF recommends monthly BSE, the majority of physicians in the USA report that they recommend mammography, CBE, and BSE to women aged 40 years and older (Meissner et al., 2011). In addition, considerable deviation from guidelines by health-care professionals is also seen, with either overuse or underuse of mammography (Bynum et al., 2005; Kapp et al., 2010; Leach et al., 2012).

In 2007, the ACS issued guidelines for high-risk women and recommended annual screening mammography and MRI starting at age 30 years for women with a known *BRCA* mutation, women who are untested but have a first-degree relative with a *BRCA* mutation, women with a 20–25% or greater lifetime risk of breast cancer as estimated mainly by family history, or women who had been treated with radiation to the chest for Hodgkin lymphoma between age 10 years and age 30 years (Saslow et al., 2007).

In the USA, mammography quality assurance is governed by the United States Food and Drug Administration under the MQSA (FDA, 1992). Early quality assurance efforts in the USA were strongly influenced by the American College of Radiology's Mammography Accreditation Program, which had the goal of establishing quality standards for mammography and began to accredit mammography facilities in August 1987 (McLelland et al., 1991). To ensure that women could depend on a uniform set of quality standards in all mammography facilities, Congress passed the MQSA in 1992. Under the MQSA, all facilities offering mammography services are required to be accredited by an approved accrediting body, undergo an annual on-site inspection, and be certified by an agency designated by the Secretary of Health and Human Services. The Food and Drug Administration was assigned the task of enforcing the MQSA by establishing standards for personnel, equipment, quality control, record-keeping, regulations, inspection processes, compliance mechanisms, and penalties for failure to comply with the regulations (Fintor et al., 1995). Accreditation must be renewed every 3 years, and on-site inspections by the state health department occur annually. Interpreting physicians must be board-certified in radiology or board-certified with extensive additional training related to radiology, and are required to interpret 960 mammograms over a 24-month period and to receive continuing medical education related to mammography over a 36-month period (FDA, 1992, 2014).

Under MQSA regulations, referring physicians and women undergoing screening must receive a report of the mammography results, and the woman's report should be written in lay language. Recently, 21 states have passed legislation mandating that mammography reports also include communication about breast density if a woman has heterogeneously dense or very dense breast tissue (Are You Dense?, 2013). The legislation is being promoted by the advocacy group Are You Dense? and commonly requires that women with significant breast density be informed on their mammography reports about their breast density, and that women with significant breast density should consider supplemental imaging. Federal legislation has also been introduced, and the National Mammography Quality Assurance Advisory Committee has endorsed adding similar language to the current federal requirements for reporting the results of mammography examinations (National Mammography Quality Assurance Advisory Committee, 2011).

(ii) Participation

In the USA, nearly all breast cancer screening is opportunistic, but it shares various programme elements commonly found in organized screening programmes. Some screening programmes, such as those operated by more integrative health plans and, in particular, the Centers for Disease Control and Prevention's National Breast and Cervical Cancer Early Detection Programme, have a greater degree of organization, but neither meets the level of integration of key elements that distinguishes organized programmes from opportunistic models (NBCCEDP, 2014). In the absence of central registers to provide invitations to screening, a referral from a health-care professional has remained the main reason that women report for having had a recent mammogram (MacDowell et al., 2000).

Mammography is widely available in the USA, although access may be limited by geography in rural and frontier areas and by shortages of units and personnel in some urban areas (D'Orsi et al., 2005; Coughlin et al., 2008; Leung et al., 2014). Availability of mammography is not governed by any central authority, and despite an increasing population, the number of mammography facilities has been declining in recent years. Between 2000 and 2010, the number of mammography facilities and mammography units in the USA declined by 10%, and the median county mammography capacity declined by 20%, from 1.77 to 1.42 mammography machines per 10 000 women aged 40 years and older (Elkin et al., 2013). Geographical variation in capacity and declines in capacity were associated with demographic, socioeconomic, and health-care market characteristics. Specifically, counties with a higher percentage of uninsured population, lower education levels, and higher population density had a lower mammography capacity.

Uptake of mammography was fairly rapid in the period from 1985 to 1989, and by 1990 a summary of seven studies demonstrated that between 25% and 41% of non-Hispanic White women aged 50–74 years reported having had a mammogram in the previous year (NCI, 1990). Data from the National Health Interview Survey in 2013 showed that 51.3% of American women aged 40 years and older reported having had a mammogram in the previous 12 months, revealing that there had been little change in breast cancer screening rates among American women since 2005, when 51.2% of women aged 40 years and older reported having had a mammogram in the previous year (Smith et al., 2015). Breast cancer screening rates differed by ethnicity, ranging from 45.9% in Hispanic women to 52.6% in non-Hispanic Black women, and screening rates among the insured (54.8%) were more than twice those among the uninsured (22.3%).

(iii) Information and breast cancer awareness

In the USA there are numerous opportunities for women to acquire information in various forms (websites, educational materials, public service announcements, etc.) about the benefits, limitations, and harms associated with breast cancer screening. Educational efforts are supported by federal and state health agencies, nongovernmental organizations (NGOs), health plans, and health service providers (American Cancer Society, 2014; CDC, 2014; Susan G. Komen, 2014). Guidelines commonly recommend mammography but also emphasize that women should be informed about screening mammography and that referring physicians should support shared and informed decision-making. However, the content of this information commonly differs in terms of the detail and thoroughness on key aspects of the benefits, limitations, and harms associated with breast cancer screening.

3.2.3 Latin America

Latin America includes Central America, South America, and the Spanish-speaking countries of the Caribbean. It is characterized by disparities in social and health service development, not only between countries but also within countries. These conditions, and particularly contextual factors related to health system organization and financing, strongly influence the implementation and performance of breast cancer screening (Akinyemiju, 2012).

Some of the countries with the highest per capita gross domestic product (GDP) in the region, such as Argentina, Brazil, and Uruguay, have high breast cancer incidence rates (age-standardized rate, ≥ 60 per 100 000), whereas countries with similar GDPs, such as Chile, Mexico, and Venezuela, have lower incidence rates (age-standardized rate, 35–41 per 100 000) (Ferlay et al., 2012; PAHO, 2012). There are large differences between countries in health system development; in some countries, such as Paraguay, about 80% of the population is without health coverage or insurance, whereas other countries, such as Cuba, report 100% health coverage (PAHO, 2012).

Despite differences in the definition of health system coverage, most countries in the region report social security systems with coverage for workers and their relatives, but only a few countries have implemented substantial complementary health-care coverage through insurance plans not only for workers but for the entire population; Chile, Colombia, Costa Rica, and Puerto Rico have reached more than 90% of their citizens, Peru about 60%, and Mexico about 40% (PAHO, 2012). However, the package of services included in these insurance plans varies enormously; consequently, specific insurance plans for cancer treatment have been implemented in some countries, such as Mexico, Peru, and Uruguay, but not in all countries (PAHO, 2012).

(a) Systems, policies, and guidelines

With the exception of Venezuela, all of the Latin American countries in which breast cancer is the leading cause of cancer mortality among women have developed recommendations or guidelines for early detection; however, currently no country in the region meets all the criteria of organized programmes. Cuba, El Salvador, and Peru have also developed national recommendations, despite the fact that breast cancer is not the leading cause of cancer mortality among women in those countries (Ferlay et al., 2012; PAHO, 2013). The available recommendations are summarized in Table 3.3.

Of the 13 countries with national recommendations, 6 include BSE as one of the strategies for breast cancer control, 10 include CBE, and 12 include mammography as the basic component for screening, but only 3 (Colombia, El Salvador, and Peru) specify two-view mammography in the available guidelines.

Although the basic screening strategies are similar, there are some differences between the Latin American countries in the age range and the frequency of examination. El Salvador, Panama, and Peru recommend BSE to all women after menarche, whereas the remaining countries recommend BSE for adult women, except for Cuba, which recommends starting BSE at age 30 years. The largest variability is seen for CBE: three countries recommend starting CBE at age 40 years, three recommend starting during the thirties, two recommend starting during the twenties, and the remaining two countries recommend CBE for all women after menarche. The observed differences between countries, and particularly the recommendation of BSE and CBE for all women, may indicate that those strategies

Table 3.3 Policies and practice for breast cancer screening in Latin America

Country	National recommendation or guideline[a]			Mammography units per million women aged 50–69 years in 2013[b]
	Screening practice	Target age (years)	Interval (years)	
Argentina	CBE	40–50	1	
	Mammography	50–70	2	—
Brazil	CBE	40–69	1	
	Mammography[c]	50–69	2	—
Chile	Mammography	50–74	2	32.2[d]
Colombia[e]	CBE	≥ 40	1	
	Mammography	50–69	2	—
Costa Rica	Mammography	≥ 40	1	150.3
Cuba	BSE[f]	≥ 30	—	
	CBE	≥ 30	1	
	Mammography	50–64	3	15.6[b]
Dominican Republic	BSE	≥ 18	Monthly	
	CBE	≥ 35	Any contact with health provider	
	Mammography	≥ 35	35–40: 2 > 40: 1	—
El Salvador	BSE	All women	Monthly	70
	CBE	All women	Any contact with health provider	
Mexico	BSE	≥ 20	Monthly	
	CBE	≥ 25	1	
	Mammography	40–69	2	74.5
Panama	BSE	All women	Monthly	
	CBE	All women	Any contact with health provider	
	Mammography	≥ 35	35: baseline 40–50: 1–2 > 50: 1	278.5
Peru[g]	BSE	All women	Monthly	
	CBE	≥ 30	1	
	Mammography	≥ 40	1	—
Puerto Rico	Mammography	50–74	2	—
Uruguay	CBE	≥ 20	20–39: 3 ≥ 40: 1	
	Mammography	≥ 40	1–2	172.4

[a] PAHO (2013).
[b] WHO (2014).
[c] In women with a family history of breast cancer, mammography is annual, starting at age 35 years.
[d] Restricted to the public sector.
[e] Updated from Ministerio de Salud y Protección Social (2013).
[f] Ortíz-Martínez et al. (2005).
[g] INEN (2008).
BSE, breast self-examination; CBE, clinical breast examination.

are not necessarily considered as screening techniques with false-positive and false-negative results but rather as complementary actions for general women's health care, a hypothesis that is reinforced by the fact that no specific indications about quality control or impact evaluation were found.

For mammography, six countries recommend beginning screening at age 50 years, four at age 40 years, and two during the thirties. The recommendation to provide mammography screening for women before age 50 years, and before age 40 years in the Dominican Republic and Panama, may be influenced by the relevant percentage of cases in this age group in most Latin American countries. Like for BSE and CBE, despite the widespread existence of recommendations, not all countries seem to have developed evidence-based guidelines, and even among those with this tool, such as Chile, Colombia, and Mexico, the final indication for mammography screening differs, with only Colombia including an economic evaluation to establish recommendations (Secretaría de Salud de México, 2008; Ministerio de Salud de Chile, 2011; Ministerio de Salud y Protección Social, 2013). The situation described here does not take into account guidelines developed by scientific societies and other organizations outside of national governments.

With regard to high-risk women, Colombia and Mexico provide specific recommendations in the available guidelines, with a clear definition of risk categories and screening based on MRI (Secretaría de Salud de México, 2008; Ministerio de Salud y Protección Social, 2013). Peru describes risk factors for breast cancer, but no specific definition of high-risk women is presented; in addition, recommendations for high-risk women aged 35 years and older are the same as those for women at average risk aged 40 years and older (INEN, 2008). In contrast, Chile recommends using validated risk scales, but no specific recommendation for screening of high-risk women is presented (Ministerio de Salud de Chile, 2011).

Information on health service availability and supply is scarce in Latin American countries. Some data show the highest rates of mammography units per million women aged 50–69 years in Panama, Uruguay, and Costa Rica (278.5, 172.4, and 150.3, respectively) and the lowest in Cuba and Paraguay (15.6 and 7.3, respectively; information restricted to the public sector) (WHO, 2014); the low availability of mammography units in some countries may be related to low participation rates despite the declaration of universal health coverage, such as in Cuba. A survey conducted among 30 surgical associations and breast surgery societies in 18 Latin American countries showed that more than 53% of surgeons lack specific training in breast care and that less than 50% have a sufficient number of cases per month to warrant proper expertise (Acuna et al., 2014).

Latin American countries have made progress in policy definition for breast cancer control, mainly concerning technical standards, access to screening, diagnosis and treatment, resource allocation, and training of personnel (González-Robledo et al., 2010, 2013). Progress on this issue does not necessarily result in programme implementation and performance; indeed, although Uruguay has better indicators for breast care access, more structured policies and regulations are seen in Argentina, Brazil, Colombia, and Mexico (González-Robledo et al., 2010). Similarly, although Chile does not have strong indicators (mammography units per million women, 32.2) (WHO, 2014), it has implemented one of the most comprehensive policies in Latin America, including a law on guarantees for health that defines, among other health conditions, specific ages and conditions for access to breast cancer diagnosis and treatment (González Robledo et al., 2010).

All of the above-mentioned screening guidelines and recommendations include general indications about mammography quality assurance, but no specific guidance is provided and no mention of CBE is made. Argentina, Brazil, and Colombia have published guidelines for mammography quality control (INCA, 2007; Blanco et al., 2010; INC, 2011), and the International Atomic Energy Agency has designed a quality control programme for mammography oriented specifically to Latin American countries (IAEA, 2006). No quality control programme has yet been implemented in Argentina (Viniegra et al., 2010).

A report from Colombia showed results from 39 centres in 6 capital cities where the quality control protocol was implemented. The evaluation included equipment and facilities, processes, and film quality. On average, general compliance with standards for screen-film mammography was 59.4%, with the highest compliance for glandular dose (94.7%) and the lowest compliance for image quality and facility conditions for image reading (Alejo-Martínez et al., 2013). In the same way, data from 35 mammography centres in Goiânia, Brazil, revealed an improvement in compliance with quality standards from 64.1% in 2007 to 77.1% in 2009; 80% of centres met the standard for glandular dose, thus indicating a positive effect of the quality control programme (Corrêa et al., 2012). Another evaluation, carried out in five mammography services in Mexico City, showed general compliance of between 52% and 82%, with critical failure points in the film-processing darkroom and viewboxes but 100% compliance in glandular dose. The clinical image reviewed by an external expert panel showed poor quality and low reading agreement (Brandan et al., 2004). Despite the satisfactory results for glandular dose, a recent study by the International Atomic Energy Agency in 13 Latin American countries that analysed more than 2000 patient doses found that 15–19% of craniocaudal views and 23–26% of mediolateral oblique views reported values above the 3 mGy standard; in addition, five countries had diagnostic levels above this limit, suggesting that improvement in process safety, monitoring, and evaluation is highly desirable (Mora et al., 2014).

(b) Participation

During the past decade, at least five countries have reported information on breast cancer screening uptake from national probabilistic surveys, and five more were included in the World Health Survey of 2003 (Table 3.4; WHO, 2005; Gobierno de El Salvador, 2009; Gobierno de Chile, 2011; Minsal, 2011; Profamilia, 2011; INSP, 2012; Torres-Mejía et al., 2013).

Most surveys have been focused on mammography, with only two countries that collected information on BSE, and only one on CBE. Data on mammography use differ in terms of year of collection, age of surveyed population, and definition of coverage. The World Health Survey conducted in 2003 obtained information from six Latin American countries (the report on the topic for Guatemala is not available) (WHO, 2005). Brazil and Uruguay presented the highest uptake in the region, and, similarly, Argentina reported 54.2% coverage in 2011 (Minsal, 2011). According to the available information, the coverage of mammography screening in these three countries is more than twice that observed for other countries with existing data, except for Chile, which has an intermediate coverage of 36.2% (Gobierno de Chile, 2011). As previously stated, these countries have the highest breast cancer incidence rates in the region, and Chile has one of the most organized health systems in Latin America, as well as suitable development of policies for cancer control.

Across all Latin American countries, about 80% of the population is urban, and, in general, women living in urban areas have a higher participation rate in screening than those living in rural areas (Table 3.4), probably due to deficiencies in health system development (Goss et al., 2013). In addition, data from Colombia show that breast cancer mortality is concentrated in large urban centres, indicating a greater need for action in

Table 3.4 Coverage of breast cancer screening in Latin America

Country	Target age (years)	Coverage definition[a]	Year of survey	Examination coverage[b] (%)			Richest-to-poorest ratio[c]
				Urban	Rural	Total	
Mammography alone							
Argentina	≥ 40	Within past 2 years	2011	NR	NR	54.2	1.5
Chile	45–64	Within past 5 years	2010	NR	NR	36.2	
Colombia	40–69	Within past 2 years	2010	21.3	5.4	18.0	15.5
Mexico	50–69	Within past 2 years	2012	32.3	17.7	21.0	
Mammography or CBE							
Brazil	40–69	Within past 3 years	2003	50.4	28.8	47.1	3.4
Dominican Republic	40–69	Within past 3 years	2003	19.1	15.2	17.6	1.9
Ecuador	40–69	Within past 3 years	2003	13.4	5.6	10.8	1.8
Paraguay	40–69	Within past 3 years	2003	18.9	6.2	13.7	12.3
Uruguay	40–69	Within past 3 years	2003	55.8	41.4	54.7	2.1
Mammography or ultrasonography							
El Salvador	40–49	Within past 2 years	2008	32.4	12.4	24.3	11.7
CBE only							
Colombia	≥ 35	Within past year	2010	24.0	14.6	24.3	2.6
BSE only							
Colombia	18–69	Monthly practice within past year	2010	25.8	18.0	24.2	2.2
El Salvador	15–49	Monthly practice	2008	17.9	8.8	14.0	

[a] Definition of coverage indicates the history of screening activities within a given period preceding the corresponding survey.

[b] Number of women reporting undergoing screening examination within the coverage period as percentage of total number of women in the target population.

[c] Differential coverage between the highest income level and the lowest income level. Caution is advised when comparing ratios, as the definition of income levels varies between countries.

BSE, breast self-examination; CBE, clinical breast examination; NR, not reported.

Compiled by the Working Group. Data adapted from WHO (2005), Gobierno de El Salvador (2009), Gobierno de Chile (2011), Minsal (2011), Profamilia (2011), INSP (2012), Torres-Mejía et al. (2013).

these zones (Piñeros-Petersen et al., 2010); as the data were adjusted and breast cancer is the only malignant neoplasm with such a geographical distribution, this suggests that the finding is due not to registration bias but rather to a lack of proper response from the health system.

Uruguay reports comparable coverage for women aged 40–49 years and those aged 50–69 years (57.1% and 52.7%, respectively) (WHO, 2005), but Mexico shows a significantly lower coverage for women aged 40–49 years than for those aged 50–69 years (17.2% and 29.4%, respectively) (INSP, 2012; Torres-Mejía et al., 2013).

The richest-to-poorest ratio as an indicator of social disparities in access to breast cancer early detection deserves special mention. Comparisons merit cautious analysis since definitions of income strata differ between country reports, both in number and in interval limits; however, the large gap between the highest and lowest income strata for Colombia, El Salvador, and Paraguay clearly indicates important social inequalities in access to screening, in spite of the expected gradient between income levels (Table 3.4). Additional studies in Colombia found similar results regarding income and education, but data on the effect of insurance plan or type of affiliation to the health system are contradictory (Charry et al., 2008; Piñeros et al., 2011). Reports from Brazil and Mexico reveal similar results, but in the case of Brazil, racial inequalities have been observed in local analysis (Dias-da-Costa et al., 2007; Lages et al., 2012), and in Mexico affiliation to the health system is associated with better access (Agudelo Botero, 2013). From a different perspective, a report from Argentina showed a reduction in social disparities when data from the 2005 and 2009 National Surveys of Risk Factors were compared (De Maio et al., 2012).

National surveys from Chile and Colombia reported relevant information on the issue of access to diagnosis and treatment after screening. In 2010, almost 98% of Colombian women received mammography results and about one half of women with abnormal mammography findings underwent biopsy (Profamilia, 2011); since no information is available on specific mammography findings, it is not possible to establish whether these data represent improper access or overuse of confirmatory diagnosis. In 2011, Chile reported that about 17% of screen-positive women had no diagnostic follow-up procedures or treatment (Gobierno de Chile, 2011). In addition, two reports from different cities in Brazil showed a significant delay between clinical suspicion and confirmatory diagnosis, with a median time of 3–6 months (Trufelli et al., 2008; Soares et al., 2012); furthermore, a significant correlation was found between stage IV disease and longer elapsed time between mammography and final biopsy results. Likewise, two reports from Colombia showed that the majority of women (65.9%) sought medical attention within 1 month after initial symptoms or abnormal mammography, whereas the median time between initial consultation and beginning of treatment was 137 days (Piñeros et al., 2009, 2011). A report from Mexico showed median times of 4.6 months from consultation to diagnosis and 5.2 months from diagnosis to beginning of treatment (Bright et al., 2011). Despite the fact that the study population may not be representative of the entirety of breast cancer cases for the given countries, data were obtained from reference institutions in Brazil and Mexico, and the study in Colombia recruited more than 1000 cases in 17 oncology centres in Bogotá.

(c) *Information and breast cancer awareness*

Among countries with data on BSE, El Salvador reported that 81.5% of women aged 15–49 years received information about breast cancer and that 44.7% of them were thought to perform BSE (Gobierno de El Salvador, 2009); the knowledge level and teaching activity were higher among women living in urban areas and among older women. Similarly, Colombia reported that 90.3% of women aged 50–69 years had knowledge of BSE, particularly those living in urban areas and those with higher education levels, with no major differences within that age range (Profamilia, 2011).

Numerous initiatives aimed at increasing knowledge of breast cancer and screening, as well as initiatives led by NGOs, may be identified in the media (particularly in Brazil); however, scarce information on the impact of these efforts was found in the scientific literature. A study conducted in a municipality in Brazil found that the mass media was the most frequent source of information about BSE; the level of knowledge on the topic (> 68%) was similar to that found in other surveys conducted in different cities in Brazil (Brito et al., 2010).

Most recommendations and guidelines in the region mention the necessity of information, communication, and education to encourage participation in breast cancer screening; however, none of them develops specific guidance on the topic, and only the Mexican guidelines explicitly recommend providing information on adverse events to all women undergoing screening (Secretaría de Salud de México, 2008).

Several actions have been implemented in Latin American countries in an attempt to improve breast cancer screening. Besides programme development, research on factors associated with screening uptake and adherence as well as intervention studies have increased in number and quality in the region.

In Peru, a pilot study is being conducted in a northern region with community health workers educating women aged 40–64 years about awareness of breast cancer symptoms, trained midwives performing CBE, and local trained physicians conducting fine-needle aspiration biopsy. Women with positive biopsies are referred for full evaluation and treatment (Goss et al., 2013). In Colombia, a pilot study has been implemented in a cluster randomized trial comparing organized hospital-based screening with regular care; for the intervention arm, all women aged 50–69 years attending health services on their own were invited to breast cancer screening, general practitioners were trained on CBE and mammography screening, and a quality control programme and follow-up were implemented for both CBE and mammography (Murillo et al., 2008). In Brazil, a centralized model of multidisciplinary and comprehensive breast care was implemented in Porto Alegre, where control of screening adherence and strict follow-up of positive results are crucial components of the intervention (Caleffi et al., 2009). No results from these studies have yet been reported, but preliminary data from Colombia showed a higher screening uptake and a higher proportion of early breast cancer in the intervention group (Thomas et al., 2013).

3.2.4 Sub-Saharan Africa

Cancer remains a low priority for much of the population in sub-Saharan Africa, an area that refers to the combined regions of Central Africa, East Africa, Southern Africa, and West Africa. In many countries in sub-Saharan Africa, many barriers to breast cancer screening exist, such as lack of infrastructure, inadequate training and expertise, inequitable distribution of services in urban versus rural areas, and poverty. Sociocultural influences, including use of traditional medicines, also work against the development of population-based breast cancer screening programmes.

NGOs are important resources for many countries in this region, as they partner with governments with the goal of reducing cancer mortality, often by promoting early detection, diagnosis, and treatment, and reducing the stigma that often surrounds a cancer diagnosis (Oluwole & Kraemer, 2013).

This section discusses systems, policies, and guidelines within the four regions, where data were available (Table 3.5). Data on participation

Table 3.5 Policies and practice for breast cancer screening in sub-Saharan Africa

Country	National recommendation or guideline			Mammography units per million women aged 50–69 years in 2013[a]	Support organization	References
	Screening practice	Target age (years)	Interval (years)			
Kenya	Awareness	All women	Not stated	6.8[b]	Kenyan Ministry of Health	Kenyan Ministry of Health (2014)
Mauritius	BSE CBE	All women ≥ 30	Not stated Not stated	49.7	Mauritius Ministry of Health	Republic of Mauritius (2014)
South Africa	BSE CBE Mammography	All women All women ≥ 40	Monthly "Regular" (unspecified) 1	7.8	NGO: Cancer Association of South Africa	CANSA (2014a)
Swaziland	BSE CBE Mammography	All women All women ≥ 40	Monthly Not stated 1	33.6	NGO: Swaziland Breast Cancer Network	Swaziland Breast Cancer Network (2008)
Zimbabwe	BSE	≥ 18	Monthly	6.9	NGO: Cancer Association of Zimbabwe	Cancer Association of Zimbabwe (2014)

[a] WHO (2014).
[b] Restricted to the public sector.
BSE, breast self-examination; CBE, clinical breast examination; NGO, nongovernmental organization.

rates in screening programmes are non-existent; where available, cross-sectional studies of any screening or early detection behaviours are discussed.

(a) *Central Africa*

Central Africa includes Angola, Cameroon, the Central African Republic, Chad, Congo, the Democratic Republic of the Congo, Equatorial Guinea, and Gabon.

(i) *Systems, policies, and guidelines*

No data were found on breast screening policies or practices for these countries.

(ii) *Participation*

In Cameroon, a 2011 retrospective study examined the medical records of 531 breast cancer patients diagnosed at Yaoundé Medical Hospital between 1989 and 2009. Self-detection was the mode of detection in 95.3% of patients, and only 2.9% of patients were diagnosed via mammography or CBE (Kemfang Ngowa et al., 2011). A study that interviewed 20 women presenting with late-stage cancer at Yaoundé General Hospital found that the main reasons for delay in seeking medical care were inability to pay, inadequate diagnosis by general doctors, cultural factors including a fatalistic attitude after a diagnosis of cancer, and lack of knowledge about breast cancer (Ekortarl et al., 2007). Compounding these issues is the fact that treatment for breast cancer is often inaccessible for many women (Price et al., 2012). A cross-sectional survey in Cameroon of 120 women in 2012 reported that although 74.2% of women had heard of BSE, 40% had never performed it (Suh et al., 2012).

(iii) *Information and breast cancer awareness*

Although there are no government guidelines on breast screening in Cameroon, periodic mass campaigns for breast health awareness and CBE are organized by the Ministry of Health (Kemfang Ngowa et al., 2011). A cross-sectional survey of women in Cameroon found that knowledge of preventive measures and risk factors was poor (Suh et al., 2012). Solidarité Chimiothérapie

(SOCHIMIO), a Cameroonian NGO affiliated with the Union for International Cancer Control (UICC), has initiated several cancer research projects in Cameroon. These are aimed primarily at providing therapeutic care to cancer patients, but educational outreach programmes have also been implemented (SOCHIMIO, 2014).

A recent publication from the Democratic Republic of the Congo reported use of the Breast Health Global Initiative guidelines in implementing a breast cancer awareness campaign in Kinshasa in 2010–2012, based on BSE and CBE by trained health-care workers (Luyeye Mvila et al., 2014). Participating women underwent CBE; in the case of suspicious findings, they underwent mammography and ultrasonography, and where necessary a needle biopsy. This campaign increased the awareness of breast cancer diagnosis and treatment.

(b) East Africa

East Africa comprises Burundi, Comoros, Djibouti, Eritrea, Ethiopia, Kenya, Madagascar, Malawi, Mauritius, Mozambique, Rwanda, Somalia, Uganda, the United Republic of Tanzania, Zambia, and Zimbabwe.

(i) Systems, policies, and guidelines

No data were found on breast screening policies or practices for the majority of countries in East Africa. Historically, medical resources have been focused on infectious diseases, and the resources allocated to breast cancer detection, diagnosis, and treatment have been very limited (Dye et al., 2010). It has been suggested that BSE could be promoted as a screening method for early detection of breast cancer (Azage et al., 2013).

In recognition of the need to develop formal guidelines, a report by the Kenyan Ministry of Health called for enhanced health promotion and education as well as improved early detection by introducing or expanding screening programmes and by developing guidelines for screening and early cancer detection (Kenyan Ministry of Health, 2014). However, many of these initiatives have yet to be implemented (Matheka, 2014). Health workers have been proposed as a link between the general population and access to care, especially in rural areas (Mutebi et al., 2013).

In Madagascar, breast screening is implemented primarily by NGOs. In 2010, the Akbaraly Foundation launched the 4aWomen project, which aims to improve the management of breast cancer screening and treatment (Akbaraly Foundation, 2014).

In Malawi, there are no government guidelines on breast cancer screening, and mammography screening is available in only one private hospital (Msyamboza et al., 2012).

Mauritius is one of the few countries in the region with formal guidelines on breast cancer screening. Mauritius developed a National Cancer Control Programme for 2010–2014 and recommended breast health awareness campaigns encouraging BSE for all women and CBE for women aged 30 years and older. Population-based screening mammography was not thought to be advisable, given the relatively high proportion of cancers in women younger than 45 years (Republic of Mauritius, 2014).

In Uganda, the limited health-care budget and resources are directed towards fighting communicable diseases (Galukande & Kiguli-Malwadde, 2010). In addition, the average age of onset of breast cancer is low, and there is a lack of mammography units (only two in government and two in private health units) and of trained personnel (42 radiologists) (Monu et al., 2012). Galukande & Kiguli-Malwadde (2010) thus commented on the greater availability and lower cost of ultrasonography as a potential breast cancer screening tool (Galukande & Kiguli-Malwadde, 2010). Although there is some government-subsidized health care, the majority of the population has to self-fund care. Consequently, the Breast Cancer Guidelines for Uganda (written by a team of oncologists, surgeons, and radiologists from Kampala) recommended BSE for its practicability and affordability (Gakwaya et al., 2008).

There are no formal screening guidelines in Zimbabwe, but several non-profit organizations such as the Cancer Association of Zimbabwe recommend breast health awareness and monthly BSE for women aged 18 years and older (Cancer Association of Zimbabwe, 2014). The Zimbabwean Ministry of Health set national goals for cancer prevention and control for 2014–2018, including a reduction of late-stage breast cancer presentation from 80% to 50% by 2018 (Ministry of Health and Child Care of Zimbabwe, 2013).

(ii) Participation

As in other countries in sub-Saharan Africa, in this region women with symptoms of breast cancer do not seek medical attention, leading to late-stage presentation and poor prognosis. Qualitative studies of women in this region report a variety of barriers to seeking early diagnosis or participating in screening.

Data from 69 breast cancer patients in Ethiopia showed that even among women who are aware of breast cancer, early signs and symptoms are frequently ignored and traditional healers are preferred; study participants indicated that stigmatization and social isolation complicate discussion and action around breast cancer (De Ver Dye et al., 2011).

A 2012 study of 390 health workers in northwestern Ethiopia found that 37% of respondents had ever practised BSE and that 14.4% practised it regularly. The main reasons for not performing regular BSE were not having problems with breasts (53.2%), not knowing the technique (30.6%), and not knowing its importance (21.4%); having knowledge of the importance of BSE was a predictor of BSE practice (Azage et al., 2013).

A qualitative study of women in Kenya reported differences between rural and urban women with respect to knowledge of symptoms and the importance of breast screening. The majority of women were fatalistic about the disease and assumed it to be incurable (Muthoni & Miller, 2010).

In Zimbabwe, a series of barriers to breast cancer screening and other cancer screening were identified. These included lack of access to early detection; inadequate resources, equipment, and technology; lack of education and awareness of the importance of regular cancer screening; prohibitive costs of screening services; and lack of referral of patients (Ministry of Health and Child Care of Zimbabwe, 2013).

(iii) Information and breast cancer awareness

A study in Kenya, designed to improve knowledge and awareness among health workers in a hospital in Nairobi using an abbreviated training intervention, reported that knowledge and practical skills related to CBE were low initially but improved significantly after the intervention (Mutebi et al., 2013). Several NGOs in Kenya, such as Cancer Free Women, support a variety of awareness and education campaigns, including teaching BSE and symptoms of breast cancer to Kenyan women (Cancer Free Women, 2013).

In Madagascar, a variety of NGOs provide preventive care initiatives and education and awareness campaigns (Akbaraly Foundation, 2014).

In Rwanda, the NGO Breast Cancer Initiative East Africa launched a month-long campaign in Kigali to provide free CBE to women and to educate both women and their partners about the importance of cancer awareness (Republic of Rwanda Ministry of Health, 2014).

In Zimbabwe, NGOs run a variety of awareness programmes to inform women about cancer prevention strategies and cancer screening procedures (Cancer Association of Zimbabwe, 2014).

(c) Southern Africa

This area comprises Botswana, Lesotho, Namibia, South Africa, and Swaziland.

(i) Systems, policies, and guidelines

No data were found on breast screening policies or practices for Southern African countries, with the exception of South Africa and Swaziland. In South Africa, the public sector health service emphasizes community-level health care, complemented by a hierarchical referral system through district hospitals. Breast cancer symptoms are usually detected by cancer patients rather than via screening. Patients attend primary health-care clinics and are then referred to secondary- and tertiary-level clinics and hospitals for diagnosis and treatment. Residential distance from hospitals has been shown to be negatively associated with risk of late-stage diagnosis (Dickens et al., 2014). The NGO Cancer Association of South Africa (CANSA) recommends monthly BSE for all women and regular CBE, and performs CBE through mobile health clinics and CANSA care clinics throughout South Africa (CANSA, 2014b). Annual mammograms are recommended for women older than 40 years, and mammograms are offered though public hospital breast clinics; however, these are not free. The Radiological Society of South Africa provides reduced-rate mammograms during October. Results from a pilot screening programme using a mobile mammography unit in the Western Cape in women aged 40 years and older in 2011–2012 reported multiple problems, both technical (e.g. poor-quality images) and administrative (e.g. images not reaching the referral centre), and a low cancer detection rate, concluding that commencement of a screening programme using this model was not justified in this setting (Apffelstaedt et al., 2014).

The Swaziland Breast Cancer Network (SBCN) operates two breast cancer clinics, which offer free consultations, examinations, diagnosis, and referrals. The SBCN recommends monthly BSE, and CBE by a trained provider, and has developed a referral tool for further diagnostic work for patients who report suspicious findings (Swaziland Breast Cancer Network, 2008). It is unclear whether the SBCN is affiliated with the Swaziland Ministry of Health; no formal guidelines on breast screening were found on the website of the Swaziland Ministry of Health. The SBCN recommends that all women older than 40 years should undergo annual mammography; however, it recognizes that mammography is used only very occasionally, by those who can afford this service.

(ii) Participation

A national population-based cross-sectional study of 2202 women in South Africa found that only 15.5% reported ever having had a mammogram; screening was associated with being from the White or Indian/Asian population group, having a higher education level, having greater wealth, and having health insurance (Peltzer & Phaswana-Mafuya, 2014). Participation rates are unavailable for other countries in this region.

(iii) Information and breast cancer awareness

In South Africa, the government and a variety of NGOs provide community outreach and educational materials to increase awareness of breast cancer signs and symptoms. Initiatives include mobile breast check units, which travel to semi-urban and urban areas offering free CBE, education about BSE, and other awareness campaigns (CANSA, 2014a). In Swaziland, the SBCN's education programmes aim to increase awareness of aspects of breast cancer, including the promotion of BSE, medical examinations, and the importance of early diagnosis and treatment (Swaziland Breast Cancer Network, 2008).

(d) West Africa

West Africa comprises the countries of Benin, Burkina Faso, The Gambia, Ghana, Guinea, Guinea-Bissau, Liberia, Mali, Niger, Nigeria,

Senegal, Sierra Leone, and Togo. In many of these countries, life expectancy is low and there is a high burden of infectious diseases. In this region, breast cancer patients are predominantly premenopausal, present at late stages, and have poor prognosis (Sighoko et al., 2013).

(i) Systems, policies, and guidelines

Data on breast screening policies and practices in this region are either sparse or non-existent. No data were found for Benin, Burkina Faso, The Gambia, Guinea, Guinea-Bissau, Liberia, Niger, or Togo. Limited data are available from other West African countries. There are no national programmes for breast screening in Ghana, Mali, Nigeria, or Senegal. The Ministry of Health of Sierra Leone is attempting to implement a variety of interventions, including a free health-care initiative, but it has no specific policy or plan for the prevention or control of breast cancer (WHO African Health Observatory, 2014).

(ii) Participation

A small cross-sectional study in Ghana reported that breast screening practices were poor; self-reported rates were 32% for BSE, 12% for CBE, and 2% for mammography, and a higher education level was strongly associated with screening behaviours (Opoku et al., 2012). A study of 66 breast cancer patients found that whereas 14 (21.2%) of the breast cancers were discovered through breast education and CBE as offered through outreach programmes, women commonly waited between 6 weeks and 2 years before seeking formal diagnosis and treatment (Clegg-Lamptey et al., 2009).

In Nigeria, the Lagos State Ministry of Health reported that there are only four functional mammography units in Lagos, that use of mammography is rare, and that most women are unaware of its use as a screening tool (Lagos State Ministry of Health, 2014).

In a cross-sectional study in Senegal in 2006, 300 patients attending five hospitals in Dakar for a medical or surgical consultation were interviewed about knowledge and practice of BSE. Study participants were young (average age, 34 years), uneducated, and living in poverty. Of the participants, 43% were aware of BSE and 29% regularly practised BSE. Practice of BSE was associated with income and education level (Gueye et al., 2009).

In Sierra Leone, a study of 3645 women identified minimal education, poverty, and reliance on traditional healers as barriers to medical care for women with breast masses (Ntirenganya et al., 2014).

(iii) Information and breast cancer awareness

In the absence of formal guidelines in West African countries, several awareness and education campaigns have been initiated. In Ghana, a cross-sectional survey assessed the impact of education programmes on knowledge and attitudes about breast cancer and breast cancer prevention as well as practices among women in rural communities and found that knowledge about breast cancer symptoms had improved and that the number of women who reported beginning BSE had increased (Mena et al., 2014).

Multiple studies of awareness, attitude, and practice of breast examination in women in Nigeria have shown a low knowledge and practice of BSE and CBE. The Breast Cancer Awareness and Free Screening programme, launched in Nigeria in 2006 in collaboration with the Ministry of Women Affairs and Poverty Alleviation, educates women about BSE and provides free counselling and referral services (Lagos State Ministry of Health, 2011). At community events, women were shown videos about how to perform BSE and received counselling and referral, where applicable. Those diagnosed through the programme were treated for free. A study in Nigeria identified several economic and cultural barriers to implementing education about basic screening programmes, including a lack of both specialized health personnel and breast cancer screening facilities, the absence of biomedical terminology in local languages, gender inequality, and the prevailing influence of traditional health practitioners (Asobayire & Barley, 2014).

In Sierra Leone, some efforts have been made to provide education to women about breast cancer and the importance of breast health (Shepherd & McInerney, 2006).

3.2.5 Central and West Asia and North Africa

The region of Central and West Asia includes Afghanistan, Armenia, Azerbaijan, Bahrain, Cyprus, Georgia, Iraq, Israel, the Islamic Republic of Iran, Jordan, Kazakhstan, Kuwait, Kyrgyzstan, Lebanon, Oman, Qatar, Saudi Arabia, the Syrian Arab Republic, Tajikistan, Turkey, Turkmenistan, the United Arab Emirates, Uzbekistan, the West Bank and Gaza Strip, and Yemen. North Africa includes the Maghreb countries (Algeria, Libya, Mauritania, Morocco, and Tunisia), Egypt, and Sudan.

These countries are heterogeneous in terms of access to screening. While high-income countries such as Israel, Kuwait, and Qatar have well-developed health services, most countries in this area are classified as low- and middle-income countries, with limited resources allocated to health care. Large population-based screening programmes do not exist in the majority of these countries, and screening is primarily opportunistic. Some countries, such as Egypt and Turkey, have active and ongoing efforts to implement population-based screening via a series of pilot projects. Breast screening costs are covered in countries in a variety of ways, including through government funding, through partnerships with NGOs, or via patients' out-of-pocket expenditure. Available data on screening policies and practice are summarized in Table 3.6.

(a) Armenia, Kazakhstan, Kyrgyzstan, and Turkey

(i) Systems, policies, and guidelines

In Armenia, the ability of the health-care system to detect and treat breast cancer has been augmented through the efforts of NGOs and private organizations, most importantly the Armenian American Wellness Center in Yerevan, which provides mammography and free teaching of BSE (AAWC, 2014). There are no formal government guidelines, but awareness campaigns from the Armenian American Wellness Center stress the importance of annual mammograms and monthly BSE.

In Kazakhstan, recommendations for breast screening are biennial mammography for women aged 50–60 years (Beysebayev et al., 2015). The NGO Together Against Cancer with the support of UICC launched the National Breast Cancer Awareness programme in 2008, based on mobile units screening women in an opportunistic fashion using diagnostic ultrasonography, and at the same time instructing women about how to perform BSE (CIS Anti-Cancer Association, 2013a).

In Kyrgyzstan, an NGO-led programme for prevention and early diagnosis of breast cancer was developed in 2006 (CIS Anti-Cancer Association, 2013b). It is unclear whether active opportunistic screening has been implemented.

Turkey has had a national breast screening programme since 2008 and has the most established screening services of these countries. Since 2012, the recommendations of the Ministry of Health's Cancer Control Department are annual mammography for women aged 40 years and older and CBE for women participating in the screening (Republic of Turkey, Ministry of Health, Department of Cancer Control, 2009; Kayhan et al., 2014). By 2012, 125 Cancer Early Diagnosis, Screening, and Training Centers (KETEM) had been established in 81 provinces in Turkey, with the aim of establishing 280 centres

Table 3.6 Policies and practice for breast cancer screening in Central/West Asia and North Africa

Country	National recommendation or guideline			Mammography units per million women aged 50–69 years in 2013[a]	Support organization	References
	Screening practice	Target age (years)	Interval (years)			
Armenia	BSE	All women	Monthly		NGO: Armenian American Wellness Center	AAWC (2014)
	Mammography	Not stated	1	22.5		
Bahrain	BSE	30–64	Not stated		Bahrain Ministry of Health	Bahrain Cancer Society (2012)
	CBE	30–64	Not stated			
	Mammography	≥ 40	2	Not stated		
Egypt	BSE	≥ 20	Monthly		Egypt Ministry of Health	Women's Health Outreach Program (2014)
	Mammography	≥ 45	1	Not stated		
Israel	Mammography	50–74	2	112.3	Israel Ministry of Health	Israel Cancer Association (2014)
		≥ 40, familial risk	1			
	MRI	≥ 40, *BRCA1/2*	1			
Jordan	BSE	All women	Monthly		Jordan Ministry of Health	JBCP (2014a)
	CBE	20–39	1–3			
		≥ 40	1			
	Mammography	40–49	2	129.1		
		≥ 50	1			
Kazakhstan	Mammography	50–60	2	22.1	NGO: Together Against Cancer	Beysebayev et al. (2015)
Kuwait	CBE	≥ 40	Not stated		Kuwait Ministry of Health	Kuwait Ministry of Health (2014)
	Mammography	≥ 40	Not stated	Not stated		
Lebanon	BSE	≥ 20	Monthly		Lebanese Breast Cancer National Task Force/Ministry of Health	Adib et al. (2009)
	CBE	20–40	3			
		≥ 40	1			
	Mammography	≥ 40	1	370.2		
Morocco	CBE	45–69	1–2	18.5	Moroccan Ministry of Health	Lalla Salma Foundation (2014)
Oman	BSE	All women	Monthly		NGO: Oman Cancer Association	Oman Cancer Association (2015)
	Mammography	≥ 40	1–2	149.8		
Qatar	BSE	≥ 20	Monthly		Qatar Supreme Council of Health	College of the North Atlantic Qatar (2012)
	CBE	≥ 35	1			
	Mammography	40–69	1	225.1		
Tunisia	CBE	40–69	1		Tunisian Ministry of Health	ATREP (2014)
	Mammography	"High-risk" women	Not stated	22.6		
Turkey	CBE	≥ 40	1		Turkish Ministry of Health	Kayhan et al. (2014)
	Mammography	≥ 40	1	230.4		
United Arab Emirates	BSE	All women	Monthly		United Arab Emirates Ministry of Health	HAAD (2013)
	CBE	≥ 40	1			
	Mammography	≥ 40	2	Not stated		

[a] WHO (2014).

BSE, breast self-examination; CBE, clinical breast examination; MRI, magnetic resonance imaging; NGO, nongovernmental organization.

by 2015 (Republic of Turkey, Ministry of Health, Department of Cancer Control, 2009; Güllüoğlu et al., 2012). Multiple pilot screening programmes have been carried out, including a 10-year population-based screening programme for women aged 40–69 years living in a large urban region of Istanbul with a well-organized address-based population registration system (Kayhan et al., 2014). In addition to these publicly administered screening projects, some municipalities and NGOs also organize screening programmes on their own initiative. All of these screenings are provided free of charge (Holland et al., 2006).

(ii) Participation

In Armenia, a cross-sectional study found that the proportion of women who practised BSE was 20% and that the proportion of women who had had at least one mammogram was 6% (Harutyunyan, 1999).

Since 2008, mobile ultrasonography units have screened about 78 000 women in Kazakhstan (CIS Anti-Cancer Association, 2013a). A study of knowledge, attitudes, and practices of women for breast screening found that the majority of the women sampled (82.6%) performed BSE, an average of 9.5 times per year; about two thirds of the women (62.9%) had had CBE performed by a physician, and only 12.4% indicated that they had previously had a mammogram (Chukmaitov et al., 2008).

(iii) Information and breast cancer awareness

The majority of education and awareness campaigns in this region are carried out by NGOs.

(b) Arab countries in West Asia

As in other countries with previously low incidence rates of breast cancer, in this region breast cancer incidence and mortality rates are rapidly increasing. Breast cancer in Arab women is often diagnosed at a younger age and at a more advanced stage compared with other populations (Ezzat et al., 1999; El Saghir et al., 2002, 2006; Salhia et al., 2011). In response, several countries in the region have developed recommendations for breast cancer screening.

(i) Systems, policies, and guidelines

The World Health Organization (WHO) Regional Office for the Eastern Mediterranean published guidelines on breast cancer screening in 2006, and, in line with the Breast Health Global Initiative guidelines, suggested that screening could be implemented in centralized cancer facilities where breast cancer treatment is available (Khatib & Modjtabai, 2006). These programmes would provide screening to only a limited proportion of the population, but they could act as pilot programmes, with the ultimate aim of expanding them to cover the entire population as more resources become available. Recommendations for screening frequency vary considerably in this region.

In Bahrain, breast cancer screening began in December 1992 for women aged 30–64 years and included education activities about CBE and BSE (Hamadeh et al., 2014). Mammography screening was performed only for suspected breast cancer cases and high-risk women after referral. Since 2005, biennial mammography screening is recommended for women aged 40 years and older, and it is provided free of charge (Bahrain Cancer Society, 2012).

The Jordan Breast Cancer Program was established in 2007 (JBCP, 2008) and recommends monthly BSE for all women, CBE once every 1–3 years for women aged 20–39 years and annually thereafter, and mammography once every 2 years for women aged 40–49 years and annually for women aged 50 years and older (JBCP, 2014a). In 2010, a programme of free mammography and CBE was implemented, which is expected to increase participation rates (JBCP, 2010).

The Kuwait National Mammography Screening Program was launched in 2014; it is designed to provide mammography and CBE to women aged 40 years and older in several governmental clinics (Kuwait Ministry of Health, 2014). It does not recommend BSE but does promote breast cancer awareness.

The Lebanese Ministry of Public Health and the Lebanese Breast Cancer National Task Force recommend monthly BSE starting at age 20 years and CBE every 3 years for women aged 20–40 years; for women aged 40 years and older, annual mammography and CBE are recommended (Adib et al., 2009).

In Oman, mammography screening is conducted at government hospitals free of charge. The Oman Cancer Association recommends annual or biennial mammography screening for women aged 40 years and older, and monthly BSE (Oman Cancer Association, 2015).

The State of Palestine Ministry of Health has no formal guidelines or policies for breast screening but emphasizes the importance of regular breast screening (State of Palestine Ministry of Health, 2014). A variety of health centres provide opportunistic screening and diagnostic mammography, but many territories have no screening centres (Khaleel Abu Shmais, 2010). There are four mammography facilities in the entire West Bank and Gaza Strip, and whereas screening is free for insured women, uninsured women are required to pay a fee (Azaiza et al., 2010).

Qatar released a National Cancer Strategy in 2011 (Supreme Council of Health of Qatar, 2014) and later developed a National Cancer Control Program (National Cancer Program Qatar, 2014). It recommends monthly BSE starting at age 20 years, annual CBE for women aged 35 years and older, and annual mammography for women aged 40–69 years, unless otherwise advised by a physician (College of the North Atlantic Qatar, 2012).

Although regional screening initiatives exist in Saudi Arabia, there are no national guidelines, and data from these initiatives are not available (Abulkhair et al., 2010).

The United Arab Emirates implemented a National Breast Screening Program in 1995 and recommends a combination of monthly BSE, annual CBE, and mammography every 2 years aged 40 years and older (HAAD, 2013). Screening services are provided free of charge and are widely available but are opportunistic in nature (Elobaid et al., 2014).

In Yemen, mammography screening has been in place since the 1990s, but there are no policies or recommendations for breast cancer screening, and few data are available on breast screening practices in the country.

(ii) Participation

Despite awareness campaigns and efforts to reduce costs and improve accessibility of screening mammography, participation tends to be low among women in this region. Data on participation in screening programmes are taken primarily from the peer-reviewed literature and are usually from cross-sectional studies. Studies report low participation rates in breast screening programmes and low awareness of BSE (Bener et al., 2002; Azaiza & Cohen, 2006; Dündar et al., 2006; Soskolne et al., 2007; Taha et al., 2010; Donnelly et al., 2013a, b; Elobaid et al., 2014). Screening programmes are opportunistic and are relatively new to the region, and there are no centrally organized invitation or follow-up systems (Donnelly et al., 2013a).

In 2008–2010, only 12.7% of breast cancers in Bahrain were screen-detected, and primary health-care centres in Bahrain reported CBE coverage rates of 6.6%, 7.1%, and 6.9% in women aged 30 years and older (Hamadeh et al., 2014).

A study of female schoolteachers in Kuwait found that 81.9% had never had CBE performed by a health professional and 85.7% did not know what mammography was (Alharbi et al., 2012). A study of 510 women attending a public health clinic found that only 21% of the women practised BSE regularly, and these women had a sufficient level of knowledge about BSE, CBE, and mammography (Al-Azmy et al., 2013).

In Lebanon, a 3-month national mammography campaign in 2009, targeted at women older than 40 years, implemented free mammography screening subsidized by the Ministry of Public Health in participating public radiology centres, and mammography screening at a reduced cost in private centres. The campaign successfully screened 10 953 women; 68.2% of the women who participated did so for the first time, and 97.8% of the women indicated their willingness to undergo the examination again the following year (Kobeissi et al., 2012).

A study of 397 women aged 30–65 years residing in the West Bank and Gaza Strip reported that more than 70% of the women had never had a mammogram or CBE and that 62% of the women performed BSE (Azaiza et al., 2010). A 2011 study of 100 women living in Gaza reported that only 27% of the women were willing to undergo screening mammography; the barriers identified included limited financial resources, lack of resources to treat breast cancer if diagnosed, lack of access to screening facilities, and concern about personal safety while travelling to medical centres (Shaheen et al., 2011).

A 2009 study of 1200 Qatari women aged 30–55 years reported that despite an adequate knowledge of breast cancer, only 24.9% had performed BSE, 23.3% had undergone CBE, and 22.5% had had a mammogram (Bener et al., 2009).

In 2011, a study of 719 Saudi Arabian women reported that 23.1% of the women practised BSE, 14.2% had undergone CBE, and 8.1% had had a mammogram (Ravichandran et al., 2011).

In the United Arab Emirates, a cross-sectional study of 247 women in 2013 found rates of 48.6% for self-reported BSE, 49.4% for CBE, and 44.9% for mammography (Elobaid et al., 2014). These rates represent an improvement on those reported in an earlier study, in 2001, when 12.7% of the study population practised BSE, 13.8% had undergone CBE, and 10.3% had had a mammogram (Bener et al., 2001).

A study of 425 female Yemeni university students found that although 76.9% of the participants had heard about BSE, only 17.4% had performed it, and 55.9% cited a lack of knowledge about BSE technique as a barrier (Ahmed, 2010). A cross-sectional study of 105 female Yemeni doctors about attitudes and practice of mammography screening found that only 24.7% sent patients for mammography screening every year regardless of the patients' history or symptoms (Al-Naggar et al., 2009).

(iii) Information and breast cancer awareness

Several cross-sectional studies across the region reported lack of knowledge of BSE and CBE, a mainstay of screening programmes in many low-resource settings.

A variety of NGOs and government bodies in this region run awareness campaigns emphasizing the importance of regular breast screening, disseminate information about the availability of mammography screening where these facilities exist, and promote awareness of breast health (Adib et al., 2009; Kobeissi et al., 2012; JBCP, 2014b; State of Palestine Ministry of Health, 2014).

(c) Islamic Republic of Iran and Israel

(i) Systems, policies, and guidelines

In the Islamic Republic of Iran, there is no formal breast screening programme, and no national guidelines exist; efforts for breast cancer prevention have focused on educating women, teaching BSE, and encouraging opportunistic screening. The most widely available forms of breast screening in the Islamic Republic of Iran are CBE and BSE (Babu et al., 2011).

In Israel, the National Mammography Screening Program was implemented in the early 1990s. Current screening policy recommendations include biennial mammography for women aged 50–74 years, annual mammography for women at increased familial risk aged 40 years and older, and annual MRI for *BRCA1/2* mutation carriers aged 40 years and older (Israel Cancer Association, 2014).

(ii) Participation

A study of 318 Iranian health-care providers found that 48% of female providers had not carried out any method of breast cancer screening for themselves during the previous year, 81.5% did not perform CBE for the majority of their female patients, and only 5.1% recommended BSE to more than 70% of their female patients (Harirchi et al., 2009). The percentage of women who had ever had a mammogram ranged from 1.3% to 28% (Donnelly et al., 2013a), and the percentage who performed BSE was estimated to be between 3% and 17% (Babu et al., 2011; Donnelly et al., 2013a). A variety of regional studies in the Islamic Republic of Iran found that knowledge of screening practices and rates of BSE were inadequate, including among health-care workers (Haji-Mahmoodi et al., 2002; Harirchi et al., 2009; Yadollahie et al., 2011; Akhtari-Zavare et al., 2014; Tazhibi & Feizi, 2014).

Data from the Israel Cancer Association showed that in 2009, of 181 429 women aged 50–74 years, 85.6% had ever been screened by mammography (Israel Cancer Association, 2014). Screening rates for Israeli Jews and Arabs were broadly similar (Keinan-Boker et al., 2013; Israel Cancer Association, 2014). There were no significant differences in the percentages of women reporting having had a mammogram in the previous 2 years, which increased by 16% in Jewish women and by 17% in Arab women from 2002 to 2008 (Keinan-Boker et al., 2013).

(iii) Information and breast cancer awareness

Few data are available on awareness campaigns in this region.

(d) North Africa

The age-standardized incidence rate of breast cancer in North Africa is currently one quarter to one half that in Europe and the USA (Corbex et al., 2014), but it is expected to double in the next 15 years as exposure to risk factors increases (including those related to population ageing).

(i) Systems, policies, and guidelines

Cancer has become a national priority in Algeria, with the preparation of the 2015–2019 National Cancer Plan (Hamdi Cherif et al., 2014), but no data on breast screening policies or practices were found. Some opportunistic pilot projects are in place; for example, a mobile mammography unit was launched in 2013 through a partnership between the Algerian government, mobile phone operator Mobilis, Roche, and the patient advocacy group El Amel (Hope) (Roche, 2014).

Similar to the situation in other countries in the area, women in Egypt present with advanced breast cancer (Omar et al., 2003; Salhia et al., 2011). The Egyptian national screening programme, the Women's Health Outreach Programme, was launched in 2007; it recommends monthly BSE starting at age 20 years and offers free annual breast screening for all Egyptian women aged 45 years and older (Salem et al., 2008; Women's Health Outreach Program, 2014). The programme consists of five phases, with a 1-year pilot phase (2007–2008) to identify barriers in implementation. Each implementation phase will address several governorates. The goal of the 5-year implementation plan is to provide coverage for the entire population.

There were no data in the literature about screening guidelines in Libya or about breast screening practices among Libyan women.

In Mauritania, a 2012 review of the health-care service found that it was underfunded, underdeveloped, and disorganized. Cancer prevention campaigns or implementation of screening policies are absent, and they are unlikely to be implemented in the near future (Global Centre for Renewal and Guidance, 2012).

Morocco set up a National Cancer Prevention and Control Plan in 2010, comprising a coordinated breast cancer awareness campaign and a programme aimed at developing breast cancer screening in half a million women. Breast cancer screening with CBE is recommended for women aged 45–69 years, at least every 2 years (Lalla Salma Foundation, 2014). A new breast and uterine cancer screening and early detection centre was opened in 2013 in Mohammedia, which provides screening facilities for more than 40 000 eligible women (Morocco World News, 2013). Mobile mammography units travel to remote areas to provide opportunistic screening to those without access to centralized screening facilities. The National Cancer Prevention and Control Plan in Morocco has developed a three-tiered system for increasing screening coverage: level 1, health-care clinics with general practitioners and nurses who provide breast health education and CBE to women; level 2, specific reproductive health clinics, which receive referrals from level 1 clinics and perform diagnostic ultrasonography and mammography; and level 3, oncology centres (Lalla Salma Foundation, 2014).

Sudan established its National Cancer Control Programme with CBE in 1982; the programme focuses on prevention, early detection and screening, diagnosis, and treatment (Hamad, 2006). However, a lack of resources has hampered implementation of breast cancer screening, and the majority of efforts have been focused on public awareness campaigns and education of medical professionals (Abuidris et al., 2013).

The Tunisian Ministry of Health has stated goals of focusing on prevention and early detection of cancer as part of the 2010–2014 National Strategy of the Fight against Cancer, and currently recommends annual CBE for women aged 40–69 years, with mammography reserved for high-risk women and those referred after primary screening via CBE (ATREP, 2014). Tunisia has implemented several pilot programmes examining the efficacy and feasibility of mammography screening in the general population. Based on the results of these programmes, the Tunisian government will consider moving towards population-based mammography screening.

(ii) Participation

In Egypt, mammography is delivered in an opportunistic fashion through mobile units equipped with digital mammography units (Women's Health Outreach Program, 2014); as of 2013, 107 193 women had been screened (Philips Healthcare, 2014). Despite these mobile units, which increase the presence in rural areas and less affluent areas, barriers to accessing mammography still exist, and other methods of breast screening have been explored, including training women living in a slum in Cairo about breast health awareness and BSE (Kharboush et al., 2011). A randomized study, with women who received CBE versus a control arm of women who received only health education, demonstrated high acceptance, with 85–91% of the women in the target population enrolling in the study. Initial results demonstrated that stage distribution was significantly better in the intervention arm compared with the control arm (Miller, 2008). A study in 2000 reported that of 565 newly diagnosed breast cancer patients, only 10.4% had practised BSE, and 2.7% reported performing BSE monthly (Abdel-Fattah et al., 2000).

In Morocco, a study of 136 female doctors and nurses found that 75% of study participants practised BSE monthly, but only 15% had ever had a mammogram (Ghanem et al., 2011).

In Tunisia, one of the first pilot studies, started in 2003, was large-scale population-based mammography screening in urban areas, but participation rates have tended to be low (Bouchlaka et al., 2009; Zaanouni et al., 2009).

The most recent study evaluated three rounds of mammography screening as part of a pilot programme, carried out in 2004–2010 in Sfax. Biennial screening was offered to women aged 45 years and older, and 17.4% of the target population underwent screening, resulting in 12 657 mammograms (Frikha et al., 2013). A cross-sectional study in Tunisia of 900 women reported poor knowledge of specific risk factors for breast cancer and of breast screening modalities; only 14% of women performed any type of breast screening (El Mhamdi et al., 2013).

(iii) Information and breast cancer awareness

Awareness campaigns and training of health-care workers are part of national screening programmes in these regions, including in Algeria (Roche, 2014), Morocco (Lalla Salma Foundation, 2014), and Tunisia (ATREP, 2014).

3.2.6 South-East Asia

During the past decade, the Republic of Korea, Singapore, and Taiwan, China, have started national organized screening programmes with mammography (Table 3.7). Although Japan was the first country to introduce a national screening programme with CBE, in 1987, and later also included mammography, organized screening remains insufficient in Japan. Eleven other countries in South-East Asia have partial programmes supported by governments or NGOs in local areas, and screening systems have not been standardized. All 15 countries in this region have breast cancer awareness programmes, which are often included in national programmes for cancer control and prevention of noncommunicable diseases.

(a) Republic of Korea

(i) Systems, policies, and guidelines

The National Cancer Screening Program, launched in 1999, recommends mammography with and without CBE as the screening method (Kim et al., 2011). The target group for screening is women aged 40 years and older, with no upper age limit, and the screening interval is 2 years. Although CBE is recommended when mammography screening is performed, the fee is not covered by the National Cancer Screening Program.

The national programme provides breast cancer screening with different fees; women are divided into three groups, based on their insurance premium (Kim et al., 2011). The lowest-income beneficiaries (those exempted from premium payment) are supported directly by the national government. For people whose insurance premium is less than the 50th percentile, a free programme is provided by the National Health Insurance system (National Cancer Screening Program), supported also by national and local governments. People whose premium is more than the 50th percentile, although they are supported by the National Health Insurance Corporation cancer screening programme, are required to make a 10% co-payment.

Based on the Cancer Control Act of 2003, the Ministry of Health and Welfare organized the cancer screening programme systematically by cooperating with public institutions (Kim et al., 2011). The National Health Insurance Corporation selects the target population and sends invitation letters. Women can visit hospitals or clinics that have been approved for cancer screening and then receive the screening results within 15 days. Women who have positive results on their primary screening undergo follow-up examinations, and the diagnostic evaluation is available with co-payment from their health insurance (Goto et al., 2015). However, co-payment for treatment is supported only when breast cancer is diagnosed by the National Cancer Screening Program.

The certification of screening providers and quality management are conducted mainly by the National Cancer Center (Goto et al., 2015). Private hospitals provide multiphasic health

Table 3.7 Policies and practice for breast cancer screening in South-East Asia

Country	Type of programme[a]	Start year	Screening practice	Target age (years)	Interval (years)	Examination coverage[b] (%)	Mammography units per million women aged 50–69 years in 2013[c]	References
Bangladesh	Partial programme	Unclear	CBE	40–69	Unclear	Unclear	—	Ministry of Health and Family Welfare, Bangladesh (2008)
Brunei Darussalam	Partial programme	Unclear	Unclear	Unclear	Unclear	Unclear	91.9	Ministry of Health, Brunei Darussalam (2007)
China	Partial programme	Unclear	Unclear	Unclear	Unclear	21.7[d]	—	Mo et al. (2013), Pan et al. (2013), Wang et al. (2013)
Hong Kong Special Administrative Region, China	Partial programme	Unclear	Unclear	Unclear	Unclear	Unclear	—	Lui et al. (2007), Centre for Health Protection (2012)
India	Partial programme	Unclear	Unclear	Unclear	Unclear	Unclear	—	Ministry of Health and Family Welfare, Government of India (2005), Agarwal & Ramakant (2008), Reddy et al. (2012)
Indonesia	Partial programme	2007	CBE	Unclear	Unclear	Unclear	—	WHO (2008a)
Japan	National programme	1987[e]	Mammography + CBE	≥ 40	2	18.3	227.3	Oshima (1994), Ministry of Health, Labour and Welfare, Japan (2013b), National Cancer Center, Japan (2013), Goto et al. (2015), Hamashima, 2016
Malaysia	Partial programme	Unclear	CBE Mammography	Unclear	Unclear	51.8 7.6	86.7	Ministry of Health Malaysia (2010), Dahlui et al. (2011)
Pakistan	Partial programme	Unclear	Unclear	Unclear	Unclear	Unclear	1.6	WHO (2008b)
Philippines	Partial programme	Unclear	Unclear	Unclear	Unclear	Unclear	13.1	National Statistics Office (2009)

Table 3.7 (continued)

Country	Type of programme[a]	Start year	Screening practice	Target age (years)	Interval (years)	Examination coverage[b] (%)	Mammography units per million women aged 50–69 years in 2013[c]	References
Republic of Korea	National organized programme	1999	Mammography ± CBE	≥ 40	2	49.5	402.3	Kim et al. (2011), National Cancer Center of Korea (2013)
Singapore	National organized programme	2002	Mammography	50–69	2	39.6[f]	127.6	Ministry of Health Singapore (2010, 2011)
Taiwan, China	National organized programme	2004	Mammography	45–69	2	36.0	—	Health Promotion Administration, Ministry of Health and Welfare (2014)
Thailand	Partial programme	Unclear	Unclear	Unclear	Unclear	Unclear	27.9	National Cancer Control Programme, Thailand (2013)
Viet Nam	Partial programme	2008	CBE	Unclear	Unclear	15–20	—	Nguyen et al. (2013)

[a] Partial programmes are supported by government and nongovernmental organizations and are conducted mainly in local areas, and screening systems have not been standardized.
[b] Annual examinations as percentage of annual target population, with the screening method and within the age range reported in the policy.
[c] WHO (2014).
[d] Coverage refers to any breast cancer examination in women older than 18 years.
[e] Current policy started in 2005.
[f] Coverage refers to the previous 2 years.
±, with or without; CBE, clinical breast examination.

check-ups, including cancer screenings. Some private companies provide subsidies for these health check-ups.

(ii) Participation

The participation rate in breast cancer screening increased from 14.1% in 2002 to 49.5% in 2011, and in 2012 the participation rate including opportunistic screening was 71.0% (National Cancer Center of Korea, 2013).

(iii) Information and breast cancer awareness

To increase participation in cancer screening, awareness campaigns have been actively promoted in the media by the National Health Insurance Corporation. BSE is well known among Korean women through television, radio, and newspapers (Yoo et al., 2012). Community-based intervention also seems to be effective in increasing participation in mammography screening (Park et al., 2011).

(b) Singapore

(i) Systems, policies, and guidelines

BreastScreen Singapore was adopted as a national screening programme in 2002, and the Ministry of Health Singapore revised the guidelines in 2010. The ministry recommended stand-alone mammography every 2 years for asymptomatic women at average risk aged 50–69 years (Ministry of Health Singapore, 2010). Women at average risk aged 40–49 years are given information describing the benefits and harms of mammography screening, and can therefore make an informed choice. Ultrasonography and CBE are not included in the programme.

BreastScreen Singapore provides subsidized mammograms at many government centres (Teo & Soo, 2013). Service partnerships were established with health service providers of two public health clusters and a private service provider (Yeoh et al., 2006). They have cooperated to select and assess mammography screening centres. After the first screening, all women in the target population are sent reminders for the subsequent screening at the appropriate interval for their age group. Multidisciplinary assessment is performed and completed until a final diagnosis is obtained (Yeoh et al., 2006). Women who have a diagnosis of breast cancer are given the choice of either seeing a breast surgeon at any centre in Singapore or remaining at the assessment centre hospital for further treatment.

To ensure that patients undergo high-quality screening, health-care providers must adhere to a common quality assurance framework for the screenings (Yeoh et al., 2006). Standards and target requirements for screening, reading, and assessment centres were established, and audit teams including trained multidisciplinary clinical professionals carry out audit visits every 2 years (Yeoh et al., 2006). Every set of films is interpreted by two radiologists; their performance is monitored, and feedback is given to individuals and to the centre to facilitate the taking of appropriate action. Although private clinics provide mammography screening to women individually, the women are charged fees (Yeoh et al., 2006).

(ii) Participation

In 2010, about 66% of Singaporean women aged 50–69 years had undergone mammography at least once, and 39.6% of Singaporean women aged 50–69 years had undergone mammography within the previous 2 years (Ministry of Health Singapore, 2011).

(iii) Information and breast cancer awareness

In 2010, 90.9% of Singaporean women aged 50–69 years were aware of mammography as a screening method for breast cancer (Ministry of Health Singapore, 2011). Women with higher education levels tended to be more aware of mammography compared with women with lower education levels.

(c) Taiwan, China

(i) Systems, policies, and guidelines

In accordance with the Cancer Prevention Act of 2003, national screening for breast cancer was started in 2004 (Health Promotion Administration, Ministry of Health and Welfare, 2014). The Taiwan, China, government currently offers free mammography screening every 2 years for women aged 45–69 years. For women aged 40–44 years, mammography screening is limited to those with a second-degree relative with breast cancer. Women in the target population can be examined at community health centres, clinics, or hospitals. To further improve accessibility of breast cancer screening services, the national government subsidized provinces and cities to provide mobile mammography services or mammography equipment.

The health insurance covers the screening fee and the cost of further examinations. To increase cancer screening coverage, the national government has provided special funding for cancer prevention and control after raising the tobacco tax (Health Promotion Administration, Ministry of Health and Welfare, 2014).

Hospitals in Taiwan, China, are required to establish an outpatient screening reminder system and a referral system for positive test results. The national government has also commissioned the Radiography Society to certify medical institutions for mammography based on requirements (Health Promotion Administration, Ministry of Health and Welfare, 2014). The degree of appropriateness of mammography equipment, including radiation exposure levels, showed a significant improvement after the enforcement of quality assurance (Hwang et al., 2013). In further efforts to improve the quality of cancer screening, the national government launched a project to build a nationwide database for quality assurance. The database is interconnected with all screening-related databases (the Taiwan Cancer Registry, the Taiwan Mortality Registry, and the Taiwan Household Registration).

(ii) Participation

In 2013, mammography was conducted in 694 000 women aged 45–69 years. The coverage rate over the past 2 years was 36% (Health Promotion Administration, Ministry of Health and Welfare, 2014).

(iii) Information and breast cancer awareness

The national government supported local health departments to conduct community screenings, introduced on-site education programmes, and followed the WHO Health Promoting Hospitals model in assisting local hospitals to promote cancer screening (Health Promotion Administration, Ministry of Health and Welfare, 2014).

(d) Japan

(i) Systems, policies, and guidelines

In 1987, national cancer screening using annual CBE was introduced in Japan for women aged 30 years and older (Oshima, 1994). In 2000, mammography screening was added for women aged 50 years and older, and in 2005 the protocol was changed to biennial mammography screening with CBE for women aged 40 years and older, with no upper age limit. In 2013, the National Cancer Center published new guidelines for organized and opportunistic breast cancer screening, in which mammography with or without CBE was recommended (National Cancer Center, Japan, 2013). [Note post-meeting: the guidelines have been further updated (Hamashima, 2016).] Use of ultrasonography as a screening tool is currently under investigation (Ishida et al., 2014).

There are two types of opportunistic screening in Japan; one is individual-based screening, and the other is provided as a premium by large health insurance associations or large companies at workplaces, but there is no obligatory monitoring or quality assurance for these types of screening (Goto et al., 2015).

Local governments are responsible for cancer screening and make decisions about the screening method, screening fee, provision of primary screening, quality assurance for primary screening, and monitoring; most of these local governments do not have a call–recall system (Goto et al., 2015). The national government provides some funding, although non-specific, for cancer screening, and the local governments pay the remaining portion of the cancer screening fees. The women's fees for the screening examination and management differ among municipalities (about US$ 5–20); 8.5% of municipalities provide free screening as part of mass screening programmes (Ministry of Health, Labour and Welfare, Japan, 2013a).

Local governments do not support follow-up examinations for women with positive results at the primary screening; therefore, the participation rate at follow-up examinations has remained at approximately 80% (Ministry of Health, Labour and Welfare, Japan, 2013b). Diagnosis and treatment are covered by health insurance, and the co-payment is usually 30%. Women can access any clinic or hospital, including university hospitals, without a referral from a general physician.

Although there is an insufficient quality assurance system for breast cancer screening in Japan, technical support for mammography has been actively promoted by the Central Committee on Quality Control of Mammographic Screening (Japan Central Organization on Quality Assurance of Breast Cancer Screening, 2014). The committee has approved technical skills for mammography screening for physicians. Several public information programmes, including for the management of mammography equipment, have been made available through the committee's website.

(ii) Participation

Although participation rates have increased since 2009, they have remained at approximately 20%. In 2011, 2 511 299 women participated in breast cancer screening, at a rate of 18.3% (Ministry of Health, Labour and Welfare, Japan, 2013b). When opportunistic screening is included, the participation rate is 43.4% (National Cancer Center, Japan, 2014).

(iii) Information and breast cancer awareness

To improve screening rates, the Japanese government implemented an intervention aimed at reducing out-of-pocket costs, and offered vouchers for free screening accompanied by information leaflets to women in specific age groups to undergo breast cancer screening nationwide (Tabuchi et al., 2013). The vouchers increased the participation rate and decreased inequalities in screening (Sano et al., 2014).

(e) Other countries in South-East Asia

(i) Bangladesh

The National Cancer Control Strategy and Plan of Action 2009–2015 in Bangladesh has promoted breast awareness among all women and CBE for women aged 40–69 years (Ministry of Health and Family Welfare, Bangladesh, 2008). However, because resources are extremely limited, the most cost-effective strategy for screening needed to be sought (Hussain & Sullivan, 2013). General health education in the country is poor; only few people are aware of cancer, and most patients are diagnosed at an advanced stage (Hossain et al., 2014). Studies have suggested that women have insufficient knowledge of breast cancer (Chowdhury & Sultana, 2011), but women with higher education levels were more likely to know about BSE (Rasu et al., 2011).

(ii) Brunei Darussalam

In 2007, the Ministry of Health developed the Integrated Health Screening and Health Promotion Programme, which includes screening for colorectal, cervical, and breast cancer for all people in Brunei Darussalam, i.e. approximately 46 000 people in 2009 (Ministry of Health, Brunei Darussalam, 2007). The programme includes mammography for women at a certain age; the national government has made efforts to collaborate with volunteer associations and has promoted breast cancer awareness.

(iii) China

China does not currently have a national screening programme or national screening guidelines (Wang et al., 2013). Although screening programmes exist in local areas, the screening method used and the target population are not standardized (Mo et al., 2013; Pan et al., 2013; Wang et al., 2013). Based on the China Chronic Disease and Risk Factor Surveillance System, in 2010, 21.7% of women aged 18 years and older had ever had any breast cancer examination (Wang et al., 2013). The participation rate for breast cancer screening was higher in the eastern region of China than in the western region, and was higher in women with higher education levels. The highest participation rate was observed among women aged 30–49 years, and the participation rate decreased with increasing age. To increase the participation rate, free breast cancer examination programmes have been offered by local governments in some rural districts (Wang et al., 2013). These programmes cover CBE, mammography, and ultrasonography. Between 2009 and 2011, such programmes facilitated the screening of 1.46 million women living in rural areas. Overall, awareness of breast cancer is low, but differences exist by location, age group, and education level (Huang et al., 2011, Liu et al., 2014). The national government has promoted the China National Plan for Noncommunicable and Chronic Diseases Prevention and Treatment, 2012–2015 (Chinese Center for Disease Control and Prevention, 2012).

(iv) Hong Kong Special Administrative Region, China

In 2012, the Cancer Expert Working Group on Prevention and Screening revised the guidelines for breast cancer screening that had been developed in 2002 and 2008 (Centre for Health Protection, 2012). BSE, CBE, and mammography were not recommended in women at average risk, but women were advised to be aware of early symptoms of breast cancer and to consult a doctor if these occur. Opportunistic screening (CBE, mammography, and ultrasonography) is available in private hospitals (Lui et al., 2007). A community-based outreach programme has increased knowledge of breast cancer and screening (Chan et al., 2007). Although most women were aware of the benefits of mammography, they were reluctant to participate in mammography screening and CBE because of screening fees and lack of time (Chua et al., 2005).

(v) India

The National Cancer Control Programme was started in 1975 and revised in 1984–1985. Although the programme promotes education for primary prevention and early detection, it is not specific for breast cancer (Ministry of Health and Family Welfare, Government of India, 2005). Breast cancer screening by CBE or mammography is available only within research studies conducted at a few institutions or to women who refer themselves to specialty hospitals to have the screening provided for a fee (Agarwal & Ramakant 2008; Reddy et al., 2012). A recent study assessed cancer awareness among women of low socioeconomic status in Mumbai. Among 182 participants, of which the majority (90.5%) were from lower socioeconomic groups, knowledge about cancer was good (84.6%) compared with knowledge about cancer screening (35.1%); awareness was higher among the richer and more educated women. Major sources of information were friends or relatives (46.1%) and the media (35.2%). Only 6.6% of the participants had undergone screening (Kumar et al., 2011). Among the 52 011 women in the intervention group of a breast cancer screening trial in Trivandrum District, 23.2% reported practicing BSE, 96.8% had attended CBE, and 49.1% of 2880 screen-positive women attended referral. Women who were not currently married or who had no family history of cancer were significantly less likely to attend the screening process at any level (Grosse Frie et al., 2013).

(vi) Indonesia

Since 1996, 8 out of 33 provinces in Indonesia have adopted the Integrated Comprehensive Cancer Control Programme and have implemented the Population-Based Cancer Control (PBCC) Program (WHO, 2008a). The PBCC Program aims to improve people's knowledge through education, focusing mainly on prevention, early detection of the most common cancers, and home-based palliative care. The PBCC Program is well established in several provinces, and all of the established programmes have a network to monitor their training activities. These activities are carried out by primary care providers and supported by the PBCC Program team. More than 74 million people are being served by the PBCC Program, and cancer awareness has increased significantly. The Ministry of Health established the National Comprehensive Cancer Plan in 2005, and in 2007 provided services for the early detection of breast cancer in six districts as pilot projects (WHO, 2008a). A preliminary result of the breast cancer screening with CBE was reported from the project conducted in Jakarta (Kardinah et al., 2014).

(vii) Malaysia

In 2010, the Ministry of Health revised the clinical practice guidelines for the management of breast cancer, including screening for the general population (Ministry of Health Malaysia, 2010). For women aged 50–74 years, biennial mammography screening was recommended. Routine mammography screening was not recommended for women aged 40–49 years, but it could be provided upon request. BSE was recommended for raising awareness but not as a screening method. The Ministry of Health has been promoting BSE and CBE by trained health workers as part of a breast care awareness campaign since 1995 (Dahlui et al., 2011). CBE by a trained health-care professional has been offered to Malaysian women aged 20–65 years attending primary health-care services since 2009 (Bhoo-Pathy et al., 2014). At the same time, women are taught the BSE technique. Since 2012, a targeted mammography screening programme has been made available for women at high risk of breast cancer, namely those with a family history of breast cancer or with breast abnormalities (Bhoo-Pathy et al., 2014). According to the Third National Health Morbidity Survey, in 2006 the breast examination rates were 57.1% for BSE, 51.8% for CBE, and 7.6% for mammography (Dahlui et al., 2011). Knowledge of breast cancer and screening is reported to be low in Malaysia (Parsa et al., 2008; Hadi et al., 2010).

(viii) Pakistan

The Lady Health Worker Programme, a unique system in Pakistan, was developed by the national government in 1994 to provide essential primary health services (WHO, 2008b). The programme selected, trained, and deployed 100 000 female community health workers throughout the country by 2005. Through monthly visits to the female community in their assigned areas, the Lady Health Workers teach BSE and highlight the importance of breast cancer screening (Baig & Ali, 2006). In urban areas, knowledge of breast cancer has spread among educated women who are employed by large companies, and 55% of these women had the experience of learning BSE (Banning & Hafeez, 2009).

(ix) Philippines

Although more than half of the female population does not have any health insurance, women in the Philippines undergo breast cancer screening even if it is at their own expense (National Statistics Office, 2009). The Breast Cancer Control Programme of the Philippines includes nationwide programmes for breast cancer prevention as follows: public information, health education, case finding, and treatment integrated into the community health structure (Ngelangel & Wang, 2002).

(x) Thailand

A National Cancer Control Programme, including breast cancer screening, was developed in Thailand in 1998 (National Cancer Control Programme, Thailand, 2013). Thailand also has opportunistic screening and some pilot studies in local areas. Because provision of universal access to mammography is not currently possible in Thailand, risk-prediction models are being developed in order to target mammography screening only at women at higher risk of breast cancer (Anothaisintawee et al., 2012, 2014). Knowledge and uptake of screening are low, and campaigns for increasing public awareness and teaching BSE have been recommended (Mukem et al., 2014).

(xi) Viet Nam

The National Cancer Control Programme was introduced in selected regions of Viet Nam in 2008. The objectives of the programme were to decrease cancer morbidity and mortality and to improve the quality of life of cancer patients (Nguyen et al., 2013). To realize these objectives, six regions in which cancer registries had been established initiated an organized screening programme with CBE. Although the screening policy focused on women aged 40–55 years, there were differences in the target age range of women among the regions, as follows: 35–60 years in Hanoi, 40–55 years in Hai Phong, 30–50 years in Thừa Thiên-Huế, and 40–54 years in Thái Nguyên. Because of the fiscal constraints of the National Cancer Control Programme, only about 15–20% of the total population in each region participated in 2008 (Nguyen et al., 2013).

3.2.7 Oceania

In Australia and New Zealand, organized breast cancer screening has been established nationwide, as well as breast awareness programmes.

(a) Australia

(i) Systems, policies, and guidelines

In Australia, organized screening was established in 1991 by the national government, and BreastScreen Australia is the national breast cancer screening programme (Australian Government, Department of Health, 2014). The Australian government performs the overall coordination in terms of policy-making, national data collection, quality control, monitoring, and evaluation. The responsibility of implementing the programmes lies with the governments of each state and territory. In 2013, BreastScreen Australia operated in more than 600 locations, including fixed and mobile screening units. Recruitment and reminder systems by mail ensure that women in the target group are screened and rescreened in accordance with the programme policy. The screening is provided free of charge for all Australian women.

The screening method for breast cancer is mammography without CBE (AIHW, 2013; Australian Government, Department of Health, 2014). The target group for screening is women aged 50–74 years (Table 3.8). Nevertheless, free mammography screening is available for

Table 3.8 Policies and practice for breast cancer screening in Oceania

Country	Type of programme[a]	Start year	Screening practice	Target age (years)	Interval (years)	Examination coverage[b] (%)	Mammography units per million women aged 50–69 years in 2013[c]	References
Australia	National organized programme	1991	Mammography	50–74	2	55.0[d]	—	AIHW (2014), Australian Government, Department of Health (2014)
Fiji	Partial programme	Unclear	Unclear	Unclear	Unclear	Unclear	28.8	Ministry of Health, Fiji (2009)
New Zealand	National organized programme	1998	Mammography	45–69	2	70.2[e]	—	BreastScreen Aotearoa (2014)

[a] Partial programmes are supported by government and nongovernmental organizations and are conducted mainly in local areas, and screening systems have not been standardized.

[b] Annual examinations as percentage of annual target population, with the screening method and within the age range reported in the policy.

[c] WHO (2014).

[d] Coverage refers to women aged 50–69 years, as this was the target age until 2012.

[e] Coverage refers to 2010–2012.

asymptomatic women aged 40–49 years, or for women aged 75 years and older who have decided to participate based on current knowledge and personal choice. The screening interval is 2 years. All women are screened using two-view mammography, and results are read by at least two professionals.

The screening results are provided by letters directly to women who have undergone the screening (Australian Government, Department of Health, 2014). If any suspicious diagnostic images are found, further investigation, including clinical examination, mammography, ultrasonography, and biopsy, is provided free of charge by BreastScreen Australia. Women with histologically confirmed breast cancer are actively involved in the decision-making process about management of the cancer and are given the option of referral to a specialized treatment clinic for breast cancer or returning to their nominated general practitioner for referral to the appropriate surgeon.

BreastScreen Australia has rigorously monitored and assessed the performance of breast cancer screening (Australian Government, Department of Health, 2014). At the national level, the screening results have been evaluated based on the following performance indicators: participation, rescreening, recall to assessment, invasive breast cancer detection, DCIS detection, sensitivity, morbidity, and mortality. A comprehensive system of accreditation ensures that all BreastScreen Australia services operate under a common set of standards (BreastScreen Australia, 2008; Australian Government, Department of Health, 2014). Each service is assessed on a regular basis by an independent team to ensure that the services provided comply with the national standards.

(ii) Participation

The programme's aim was to achieve a participation rate of at least 70% among women aged 50–69 years. In 2011–2012, the programme was able to screen about 55% of women in this age group (Table 3.8; AIHW, 2014). The participation of Aboriginal and Torres Strait Islander women aged 50–69 years was 38%, compared with participation of non-Indigenous women of 54%.

(iii) Information and breast cancer awareness

Extensive efforts, including public awareness campaigns, have improved the knowledge of breast cancer and the need to seek medical advice when symptoms occur (Jones et al., 2010). In many of the states and territories, BreastScreen Australia programmes have continued to develop strategies and initiatives, including the use of appropriate communication, to encourage greater participation by Aboriginal and Torres Strait Islander women (AIHW, 2013). These strategies include group bookings for breast cancer screening for Aboriginal and Torres Strait Islander women. Non-English-speaking women generally participate in breast cancer screening less frequently than English-speaking women; special programmes based on cultural background were adopted to promote awareness of breast cancer among immigrant Chinese women (Koo et al., 2012).

(b) Fiji

The Fiji national government has developed a national strategy plan for noncommunicable disease prevention and control (Ministry of Health, Fiji, 2009). The programme includes improvement of public education on breast cancer.

(c) New Zealand

BreastScreen Aotearoa was established as a national breast cancer screening programme in 1998, to provide free mammograms and follow-up for asymptomatic women (BreastScreen Aotearoa, 2014). This programme is part of the National Screening Unit of the Ministry of Health and provides breast screening services throughout New Zealand.

(i) Systems, policies, and guidelines

The eligible age range for free breast cancer screening was first set at 50–64 years and then extended to 45–69 years in 2004, following the recommendations of a multidisciplinary Expert Advisory Group (Table 3.8). Women aged 70 years and older are not eligible for free mammograms provided by BreastScreen Aotearoa (Baker et al., 2005a, b). The screening interval is 2 years, and all women are screened using two-view mammography (BreastScreen Aotearoa, 2014).

The programme identifies the target population and then sends invitation letters (BreastScreen Aotearoa, 2014). BreastScreen Aotearoa provides clinics for breast cancer screening throughout New Zealand, including clinics in communities, public hospitals, and mobile units. Women who have undergone screening usually receive the results within 2 weeks after the mammography and, upon consent, the general practitioner can also be informed of the results. The assessment of breast cancer is made by a multidisciplinary team of experts. Treatment of breast cancer is provided free of charge in public hospitals and clinics, but a certain amount must be paid for private treatment.

All BreastScreen Aotearoa facilities must meet the BreastScreen Aotearoa National Policy and Quality Standards (BreastScreen Aotearoa, 2014). These standards determine the minimum requirements for any provider of BreastScreen Aotearoa services. Regular audits of BreastScreen Aotearoa are performed to assess how the quality standards are met.

(ii) Participation

In 2010–2012, the coverage rate was 70.2% (Table 3.8): 62.7% for Māori women and 71.1% for non-Māori women (BreastScreen Aotearoa, 2014).

The coverage rate for women aged 50–69 years has increased steadily in Māori women, who have a higher breast cancer mortality rate compared with non-Māori women.

(iii) Information and breast cancer awareness

BreastScreen Aotearoa provides information in various forms, such as leaflets for breast cancer awareness and screening, including specific messages for Māori women (BreastScreen Aotearoa, 2014). The Te Whanau a Apanui Community Health Services have provided education and information about breast cancer screening for Māori and Pacific women (Thomson et al., 2009). The programme also provides mammography screening by a mobile unit, which has increased the participation rate. Although the number of migrant Chinese women has increased, their participation rate has remained lower than that of other New Zealanders because of insufficient knowledge of the national cancer screening programmes and limited engagement with preventive primary care services (Zhang et al., 2014).

References

AAWC (2014). Breast cancer is the leading cause of cancer deaths among women in Armenia. Armenian American Wellness Center, Armenian American Cultural Association. Available from: http://healthiernation.org/services/radiology/.

Abdel-Fattah M, Zaki A, Bassili A, el-Shazly M, Tognoni G (2000). Breast self-examination practice and its impact on breast cancer diagnosis in Alexandria, Egypt. *East Mediterr Health J*, 6(1):34–40. PMID:11370338

Abhyankar P, Volk RJ, Blumenthal-Barby J, Bravo P, Buchholz A, Ozanne E et al. (2013). Balancing the presentation of information and options in patient decision aids: an updated review. *BMC Med Inform Decis Mak*, 13(Suppl 2):S6. doi:10.1186/1472-6947-13-S2-S6 PMID:24625214

Abraído-Lanza AF, Chao MT, Gates CY (2005). Acculturation and cancer screening among Latinas: results from the National Health Interview Survey. *Ann Behav Med*, 29(1):22–8. doi:10.1207/s15324796abm2901_4 PMID:15677297

Abuidris DO, Elsheikh A, Ali M, Musa H, Elgaili E, Ahmed AO et al. (2013). Breast-cancer screening with trained volunteers in a rural area of Sudan: a pilot study. *Lancet Oncol*, 14(4):363–70. doi:10.1016/S1470-2045(12)70583-1 PMID:23375833

Abulkhair OA, Al Tahan FM, Young SE, Musaad SM, Jazieh AR (2010). The first national public breast cancer screening program in Saudi Arabia. *Ann Saudi Med*, 30(5):350–7. PMID:20697170

Acuna SA, Angarita FA, Escallon J (2014). Assessing patterns of practice of sentinel lymph node biopsy for breast cancer in Latin America. *World J Surg*, 38(5):1077–83. doi:10.1007/s00268-013-2382-1 PMID:24305934

Adib SM, El Saghir NS, Ammar W (2009). Guidelines for breast cancer screening in Lebanon Public Health Communication. *J Med Liban*, 57(2):72–4. PMID:19623881

Agarwal G, Ramakant P (2008). Breast cancer care in India: the current scenario and the challenges for the future. *Breast Care (Basel)*, 3(1):21–7. doi:10.1159/000115288 PMID:20824016

Agudelo Botero M (2013). Sociodemographic determinants of access to breast cancer screening in Mexico: a review of national surveys [in Spanish]. *Salud Colect*, 9(1):79–90. doi:10.1590/S1851-82652013000100007 PMID:23680751

Ahmed BA (2010). Awareness and practice of breast cancer and breast-self examination among university students in Yemen. *Asian Pac J Cancer Prev*, 11(1):101–5. PMID:20593937

Ahmed NU, Smith GL, Haber G, Belcon MC (2009). Are women with functional limitations at high risk of underutilization of mammography screening? *Womens Health Issues*, 19(1):79–87. doi:10.1016/j.whi.2008.09.001 PMID:19111790

AIHW (2013). Cancer in Aboriginal and Torres Strait Islander people of Australia: an overview. Cancer Series No. 78. Canberra: Australian Institute of Health and Welfare, Australian Government. Available from: http://www.aihw.gov.au/publication-detail/?id=60129544700.

AIHW (2014). BreastScreen Australian monitoring report 2011-2012. Cancer Series No. 72. Cat. No. CAN 68. Canberra: Australian Institute of Health and Welfare, Australian Government. Available from: http://www.aihw.gov.au/publication-detail/?id=60129548886/.

Akbaraly Foundation (2014). Care for a woman life for a country. Available from: http://www.fondationakbaraly.org/.

Akhtari-Zavare M, Ghanbari-Baghestan A, Latiff LA, Matinnia N, Hoseini M (2014). Knowledge of breast cancer and breast self-examination practice among Iranian women in Hamedan, Iran. *Asian Pac J Cancer Prev*, 15(16):6531–4. doi:10.7314/APJCP.2014.15.16.6531 PMID:25169482

Akinyemiju TF (2012). Socio-economic and health access determinants of breast and cervical cancer screening in low-income countries: analysis of the World Health Survey. *PLoS ONE*, 7(11):e48834. doi:10.1371/journal.pone.0048834 PMID:23155413

Al-Azmy SF, Alkhabbaz A, Almutawa HA, Ismaiel AE, Makboul G, El-Shazly MK (2013). Practicing breast self-examination among women attending primary health care in Kuwait. *Alexandria J Med*, 49(3):281–6. doi:10.1016/j.ajme.2012.08.009

Al-Naggar RA, Isa ZM, Shah SA, Chen R, Kadir SY (2009). Mammography screening: Female doctors' attitudes and practice in Sana'a, Yemen. *Asian Pac J Cancer Prev*, 10(5):743–6. PMID:20104962

Albada A, Ausems MG, Bensing JM, van Dulmen S (2009). Tailored information about cancer risk and screening: a systematic review. *Patient Educ Couns*, 77(2):155–71. doi:10.1016/j.pec.2009.03.005 PMID:19376676

Alejo-Martínez H, Wiesner-Ceballos C, Arciniegas-Álvarez MA, Poveda-Suárez CA, Puerto-Jiménez DN, Ardila-Hernández IT et al. (2013). La calidad de la mamografía en Colombia: análisis de un estudio piloto *Anales de Radiología México*, 2013(3):164–74. Available from: http://www.medigraphic.com/pdfs/anaradmex/arm-2013/arm133e.pdf.

Alharbi NA, Alshammari MS, Almutairi BM, Makboul G, El-Shazly MK (2012). Knowledge, awareness, and practices concerning breast cancer among Kuwaiti female school teachers. *Alexandria J Med*, 48(1):75–82. doi:10.1016/j.ajme.2011.10.003

American Cancer Society (2014). Breast cancer prevention and early detection. Available from: http://www.cancer.org/cancer/breastcancer/moreinformation/breastcancerearlydetection/breast-cancer-early-detection-toc.

Andersen MR, Smith R, Meischke H, Bowen D, Urban N (2003). Breast cancer worry and mammography use by women with and without a family history in a population-based sample. *Cancer Epidemiol Biomarkers Prev*, 12(4):314–20. PMID:12692105

Andersen SB, Vejborg I, von Euler-Chelpin M (2008). Participation behaviour following a false positive test in the Copenhagen mammography screening programme. *Acta Oncol*, 47(4):550–5. doi:10.1080/02841860801935483 PMID:18465321

Andresen EM, Peterson-Besse JJ, Krahn GL, Walsh ES, Horner-Johnson W, Iezzoni LI (2013). Pap, mammography, and clinical breast examination screening among women with disabilities: a systematic review. *Womens Health Issues*, 23(4):e205–14. doi:10.1016/j.whi.2013.04.002 PMID:23816150

Anothaisintawee T, Teerawattananon Y, Wiratkapun C, Kasamesup V, Thakkinstian A (2012). Risk prediction models of breast cancer: a systematic review of model performances. *Breast Cancer Res Treat*, 133(1):1–10. doi:10.1007/s10549-011-1853-z PMID:22076477

Anothaisintawee T, Teerawattananon Y, Wiratkapun C, Srinakarin J, Woodtichartpreecha P, Hirunpat S et al. (2014). Development and validation of a breast cancer risk prediction model for Thai women: a cross-sectional study. *Asian Pac J Cancer Prev*, 15(16):6811–7. doi:10.7314/APJCP.2014.15.16.6811 PMID:25169530

Apffelstaedt JP, Hattingh R, Baatjes K, Wessels N (2014). Results of a pilot programme of mammographic breast cancer screening in the Western Cape. *S Afr Med J*, 104(4):297–8. doi:10.7196/samj.7242 PMID:25118557

Are You Dense? (2013). Exposing the best-kept secret. Available from: http://www.areyoudense.org, http://areyoudenseadvocacy.org.

Aro AR, de Koning HJ, Absetz P, Schreck M (2001). Two distinct groups of non-attenders in an organized mammography screening program. *Breast Cancer Res Treat*, 70(2):145–53. doi:10.1023/A:1012939228916 PMID:11768605

Aro AR, Pilvikki Absetz S, van Elderen TM, van der Ploeg E, van der Kamp LJ (2000). False-positive findings in mammography screening induces short-term distress - breast cancer-specific concern prevails longer. *Eur J Cancer*, 36(9):1089–97. doi:10.1016/S0959-8049(00)00065-4 PMID:10854941

Asobayire A, Barley R (2014). Women's cultural perceptions and attitudes towards breast cancer: Northern Ghana. *Health Promot Int*, 30(3):647–57. doi:10.1093/heapro/dat087 PMID:24474424

ATREP (2014). Stratégie nationale de lutte contre le cancer, 2010–2014. Association Tunisienne pour la Recherche et les Etudes en Pharmacie, Ministère de la Santé, Tunisia. Available from: http://www.insp.rns.tn/doc/cancer/plan_cancer_monastir_13_04_2014.pdf.

Austoker J (1999). Gaining informed consent for screening. Is difficult–but many misconceptions need to be undone. *BMJ*, 319(7212):722–3. doi:10.1136/bmj.319.7212.722 PMID:10487983

Australian Government, Department of Health (2014). BreastScreen Australian Program. Available from: http://www.cancerscreening.gov.au/internet/screening/publishing.nsf/Content/about-breastscancer.

Avila IYC, Triana LFB, Martelo LC, Villadiego GM, Payares WPO, Medrano EMV et al. (2014). Factores asociados al uso de mamografía en mujeres mayores de 50 años: Cartagena. *Rev Cienc Salud*, 12(2):183–93. doi:10.12804/revsalud12.2.2014.04

Azage M, Abeje G, Mekonnen A (2013). Assessment of factors associated with breast self-examination among health extension workers in West Gojjam Zone, Northwest Ethiopia. *Int J Breast Cancer*, 2013:814395. doi:10.1155/2013/814395 PMID:24298389

Azaiza F, Cohen M (2006). Health beliefs and rates of breast cancer screening among Arab women. *J Womens Health (Larchmt)*, 15(5):520–30. doi:10.1089/jwh.2006.15.520 PMID:16796479

Azaiza F, Cohen M, Awad M, Daoud F (2010). Factors associated with low screening for breast cancer in the Palestinian Authority: relations of availability, environmental barriers, and cancer-related fatalism. *Cancer*, 116(19):4646–55. doi:10.1002/cncr.25378 PMID:20589933

Babu GR, Samari G, Cohen SP, Mahapatra T, Wahbe RM, Mermash S et al. (2011). Breast cancer screening among females in Iran and recommendations for improved practice: a review. *Asian Pac J Cancer Prev*, 12(7):1647–55. PMID:22126539

Bahrain Cancer Society (2012). Breast screening. Available from: http://www.bahraincancer.com/bcs_cancer_national_campaign.asp.

Baig S, Ali TS (2006). Evaluation of efficacy of self breast examination for breast cancer prevention: a cost effective screening tool. *Asian Pac J Cancer Prev*, 7(1):154–6. PMID:16629536

Baines CJ, To T, Wall C (1990). Women's attitudes to screening after participation in the National Breast Screening Study. A questionnaire survey. *Cancer*, 65(7):1663–9. doi:10.1002/1097-0142(19900401)65:7<1663::AID-CNCR2820650735>3.0.CO;2-A PMID:2311075

Baker LH (1982). Breast Cancer Detection Demonstration Project: five-year summary report. *CA Cancer J Clin*, 32(4):194–225. doi:10.3322/canjclin.32.4.194 PMID:6805867

Baker S, Wall M, Bloomfield A (2005a). Breast cancer screening for women aged 40 to 49 years–what does the evidence mean for New Zealand? *N Z Med J*, 118(1221):U1628. PMID:16138166

Baker S, Wall M, Bloomfield A (2005b). What is the most appropriate breast-cancer screening interval for women aged 45 to 49 years in New Zealand? *N Z Med J*, 118(1221):U1636. PMID:16138174

Bakker DA, Lightfoot NE, Steggles S, Jackson C (1998). The experience and satisfaction of women attending breast cancer screening. *Oncol Nurs Forum*, 25(1):115–21. PMID:9460779

Banks E, Beral V, Cameron R, Hogg A, Langley N, Barnes I et al. (2002). Comparison of various characteristics of women who do and do not attend for breast cancer screening. *Breast Cancer Res*, 4(1):R1. doi:10.1186/bcr418 PMID:11879559

Banning M, Hafeez H (2009). Perceptions of breast health practices in Pakistani Muslim women. *Asian Pac J Cancer Prev*, 10(5):841–7. PMID:20104976

Barker KK, Galardi TR (2011). Dead by 50: lay expertise and breast cancer screening. *Soc Sci Med*, 72(8):1351–8. doi:10.1016/j.socscimed.2011.02.024 PMID:21440969

Baron-Epel O (2010). Attitudes and beliefs associated with mammography in a multiethnic population in Israel. *Health Educ Behav*, 37(2):227–42. doi:10.1177/1090198109339460 PMID:19690289

Barratt A (2008). Evidence based medicine and shared decision making: the challenge of getting both evidence and preferences into health care. *Patient Educ Couns*, 73(3):407–12. doi:10.1016/j.pec.2008.07.054 PMID:18845414

Bello TO, Olugbenga-Bello AI, Oguntola AS, Adeoti ML, Ojemakinde OM (2011). Knowledge and practice of breast cancer screening among female nurses and lay women in Osogbo, Nigeria. *West Afr J Med*, 30(4):296–300. PMID:22669837

Bener A, Alwash R, Miller CJ, Denic S, Dunn EV (2001). Knowledge, attitudes, and practices related to breast cancer screening: a survey of Arabic women. *J Cancer Educ*, 16(4):215–20. PMID:11848670

Bener A, El Ayoubi HR, Moore MA, Basha B, Joseph S, Chouchane L (2009). Do we need to maximise the breast cancer screening awareness? Experience with an endogamous society with high fertility. *Asian Pac J Cancer Prev*, 10(4):599–604. PMID:19827877

Bener A, Honein G, Carter AO, Da'ar Z, Miller C, Dunn EV (2002). The determinants of breast cancer screening behavior: a focus group study of women in the United Arab Emirates. *Oncol Nurs Forum*, 29(9):E91–8. doi:10.1188/02.ONF.E91-E98 PMID:12370705

Beysebayev E, Tulebayev K, Meymanalyev T (2015). Breast cancer diagnosis by mammography in Kazakhstan - staging results of breast cancer with double reading. *Asian Pac J Cancer Prev*, 16(1):31–4. doi:10.7314/APJCP.2015.16.1.31 PMID:25640371

Bhoo-Pathy N, Subramaniam S, Taib NA, Hartman M, Alias Z, Tan GH et al. (2014). Spectrum of very early breast cancer in a setting without organised screening. *Br J Cancer*, 110(9):2187–94. doi:10.1038/bjc.2014.183 PMID:24736587

Biesecker BB, Schwartz MD, Marteau TM (2013). Enhancing informed choice to undergo health screening: a systematic review. *Am J Health Behav*, 37(3):351–9. doi:10.5993/AJHB.37.3.8 PMID:23985182

Bird JA, McPhee SJ, Ha NT, Le B, Davis T, Jenkins CN (1998). Opening pathways to cancer screening for Vietnamese-American women: lay health workers hold a key. *Prev Med*, 27(6):821–9. doi:10.1006/pmed.1998.0365 PMID:9922064

Black ME, Stein KF, Loveland-Cherry CJ (2001). Older women and mammography screening behavior: do possible selves contribute? *Health Educ Behav*, 28(2):200–16. doi:10.1177/109019810102800206 PMID:11265829

Blanco S, Buffa R, Gamarra S, Pesce V, Viniegra M (2010). Guía técnica de procedimientos mínimos de control de calidad en mamografía analógica. Buenos Aires, Argentina: Programa Nacional de Cáncer de Mama, Instituto Nacional del Cáncer. Available from: http://www.msal.gob.ar/inc/images/stories/downloads/publicaciones/equipo_medico/Cancer_de_mama/

Guia_Tecnicos_en_mamografia_analogica_cancer_de_mama.pdf.

Blumenthal D, Collins SR (2014). Health care coverage under the Affordable Care Act–a progress report. *N Engl J Med*, 371(3):275–81. doi:10.1056/NEJMhpr1405667 PMID:24988300

Blumenthal-Barby JS, Cantor SB, Russell HV, Naik AD, Volk RJ (2013). Decision aids: when 'nudging' patients to make a particular choice is more ethical than balanced, nondirective content. *Health Aff (Millwood)*, 32(2):303–10. doi:10.1377/hlthaff.2012.0761 PMID:23381523

Bodapati SL, Babu GR (2013). Oncologist perspectives on breast cancer screening in India- results from a qualitative study in Andhra Pradesh. *Asian Pac J Cancer Prev*, 14(10):5817–23. doi:10.7314/APJCP.2013.14.10.5817 PMID:24289583

Borrayo EA (2004). Where's Maria? A video to increase awareness about breast cancer and mammography screening among low-literacy Latinas. *Prev Med*, 39(1):99–110. doi:10.1016/j.ypmed.2004.03.024 PMID:15207991

Borrayo EA, Buki LP, Feigal BM (2005). Breast cancer detection among older Latinas: is it worth the risk? *Qual Health Res*, 15(9):1244–63. doi:10.1177/1049732305281337 PMID:16204403

Bouchlaka A, Ben Abdallah M, Ben Aissa R, Smida S, Ouechtati A, Boussen H et al. (2009). Practice of large scale mammography in the Ariana area of Tunisia: prelude to a mass screening? [in French]. *Tunis Med*, 87(7):426–31. PMID:20063674

Brandan ME, Ruiz-Trejo C, Verdejo-Silva M, Guevara M, Lozano-Zalce H, Madero-Preciado L et al. (2004). Evaluation of equipment performance, patient dose, imaging quality, and diagnostic coincidence in five Mexico City mammography services. *Arch Med Res*, 35(1):24–30. doi:10.1016/j.arcmed.2003.06.008 PMID:15036796

BreastScreen Aotearoa (2014). Independent Māori Monitoring Report 4; New Times Series Report: Screening and Assessment, July 2010 to June 2012: Ages 45 to 69 years. Wellington, New Zealand: University of Otago. Available from: http://www.nsu.govt.nz/system/files/page/independent_maori_monitoring_report_screening_and_assessment_july_2010_to_june_2012.pdf.

BreastScreen Australia (2008). National Accreditation Standards: BreastScreen Australia Quality Improvement Programs. Available from: http://www.cancerscreening.gov.au/internet/screening/publishing.nsf/Content/br-accreditation/$File/standards.pdf.

Brett J, Austoker J (2001). Women who are recalled for further investigation for breast screening: psychological consequences 3 years after recall and factors affecting re-attendance. *J Public Health Med*, 23(4):292–300. doi:10.1093/pubmed/23.4.292 PMID:11873891

Brett J, Bankhead C, Henderson B, Watson E, Austoker J (2005). The psychological impact of mammographic screening. A systematic review. *Psychooncology*, 14(11):917–38. doi:10.1002/pon.904 PMID:15786514

Brewer NT, Salz T, Lillie SE (2007). Systematic review: the long-term effects of false-positive mammograms. *Ann Intern Med*, 146(7):502–10. doi:10.7326/0003-4819-146-7-200704030-00006 PMID:17404352

Bright K, Barghash M, Donach M, de la Barrera MG, Schneider RJ, Formenti SC (2011). The role of health system factors in delaying final diagnosis and treatment of breast cancer in Mexico City, Mexico. *Breast*, 20(Suppl 2):S54–9. doi:10.1016/j.breast.2011.02.012 PMID:21371885

Brito LM, Chein MB, Brito LG, Amorim AM, Marana HR (2010). Knowledge, practice and attitude about breast self-exam from women of a Northeastern municipality, Brazil [in Portuguese]. *Rev Bras Ginecol Obstet*, 32(5):241–6. PMID:21085754

Brodersen J, Siersma V, Ryle M (2011). Breast cancer screening: "reassuring" the worried well? *Scand J Public Health*, 39(3):326–32. doi:10.1177/1403494810396558 PMID:21273225

Brodersen J, Thorsen H, Cockburn J (2004). The adequacy of measurement of short and long-term consequences of false-positive screening mammography. *J Med Screen*, 11(1):39–44. doi:10.1258/096914104772950745 PMID:15006113

Bulliard JL, de Landtsheer JP, Levi F (2004). Profile of women not attending in the Swiss Mammography Screening Pilot Programme. *Breast*, 13(4):284–9. doi:10.1016/j.breast.2004.03.001 PMID:15325662

Burkell J, Campbell DG (2005). "What does this mean?" How Web-based consumer health information fails to support information seeking in the pursuit of informed consent for screening test decisions. *J Med Libr Assoc*, 93(3):363–73. PMID:16059426

Burton MV, Warren R, Price D, Earl H (1998). Psychological predictors of attendance at annual breast screening examinations. *Br J Cancer*, 77(11):2014–9. doi:10.1038/bjc.1998.335 PMID:9667685

Bynum JP, Braunstein JB, Sharkey P, Haddad K, Wu AW (2005). The influence of health status, age, and race on screening mammography in elderly women. *Arch Intern Med*, 165(18):2083–8. doi:10.1001/archinte.165.18.2083 PMID:16216997

Caleffi M, Ribeiro RA, Duarte Filho DL, Ashton-Prolla P, Bedin AJ Jr, Skonieski GP et al. (2009). A model to optimize public health care and downstage breast cancer in limited-resource populations in southern Brazil. (Porto Alegre Breast Health Intervention Cohort). *BMC Public Health*, 9(1):83. doi:10.1186/1471-2458-9-83 PMID:19284670

Canadian Breast Cancer Foundation (2014). Benefits and limitations of mammography. Available from:

http://www.cbcf.org/central/AboutBreastHealth/GetScreened, accessed 13 January 2015.

Canbulat N, Uzun O (2008). Health beliefs and breast cancer screening behaviors among female health workers in Turkey. *Eur J Oncol Nurs*, 12(2):148–56. doi:10.1016/j.ejon.2007.12.002 PMID:18314391

Cancer Association of Zimbabwe (2014). Cancer Association of Zimbabwe. Harare, Zimbabwe. Available from: http://www.cancerzimbabwe.org/index.html, accessed 26 October 2014.

Cancer Free Women (2013). Breast cancer war fronts. Available from: http://cancerfreewomen.org/.

Cancer Quality Council of Ontario (2014). Breast cancer screening participation. Available from: http://www.csqi.on.ca/by_patient_journey/screening/breast_screening_participation/.

CANSA (2014a). Get screened – early detection is key. Cancer Association of South Africa. Available from: http://www.cansa.org.za/get-screened-early-detection/.

CANSA (2014b). Screening and cancer control. Cancer Association of South Africa. Available from: http://www.cansa.org.za/screening-and-cancer-control/, accessed 14 April 2015.

CDC (2000). State laws relating to breast cancer. Atlanta (GA), USA: Centers for Disease Control and Prevention.

CDC (2014). What is a mammogram and when should I get one? Atlanta (GA), USA: Centers for Disease Control and Prevention. Available from: http://www.cdc.gov/cancer/breast/basic_info/mammograms.htm.

CDC (1989). Trends in screening mammograms for women 50 years of age and older–Behavioral Risk Factor Surveillance System, 1987. *MMWR Morb Mortal Wkly Rep*, 38(9):137–40. PMID:2493130

Centre for Health Protection (2012). Cancer Expert Working Group on Cancer Prevention and Screening: Recommendation on breast cancer screening. Available from: http://www.chp.gov.hk/files/pdf/recommendations_on_breast_cancer_screening_2012.pdf.

Chamot E, Charvet AI, Perneger TV (2001). Predicting stages of adoption of mammography screening in a general population. *Eur J Cancer*, 37(15):1869–77. doi:10.1016/S0959-8049(01)00234-9 PMID:11576843

Chamot E, Charvet AI, Perneger TV (2005). Variability in women's desire for information about mammography screening: implications for informed consent. *Eur J Cancer Prev*, 14(4):413–8. doi:10.1097/00008469-200508000-00015 PMID:16030433

Chamot E, Charvet AI, Perneger TV (2007). Who gets screened, and where: a comparison of organised and opportunistic mammography screening in Geneva, Switzerland. *Eur J Cancer*, 43(3):576–84. doi:10.1016/j.ejca.2006.10.017 PMID:17223542

Champion V, Foster JL, Menon U (1997). Tailoring interventions for health behavior change in breast cancer screening. *Cancer Pract*, 5(5):283–8. PMID:9341350

Chan SS, Chow DM, Loh EK, Wong DC, Cheng KK, Fung WY et al. (2007). Using a community-based outreach program to improve breast health awareness among women in Hong Kong. *Public Health Nurs*, 24(3):265–73. doi:10.1111/j.1525-1446.2007.00633.x PMID:17456128

Charry LC, Carrasquilla G, Roca S (2008). Equity regarding early breast cancer screening according to health insurance status in Colombia [in Spanish]. *Rev Salud Publica (Bogota)*, 10(4):571–82. doi:10.1590/S0124-00642008000400007 PMID:19360207

Chiarelli AM, Edwards SA, Prummel MV, Muradali D, Majpruz V, Done SJ et al. (2013). Digital compared with screen-film mammography: performance measures in concurrent cohorts within an organized breast screening program. *Radiology*, 268(3):684–93. doi:10.1148/radiol.13122567 PMID:23674784

Chinese Center for Disease Control and Prevention (2012). China National Plan for NCD Prevention and Treatment (2012-2015). Available from: http://www.chinacdc.cn/en/ne/201207/t20120725_64430.html.

Chowdhury S, Sultana S (2011). Awareness on breast cancer among the women of reproductive age. *J Family Report Health*, 5:125–32.

Chua MS, Mok TS, Kwan WH, Yeo W, Zee B (2005). Knowledge, perceptions, and attitudes of Hong Kong Chinese women on screening mammography and early breast cancer management. *Breast J*, 11(1):52–6. doi:10.1111/j.1075-122X.2005.21480.x PMID:15647079

Chukmaitov A, Wan TT, Menachemi N, Cashin C (2008). Breast cancer knowledge and attitudes toward mammography as predictors of breast cancer preventive behavior in Kazakh, Korean, and Russian women in Kazakhstan. *Int J Public Health*, 53(3):123–30. doi:10.1007/s00038-008-7001-9 PMID:19127885

CIS Anti-Cancer Association (2013a). The CIS Anti-Cancer Association: Kazakhstan. Available from: http://oncologyngo-cis.org/en/participants/kazakhstan/.

CIS Anti-Cancer Association (2013b). The CIS Anti-Cancer Association: Kyrgyzstan. Available from: http://oncologyngo-cis.org/en/participants/Kyrgyzstan.

Clegg-Lamptey J, Dakubo J, Attobra YN (2009). Why do breast cancer patients report late or abscond during treatment in Ghana? A pilot study. *Ghana Med J*, 43(3):127–31. PMID:20126325

Cockburn J, De Luise T, Hurley S, Clover K (1992). Development and validation of the PCQ: a questionnaire to measure the psychological consequences of screening mammography. *Soc Sci Med*, 34(10):1129–34. doi:10.1016/0277-9536(92)90286-Y PMID:1641674

Cockburn J, Staples M, Hurley SF, De Luise T (1994). Psychological consequences of screening mammography. *J Med Screen*, 1(1):7–12. PMID:8790480

Coleman EA, Coon S, Mohrmann C, Hardin S, Stewart B, Gibson RS et al. (2003a). Developing and testing lay literature about breast cancer screening for African

American women. *Clin J Oncol Nurs*, 7(1):66–71. doi:10.1188/03.CJON.66-71 PMID:12629937

Coleman EA, Lord J, Heard J, Coon S, Cantrell M, Mohrmann C et al. (2003b). The Delta project: increasing breast cancer screening among rural minority and older women by targeting rural healthcare providers. *Oncol Nurs Forum*, 30(4):669–77. doi:10.1188/03.ONF.669-677 PMID:12861326

College of the North Atlantic Qatar (2012). Breast cancer awareness. Available from: https://www.cna-qatar.com/breastcancerawareness/Pages/Calendar-of-Events.aspx.

Consedine NS (2012). The demographic, system, and psychosocial origins of mammographic screening disparities: prediction of initiation versus maintenance screening among immigrant and non-immigrant women. *J Immigr Minor Health*, 14(4):570–82. doi:10.1007/s10903-011-9524-z PMID:21904869

Corbex M, Bouzbid S, Boffetta P (2014). Features of breast cancer in developing countries, examples from North-Africa. *Eur J Cancer*, 50(10):1808–18. doi:10.1016/j.ejca.2014.03.016 PMID:24767469

Corrêa RdaS, Freitas-Junior R, Peixoto JE, Rodrigues DC, Lemos ME, Dias CM et al. (2012). Effectiveness of a quality control program in mammography for the Brazilian National Health System [in Portuguese]. *Rev Saude Publica*, 46(5):769–76. PMID:23128252

Coughlin SS, Leadbetter S, Richards T, Sabatino SA (2008). Contextual analysis of breast and cervical cancer screening and factors associated with health care access among United States women, 2002. *Soc Sci Med*, 66(2):260–75. doi:10.1016/j.socscimed.2007.09.009 PMID:18022299

Council of Europe (2003). Council recommendation of 2 December 2003 on cancer screening (2003/878/EC). *Off J Eur Union L*, 327:34–8. Available from: http://eur-lex.europa.eu/LexUriServ/LexUriServ.do?uri=OJ:L:2003:327:0034:0038:EN:PDF.

CPAC (2013). Organized breast cancer screening programs in Canada: report on program performance in 2007 and 2008. Toronto: Canadian Partnership Against Cancer.

CPAC (2014). Breast cancer screening guidelines across Canada: environmental scan. Toronto: Canadian Partnership Against Cancer. Available from: www.cancerview.ca, accessed 13 January 2015.

Crossley ML (2002). 'Could you please pass one of those health leaflets along?': exploring health, morality and resistance through focus groups. *Soc Sci Med*, 55(8):1471–83. doi:10.1016/S0277-9536(01)00265-9 PMID:12231023

Crump SR, Mayberry RM, Taylor BD, Barefield KP, Thomas PE (2000). Factors related to noncompliance with screening mammogram appointments among low-income African-American women. *J Natl Med Assoc*, 92(5):237–46. PMID:10881473

Crump SR, Shipp MP, McCray GG, Morris SJ, Okoli JA, Caplan LS et al. (2008). Abnormal mammogram follow-up: do community lay health advocates make a difference? *Health Promot Pract*, 9(2):140–8. doi:10.1177/1524839907312806 PMID:18340089

D'Orsi C, Tu SP, Nakano C, Carney PA, Abraham LA, Taplin SH et al. (2005). Current realities of delivering mammography services in the community: do challenges with staffing and scheduling exist? *Radiology*, 235(2):391–5. doi:10.1148/radiol.2352040132 PMID:15798153

Dahlui M, Ramli S, Bulgiba AM (2011). Breast cancer prevention and control programs in Malaysia. *Asian Pac J Cancer Prev*, 12(6):1631–4. PMID:22126511

Davey C, White V, Gattellari M, Ward JE (2005). Reconciling population benefits and women's individual autonomy in mammographic screening: in-depth interviews to explore women's views about 'informed choice'. *Aust N Z J Public Health*, 29(1):69–77. doi:10.1111/j.1467-842X.2005.tb00752.x PMID:15782876

Davis TC, Arnold CL, Rademaker A, Bailey SC, Platt DJ, Reynolds C et al. (2012). Differences in barriers to mammography between rural and urban women. *J Womens Health (Larchmt)*, 21(7):748–55. doi:10.1089/jwh.2011.3397 PMID:22519704

De Maio FG, Linetzky B, Ferrante D (2012). Changes in the social gradients for Pap smears and mammograms in Argentina: evidence from the 2005 and 2009 National Risk Factor Surveys. *Public Health*, 126(10):821–6. doi:10.1016/j.puhe.2012.05.011 PMID:23083845

de Munck L, Kwast A, Reiding D, de Bock GH, Otter R, Willemse PH et al. (2013). Attending the breast screening programme after breast cancer treatment: a population-based study. *Cancer Epidemiol*, 37(6):968–72. doi:10.1016/j.canep.2013.09.003 PMID:24075800

De Ver Dye T, Bogale S, Hobden C, Tilahun Y, Hechter V, Deressa T et al. (2011). A mixed-method assessment of beliefs and practice around breast cancer in Ethiopia: implications for public health programming and cancer control. *Glob Public Health*, 6(7):719–31. doi:10.1080/17441692.2010.510479 PMID:20865612

Dean C, Roberts MM, French K, Robinson S (1986). Psychiatric morbidity after screening for breast cancer. *J Epidemiol Community Health*, 40(1):71–5. doi:10.1136/jech.40.1.71 PMID:3711771

Defrank JT, Brewer N (2010). A model of the influence of false-positive mammography screening results on subsequent screening. *Health Psychol Rev*, 4(2):112–27. doi:10.1080/17437199.2010.500482 PMID:21874132

DeFrank JT, Rimer BK, Bowling JM, Earp JA, Breslau ES, Brewer NT (2012). Influence of false-positive mammography results on subsequent screening: do physician recommendations buffer negative effects? *J Med Screen*, 19(1):35–41. doi:10.1258/jms.2012.011123 PMID:22438505

Denberg TD, Wong S, Beattie A (2005). Women's misconceptions about cancer screening: implications for informed decision-making. *Patient Educ Couns*, 57(3):280–5. doi:10.1016/j.pec.2004.07.015 PMID:15893209

Department of Health (2013). Public health functions to be exercised by NHS England – Service Specification No. 24 – Breast Screening Programme. Available from: https://www.gov.uk/government/uploads/system/uploads/attachment_data/file/192975/24_Breast_Screening_Programme__service_specification_VARIATION__130422_-NA.pdf.

Dias-da-Costa JS, Olinto MT, Bassani D, Marchionatti CR, de Bairros FS, de Oliveira ML et al. (2007). Inequalities in clinical breast examination in São Leopoldo, Rio Grande do Sul, Brazil [in Portuguese]. *Cad Saude Publica*, 23(7):1603–12. doi:10.1590/S0102-311X2007000700011 PMID:17572809

Dickens C, Joffe M, Jacobson J, Venter F, Schüz J, Cubasch H et al. (2014). Stage at breast cancer diagnosis and distance from diagnostic hospital in a periurban setting: a South African public hospital case series of over 1,000 women. *Int J Cancer*, 135(9):2173–82. doi:10.1002/ijc.28861 PMID:24658866

Dinshaw K, Mishra G, Shastri S, Badwe R, Kerkar R, Ramani S et al. (2007). Determinants of compliance in a cluster randomised controlled trial on screening of breast and cervix cancer in Mumbai, India. 1. Compliance to screening. *Oncology*, 73(3-4):145–53. doi:10.1159/000126497 PMID:18408401

Domenighetti G, D'Avanzo B, Egger M, Berrino F, Perneger T, Mosconi P et al. (2003). Women's perception of the benefits of mammography screening: population-based survey in four countries. *Int J Epidemiol*, 32(5):816–21. doi:10.1093/ije/dyg257 PMID:14559757

Donnelly TT, Al Khater AH, Al-Bader SB, Al Kuwari MG, Al-Meer N, Malik M et al. (2013b). Beliefs and attitudes about breast cancer and screening practices among Arab women living in Qatar: a cross-sectional study. *BMC Womens Health*, 13(1):49. doi:10.1186/1472-6874-13-49 PMID:24330708

Donnelly TT, Khater AH, Al-Bader SB, Al Kuwari MG, Al-Meer N, Malik M et al. (2013a). Arab women's breast cancer screening practices: a literature review. *Asian Pac J Cancer Prev*, 14(8):4519–28. doi:10.7314/APJCP.2013.14.8.4519 PMID:24083695

Dreier M, Borutta B, Töppich J, Bitzer EM, Walter U (2012). Mammography and cervical cancer screening–a systematic review about women's knowledge, attitudes and participation in Germany [in German]. *Gesundheitswesen*, 74(11):722–35. PMID:22012563

Dündar PE, Ozmen D, Oztürk B, Haspolat G, Akyildiz F, Coban S et al. (2006). The knowledge and attitudes of breast self-examination and mammography in a group of women in a rural area in western Turkey. *BMC Cancer*, 6(1):43. doi:10.1186/1471-2407-6-43 PMID:16504119

Duport N, Ancelle-Park R (2006). Do socio-demographic factors influence mammography use of French women? Analysis of a French cross-sectional survey. *Eur J Cancer Prev*, 15(3):219–24. doi:10.1097/01.cej.0000198902.78420.de PMID:16679864

Dye TD, Bogale S, Hobden C, Tilahun Y, Hechter V, Deressa T et al. (2010). Complex care systems in developing countries: breast cancer patient navigation in Ethiopia. *Cancer*, 116(3):577–85. doi:10.1002/cncr.24776 PMID:20029968

Edgar L, Glackin M, Hughes C, Rogers KM (2013). Factors influencing participation in breast cancer screening. *Br J Nurs*, 22(17):1021–6. doi:10.12968/bjon.2013.22.17.1021 PMID:24067312

Edwards NI, Jones DA (2000). Uptake of breast cancer screening in older women. *Age Ageing*, 29(2):131–5. doi:10.1093/ageing/29.2.131 PMID:10791447

Ekortarl A, Ndom P, Sacks A (2007). A study of patients who appear with far advanced cancer at Yaounde General Hospital, Cameroon, Africa. *Psychooncology*, 16(3):255–7. doi:10.1002/pon.1144 PMID:17310465

El Mhamdi S, Bouanene I, Mhirsi A, Sriha A, Ben Salem K, Soltani MS (2013). Women's knowledge, attitudes and practice about breast cancer screening in the region of Monastir (Tunisia). *Aust J Prim Health*, 19(1):68–73. doi:10.1071/PY11123 PMID:22951080

El Saghir NS, Seoud M, Khalil MK, Charafeddine M, Salem ZK, Geara FB et al. (2006). Effects of young age at presentation on survival in breast cancer. *BMC Cancer*, 6(1):194. doi:10.1186/1471-2407-6-194 PMID:16857060

El Saghir NS, Shamseddine AI, Geara F, Bikhazi K, Rahal B, Salem ZM et al. (2002). Age distribution of breast cancer in Lebanon: increased percentages and age adjusted incidence rates of younger-aged groups at presentation. *J Med Liban*, 50(1-2):3–9. PMID:12841305

Elkin EB, Atoria CL, Leoce N, Bach PB, Schrag D (2013). Changes in the availability of screening mammography, 2000–2010. *Cancer*, 119(21):3847–53. doi:10.1002/cncr.28305 PMID:23943323

Elobaid YE, Aw TC, Grivna M, Nagelkerke N (2014). Breast cancer screening awareness, knowledge, and practice among arab women in the United Arab Emirates: a cross-sectional survey. *PLoS ONE*, 9(9):e105783. doi:10.1371/journal.pone.0105783 PMID:25265385

Espinosa de Los Monteros K, Gallo LC (2011). The relevance of fatalism in the study of Latinas' cancer screening behavior: a systematic review of the literature. *Int J Behav Med*, 18(4):310–8. doi:10.1007/s12529-010-9119-4 PMID:20953916

Ezzat AA, Ibrahim EM, Raja MA, Al-Sobhi S, Rostom A, Stuart RK (1999). Locally advanced breast cancer in Saudi Arabia: high frequency of stage III in a young population. *Med Oncol*, 16(2):95–103. doi:10.1007/BF02785842 PMID:10456657

Farmer D, Reddick B, D'Agostino R, Jackson SA (2007). Psychosocial correlates of mammography screening in older African American women. *Oncol Nurs Forum*, 34(1):117–23. doi:10.1188/07.ONF.117-123 PMID:17562638

Fayanju OM, Kraenzle S, Drake BF, Oka M, Goodman MS (2014). Perceived barriers to mammography among underserved women in a Breast Health Center Outreach Program. *Am J Surg*, 208(3):425–34. doi:10.1016/j.amjsurg.2014.03.005 PMID:24908357

FDA (1992). The Mammography Quality Standards Act final regulations: preparing for MQSA inspections; final guidance for industry and FDA. United States Food and Drug Administration. Available from: http://www.fda.gov/downloads/MedicalDevices/DeviceRegulationandGuidance/GuidanceDocuments/ucm094441.pdf.

FDA (2014). Mammography Quality Standards Act and Program. United States Food and Drug Administration. Available from: http://www.fda.gov/Radiation-EmittingProducts/MammographyQualityStandardsActandProgram/default.htm, accessed 13 January 2015.

Ferlay J, Soerjomataram I, Ervik M, Dikshit R, Eser S, Mathers C et al. (2012). GLOBOCAN 2012 v1.0. Cancer Incidence and Mortality Worldwide: IARC CancerBase No. 11 [Internet]. Lyon, France: International Agency for Research on Cancer. Available from: http://www.iarc.fr/en/publications/eresources/cancerbases/.

Fernández ME, Gonzales A, Tortolero-Luna G, Williams J, Saavedra-Embesi M, Chan W et al. (2009). Effectiveness of Cultivando la Salud: a breast and cervical cancer screening promotion program for low-income Hispanic women. *Am J Public Health*, 99(5):936–43. doi:10.2105/AJPH.2008.136713 PMID:19299678

Finnish Cancer Registry (2014). Breast cancer screening. Institute for Statistical and Epidemiological Cancer, Finnish Cancer Registry. Available from: http://www.cancer.fi/syoparekisteri/en/mass-screening-registry/breast_cancer_screening/screening_programme.

Fintor L, Alciati MH, Fischer R (1995). Legislative and regulatory mandates for mammography quality assurance. *J Public Health Policy*, 16(1):81–107. doi:10.2307/3342978 PMID:7738160

Flores YN, Davidson PL, Nakazono TT, Carreon DC, Mojica CM, Bastani R (2013). Neighborhood socio-economic disadvantage and race/ethnicity as predictors of breast cancer stage at diagnosis. *BMC Public Health*, 13(1):1061. doi:10.1186/1471-2458-13-1061 PMID:24209733

Forss A, Tishelman C, Widmark C, Lundgren E, Sachs L, Törnberg S (2001). 'I got a letter...' a qualitative study of women's reasoning about attendance in a cervical cancer screening programme in urban Sweden. *Psychooncology*, 10(1):76–87. doi:10.1002/1099-1611(200101/02)10:1<76::AID-PON496>3.0.CO;2-P PMID:11180579

Fowler BA (2006). Social processes used by African American women in making decisions about mammography screening. *J Nurs Scholarsh*, 38(3):247–54. doi:10.1111/j.1547-5069.2006.00110.x PMID:17044342

Fox SA, Pitkin K, Paul C, Carson S, Duan N (1998). Breast cancer screening adherence: does church attendance matter? *Health Educ Behav*, 25(6):742–58. doi:10.1177/109019819802500605 PMID:9813745

Fricker J (2009). Helping women make the right choices: Europa Donna launches Breast Health Day. *Cancer World*, 2:32–34. Available from: http://www.cancerworld.org/Articles/Issues/29/March-April-2009/Spotlight-on/51/Helping-women-make-the-right-choices-Europa-Donna-launches-Breast-Health-Day.html.

Frikha M, Yaiche O, Elloumi F, Mnejja W, Slimi L, Kassis M et al. (2013). Results of a pilot study for breast cancer screening by mammography in Sfax region, Tunisia [in French]. *J Gynecol Obstet Biol Reprod (Paris)*, 42(3):252–61. doi:10.1016/j.jgyn.2013.01.007 PMID:23478043

Gakwaya A, Galukande M, Luwaga A, Jombwe J, Fualal J, Kiguli-Malwadde E et al.; Uganda Breast Cancer Working Group (2008). Breast cancer guidelines for Uganda (2nd edition 2008). *Afr Health Sci*, 8(2):126–32.

Galukande M, Kiguli-Malwadde E (2010). Rethinking breast cancer screening strategies in resource-limited settings. *Afr Health Sci*, 10(1):89–92. PMID:20811531

Garbers S, Chiasson MA (2004). Patterns of agreement on breast cancer screening knowledge and practices among women in Dominican and Mexican families in New York City. *Med Sci Monit*, 10(11):CR628–34. PMID:15507855

George SA (2000). Barriers to breast cancer screening: an integrative review. *Health Care Women Int*, 21(1):53–65. doi:10.1080/073993300245401 PMID:11022449

Ghanem S, Glaoui M, Elkhoyaali S, Mesmoudi M, Boutayeb S, Errihani H (2011). Knowledge of risk factors, beliefs and practices of female healthcare professionals towards breast cancer, Morocco. *Pan Afr Med J*, 10(0):21. doi:10.4314/pamj.v10i0.72231 PMID:22187603

Giordano L, Cogo C, Patnick J, Paci E; Euroscreen Working Group (2012b). Communicating the balance sheet in breast cancer screening. *J Med Screen*, 19(Suppl 1):67–71. doi:10.1258/jms.2012.012084 PMID:22972812

Giordano L, Rowinski M, Gaudenzi G, Segnan N (2005). What information do breast cancer screening programmes provide to Italian women? *Eur J Public Health*, 15(1):66–9. doi:10.1093/eurpub/cki117 PMID:15788806

Giordano L, Stefanini V, Senore C, Frigerio A, Castagno R, Marra V et al. (2012c). The impact of different communication and organizational strategies on mammography screening uptake in women aged 40–45 years. *Eur J Public Health*, 22(3):413–8. doi:10.1093/eurpub/ckr090 PMID:21746751

Giordano L, von Karsa L, Tomatis M, Majek O, de Wolf C, Lancucki L et al.; Eunice Working Group (2012a). Mammographic screening programmes in Europe: organization, coverage and participation. *J Med Screen*, 19(Suppl 1):72–82. doi:10.1258/jms.2012.012085 PMID:22972813

Giroux J, Welty TK, Oliver FK, Kaur JS, Leonardson G, Cobb N (2000). Low national breast and cervical cancer-screening rates in American Indian and Alaska Native women with diabetes. *J Am Board Fam Pract*, 13(4):239–45. doi:10.3122/15572625-13-4-239 PMID:10933287

Global Centre for Renewal and Guidance (2012). The Mauritanian Health Care System: overview and recommendations. Available from: http://diringerassociates.com/wp-content/uploads/2012/06/Mauritanian-Health-System-GCRG-Report-Final.pdf.

Gobierno de Chile (2011). Encuesta Nacional de Salud 2009–2010. Santiago, Chile: Ministerio de Salud, Gobierno de Chile. Available from: http://web.minsal.cl/portal/url/item/bcb03d7bc28b64dfe040010165012d23.pdf.

Gobierno de El Salvador (2009). Encuesta Nacional de Salud Familiar – FESAL 2008. San Salvador, El Salvador: Asociación Demográfica Salvadoreña. Available from: http://www.fesal.org.sv/.

González-Robledo LM, González-Robledo MC, Nigenda G, López-Carrillo L (2010). Government actions for the early detection of breast cancer in Latin America. Future challenges [in Spanish]. *Salud Publica Mex*, 52(6):533–43. PMID:21271013

González-Robledo MC, González-Robledo LM, Nigenda G (2013). Public policy-making on breast cancer in Latin America [in Spanish]. *Rev Panam Salud Publica*, 33(3):183–9. PMID:23698137

Goss PE, Lee BL, Badovinac-Crnjevic T, Strasser-Weippl K, Chavarri-Guerra Y, St Louis J et al. (2013). Planning cancer control in Latin America and the Caribbean. *Lancet Oncol*, 14(5):391–436. doi:10.1016/S1470-2045(13)70048-2 PMID:23628188

Goto R, Hamashima C, Mun S, Lee WC (2015). Why screening rates vary between Korea and Japan–differences between two national healthcare systems. *Asian Pac J Cancer Prev*, 16(2):395–400. doi:10.7314/APJCP.2015.16.2.395 PMID:25684461

Graham A, Savic G, Gardner B (1998). Cervical and breast cancer screening in wheelchair dependent females. *Spinal Cord*, 36(5):340–4. doi:10.1038/sj.sc.3100613 PMID:9601114

Griffiths F, Bendelow G, Green E, Palmer J (2010). Screening for breast cancer: medicalization, visualization and the embodied experience. *Health (London)*, 14(6):653–68. doi:10.1177/1363459310361599 PMID:20974697

Grosse Frie K, Ramadas K, Anju GA, Mathew BS, Muwonge R, Sauvaget CS et al. (2013). Determinants of participation in a breast cancer screening trial in Trivandrum District, India. *Asian Pac J Cancer Prev*, 14(12):7301–7. doi:10.7314/APJCP.2013.14.12.7301 PMID:24460292

Grunfeld EA, Ramirez AJ, Hunter MS, Richards MA (2002). Women's knowledge and beliefs regarding breast cancer. *Br J Cancer*, 86(9):1373–8. doi:10.1038/sj.bjc.6600260 PMID:11986766

Gueye SM, Bawa KD, Ba MG, Mendes V, Toure CT, Moreau JC (2009). Breast cancer screening in Dakar: knowledge and practice of breast self examination among a female population in Senegal [in French]. *Rev Med Brux*, 30(2):77–82. PMID:19517903

Güllüoğlu UBM, Urgulu O, Zafer N, Gültekin M, Tuncer M (2012). Breast cancer in Turkey. In: Boyle P, Autier P, Adebamowo C, Anderson B, Pinillos Aston L, Badwe RA et al., editors. World breast cancer report 2012. Lyon, France: International Prevention Research Institute.

Gummersbach E, Piccoliori G, Zerbe CO, Altiner A, Othman C, Rose C et al. (2010). Are women getting relevant information about mammography screening for an informed consent: a critical appraisal of information brochures used for screening invitation in Germany, Italy, Spain and France. *Eur J Public Health*, 20(4):409–14. doi:10.1093/eurpub/ckp174 PMID:19892852

HAAD (2013). Live healthy and simply check. Health Authority of Abu Dhabi. Available from: http://www.haad.ae/simplycheck/tabid/58/Mid/387/ItemID/8/ctl/Details/Default.aspx.

Hadi M, Hassali MA, Shafie AA, Awaisu A (2010). Knowledge and perception of breast cancer among women of various ethnic groups in the state of Penang: a cross-sectional survey. *Med Princ Pract*, 19(1):61–7. doi:10.1159/000252837 PMID:19996622

Hafslund B, Nortvedt MW (2009). Mammography screening from the perspective of quality of life: a review of the literature. *Scand J Caring Sci*, 23(3):539–48. doi:10.1111/j.1471-6712.2008.00634.x PMID:19170959

Haji-Mahmoodi M, Montazeri A, Jarvandi S, Ebrahimi M, Haghighat S, Harirchi I (2002). Breast self-examination: knowledge, attitudes, and practices among female health care workers in Tehran, Iran. *Breast J*, 8(4):222–5. doi:10.1046/j.1524-4741.2002.08406.x PMID:12100114

Hamad HM (2006). Cancer initiatives in Sudan. *Ann Oncol*, 17(Suppl 8):viii32, viii36. PMID:16801337

Hamadeh RR, Abulfatih NM, Fekri MA, Al-Mehza HE (2014). Epidemiology of breast cancer among Bahraini women: data from the Bahrain Cancer Registry. *Sultan Qaboos Univ Med J*, 14(2):e176–82. PMID:24790739

Hamashima C (2016). The Japanese Guidelines for Breast Cancer Screening. *Jpn J Clin Oncol*, 2016:1–11. doi:10.1093/jjco/hyw008

Hamdi Cherif M, Serraino D, Mahnane A, Laouamri S, Zaidi Z, Boukharouba H et al. (2014). Time trends of cancer incidence in Setif, Algeria, 1986–2010:

an observational study. *BMC Cancer*, 14(1):637. doi:10.1186/1471-2407-14-637 PMID:25175348

Han HR, Lee H, Kim MT, Kim KB (2009). Tailored lay health worker intervention improves breast cancer screening outcomes in non-adherent Korean-American women. *Health Educ Res*, 24(2):318–29. doi:10.1093/her/cyn021 PMID:18463411

Hanson K, Montgomery P, Bakker D, Conlon M (2009). Factors influencing mammography participation in Canada: an integrative review of the literature. *Curr Oncol*, 16(5):65–75. PMID:19862363

Harirchi I, Mousavi SM, Mohagheghi MA, Mousavi-Jarrahi A, Ebrahimi M, Montazeri A et al. (2009). Early detection for breast cancer in iran. *Asian Pac J Cancer Prev*, 10(5):849–51. PMID:20104977

Harutyunyan TS (1999). Breast self-examination practice in Yerevan women: cross-sectional KAP (knowledge-attitude-practice) survey [dissertation]. Yerevan, Armenia: American University of Armenia. Available from: aua.am/chsr/PDF/MPH/1999/TsovinarHarutyunyan.pdf.

Hatefnia E, Niknami S, Bazargan M, Mahmoodi M, Lamyianm M, Alavi N (2010). Correlates of mammography utilization among working Muslim Iranian women. *Health Care Women Int*, 31(6):499–514. doi:10.1080/07399331003725507 PMID:20461601

Hay JL, McCaul KD, Magnan RE (2006). Does worry about breast cancer predict screening behaviors? A meta-analysis of the prospective evidence. *Prev Med*, 42(6):401–8. doi:10.1016/j.ypmed.2006.03.002 PMID:16626796

Health Promotion Administration, Ministry of Health and Welfare (2014). Health Promotion Administration Annual Report: promoting your health. Taipei, Taiwan, China: Taiwan Health Promotion Administration, Ministry of Health and Welfare. Available from: http://www.hpa.gov.tw/BHPNet/English/Index.aspx.

Hersch J, Barratt A, Jansen J, Houssami N, Irwig L, Jacklyn G et al. (2014). The effect of information about overdetection of breast cancer on women's decision-making about mammography screening: study protocol for a randomised controlled trial. *BMJ Open*, 4(5):e004990. doi:10.1136/bmjopen-2014-004990 PMID:24833692

Hersch J, Jansen J, Barratt A, Irwig L, Houssami N, Howard K et al. (2013). Women's views on overdiagnosis in breast cancer screening: a qualitative study. *BMJ*, 346(1):f158. doi:10.1136/bmj.f158 PMID:23344309

Hersch J, Jansen J, Irwig L, Barratt A, Thornton H, Howard K et al. (2011). How do we achieve informed choice for women considering breast screening? *Prev Med*, 53(3):144–6. doi:10.1016/j.ypmed.2011.06.013 PMID:21723312

Holland WW, Stewart S, Masseria C (2006). Policy Brief: Screening in Europe. Brussels, Belgium: World Health Organization, European Observatory on Health Systems and Policies. Available from: http://www.euro.who.int/__data/assets/pdf_file/0007/108961/E88698.pdf.

Hossain MS, Ferdous S, Karim-Kos HE (2014). Breast cancer in South Asia: a Bangladeshi perspective. *Cancer Epidemiol*, 38(5):465–70. doi:10.1016/j.canep.2014.08.004 PMID:25182670

Huang Y, Zhou K, Li H, Wang A, Li J, Pang Y et al. (2011). Knowledge, attitudes, and behaviour regarding breast cancer screening among women from different socio-economic regions in southwest China: a cross-sectional study. *Asian Pac J Cancer Prev*, 12(1):203–9. PMID:21517258

Hur HK, Kim GY, Park SM (2005). Predictors of mammography participation among rural Korean women age 40 and over. *Taehan Kanho Hakhoe Chi*, 35(8):1443–50. PMID:16415625

Hussain SA, Sullivan R (2013). Cancer control in Bangladesh. *Jpn J Clin Oncol*, 43(12):1159–69. doi:10.1093/jjco/hyt140 PMID:24163419

Hwang YS, Tsai HY, Chen CC, Tsay PK, Pan HB, Hsu GC et al. (2013). Effects of quality assurance regulatory enforcement on performance of mammography systems: evidence from large-scale surveys in Taiwan. *AJR Am J Roentgenol*, 201(2):W307-12. doi:10.2214/AJR.12.9614 PMID:23883245

IAEA (2006). Control de calidad en mamografía – protocolo elaborado en el marco de dos proyectos regionales ARCAL/OIEA. IAEA-TECDOC-1517. Vienna, Austria: International Atomic Energy Agency. Available from: http://www-pub.iaea.org/books/IAEABooks/7569/Control-de-Calidad-en-Mamografa.

INC (2011). Control de calidad para los servicios de mamografía analógica. Bogotá, Colombia: Instituto Nacional de Cancerología.

INCA (2007). Mamografía: da prática ao controle – recomendações para professioais de sáude. Rio de Janeiro, Brazil: Instituto Nacional do Cáncer.

INEN (2008). Norma técnica oncólogica para la prevención, detección y diagnóstico temprano del cáncer de mama a nivel nacional. Lima, Peru: Instituto Nacional de Enfermedades Neoplásicas. Available from: bvs.minsa.gob.pe/local/minsa/1786.pdf.

INSP (2012). Encuesta nacional de salud y nutrición. Cuernavaca, Mexico: Instituto Nacional de Salud Pública.

Ishida T, Suzuki A, Kawai M, Narikawa Y, Saito H, Yamamoto S et al. (2014). A randomized controlled trial to verify the efficacy of the use of ultrasonography in breast cancer screening aged 40–49 (J-START): 76 196 women registered. *Jpn J Clin Oncol*, 44(2):134–40. doi:10.1093/jjco/hyt199 PMID:24407835

Israel Cancer Association (2014). The National Mammography Screening Program, Israel. Available from: http://en.cancer.org.il/template_e/default.aspx?PageId=7645.

Ivanov LL, Hu J, Leak A (2010). Immigrant women's cancer screening behaviors. *J Community Health Nurs*, 27(1):32–45. doi:10.1080/07370010903466163 PMID:20131135

Japan Central Organization on Quality Assurance of Breast Cancer Screening (2014). The Japan Central Organization on Quality Assurance of Breast Cancer Screening [in Japanese]. Available from: http://www.qabcs.or.jp.

JBCP (2008). Annual Newsletter of the Jordan Breast Cancer Program. Issue 1. Amman: Jordan Breast Cancer Program. Available from: http://www.jbcp.jo/files/newsletter.pdf.

JBCP (2010). Our voice has been heard: MOH new law for early detection of breast cancer. Issue 3, p. 9. Amman: Jordan Breast Cancer Program. Available from: http://www.jbcp.jo/files/JBCP%20Newsletter%202010.pdf.

JBCP (2014a). Jordan Breast Cancer Program. Available from: http://www.khcc.jo/section/recommended-screening-checklists.

JBCP (2014b). Early detection plan. Jordan Breast Cancer Program. Available from: http://www.uicc.org/jordan-breast-cancer-program-2014-campaign.

Jepson RG, Hewison J, Thompson A, Weller D (2007). Patient perspectives on information and choice in cancer screening: a qualitative study in the UK. *Soc Sci Med*, 65(5):890–9. doi:10.1016/j.socscimed.2007.04.009 PMID:17507131

Johnston K, Brown J, Gerard K, O'Hanlon M, Morton A (1998). Valuing temporary and chronic health states associated with breast screening. *Soc Sci Med*, 47(2):213–22. doi:10.1016/S0277-9536(98)00065-3 PMID:9720640

Jones SC, Gregory P, Nehill C, Barrie L, Luxford K, Nelson A et al. (2010). Australian women's awareness of breast cancer symptoms and responses to potential symptoms. *Cancer Causes Control*, 21(6):945–58. doi:10.1007/s10552-010-9522-9 PMID:20177964

Jørgensen KJ, Gøtzsche PC (2004). Presentation on websites of possible benefits and harms from screening for breast cancer: cross sectional study. *BMJ*, 328(7432):148. doi:10.1136/bmj.328.7432.148 PMID:14726344

Jørgensen KJ, Gøtzsche PC (2006). Content of invitations for publicly funded screening mammography. *BMJ*, 332(7540):538–41. doi:10.1136/bmj.332.7540.538 PMID:16513713

Kapp JM, Yankaskas BC, LeFevre ML (2010). Are mammography recommendations in women younger than 40 related to increased risk? *Breast Cancer Res Treat*, 119(2):485–90. doi:10.1007/s10549-008-0305-x PMID:19148745

Kardinah D, Anderson BO, Duggan C, Ali IA, Thomas DB (2014). Short report: Limited effectiveness of screening mammography in addition to clinical breast examination by trained nurse midwives in rural Jakarta, Indonesia. *Int J Cancer*, 134(5):1250–5. doi:10.1002/ijc.28442 PMID:24037942

Katapodi MC, Lee KA, Facione NC, Dodd MJ (2004). Predictors of perceived breast cancer risk and the relation between perceived risk and breast cancer screening: a meta-analytic review. *Prev Med*, 38(4):388–402. doi:10.1016/j.ypmed.2003.11.012 PMID:15020172

Katz SJ, Zemencuk JK, Hofer TP (2000). Breast cancer screening in the United States and Canada, 1994: socioeconomic gradients persist. *Am J Public Health*, 90(5):799–803. doi:10.2105/AJPH.90.5.799 PMID:10800435

Kaufert PA (1996). Women and the debate over mammography: an economic, political, and moral history. In: Sargent CF, Brettell CB, editors. Gender and health. An international perspective. New Jersey, USA: Prentice Hall; pp. 167–86.

Kayhan A, Gurdal SO, Ozaydin N, Cabioglu N, Ozturk E, Ozcinar B et al. (2014). Successful first round results of a Turkish breast cancer screening program with mammography in Bahcesehir, Istanbul. *Asian Pac J Cancer Prev*, 15(4):1693–7. doi:10.7314/APJCP.2014.15.4.1693 PMID:24641392

Keinan-Boker L, Baron-Epel O, Fishler Y, Liphshitz I, Barchana M, Dichtiar R et al. (2013). Breast cancer trends in Israeli Jewish and Arab women, 1996–2007. *Eur J Cancer Prev*, 22(2):112–20. doi:10.1097/CEJ.0b013e3283581d3c PMID:23361380

Kemfang Ngowa JD, Yomi J, Kasia JM, Mawamba Y, Ekortarh AC, Vlastos G (2011). Breast cancer profile in a group of patients followed up at the radiation therapy unit of the Yaounde General Hospital, Cameroon. *Obstet Gynecol Int*, 2011:143506. doi:10.1155/2011/143506 PMID:21785601

Kenyan Ministry of Health (2014). National Cancer Control Strategy 2011–2016. Kenya Ministry of Public Health and Sanitation and Ministry of Medical Services. Available from: http://www.ipcrc.net/pdfs/Kenya-National-Cancer-Control-strategy.pdf, accessed 14 April 2015.

Khaleel Abu Shmais F (2010). Use of mammography test pattern and percentage of breast cancer detected in Nablus District [dissertation]. Nablus, West Bank: An-Najah National University. Available from: http://scholar.najah.edu/sites/default/files/all-thesis/use_of_mammography_test_pattern_and_percentage_of_breast_cancer_detected_in_nablus_district.pdf.

Kharboush IF, Ismail HM, Kandil AA, Mamdouh HM, Muhammad YY, El Sharkawy OG et al. (2011). Raising the breast health awareness amongst women in an urban slum area in Alexandria, Egypt. *Breast Care (Basel)*, 6(5):375–9. doi:10.1159/000331311 PMID:22619648

Khatib OMN, Modjtabai A, editors (2006). Guidelines for the early detection and screening of breast cancer. EMRO Technical Publications Series 30. Cairo,

Egypt: World Health Organization Regional Office for the Eastern Mediterranean. Available from: http://applications.emro.who.int/dsaf/dsa696.pdf.

Kim Y, Jun JK, Choi KS, Lee HY, Park EC (2011). Overview of the National Cancer screening programme and the cancer screening status in Korea. *Asian Pac J Cancer Prev*, 12(3):725–30. PMID:21627372

Kirkpatrick A, Törnberg S, Thijssen MAO (1993). European guidelines for quality assurance in mammography screening. Luxembourg: European Commission.

Klawiter M (2008). The biopolitics of breast cancer. Changing cultures of disease and activism. Minneapolis (MN), USA: University of Minnesota Press.

Kobeissi L, Hamra R, Samari G, Koleilat L, Khalifeh M (2012). The 2009 Lebanese National Mammography Campaign: results and assessment using a survey design. *Epidemiol*, 2(1):1000112. doi:10.4172/2161-1165.1000112. Available from: http://omicsonline.org/the-2009-lebanese-national-mammography-campaign-results-and-assessment-using-a-survey-design-2161-1165.1000112.php?aid=3789.

Koo FK, Kwok C, White K, D'Abrew N, Roydhouse JK (2012). Strategies for piloting a breast health promotion program in the Chinese-Australian population. *Prev Chronic Dis*, 9:E03. PMID:22172170

Koval AE, Riganti AA, Foley KL (2006). CAPRELA (Cancer Prevention for Latinas): findings of a pilot study in Winston-Salem, Forsyth County. *N C Med J*, 67(1):9–15. PMID:16550986

Kumar YS, Mishra G, Gupta S, Shastri S (2011). Level of cancer awareness among women of low socioeconomic status in Mumbai slums. *Asian Pac J Cancer Prev*, 12(5):1295–8. PMID:21875285

Kuwait Ministry of Health (2014). Kuwait National Mammography Screening Program. Available from: http://ameinfo.com/finance-and-economy/economy/healthcare/ministry-health-launches-kuwait-national-mammography-screening-program/.

Lages RB, Oliveira GP, Simeão Filho VM, Nogueira FM, Teles JB, Vieira SC (2012). Inequalities associated with lack of mammography in Teresina-Piauí-Brazil, 2010–2011. *Rev Bras Epidemiol*, 15(4):737–47. doi:10.1590/S1415-790X2012000400006 PMID:23515770

Lagos State Ministry of Health (2011). Breast cancer screening and awareness programme. Nigeria. Available from: http://www.lagosstateministryofhealth.com/programmes/breast-cancer-screening-and-awareness-programme#.VSWnNZNkaNY.

Lagos State Ministry of Health (2014). Breast cancer screening and awareness programme. Lagos State Ministry of Health. Available from: http://www.lagosstateministryofhealth.com/programme_info.php?programme_id=24.

Lalla Salma Foundation (2014). Cancer prevention and treatment in Morocco. Available from: http://www.contrelecancer.ma/en/, accessed 21 October 2014.

Lampic C, Thurfjell E, Bergh J, Sjödén PO (2001). Short- and long-term anxiety and depression in women recalled after breast cancer screening. *Eur J Cancer*, 37(4):463–9. doi:10.1016/S0959-8049(00)00426-3 PMID:11267855

Lastier D, Salines E, Rogel A (2013). Programme de dépistage du cancer du sein en France: résultats 2010, évolutions depuis 2006. Saint-Maurice, France: Institut de Veille Sanitaire.

Latimer AE, Katulak NA, Mowad L, Salovey P (2005). Motivating cancer prevention and early detection behaviors using psychologically tailored messages. *J Health Commun*, 10(Suppl 1):137–55. doi:10.1080/10810730500263364 PMID:16377605

Lauver DR, Henriques JB, Settersten L, Bumann MC (2003). Psychosocial variables, external barriers, and stage of mammography adoption. *Health Psychol*, 22(6):649–53. doi:10.1037/0278-6133.22.6.649 PMID:14640864

Leach CR, Klabunde CN, Alfano CM, Smith JL, Rowland JH (2012). Physician over-recommendation of mammography for terminally ill women. *Cancer*, 118(1):27–37. doi:10.1002/cncr.26233 PMID:21681736

Lerda D, Deandrea S, Freeman C, Lopez-Alcaida J, Neamtiu L, Nicholl C et al. (2014). Report of a European survey on the organisation of breast cancer care services. Luxembourg: European Commission.

Leung J, McKenzie S, Martin J, McLaughlin D (2014). Effect of rurality on screening for breast cancer: a systematic review and meta-analysis comparing mammography. *Rural Remote Health*, 14(2):2730. PMID:24953122

Levy-Storms L, Wallace SP (2003). Use of mammography screening among older Samoan women in Los Angeles county: a diffusion network approach. *Soc Sci Med*, 57(6):987–1000. doi:10.1016/S0277-9536(02)00474-4 PMID:12878100

Lindén-Boström M, Persson C, Eriksson C (2010). Neighbourhood characteristics, social capital and self-rated health–a population-based survey in Sweden. *BMC Public Health*, 10:628. PMID:20964808

Liu LY, Wang F, Yu LX, Ma ZB, Zhang Q, Gao DZ et al. (2014). Breast cancer awareness among women in Eastern China: a cross-sectional study. *BMC Public Health*, 14(1):1004. doi:10.1186/1471-2458-14-1004 PMID:25257142

Lostao L, Joiner TE (2001). Health-oriented behaviors: their implication in attending for breast cancer screening. *Am J Health Behav*, 25(1):21–32. doi:10.5993/AJHB.25.1.3 PMID:11289725

Lowe JB, Balanda KP, Del Mar C, Hawes E (1999). Psychologic distress in women with abnormal findings in mass mammography screening. *Cancer*, 85(5):1114–8. doi:10.1002/

(SICI)1097-0142(19990301)85:5<1114::AID-CNCR15>3.0.CO;2-Y PMID:10091796

Lui CY, Lam HS, Chan LK, Tam KF, Chan CM, Leung TY et al. (2007). Opportunistic breast cancer screening in Hong Kong; a revisit of the Kwong Wah Hospital experience. *Hong Kong Med J*, 13(2):106–13. PMID:17406037

Luyeye Mvila G, Postema S, Marchal G, Van Limbergen E, Verdonck F, Matthijs G et al. (2014). From the set-up of a screening program of breast cancer patients to the identification of the first BRCA mutation in the DR Congo. *BMC Public Health*, 14(1):759. doi:10.1186/1471-2458-14-759 PMID:25070656

MacDowell NM, Nitz-Weiss M, Short A (2000). The role of physician communication in improving compliance with mammography screening among women ages 50–79 in a commercial HMO. *Manag Care Q*, 8(4):11–9. PMID:11146840

Maheswaran R, Pearson T, Jordan H, Black D (2006). Socioeconomic deprivation, travel distance, location of service, and uptake of breast cancer screening in North Derbyshire, UK. *J Epidemiol Community Health*, 60(3):208–12. doi:10.1136/jech.200X.038398 PMID:16476749

Marshall G (1994). A comparative study of re-attenders and non-re-attenders for second triennial National Breast Screening Programme appointments. *J Public Health Med*, 16(1):79–86. PMID:8037957

Matheka D (2014). Tackling cancer in Kenya. Translational Global Health (PLOS blogs). Available from: http://blogs.plos.org/globalhealth/2014/01/tackling-cancer-kenya/.

Maxwell AE, Wang JH, Young L, Crespi CM, Mistry R, Sudan M et al. (2011). Pilot test of a peer-led small-group video intervention to promote mammography screening among Chinese American immigrants. *Health Promot Pract*, 12(6):887–99. doi:10.1177/1524839909355550 PMID:20720095

Mayo RM, Ureda JR, Parker VG (2001). Importance of fatalism in understanding mammography screening in rural elderly women. *J Women Aging*, 13(1):57–72. doi:10.1300/J074v13n01_05 PMID:11217186

McDonald PA, Thorne DD, Pearson JC, Adams-Campbell LL (1999). Perceptions and knowledge of breast cancer among African-American women residing in public housing. *Ethn Dis*, 9(1):81–93. PMID:10355477

McLelland R, Hendrick RE, Zinninger MD, Wilcox PA (1991). The American College of Radiology Mammography Accreditation Program. *AJR Am J Roentgenol*, 157(3):473–9. doi:10.2214/ajr.157.3.1872231 PMID:1872231

Meissner HI, Klabunde CN, Han PK, Benard VB, Breen N (2011). Breast cancer screening beliefs, recommendations and practices: primary care physicians in the United States. *Cancer*, 117(14):3101–11. doi:10.1002/cncr.25873 PMID:21246531

Mena M, Wiafe-Addai B, Sauvaget C, Ali IA, Wiafe SA, Dabis F et al. (2014). Evaluation of the impact of a breast cancer awareness program in rural Ghana: a cross-sectional survey. *Int J Cancer*, 134(4):913–24. doi:10.1002/ijc.28412 PMID:23913595

Meystre-Agustoni G, Paccaud F, Jeannin A, Dubois-Arber F (2001). Anxiety in a cohort of Swiss women participating in a mammographic screening programme. *J Med Screen*, 8(4):213–9. doi:10.1136/jms.8.4.213 PMID:11743038

Michaels C, McEwen MM, McArthur DB (2008). Saying "no" to professional recommendations: client values, beliefs, and evidence-based practice. *J Am Acad Nurse Pract*, 20(12):585–9. doi:10.1111/j.1745-7599.2008.00372.x PMID:19120589

Michielutte R, Dignan MB, Smith BL (1999). Psychosocial factors associated with the use of breast cancer screening by women age 60 years or over. *Health Educ Behav*, 26(5):625–47. doi:10.1177/109019819902600505 PMID:10533169

Miller AB (2008). Practical applications for clinical breast examination (CBE) and breast self-examination (BSE) in screening and early detection of breast cancer. *Breast Care (Basel)*, 3(1):17–20. doi:10.1159/000113934 PMID:20824015

Ministerio de Salud de Chile (2011). Guía clínica - cáncer de mama. Serie Guías Clínicas Minsal. Santiago, Chile: Ministerio de Salud de Chile.

Ministerio de Salud y Protección Social (2013). Guía de práctica clínica (GPC) para la detección temprana, tratamiento integral, seguimiento y rehabilitación del cáncer de mama. Bogotá, Colombia: Instituto Nacional de Cancerología.

Ministry of Health Brunei Darussalam (2007). Integrated health screening and health promotion program. Available from: http://www.moh.gov.bn/hpc/programme_services02.htm.

Ministry of Health Fiji (2009). Non-communicable disease prevention and control. National strategic plan 2010–2014. Available from: http://www.health.gov.fj/wp-content/uploads/2014/05/2_National-Non-Communicable-Diseases-Strategic-Plan-2010-2014.pdf.

Ministry of Health Labour and Welfare, Japan (2013a). Survey of implementation of cancer screening, 2013 [in Japanese]. Available from: http://www.e-stat.go.jp/SG1/estat/GL08020103.do?_toGL08020103_&listID=000001106917&requestSender=dsearch.

Ministry of Health Labour and Welfare, Japan (2013b). Report of health promotion and community health 2011 [in Japanese]. Available from: http://www.e-stat.go.jp/SG1/estat/GL08020103.do?_toGL08020103_&listID=000001106953&disp=Other&requestSender=dsearch.

Ministry of Health and Child Care of Zimbabwe (2013). National cancer prevention and control strategy for

Zimbabwe 2014–2018. Available from: http://www.cancerzimbabwe.org/articles/Nat%20Cancer%20Prevention%20and%20Control%20Doc_18_3_14.pdf.

Ministry of Health and Family Welfare Bangladesh (2008). National cancer control strategy and plan of action 2009–2015. Directorate General of Health Services. Available from: http://www.iccp-portal.org/sites/default/files/plans/Publication_Cancer_Strategy.pdf.pdf.

Ministry of Health and Family Welfare, Government of India (2005). National cancer control programme guidelines.

Ministry of Health Malaysia (2010). Clinical practice guidelines: management of breast cancer. Kuala Lumpur, Malaysia. Available from: http://www.moh.gov.my/attachments/6915.pdf.

Ministry of Health Singapore (2010). Cancer screening. MOH Clinical Practice Guidelines. Available from: https://www.moh.gov.sg/content/moh_web/healthprofessionalsportal/doctors/guidelines/cpg_medical/2010/cpgmed_cancer_screening.html.

Ministry of Health Singapore (2011). National Health Survey 2010. Epidemiology and Disease Control Division, Ministry of Health Singapore. Available from: https://www.moh.gov.sg/content/moh_web/home/Publications/Reports/2011/national_health_survey2010.html.

Minsal (2011). Segunda encuesta nacional de factores de riesgo para enfermedades no transmisibles. Buenos Aires, Argentina: Ministerio de Salud de Argentina.

Mo M, Liu GY, Zheng Y, Di LF, Ji YJ, Lv LL et al. (2013). Performance of breast cancer screening methods and modality among Chinese women: a report from a society-based breast screening program (SBSP) in Shanghai. *Springerplus*, 2(1):276. doi:10.1186/2193-1801-2-276 PMID:23961381

Molina A, Moreno J, Peiró R, Salas D (2013). Social inequalities in participation in cancer screening programmes: the state of the art of the research. Valencia, Spain: Fundación para el Fomento de la Investigación Sanitaria y Biomédica de la Comunidad Valenciana (FISABIO)-CSISP. Available from: http://www.epaac.eu/images/WP_6_Screening__Early_Diagnosis/SOCIAL_INEQUALITIES_IN_PARTICIPATION_IN_CANCER_SCREENING_PROGRA.pdf.

Montgomery M (2013). Ontario to spend $25 million on new mammogram technology. Radio Canada International, 14 May 2013. Available from: http://www.rcinet.ca/en/2013/05/14/ontario-to-spend-25-million-on-new-mammogram-technology/.

Montgomery M, McCrone SH (2010). Psychological distress associated with the diagnostic phase for suspected breast cancer: systematic review. *J Adv Nurs*, 66(11):2372–90. doi:10.1111/j.1365-2648.2010.05439.x PMID:21039773

Monu JU, Muyinda Z, Taljanovic M (2012). ISS outreach sub-Saharan Africa insight: Uganda 2011. *Skeletal Radiol*, 41(11):1347–8. doi:10.1007/s00256-012-1494-2 PMID:22899548

Mora P, Blanco S, Khoury H, Leyton F, Cárdenas J, Defaz MY et al. (2014). Latin American dose survey results in mammography studies under IAEA programme: radiological protection of patients in medical exposures (TSA3). *Radiat Prot Dosimetry*, 163(4):473-9. doi:10.1093/rpd/ncu205 PMID:24993012

Morocco World News (2013). Princess Lalla Salma inaugurates in Mohammedia breast and uterine cancer center. Available from: http://www.moroccoworldnews.com/2013/10/110484/princess-lalla-salma-inaugurates-in-mohammedia-breast-and-uterine-cancer-center/.

Moser K, Patnick J, Beral V (2009). Inequalities in reported use of breast and cervical screening in Great Britain: analysis of cross sectional survey data. *BMJ*, 338(2):b2025. doi:10.1136/bmj.b2025 PMID:19531549

Moser K, Sellars S, Wheaton M, Cooke J, Duncan A, Maxwell A et al. (2011). Extending the age range for breast screening in England: pilot study to assess the feasibility and acceptability of randomization. *J Med Screen*, 18(2):96–102. doi:10.1258/jms.2011.011065 PMID:21852703

Msyamboza KP, Dzamalala C, Mdokwe C, Kamiza S, Lemerani M, Dzowela T et al. (2012). Burden of cancer in Malawi; common types, incidence and trends: national population-based cancer registry. *BMC Res Notes*, 5(1):149. doi:10.1186/1756-0500-5-149 PMID:22424105

Mukem S, Sriplung H, McNeil E, Tangcharoensathien V (2014). Breast cancer screening among women in Thailand: analyses of population-based household surveys. *J Med Assoc Thai*, 97(11):1106–18. PMID:25675674

Murillo R, Díaz S, Sánchez O, Perry F, Piñeros M, Poveda C et al. (2008). Pilot implementation of breast cancer early detection programs in Colombia. *Breast Care (Basel)*, 3(1):29–32. doi:10.1159/000114446 PMID:20824017

Mutebi M, Wasike R, Mushtaq A, Kahie A, Ntoburi S (2013). The effectiveness of an abbreviated training program for health workers in breast cancer awareness: innovative strategies for resource constrained environments. *Springerplus*, 2(1):528. doi:10.1186/2193-1801-2-528 PMID:24324920

Muthoni A, Miller AN (2010). An exploration of rural and urban Kenyan women's knowledge and attitudes regarding breast cancer and breast cancer early detection measures. *Health Care Women Int*, 31(9):801–16. doi:10.1080/07399331003628453 PMID:20677038

National Cancer Center, Japan (2013). Breast cancer screening 2013 [in Japanese]. Available from: http://canscreen.ncc.go.jp/guideline/nyugan.html.

National Cancer Center, Japan (2014). Cancer Information Service [in Japanese]. Available from: http://ganjoho.jp/professional/statistics/statistics.html.

National Cancer Center of Korea (2013). Cancer facts & figures 2013 in the Republic of Korea. National Cancer Center, Ministry of Health and Welfare. Available from: https://www.ncc.re.kr/sub07_Publications.ncc.

National Cancer Control Programme Thailand (2013). National Cancer Control Programmes (2556–2560) [in Thai]. Available from: http://www.nci.go.th/th/File_download/D_index/NCCP_2556-2560.pdf.

National Cancer Program Qatar (2014). Available from: http://www.ncp.qa/Pages/Default.aspx.

National Mammography Quality Assurance Advisory Committee (2011). Reporting breast density on mammography reports and patient lay summaries – committee discussion – pages 194–242. Available from: http://www.fda.gov/downloads/AdvisoryCommittees/CommitteesMeetingMaterials/Radiation-EmittingProducts/NationalMammographyQualityAssuranceAdvisoryCommittee/UCM282944.pdf.

National Statistics Office (2009). Philippine National Demographic and Health Survey 2008. Manila, Philippines: National Statistics Office.

NBCCEDP (2002). About the program. National Breast and Cervical Cancer Early Detection Program. Atlanta (GA), USA: Centers for Disease Control and Prevention. Available from: http://www.cdc.gov/cancer/nbccedp/about.htm, accessed 13 January 2015.

NBCCEDP (2014). National Breast and Cervical Cancer Early Detection Program. Atlanta (GA), USA: Centers for Disease Control and Prevention. Available from: http://www.cdc.gov/cancer/nbccedp/, accessed 13 January 2015.

NCI (1990). Screening mammography: a missed clinical opportunity? Results of the NCI Breast Cancer Screening Consortium and National Health Interview Survey Studies. *JAMA*, 264(1):54–8. doi:10.1001/jama.1990.03450010058030 PMID:2355430

NCI (2013). Cancer testing covered by Medicare. United States National Cancer Institute. Available from: http://appliedresearch.cancer.gov/seermedicare/considerations/testing.html, accessed 13 January 2015.

Ngelangel CA, Wang EH (2002). Cancer and the Philippine Cancer Control Program. *Jpn J Clin Oncol*, 32(Suppl 1):S52–61. doi:10.1093/jjco/hye126 PMID:11959878

Nguyen LH, Laohasiriwong W, Stewart JF, Wright P, Nguyen YTB, Coyte PC (2013). Cost-effectiveness analysis of a screening program for breast cancer in Vietnam. *Value in Health Regional Issues*, 2(1):21–8. doi:10.1016/j.vhri.2013.02.004

Nguyen TT, Le G, Nguyen T, Le K, Lai K, Gildengorin G et al. (2009). Breast cancer screening among Vietnamese Americans: a randomized controlled trial of lay health worker outreach. *Am J Prev Med*, 37(4):306–13. doi:10.1016/j.amepre.2009.06.009 PMID:19765502

NHS Choices (2014). 1 in 3 women who get breast cancer are over 70, so don't assume you're past it. Available from: http://www.nhs.uk/be-clear-on-cancer/breast-cancer, accessed 28 July 2014.

Ntirenganya F, Petroze RT, Kamara TB, Groen RS, Kushner AL, Kyamanywa P et al. (2014). Prevalence of breast masses and barriers to care: results from a population-based survey in Rwanda and Sierra Leone. *J Surg Oncol*, 110(8):903–6. doi:10.1002/jso.23726 PMID:25088235

O'Donnell S, Goldstein B, Dimatteo MR, Fox SA, John CR, Obrzut JE (2010). Adherence to mammography and colorectal cancer screening in women 50–80 years of age the role of psychological distress. *Womens Health Issues*, 20(5):343–9. doi:10.1016/j.whi.2010.04.002 PMID:20800770

Olsson P, Armelius K, Nordahl G, Lenner P, Westman G (1999). Women with false positive screening mammograms: how do they cope? *J Med Screen*, 6(2):89–93. doi:10.1136/jms.6.2.89 PMID:10444727

Oluwole D, Kraemer J; Pink Ribbon Red Ribbon (2013). Innovative public-private partnership: a diagonal approach to combating women's cancers in Africa. *Bull World Health Organ*, 91(9):691–6. doi:10.2471/BLT.12.109777 PMID:24101785

Oman Cancer Association (2015). Breast screening. Available from: http://timesofoman.com/article/46686/Oman/1547-women-screened-for-cancer-by-mobile-mammography-unit-of-Oman-Cancer-Association.

Omar S, Khaled H, Gaafar R, Zekry AR, Eissa S, el-Khatib O (2003). Breast cancer in Egypt: a review of disease presentation and detection strategies. *East Mediterr Health J*, 9(3):448–63. PMID:15751939

Opoku SY, Benwell M, Yarney J (2012). Knowledge, attitudes, beliefs, behaviour and breast cancer screening practices in Ghana, West Africa. *Pan Afr Med J*, 11:28. PMID:22514762

Ortíz-Martínez A, González-Martín A, Rodríguez-Monteagudo JL (2005). Revitalización del programa de detección preclínica precoz del cáncer de mama. *Gaceta Médica Espirituana*, 7(3). Available from: http://bvs.sld.cu/revistas/gme/pub/vol.7.%283%29_08/p8.html.

Oshima A (1994). A critical review of cancer screening programs in Japan. *Int J Technol Assess Health Care*, 10(3):346–58. doi:10.1017/S0266462300006590 PMID:8070998

Østerlie W, Solbjør M, Skolbekken JA, Hofvind S, Saetnan AR, Forsmo S (2008). Challenges of informed choice in organised screening. *J Med Ethics*, 34(9):e5. doi:10.1136/jme.2008.024802 PMID:18757624

Pace LE, Keating NL (2014). A systematic assessment of benefits and risks to guide breast cancer screening decisions. *JAMA*, 311(13):1327–35. doi:10.1001/jama.2014.1398 PMID:24691608

PAHO (2012). Health in the Americas 2012 edition. Washington (DC), USA: Pan American Health Organization.

PAHO (2013). Cancer in the Americas – country profile 2013. Washington (DC), USA: Pan American Health Organization.

Palència L, Espelt A, Rodríguez-Sanz M, Puigpinós R, Pons-Vigués M, Pasarín MI et al. (2010). Socio-economic inequalities in breast and cervical cancer screening practices in Europe: influence of the type of screening program. *Int J Epidemiol*, 39(3):757–65. doi:10.1093/ije/dyq003 PMID:20176587

Pan L, Han LL, Tao LX, Zhou T, Li X, Gao Q et al. (2013). Clinical risk factor analysis for breast cancer: 568,000 subjects undergoing breast cancer screening in Beijing, 2009. *Asian Pac J Cancer Prev*, 14(9):5325–9. doi:10.7314/APJCP.2013.14.9.5325 PMID:24175820

Papas MA, Klassen AC (2005). Pain and discomfort associated with mammography among urban low-income African-American women. *J Community Health*, 30(4):253–67. doi:10.1007/s10900-005-3704-5 PMID:15989208

Park K, Hong WH, Kye SY, Jung E, Kim MH, Park HG (2011). Community-based intervention to promote breast cancer awareness and screening: the Korean experience. *BMC Public Health*, 11(1):468. doi:10.1186/1471-2458-11-468 PMID:21669004

Parsa P, Kandiah M, Mohd Zulkefli NA, Rahman HA (2008). Knowledge and behavior regarding breast cancer screening among female teachers in Selangor, Malaysia. *Asian Pac J Cancer Prev*, 9(2):221–7. PMID:18712963

Peek ME, Sayad JV, Markwardt R (2008). Fear, fatalism and breast cancer screening in low-income African-American women: the role of clinicians and the health care system. *J Gen Intern Med*, 23(11):1847–53. doi:10.1007/s11606-008-0756-0 PMID:18751758

Peltzer K, Phaswana-Mafuya N (2014). Breast and cervical cancer screening and associated factors among older adult women in South Africa. *Asian Pac J Cancer Prev*, 15(6):2473–6. doi:10.7314/APJCP.2014.15.6.2473 PMID:24761849

Perry N, Broeders M, de Wolf C, Törnberg S, Holland R, von Karsa L et al., editors (2006). European guidelines for quality assurance in breast cancer screening and diagnosis. Fourth edition. Luxembourg: European Commission, Office for Official Publications of the European Communities. Available from: http://ec.europa.eu/health/ph_projects/2002/cancer/cancer_2002_01_en.htm.

Pfeffer N (2004). Screening for breast cancer: candidacy and compliance. *Soc Sci Med*, 58(1):151–60. doi:10.1016/S0277-9536(03)00156-4 PMID:14572928

Philips Healthcare (2014). Reaching the unreachable: addressing the challenges of breast cancer screening in Egypt. Netherlands: Philips Healthcare. Available from: http://www.healthcare.philips.com.

Piñeros M, Sánchez R, Cendales R, Perry F, Ocampo R (2009). Patient delay among Colombian women with breast cancer. *Salud Publica Mex*, 51(5):372–80. doi:10.1590/S0036-36342009000500004 PMID:19936550

Piñeros M, Sánchez R, Perry F, García OA, Ocampo R, Cendales R (2011). Delay for diagnosis and treatment of breast cancer in Bogotá, Colombia [in Spanish]. *Salud Publica Mex*, 53(6):478–85. PMID:22282140

Piñeros-Petersen M, Pardo-Ramos C, Gamboa-Garay O, Hernández-Suárez G (2010). Atlas de mortalidad por cáncer en Colombia. Bogotá, Colombia: Instituto Nacional de Cancerología, Instituto Geográfico Agustín Codazzi.

Price AJ, Ndom P, Atenguena E, Mambou Nouemssi JP, Ryder RW (2012). Cancer care challenges in developing countries. *Cancer*, 118(14):3627–35. doi:10.1002/cncr.26681 PMID:22223050

Prinjha S, Evans J, McPherson A (2006). Women's information needs about ductal carcinoma in situ before mammographic screening and after diagnosis: a qualitative study. *J Med Screen*, 13(3):110–4. doi:10.1258/096914106778440581 PMID:17007650

Profamilia (2011). Encuesta Nacional de Demografía y Salud 2010. Bogotá, Colombia: Ministerio de Salud y Protección Social. Available from: https://dhsprogram.com/pubs/pdf/FR246/FR246.pdf.

Rajaram SS, Rashidi A (1998). Minority women and breast cancer screening: the role of cultural explanatory models. *Prev Med*, 27(5 Pt 1):757–64. doi:10.1006/pmed.1998.0355 PMID:9808808

Rakowski W, Ehrich B, Goldstein MG, Rimer BK, Pearlman DN, Clark MA et al. (1998). Increasing mammography among women aged 40–74 by use of a stage-matched, tailored intervention. *Prev Med*, 27(5 Pt 1):748–56. doi:10.1006/pmed.1998.0354 PMID:9808807

Rasu RS, Rianon NJ, Shahidullah SM, Faisel AJ, Selwyn BJ (2011). Effect of educational level on knowledge and use of breast cancer screening practices in Bangladeshi women. *Health Care Women Int*, 32(3):177–89. doi:10.1080/07399332.2010.529213 PMID:21337241

Ravichandran K, Al-Hamdan NA, Mohamed G (2011). Knowledge, attitude, and behavior among Saudis toward cancer preventive practice. *J Family Community Med*, 18(3):135–42. doi:10.4103/2230-8229.90013 PMID:22175041

Rawl SM, Champion VL, Menon U, Foster JL (2000). The impact of age and race on mammography practices. *Health Care Women Int*, 21(7):583–97. doi:10.1080/07399330050151833 PMID:11813767

Reddy N, Ninan T, Tabar L, Bevers T (2012). The results of a breast cancer screening cAMP at a district level in rural India. *Asian Pac J Cancer Prev*, 13(12):6067–72. doi:10.7314/APJCP.2012.13.12.6067 PMID:23464405

Republic of Mauritius (2014). National cancer control programme. Available from: http://health.govmu.org/. English/Documents/cancer-ap.pdf, accessed 14 April 2015.

Republic of Rwanda Ministry of Health (2014). Breast cancer screening. Available from: http://www.moh.gov.rw/index.php?id=34&tx_ttnews%5Btt_news%5D=225&cHash=3d99509f1ec23e3f5a1aab2df5a5e45d.

Republic of Turkey, Ministry of Health, Department of Cancer Control (2009). National Cancer Program 2009–2015. Available from: http://www.iccp-portal.org/sites/default/files/plans/Turkey%20NATIONAL_CANCER_PROGRAM2-1.pdf.

Roche (2014). Raising awareness of breast cancer in Algeria. Available from: http://www.roche.com/sustainability/for_patients/access_to_healthcare/making_innovation_accessible/ath_bc_algeria.

Rutledge DN, Barsevick A, Knobf MT, Bookbinder M (2001). Breast cancer detection: knowledge, attitudes, and behaviors of women from Pennsylvania. *Oncol Nurs Forum*, 28(6):1032–40. PMID:11475877

Ryle M (2009). Screeningsdiagnosticeret sygdom som intervention i den personlige livsførelse. Belyst ved organiseret mammografiscreening i Danmark [dissertation]. Copenhagen, Denmark: Institut for Folkesundhedsvidenskab, Københavns Universitet.

Saadi A, Bond B, Percac-Lima S (2012). Perspectives on preventive health care and barriers to breast cancer screening among Iraqi women refugees. *J Immigr Minor Health*, 14(4):633–9. doi:10.1007/s10903-011-9520-3 PMID:21901446

Salem DS, Kamal RM, Helal MH, Hamed ST, Abdelrazek NA, Said NH et al. (2008). Women Health Outreach Program; a new experience for all Egyptian women. *J Egypt Natl Canc Inst*, 20(4):313–22. PMID:20571589

Salhia B, Tapia C, Ishak EA, Gaber S, Berghuis B, Hussain KH et al. (2011). Molecular subtype analysis determines the association of advanced breast cancer in Egypt with favorable biology. *BMC Womens Health*, 11(1):44. doi:10.1186/1472-6874-11-44 PMID:21961708

Samah AA, Ahmadian M (2012). Socio-demographic correlates of participation in mammography: a survey among women aged between 35- 69 in Tehran, Iran. *Asian Pac J Cancer Prev*, 13(6):2717–20. doi:10.7314/APJCP.2012.13.6.2717 PMID:22938447

Sano H, Goto R, Hamashima C (2014). What is the most effective strategy for improving the cancer screening rate in Japan? *Asian Pac J Cancer Prev*, 15(6):2607–12. doi:10.7314/APJCP.2014.15.6.2607 PMID:24761871

Sardanelli F, Boetes C, Borisch B, Decker T, Federico M, Gilbert FJ et al. (2010). Magnetic resonance imaging of the breast: recommendations from the EUSOMA working group. *Eur J Cancer*, 46(8):1296–316. doi:10.1016/j.ejca.2010.02.015 PMID:20304629

Saslow D, Boetes C, Burke W, Harms S, Leach MO, Lehman CD et al.; American Cancer Society Breast Cancer Advisory Group (2007). American Cancer Society guidelines for breast screening with MRI as an adjunct to mammography. *CA Cancer J Clin*, 57(2):75–89. doi:10.3322/canjclin.57.2.75 PMID:17392385

Scaf-Klomp W, Sanderman R, van de Wiel HB, Otter R, van den Heuvel WJ (1997). Distressed or relieved? Psychological side effects of breast cancer screening in The Netherlands. *J Epidemiol Community Health*, 51(6):705–10. doi:10.1136/jech.51.6.705 PMID:9519137

Schulz PJ, Meuffels B (2012). Justifying age thresholds for mammographic screening: an application of pragma-dialectical argumentation theory. *Health Commun*, 27(2):167–78. doi:10.1080/10410236.2011.571758 PMID:21823968

Schwartz LM, Woloshin S, Fowler FJ Jr, Welch HG (2004). Enthusiasm for cancer screening in the United States. *JAMA*, 291(1):71–8. doi:10.1001/jama.291.1.71 PMID:14709578

Secretaría de Salud de México (2008). Prevención y diagnóstico oportuno del cáncer de mama en el primer nivel de atención – Guía de práctica clínica. II C00–D48 Tumores (Neoplasias) – C50 Tumor maligno de la mama. Mexico City, Mexico: Secretaría de Salud de México.

Segnan N (1997). Socioeconomic status and cancer screening. *IARC Sci Publ*, 138:369–76. PMID:9353678

Shaheen R, Slanetz PJ, Raza S, Rosen MP (2011). Barriers and opportunities for early detection of breast cancer in Gaza women. *Breast*, 20(Suppl 2):S30–4. doi:10.1016/j.breast.2011.01.010 PMID:21316968

Shapiro S, Strax P, Venet L (1971). Periodic breast cancer screening in reducing mortality from breast cancer. *JAMA*, 215(11):1777–85. doi:10.1001/jama.1971.03180240027005 PMID:5107709

Shepherd JH, McInerney PA (2006). Knowledge of breast cancer in women in Sierra Leone. *Curationis*, 29(3):70–7. doi:10.4102/curationis.v29i3.1105 PMID:17131611

Sighoko D, Kamaté B, Traore C, Mallé B, Coulibaly B, Karidiatou A et al. (2013). Breast cancer in pre-menopausal women in West Africa: analysis of temporal trends and evaluation of risk factors associated with reproductive life. *Breast*, 22(5):828–35. doi:10.1016/j.breast.2013.02.011 PMID:23489760

Smith RA, Manassaram-Baptiste D, Brooks D, Doroshenk M, Fedewa S, Saslow D et al. (2015). Cancer screening in the United States, 2015: a review of current American cancer society guidelines and current issues in cancer screening. *CA Cancer J Clin*, 65(1):30–54. doi:10.3322/caac.21261 PMID:25581023

Smith RA, Saslow D, Sawyer KA, Burke W, Costanza ME, Evans WP 3rd et al.; American Cancer Society Breast Cancer Advisory Group (2003). American Cancer Society guidelines for breast cancer screening: update 2003. *CA Cancer J Clin*, 53(3):141–69. doi:10.3322/canjclin.53.3.141 PMID:12809408

Soares PB, Quirino Filho S, de Souza WP, Gonçalves RC, Martelli DR, Silveira MF et al. (2012). Characteristics of women with breast cancer seen at reference services in the North of Minas Gerais. *Rev Bras Epidemiol*, 15(3):595–604. doi:10.1590/S1415-790X2012000300013 PMID:23090306

SOCHIMIO (2014). Solidarité Chimiothérapie, Union contre le Cancer. Available from: http://sochimiocm.org/sochimio/index.php/en/actions-et-realisations, accessed 15 April 2015.

Solbjør M (2008). "You have to have trust in those pictures": a perspective to women's trust in mammography screening. In: Brownlie J, Greene A, Howson A, editors. Researching trust and health. London, UK: Routledge.

Solbjør M, Skolbekken JA, Sætnan AR, Hagen AI, Forsmo S (2012a). Mammography screening and trust: the case of interval breast cancer. *Soc Sci Med*, 75(10):1746–52. doi:10.1016/j.socscimed.2012.07.029 PMID:22906524

Solbjør M, Skolbekken JA, Sætnan AR, Hagen AI, Forsmo S (2012b). Could screening participation bias symptom interpretation? An interview study on women's interpretations of and responses to cancer symptoms between mammography screening rounds. *BMJ Open*, 2(6):e001508. doi:10.1136/bmjopen-2012-001508 PMID:23148341

Soskolne V, Marie S, Manor O (2007). Beliefs, recommendations and intentions are important explanatory factors of mammography screening behavior among Muslim Arab women in Israel. *Health Educ Res*, 22(5):665–76. doi:10.1093/her/cyl132 PMID:17138612

St-Jacques S, Philibert MD, Langlois A, Daigle JM, Pelletier E, Major D et al. (2013). Geographic access to mammography screening centre and participation of women in the Quebec Breast Cancer Screening Programme. *J Epidemiol Community Health*, 67(10):861–7. doi:10.1136/jech-2013-202614 PMID:23851149

Stamler LL, Thomas B, Lafreniere K (2000). Working women identify influences and obstacles to breast health practices. *Oncol Nurs Forum*, 27(5):835–42. PMID:10868394

State of Palestine Ministry of Health (2014). National health strategy 2014–2016. Available from: http://www.moh.ps/attach/617.pdf.

Straughan PT, Seow A (2000). Attitudes as barriers in breast screening: a prospective study among Singapore women. *Soc Sci Med*, 51(11):1695–703. doi:10.1016/S0277-9536(00)00086-1 PMID:11072888

Suarez L, Pulley L (1995). Comparing acculturation scales and their relationship to cancer screening among older Mexican-American women. *J Natl Cancer Inst Monogr*, (18):41–7. PMID:8562221

Suh MA, Atashili J, Fuh EA, Eta VA (2012). Breast self-examination and breast cancer awareness in women in developing countries: a survey of women in Buea, Cameroon. *BMC Res Notes*, 5(1):627. doi:10.1186/1756-0500-5-627 PMID:23140094

Sung JF, Blumenthal DS, Coates RJ, Alema-Mensah E (1997). Knowledge, beliefs, attitudes, and cancer screening among inner-city African-American women. *J Natl Med Assoc*, 89(6):405–11. PMID:9195801

Supreme Council of Health of Qatar (2014). National cancer strategy. Available from: http://www.sch.gov.qa/health-strategies/national-cancer-strategy.

Susan G. Komen (2014). Mammography. Available from: http://ww5.komen.org/BreastCancer/Mammography.html.

Sutton S, Saidi G, Bickler G, Hunter J (1995). Does routine screening for breast cancer raise anxiety? Results from a three wave prospective study in England. *J Epidemiol Community Health*, 49(4):413–8. doi:10.1136/jech.49.4.413 PMID:7650466

Swanson V, McIntosh IB, Power KG, Dobson H (1996). The psychological effects of breast screening in terms of patients' perceived health anxieties. *Br J Clin Pract*, 50(3):129–35. PMID:8733330

Swaziland Breast Cancer Network (2008). Swaziland Breast Cancer Network. Available from: http://www.breastcancernet.org.sz, accessed 21 October 2014.

Tabuchi T, Hoshino T, Nakayama T, Ito Y, Ioka A, Miyashiro I et al. (2013). Does removal of out-of-pocket costs for cervical and breast cancer screening work? A quasi-experimental study to evaluate the impact on attendance, attendance inequality and average cost per uptake of a Japanese government intervention. *Int J Cancer*, 133(4):972–83. doi:10.1002/ijc.28095 PMID:23400833

Taggart L, Truesdale-Kennedy M, McIlfatrick S (2011). The role of community nurses and residential staff in supporting women with intellectual disability to access breast screening services. *J Intellect Disabil Res*, 55(1):41–52. doi:10.1111/j.1365-2788.2010.01345.x PMID:21121993

Taha H, Halabi Y, Berggren V, Jaouni S, Nyström L, Al-Qutob R et al. (2010). Educational intervention to improve breast health knowledge among women in Jordan. *Asian Pac J Cancer Prev*, 11(5):1167–73. PMID:21198258

Tang TS, Patterson SK, Roubidoux MA, Duan L (2009). Women's mammography experience and its impact on screening adherence. *Psychooncology*, 18(7):727–34. doi:10.1002/pon.1463 PMID:19035468

Tazhibi M, Feizi A (2014). Awareness levels about breast cancer risk factors, early warning signs, and screening and therapeutic approaches among Iranian adult women: a large population based study using latent class analysis. *BioMed Res Int*, 2014:306352. doi:10.1155/2014/306352 PMID:25295257

Teo MCC, Soo KC (2013). Cancer trends and incidences in Singapore. *Jpn J Clin Oncol*, 43(3):219–24. doi:10.1093/jjco/hys230 PMID:23303840

Thomas DB, Murillo R, Kardinah, Anderson BO (2013). Breast cancer early detection and clinical guidelines. In: Soliman A, Schottenfeld D, Boffetta P, editors. Cancer epidemiology: low and middle income countries and special populations. New York (NY), USA: Oxford University Press; pp. 378–95. doi:10.1093/med/9780199733507.003.0022

Thomson RM, Crengle S, Lawrenson R (2009). Improving participation in breast screening in a rural general practice with a predominately Maori population. *N Z Med J*, 122(1291):39–47. PMID:19322254

Tonelli M, Connor Gorber S, Joffres M, Dickinson J, Singh H, Lewin G et al.; Canadian Task Force on Preventive Health Care (2011). Recommendations on screening for breast cancer in average-risk women aged 40–74 years. *CMAJ*, 183(17):1991–2001. doi:10.1503/cmaj.110334 PMID:22106103

Torres-Mejía G, Ortega-Olvera C, Ángeles-Llerenas A, Villalobos-Hernández AL, Salmerón-Castro J, Lazcano-Ponce E et al. (2013). Utilization patterns of prevention and early diagnosis for cancer in women [in Spanish]. *Salud Publica Mex*, 55(Suppl 2):S241–8. PMID:24626701

Trivedi AN, Rakowski W, Ayanian JZ (2008). Effect of cost sharing on screening mammography in Medicare health plans. *N Engl J Med*, 358(4):375–83. doi:10.1056/NEJMsa070929 PMID:18216358

Trufelli DC, Miranda VC, Santos MB, Fraile NM, Pecoroni PG, Gonzaga SF et al. (2008). Analysis of delays in diagnosis and treatment of breast cancer patients at a public hospital [in Portuguese]. *Rev Assoc Med Bras*, 54(1):72–6. doi:10.1590/S0104-42302008000100024 PMID:18392490

Tsunematsu M, Kawasaki H, Masuoka Y, Kakehashi M (2013). Factors affecting breast cancer screening behavior in Japan–assessment using the health belief model and conjoint analysis. *Asian Pac J Cancer Prev*, 14(10):6041–8. doi:10.7314/APJCP.2013.14.10.6041 PMID:24289622

US Preventive Services Task Force (2009). Screening for breast cancer: U.S. Preventive Services Task Force recommendation statement. *Ann Intern Med*, 151(10):716–26, W-236. doi:10.7326/0003-4819-151-10-200911170-00008 PMID:19920272

Vahabi M (2010). Verbal versus numerical probabilities: does format presentation of probabilistic information regarding breast cancer screening affect women's comprehension? *Health Educ J*, 69(2):150–63. doi:10.1177/0017896909349262

Vahabi M, Gastaldo D (2003). Rational choice(s)? Rethinking decision-making on breast cancer risk and screening mammography. *Nurs Inq*, 10(4):245–56. doi:10.1046/j.1440-1800.2003.00190.x PMID:14622371

van Agt H, Fracheboud J, van der Steen A, de Koning H (2012). Do women make an informed choice about participating in breast cancer screening? A survey among women invited for a first mammography screening examination. *Patient Educ Couns*, 89(2):353–9. doi:10.1016/j.pec.2012.08.003 PMID:22963769

Vermeer B, Van den Muijsenbergh ME (2010). The attendance of migrant women at the national breast cancer screening in the Netherlands 1997–2008. *Eur J Cancer Prev*, 19(3):195–8. doi:10.1097/CEJ.0b013e328337214c PMID:20150815

Viniegra M, Paolino M, Arrosi S (2010). Cáncer de mama en Argentina: organización, cobertura y calidad de las acciones de prevención y control. Buenos Aires, Argentina: Organización Panamericana de la Salud.

von Euler-Chelpin M, Olsen AH, Njor S, Jensen A, Vejborg I, Schwartz W et al. (2008). Does educational level determine screening participation? *Eur J Cancer Prev*, 17(3):273–8. doi:10.1097/CEJ.0b013e3282f0c017 PMID:18414200

von Karsa L, Anttila A, Ronco G, Ponti A, Malila N, Arbyn M et al. (2008). Cancer screening in the European Union: report on the implementation of the Council Recommendation on cancer screening. Luxembourg: European Communities.

Walker LG, Cordiner CM, Gilbert FJ, Needham G, Deans HE, Affleck IR et al. (1994). How distressing is attendance for routine breast screening? *Psychooncology*, 3(4):299–304. doi:10.1002/pon.2960030406

Waller J, Douglas E, Whitaker KL, Wardle J (2013). Women's responses to information about overdiagnosis in the UK breast cancer screening programme: a qualitative study. *BMJ Open*, 3(4):e002703. doi:10.1136/bmjopen-2013-002703 PMID:23610383

Waller J, Whitaker KL, Winstanley K, Power E, Wardle J (2014). A survey study of women's responses to information about overdiagnosis in breast cancer screening in Britain. *Br J Cancer*, 111(9):1831–5. doi:10.1038/bjc.2014.482 PMID:25167224

Wang B, He M, Wang L, Engelgau MM, Zhao W, Wang L (2013). Breast cancer screening among adult women in China, 2010. *Prev Chronic Dis*, 10:E183. doi:10.5888/pcd10.130136 PMID:24199736

Wee CC, McCarthy EP, Davis RB, Phillips RS (2000). Screening for cervical and breast cancer: is obesity an unrecognized barrier to preventive care? *Ann Intern Med*, 132(9):697–704. doi:10.7326/0003-4819-132-9-200005020-00003 PMID:10787362

Wells KJ, Roetzheim RG (2007). Health disparities in receipt of screening mammography in Latinas: a critical review of recent literature. *Cancer Control*, 14(4):369–79. PMID:17914337

WHO African Health Observatory (2014). Sierra Leone: non-communicable disease and conditions. World Health Organization Regional Office for Africa. Available from: http://www.aho.afro.who.int/profiles_information/index.

php/Sierra_Leone:Analytical_summary_-_Non-communicable_diseases_and_conditions.
WHO (2005). World Health Survey 2003. Geneva, Switzerland: World Health Organization. Available from: http://apps.who.int/healthinfo/systems/surveydata/index.php/catalog/whs.
WHO (2008a). Cancer control: knowledge into action: WHO guide for effective programmes. Policy and advocacy. Geneva, Switzerland: World Health Organization.
WHO (2008b). Country case study: Pakistan's Lady Health Worker Programme. Geneva, Switzerland: World Health Organization.
WHO (2014). World Health Statistics 2014. Geneva, Switzerland: World Health Organization.
Wilkinson JE, Deis CE, Bowen DJ, Bokhour BG (2011). 'It's easier said than done': perspectives on mammography from women with intellectual disabilities. *Ann Fam Med*, 9(2):142–7. doi:10.1370/afm.1231 PMID:21403141
Williams-Piehota P, Pizarro J, Schneider TR, Mowad L, Salovey P (2005). Matching health messages to monitor-blunter coping styles to motivate screening mammography. *Health Psychol*, 24(1):58–67. doi:10.1037/0278-6133.24.1.58 PMID:15631563
Willis K (2008). "I come because I am called": recruitment and participation in mammography screening in Uppsala, Sweden. *Health Care Women Int*, 29(2):135–50. doi:10.1080/07399330701738143 PMID:18350420
Women's Health Outreach Program (2014). Women's Health Outreach Program for Egypt. Available from: http://www.whop.gov.eg.
Yadollahie M, Simi A, Habibzadeh F, Ghashghaiee RT, Karimi S, Behzadi P et al. (2011). Knowledge of and attitudes toward breast self-examination in Iranian women: a multi-center study. *Asian Pac J Cancer Prev*, 12(8):1917–24. PMID:22292625
Yeoh KG, Chew L, Wang SC (2006). Cancer screening in Singapore, with particular reference to breast, cervical and colorectal cancer screening. *J Med Screen*, 13(Suppl 1):S14–9. PMID:17227636
Yoo BN, Choi KS, Jung KW, Jun JK (2012). Awareness and practice of breast self-examination among Korean women: results from a nationwide survey. *Asian Pac J Cancer Prev*, 13(1):123–5. doi:10.7314/APJCP.2012.13.1.123 PMID:22502653
Yu MY, Song L, Seetoo A, Cai C, Smith G, Oakley D (2007). Culturally competent training program: a key to training lay health advisors for promoting breast cancer screening. *Health Educ Behav*, 34(6):928–41. doi:10.1177/1090198107304577 PMID:17965228
Yu MY, Wu TY, Mood DW (2005). Cultural affiliation and mammography screening of Chinese women in an urban county of Michigan. *J Transcult Nurs*, 16(2):107–16. doi:10.1177/1043659605274745 PMID:15764633
Zaanouni E, Ben Abdallah M, Bouchlaka A, Ben Aissa R, Kribi L, M'barek F et al. (2009). Preliminary results and analysis of the feasibility of mammographic breast cancer screening in women younger than 50 years of the Ariana area in Tunisia [in French]. *Tunis Med*, 87(7):443–9. PMID:20063677
Zackrisson S, Lindström M, Moghaddassi M, Andersson I, Janzon L (2007). Social predictors of non-attendance in an urban mammographic screening programme: a multilevel analysis. *Scand J Public Health*, 35(5):548–54. doi:10.1080/14034940701291716 PMID:17852976
Zapka JG, Geller BM, Bulliard JL, Fracheboud J, Sancho-Garnier H, Ballard-Barbash R; IBSN Communications Working Group (2006). Print information to inform decisions about mammography screening participation in 16 countries with population-based programs. *Patient Educ Couns*, 63(1–2):126–37. doi:10.1016/j.pec.2005.09.012 PMID:16962910
Zhang W, Rose SB, Foster A, Pullon S, Lawton B (2014). Breast cancer and breast screening: perceptions of Chinese migrant women living in New Zealand. *J Prim Health Care*, 6(2):135–42. PMID:24892131
Zhu K, Hunter S, Bernard LJ, Payne-Wilks K, Roland CL, Levine RS (2000). Mammography screening in single older African-American women: a study of related factors. *Ethn Dis*, 10(3):395–405. PMID:11110356

4. EFFICACY OF BREAST CANCER SCREENING

4.1 Methodological and analytical issues

To evaluate the efficacy of screening, it is important to consider the definitions of efficacy and effectiveness for an intervention, to define outcome measures, and to consider potential biases.

4.1.1 Efficacy versus effectiveness

The term "efficacy" should be distinguished from the term "effectiveness". Efficacy is "the extent to which a specific intervention, procedure, regimen, or service produces a beneficial result under **ideal conditions**" (Porta, 2014), whereas effectiveness is "a measure of the extent to which a specific intervention, procedure, regimen, or service, when deployed in the field in the **usual circumstances**, does what it is intended to do for a specified population" (Porta, 2014). In practice, true efficacy [under ideal conditions] can rarely be estimated. Randomized controlled trials (RCTs), which are conducted to initially assess whether screening works, assess efficacy by estimating a primary outcome, such as reduction in breast cancer mortality in the study arm compared with the control arm. However, the measure of efficacy is limited by the implementation of the intervention and other practical issues – for instance, less than 100% compliance in the study arm and unintended screening in the control arm. Hence, an intention-to-treat analysis of RCTs, i.e. an analysis in which the data are analysed according to the original randomized design, may actually have a limited ability to address efficacy, due to non-ideal circumstances (Gulati et al., 2012).

This section focuses primarily on the assessment of efficacy; methodological issues in the assessment of effectiveness are addressed in Section 5.1.

4.1.2 Primary outcome measures

The primary outcome measure is reduction in breast cancer mortality, although increasing life expectancy or reduction of metastatic disease can also be considered efficacy measures. Given the natural history of the disease, a minimum requirement in addressing efficacy is a sufficiently long follow-up (Hanley, 2011). Some authors have suggested that the use of breast cancer mortality as the end-point of a trial may have led to unreliable estimates of the relative risk reduction, due to possible uncertainties surrounding the determination of breast cancer death (leading to misclassification of deaths), and that the use of all-cause mortality as the end-point of a trial would resolve this bias (Black et al., 2002; Gøtzsche & Jørgensen, 2013). However, others have argued that all-cause mortality is not an appropriate end-point for screening trials for a specific disease (Tabár et al., 2002; Marmot et al.,

2013; Weiss, 2014). Although using all-cause mortality avoids the need to determine cause of death precisely, breast cancer deaths reflect a small fraction of all-cause mortality, and trials of the size needed to have sufficient statistical power to detect the expected small effects of screening on all-cause mortality would be logistically and financially impracticable. A Swedish review, which incorporated all Swedish RCTs of breast cancer screening, showed a 2% non-significant reduction in all-cause mortality (Nyström et al., 2002a), which is in line with the expected 0.94% (Nyström et al., 2002b).

4.1.3 Biases

Several sources of bias have important effects on the estimation of screening efficacy.

The first important bias is lead-time bias. The general concept of screening is that by early detection of disease and subsequent treatment, prognosis is improved and the probability of death from the disease is reduced. The time between screen detection and the point at which a tumour would have presented and been clinically diagnosed (in the absence of screening) is referred to as "lead time" (Cole & Morrison, 1980). The survival time, the time from breast cancer diagnosis to death, of screen-detected cases is increased because of this lead time, even for individuals who do not benefit from screening. Lead-time bias may therefore appear to act in favour of screening, if efficacy is evaluated by survival analyses.

The second important bias is length bias (Cole & Morrison, 1980) (sometimes referred to as length-time bias). The probability of a tumour being detected at screening is (partially) dependent on the growth rate of the tumour, because slow-growing tumours have a longer preclinical detectable phase (sojourn time) and are therefore more likely to be detected than fast-growing tumours. Tumours detected at screening thus reflect a biased sample of preclinical lesions, including slower-growing tumours, which are generally thought to be associated with a better prognosis and therefore longer survival. This again leads to bias apparently in favour of screening. The most extreme form of length bias is referred to as overdiagnosis. Some ductal carcinoma in situ (DCIS) may never progress to invasive cancer or present clinically (in the absence of screening) (Yen et al., 2003), and some invasive cancers may be sufficiently indolent that they would never have presented clinically during the woman's lifetime if they had not been detected by screening (see Section 4.2.3c).

The last important bias in evaluating screening is selection bias. Women attend screening voluntarily, and participants might therefore generally be more health-conscious and have a lower baseline risk of breast cancer than non-participants, although in practice this assumption may not hold true (Paap et al., 2011). The decision to attend screening may also be influenced by certain demographic and social factors (see Section 3.1) that affect disease prognosis, for example familial risk. In RCTs with mortality as the end-point, such a selection may hamper the generalizability of the results.

Evaluations of efficacy and effectiveness must control for the above-mentioned biases if they are to provide credible estimates. To eliminate lead-time and length bias, differences in breast cancer mortality rates (between the trial arms or different populations) should be the end-point of a study rather than survival, because survival time in cancer patients is extended due to lead time and is more favourable due to length-biased sampling. Selection bias can partially be quantified by comparing non-participants with historical or recent data on mortality or risk factors and can, perhaps, be controlled for by adjusting for risk factors or their surrogates (e.g. socioeconomic status; Allgood et al., 2008) or by the application of an empirically derived adjustment factor (Paap et al., 2014). In addition, it has been argued that any bias due to selection for screening is likely to be small in organized programmes with invitation schemes based on population registries and with high attendance rates (van Schoor et al., 2011a, b).

4.1.4 Use of randomized controlled trials

Reduction in breast cancer mortality in women offered screening relative to women not offered screening is the appropriate measure of benefit of an RCT. Lead-time and length bias are then eliminated in the analyses. Women are followed up from the time of randomization instead of from the time of diagnosis, which avoids lead time, and all deaths from breast cancer that occur during the follow-up period are included in the analysis. The RCTs of breast cancer screening are evaluated in accordance with the intention-to-screen principle, taking into account in the intervention group both women who accept the invitation to screening and women who decline the invitation. The resulting point estimate of reduction in breast cancer mortality therefore does not evaluate the screened groups of individuals only.

In RCTs, participants are randomly assigned to either the intervention group or the control group to prevent confounding at baseline, accounting for both observable characteristics and unknown confounders. However, even well performed randomization schemes may not prevent potential imbalances completely. To take into account possible differences in risk factors for death from breast cancer between the intervention group and the control group, an assessment should preferably be made of the distribution of risk factors in both groups at trial entry, which would permit adjustment in the analysis (although most known risk factors for breast cancer seem to have limited predictive value). If individual randomization is not feasible, for example when the same clinician would be required to use a simple screening test in one individual and not use it in another, randomization by cluster is an alternative. Both types of randomization have been used in the RCTs of breast cancer screening. Recruitment and randomization are less complex with cluster randomization, but an equal distribution of risk factors between the intervention group and the control group is less likely to be achieved than with individual randomization. Furthermore, subjects with a previous diagnosis of breast cancer at the time of randomization are, ideally, excluded from the trial. Whereas a previous diagnosis can be determined more easily in RCTs with individual randomization, this may be more difficult to achieve beforehand with cluster randomization. An important advantage of cluster randomization is that contamination of (screening in) the control group may be reduced.

As mentioned above, the screening effect in RCTs is dependent on, among other things, the compliance in the intervention group and the limitation of contamination of the control group. Low compliance reduces the estimate of effect and must therefore be reported. Screening of controls by services outside of the trial will also dilute the effect of screening on breast cancer mortality. Possible contamination of the control group is often difficult to measure, especially because mammography is also used for clinical diagnosis of breast cancer and this use may not be easily distinguished from use for opportunistic screening. Methods to adjust for contamination and poor compliance have been proposed (Cuzick et al., 1997; Baker et al., 2002). Furthermore, unless the breast cancer mortality analysis is limited to those diagnosed with breast cancer during the screening phase of the trial period, with longer follow-up, screening of the control group can influence the observed difference between the intervention group and the control group.

The difference in outcome between the groups of subjects randomized is further determined by a large number of varying factors. The age groups at entry, screening interval, attendance

Fig. 4.1 Trajectory of a screening outcome

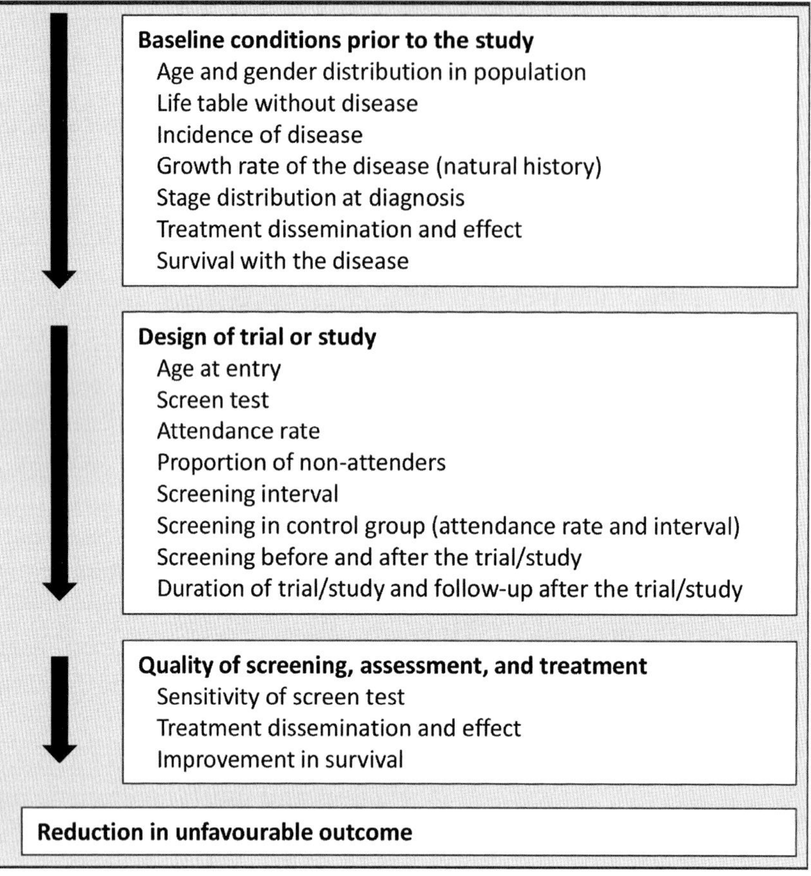

From de Koning (2009).

of trial screening, and opportunistic screening in both women randomized to screening and control women all influence the ultimate extent of the effects. Such "analyses per protocol" were not routinely conducted in the available trials. Through modelling, it has been shown that these relatively simple differences alone could make one trial exhibit a 25% greater effect than another (de Koning et al., 1995).

However, for estimating the magnitude of (true) efficacy, it is equally important to consider how much earlier the diagnosis was made as a result of screening and the effect this has. Therefore, the more important questions relate to the quality of the screening, how many women were referred for further examination, and how many tumours were detected and at which stage. The baseline conditions before the study, or in this case those of the control group, are also significant. If women in one region on average receive health care at an earlier stage, this can mean that the difference between "early" and "late" (read: intervention group compared with control group) is smaller in one region than in another, even if the quality of screening and therapy may be the same. In standard meta-analyses, all of these differences are ignored, and modelling has been proposed to estimate the impact of such effects and to lead to better estimates of "efficacy under ideal circumstances". Fig. 4.1 exemplifies the most important different steps that ultimately lead to the (reported) reduction in the unfavourable outcome of disease – for example, breast cancer mortality – that should be considered when estimating the true efficacy.

4.1.5 *Use of observational studies in assessing efficacy*

Estimates of screening efficacy from contemporary observational studies may be considered more relevant than those from the RCTs, most of which were initiated in the 1970s or early 1980s. Recent studies can take into account improvements in mammography techniques and in treatment that have occurred over the past 30 years. However, observational studies are prone to the biases discussed above, and adequate control for these biases by design or analysis is difficult. The presence of other potential biases differs between studies and is dependent on the study design, the duration and completeness of follow-up, and, in a case–control study, the definition of exposure to screening. In practice, these observational studies have been used primarily to assess the effectiveness of screening programmes (see Section 5.1.2).

4.2 Mammography

The basic characteristics of the randomized trials of the efficacy of screen-film mammography screening are shown in Table 4.1. All of these trials were considered by the previous IARC Working Group on breast cancer screening (IARC, 2002). All ages given in this section, unless otherwise stated, refer to age at entry into the trial.

4.2.1 *Description of randomized trials*

(a) Health Insurance Plan trial

In December 1963, the Health Insurance Plan of Greater New York, USA, had 85 000 female members aged 40–64 years (Shapiro et al., 1966). In 23 of the plan's 31 medical groups, women were individually randomized to annual film mammography screening and clinical breast examination (CBE) for 4 years or to a control arm receiving the usual care within the plan but no screening. Randomization was pair-matched by age, size of the insured family, and employment group through which the family had joined the plan. Of those randomized to screening, 67% attended the first screening round. Although data on risk factors were not collected from all participants, there were no differences between a 10% sample of the examined group, a 20% sample of non-attenders, and a 20% sample of controls with respect to age, socioeconomic status, and history of pregnancies (Shapiro et al., 1988).

Gøtzsche & Olsen (2000) suggested that the exclusions after randomization and the review of causes of death may have led to lack of comparability between the screened and unscreened groups. Miller (2001) advised that the decisions made on the deaths reviewed were entirely masked. [Miller was a member of the death review committee.] A difference in the numbers of women with breast cancer initially excluded from the two arms of the trial arose because previously diagnosed breast cancers were identified in women in the screened group when they attended screening, but this was not possible for the controls. However, the 18-year follow-up enabled identification of deaths from breast cancer in the two groups; determination of the date of diagnosis was then made from hospital records. Women who had died from breast cancers diagnosed before randomization were then excluded.

[The Working Group concluded that the Health Insurance Plan trial was valid and could be included in its overall evaluation of screening by mammography. The technology used produced images of comparable quality to those from screen-film mammography (see Sections 2.1.1 and 2.1.2 for details on the history of screening techniques).]

Table 4.1 Basic characteristics of randomized trials of the efficacy of screen-film mammography screening

Trial, country	Randomization	No. of women	Accrual period for screening		Age at entry (years)	Intervention	No. of mammography views	Screening interval (months)	No. of rounds	Attendance rate at first round (%)	Determination of end-point
			Invited group	Control group							
Health Insurance Plan trial, USA	Individual	60 696	December 1963–June 1966		40–64	M + CBE	2	12	4	67	Independent death review
Malmö I trial, Sweden	Individual	42 283	October 1976–August 1978	October 1992–February 1993	45–70	M	2	18–24	6–8	74	Independent death review Official statistics
Malmö II trial, Sweden	Individual	17 786	September 1978–November 1990	September 1991–April 1994	43–49	M	2	18–24	1–7	75–80	Official statistics
Two-County trial: Kopparberg County, Sweden	Cluster	57 897	July 1977–February 1980	September 1982–December 1986	40–74	M	1	24 (40–49) 33 (≥ 50)	2–4	89	Death review
Two-County trial: Östergötland County, Sweden	Cluster	76 617	May 1978–March 1981	April 1986–February 1988	40–74	M	1	24 (40–49) 33 (≥ 50)	2–4	89	Death review Official statistics
Edinburgh trial, United Kingdom	Cluster	54 643	1978–1985		45–64	M + CBE	2	24	2–4	61	Death certificates
CNBSS 1 trial, Canada	Individual	50 430	January 1980–March 1985		40–49	M + CBE	2	12	4 or 5	100	Independent death review Official statistics
CNBSS 2 trial, Canada	Individual	39 405	January 1980–March 1985		50–59	M + CBE	2	12	4 or 5	100	Independent death review Official statistics
Stockholm trial, Sweden	Cluster	60 117	March 1981–May 1983	October 1985–May 1986	40–64	M	1	28	2	81	Official statistics

Table 4.1 (continued)

Trial, country	Randomization	No. of women	Accrual period for screening		Age at entry (years)	Intervention	No. of mammography views	Screening interval (months)	No. of rounds	Attendance rate at first round (%)	Determination of end-point
			Invited group	Control group							
Gothenburg trial, Sweden	Individual Cluster	51 611	December 1982–April 1984	November 1987–June 1991	39–59	M	2	18	4 or 5	85	Official statistics
United Kingdom Age trial	Individual	160 921	1991–1997	On reaching age 50–52 years	39–41	M	2, first screen 1, subsequently	12	4–7	68	Official statistics

CBE, clinical breast examination; CNBSS, Canadian National Breast Screening Study; M, mammography.

(b) Malmö trials

In the first of two trials in Malmö, Sweden (Malmö I), starting in October 1976 all women born in 1908–1932 were identified from the population register and randomized by a computer program within each birth-year cohort. The resulting lists were divided; the 21 088 women in the first half were invited, and the 21 195 women in the second half served as controls (Andersson et al., 1988). Women were invited to screen-film mammography alone, with two views (craniocaudal and mediolateral oblique) in the first two rounds, and with either both views or only the oblique view, depending on the parenchymal pattern, in the subsequent rounds, every 18–24 months. A single mediolateral oblique view was taken for women whose breasts were mainly fatty on mammography, and both views were taken for women with dense breasts. The attendance rate was higher for the first round (74%) than for subsequent rounds (70%), and was higher among younger women than among older women.

After August 1978, the investigators aimed to continue to recruit women who reached the age of 45 years and to randomize them to either receive or not receive an invitation to mammography. In the second trial (Malmö II), 17 786 women born in 1933–1945 were recruited, with 9574 in the invited group and 8212 in the control group. The randomization and screening procedures were the same as in the first trial, and recruitment continued until 1990 (Andersson & Janzon, 1997).

(c) Two-County trial (Kopparberg and Östergötland)

In 1975, the Swedish National Board of Health and Welfare invited five county councils to start a mammography screening trial. Two counties, Kopparberg (now Dalarna) County and Östergötland County, accepted the invitation. Women in this trial were randomized by cluster within geographical areas (municipalities, parishes, tax districts). The municipalities in Östergötland County were grouped pairwise with respect to the size of the population and geographical characteristics. The more-populated municipalities of Linköping, Norrköping, and Motala were split into six, eight, and two clusters, respectively, of similar size, creating three, four, and one pairs, respectively, to increase the number of clusters. The clusters were randomly allocated to an invitation group or to a control group. A total of 76 617 women aged 40–74 years were randomized to mammography or the usual care (Nyström et al., 2002a). In Kopparberg County, the invited group was planned to be twice as large as the control group. Thus, triplets of geographical areas were identified by dividing each block into three units of roughly equal size, of which two were randomly allocated by local politicians to receive screening and one to the control group. A total of 57 897 women aged 40–74 years were included (Tabár et al., 1985). In total, 77 080 women were randomized to regular invitation to screening (active study population [ASP]) and 55 985 to no invitation (passive study population [PSP]) in 45 geographical clusters (Duffy et al., 2003a). In the ASP, women aged 40–49 years were invited to screening by single-view mammography every 24 months, and those aged 50 years and older were invited on average every 33 months. The overall compliance with the invitations for women aged 40–74 years was 89% for the first screen and 83% for the second screen. Women aged 40–49 years had the highest compliance, 93% for the first screen and 89% for the second screen, and women aged 70–74 years had the lowest compliance, 79% for the first screen and 67% for the second screen (Tabár et al., 1985). Women aged 70–74 years at randomization were not invited to a third screen. The compliance for the third screen was 88% for women aged 40–49 years, 86% for those aged 50–59 years, and 78% for those aged 60–69 years (Tabár et al., 1992).

When this trial was conducted, adjuvant chemotherapy and hormone therapy were not available in Sweden, and therefore they were not used for the treatment of breast cancer cases in the trial (Holmberg et al., 1986, Tabár et al., 1999). Furthermore, because the controls (PSP) were not contacted until a decision was made to screen them at the end of screening of the ASP, no data on breast cancer risk factors were collected to permit confirmation that balance in the distribution of risk factors was achieved by the cluster randomization.

In response to suggestions that there were various potential problems with the randomization in the Two-County trial (Olsen & Gøtzsche, 2001), Nyström et al. (2002a) reported that the breast cancer incidence and mortality rates in the clusters of the screened and control groups in Östergötland County before the trial (1968–1977) were similar. They suggested that there is no reason to believe that the cluster randomization in this component of the trial was biased, as any bias would have manifested in breast cancer incidence and mortality rates. Duffy et al. (2003a) reanalysed the available data, taking into account the cluster randomization. Although there was no significant difference in prior breast cancer mortality between the ASP and PSP clusters, the authors reported an analysis adjusting for prior mortality within clusters. This yielded a significant 27% reduction in mortality in the ASP, a minor dilution of the unadjusted estimate (30%). [This suggested that there was no substantial bias in terms of prior risk of breast cancer mortality as a result of the cluster randomization.]

Issues have been raised about the numbers of cases included in the analyses of the Two-County trial (Zahl et al., 2006). Dean (2007) advised that the analysis of Zahl et al. (2006) was inaccurate with respect to trial dates and did not take into account the staggered entry of districts into the trial (Fagerberg & Tabár, 1988).

Verification of the cause of death is crucial in any trial. Holmberg et al. (2009) characterized and quantified differences in the number of breast cancer cases and deaths identified in the Two-County trial by the local end-point committee compared with the Swedish overview committee. Of the 2615 outcomes included by the local end-point committee or the overview committee, there were 478 (18%) disagreements, of which 82% were due to differences in application of inclusion/exclusion criteria and 18% were due to disagreement with respect to cause of death or vital status at ascertainment. For Östergötland County, the overview committee-based determination of cause of death resulted in a reduction of the estimate of the effect of screening compared with the local end-point committee, but for Kopparberg County the difference was modest.

The Two-County trial was closed after completion of the first round of screening in the PSP; participants in both groups continued with service screening. All cases of breast cancer in both groups diagnosed up to and including the end of the first screen of the PSP were followed up for death from breast cancer (Holmberg et al., 2009).

(d) Edinburgh trial

In Edinburgh, United Kingdom, in 1978–1981, 87 general practitioners' practices, covering 44 268 women aged 45–64 years, were randomized for a breast cancer screening trial (Alexander et al., 1999). The 22 926 women in the practices in the intervention group were invited to participate in a screening programme, which included CBE every year and two-view mammography every 2 years. The 21 342 women in the practices in the control group received only the usual care. Subsequently, additional eligible women who joined these practices and existing patients who reached the age of 45 years were recruited into two further cohorts: 4867 women in 1982–1983 and 5499 women in 1984–1985 (Alexander et al., 1999).

Alexander et al. (1989) reported that the cluster randomization in the Edinburgh trial resulted in differences by socioeconomic category and also in rates of mortality from all causes between the two comparison groups.

[The Working Group noted concerns about the potential for bias resulting from the cluster randomization procedure. Although the authors adjusted for socioeconomic status in their analyses, it is not clear that this entirely removed the bias. Nevertheless, the Working Group concluded that this trial could be included in the evaluation.]

(e) *Canadian National Breast Screening Study trials*

The Canadian National Breast Screening Study (CNBSS) was originally designed as a single trial in women aged 40–59 years (Miller et al., 1981), and was managed as such, but after the first mortality reports (Miller et al., 1992a, b), it was regarded as two trials: CNBSS 1, in women aged 40–49 years, and CNBSS 2, in women aged 50–59 years. Women were eligible for the trials if they had not had breast cancer, had not had a mammogram in the previous 12 months, were not currently pregnant, and completed a questionnaire providing full identification and data on risk factors for breast cancer (Miller et al., 1981). Before randomization, all participants gave written informed consent after having been told that they had a 50% chance of having a mammogram. They then received CBE and instruction in breast self-examination (BSE), and the findings were recorded. While the participant remained in the examining room, the examiner went to receive the results of randomization from the centre coordinator, and then told the participant whether she would receive mammography screening. Subsequently, women randomized to screening in both trials were offered annual CBE and mammography (Miller et al., 1992a, b). Control women aged 40–49 years in the CNBSS 1 trial received a questionnaire every year. Control women aged 50–59 years in the CNBSS 2 trial were offered annual CBE.

Women were invited to volunteer to participate in the trials by several methods (Baines et al., 1989) and were recruited in 1980–1985. A total of 50 430 women aged 40–49 years were enrolled in the CNBSS 1 trial, and 39 405 women aged 50–59 years were enrolled in the CNBSS 2 trial. The distribution of breast cancer risk factors in the two groups in both trials was identical, confirming that balance was achieved by randomization (Miller et al., 1992a, b). The treatment administered to breast cancer cases in women aged 40–49 years in the CNBSS 1 trial was evaluated to be compatible with standards then applied in North America for adjuvant chemotherapy and hormone therapy (Kerr, 1991).

For women in the mammography group of the CNBSS 1 trial, full compliance with screening (mammography plus CBE) after the first screen (when compliance was 100% with CBE) varied from 89.4% (for the second screen) to 85.6% (for the fifth screen). In addition, a small proportion (1.7–2.9%) of the women accepted CBE but refused to undergo mammography. More than 90% of the participants in the control group (ranging from 93.3% to 94.9% in the various years) returned their annual questionnaire (Miller et al., 1992a). For women in the mammography group of the CNBSS 2 trial, full compliance with screening after the first screen varied from 90.4% (for the second screen) to 86.7% (for the fifth screen). In addition, a small proportion (1.8–3.2%) of the women accepted CBE but refused to undergo mammography. In the control group, compliance with annual CBE screening varied from 89.1% (for the second screen) to 85.4% (for the fifth screen); questionnaires only were obtained for 2.8–7.0% of the women (Miller et al., 1992b).

Boyd et al. (1993) criticized the process of randomization in the trials, but a systematic external review of the randomization records showed no evidence of subversion of randomization (Bailar & MacMahon, 1997). The mammography equipment used in these trials has also been criticized (Kopans, 1990, 1993, 2014; Moskowitz, 1992; Kopans & Feig, 1993; Tabár, 2014), and these criticisms have been addressed by the investigators (Miller et al., 1990, 2014a, b).

(f) Stockholm trial

A trial was performed in the south-eastern part of Greater Stockholm, Sweden, in which about 60 000 women aged 40–64 years in March 1981 were randomized by day of birth to invitation to mammography screening or to a control group (Frisell et al., 1986). Women born on days 1–10 and 21–31 of the month were invited to screening, and women born on days 11–20 constituted the control group. Attendance was 81% for the first round. In the review of Swedish trials by Nyström et al. (2002a), women born on day 31 were not included, and the totals analysed were 39 139 in the intervention group and 20 978 in the control group.

(g) Gothenburg trial

From December 1982 to April 1984, all women born in 1923–1944 and living in the city of Gothenburg, Sweden, were randomized to mammography screening or to a control group; of the 51 611 women, 25 941 were aged 39–49 years. Randomization was by cluster on the basis of date of birth for the cohorts born in 1929–1935 and by individual birth date for those born in 1936–1944 (Bjurstam et al., 1997). To enable rescreening of women every 18 months, with a limited capacity for mammography, the ratio of women randomized to the invited group and the control group was 1:1.2 in the age group 39–49 years and 1:1.6 in the age group 50–59 years. Attendance of invited women was 85% for the first round and 77% on average for subsequent rounds.

(h) United Kingdom Age trial

In 1991, a national, multicentre RCT was set up by the United Kingdom Coordinating Committee on Cancer Research (Moss, 1999). Women aged 39–41 years were randomized 1:2 to annual mammography screening for 7 years or to no screening, followed up without screening until they reached the age of 50 years, and then invited to participate in the United Kingdom National Health Service Breast Screening Programme of 3-yearly mammography. This is the only randomized screening trial that completely avoids “age creep” (the delayed benefits of screening for women randomized in their forties but diagnosed with breast cancer after their fiftieth birthday) (de Koning et al., 1995; Smith, 2000). The aim was to recruit 195 000 women, with 65 000 forming a study group and the remaining 130 000 a control group. However, recruitment was slower than anticipated, and a total of 160 921 women were randomized (Johns et al., 2010b). Attendance of women invited to routine screening was 68% for the first round and 69% for subsequent rounds. A total of 43 709 women in the intervention arm (81%) attended at least one routine screen, and 23 262 (43%) attended at least seven screens; 31 392 women attended 75% or more of all routine screens to which they were invited. To estimate the level of unscheduled screening in the control arm, Kingston et al. (2010) analysed data obtained from questionnaires sent to a random sample of 3706 women at five centres in the control arm of this trial, with a response rate of 58.8%. Overall, 24.9% of women surveyed reported having had a mammogram, but only about one third of the mammograms (8.4%) were for non-symptomatic reasons.

4.2.2 Beneficial effects

In this section, the data available from the randomized trials on breast cancer mortality, incidence of advanced breast cancer, and less-extensive therapy are summarized.

(a) Reduced breast cancer mortality

Of the 12 trials considered by the previous IARC Working Group on breast cancer screening (IARC, 2002), 11 had results on breast cancer mortality. The results from the United Kingdom Age trial were subsequently reported after 10 years of follow-up, and those for the CNBSS trials and the Two-County trial were subsequently updated.

For the Health Insurance Plan trial, the relative risk of death from breast cancer 18 years after recruitment was estimated by the previous IARC Working Group on breast cancer screening (IARC, 2002) from the data of Shapiro et al. (1988) to be 0.78 (95% confidence interval [CI], 0.61–1.00) overall.

In the Malmö I trial (women aged 45–70 years at randomization) with a follow-up of 19.2 years, the relative risk of death from breast cancer was 0.81 (95% CI, 0.66–1.00). In the Malmö II trial (women aged 43–49 years at randomization) after 9.1 years of follow-up, the corresponding relative risk was 0.65 (95% CI, 0.39–1.08) (Nyström et al., 2002a).

For the Two-County trial, after 29 years of follow-up, the relative risk of death from breast cancer among breast cancer cases diagnosed in the screening phase of both components of the trial (women aged 40–74 years at randomization) was 0.69 (95% CI, 0.56–0.84) according to data from the local end-point committee and 0.73 (95% CI, 0.59–0.89) according to consensus data from the overview committee appointed by the Swedish Cancer Society (Tabár et al., 2011).

For the Edinburgh trial, a report based on 14 years of follow-up and 577 518 person-years in the initial cohort (women aged 45–64 years at recruitment) showed a rate ratio for breast cancer mortality of 0.87 (95% CI, 0.70–1.06). After adjustment for socioeconomic status, the rate ratio was 0.79 (95% CI, 0.60–1.02) (Alexander et al., 1999).

For the CNBSS trials, after 20–24 years of follow-up, the breast cancer mortality hazard ratio based on the breast cancer cases ascertained in the 5-year screening period for both trials combined was 1.05 (95% CI, 0.85–1.30). The breast cancer mortality hazard ratio remained similar if the cancer accrual period was extended to 6 years (1.06; 95% CI, 0.87–1.29) or 7 years (1.07; 95% CI, 0.89–1.29) (Miller et al., 2014a).

In the Stockholm trial (women aged 40–64 years at assignment), the relative risk of death from breast cancer was 0.90 (95% CI, 0.63–1.28) after a median follow-up of 14.9 years. Although the possibility of double counting of controls in earlier analyses has been raised, in the most recent analysis reassurance was provided that there was no double counting (Nyström et al., 2002a).

In the Gothenburg trial (women aged 39–59 years at assignment), the overall relative risk of death from breast cancer was 0.79 (95% CI, 0.58–1.08) after a median follow-up of 14 years (Bjurstam et al., 2003).

In the United Kingdom Age trial (women aged 39–41 years at assignment), the ratio of breast cancer deaths in the study group relative to the control group was 0.83 (95% CI, 0.66–1.04) after a mean follow-up of 10.7 years (Moss et al., 2006).

(b) Age-specific effects of screening

The results from randomized trials that have published results related to mammography screening for women aged 40–49 years at entry are presented in Table 4.2. Relative risks of death from breast cancer ranged from 0.64 to 1.52, with a median of 0.76.

Limited data are available for the Health Insurance Plan trial, although Shapiro et al. (1988) noted that the benefit appeared to be restricted to women diagnosed with breast cancer after the age of 50 years, and took many years to appear.

Table 4.2 Age-specific results of randomized trials of the efficacy of mammography screening, with and without clinical breast examination – women aged 40–49 years

Trial, country References	Age (years) at enrolment/ screening	Mean duration of follow-up (years)	No. of women	Breast cancer mortality per 100 000 person-years (no. of breast cancer deaths) in screened/control group	RR	95% CI
Health Insurance Plan trial, USA Shapiro et al. (1988), IARC (2002)	40–49/40–54	18	NR	(49)/(65)	0.77	0.52–1.13
Malmö I and II trials, Sweden Andersson & Janzon (1997)	45–49/45–69	15.5 (Malmö I) 10 (Malmö II)	25 770	34 (57)/54 (78)	0.64	0.45–0.89
Malmö II trial, Sweden Nyström et al. (2002a)	43–49/43–57	9.1 (Malmö II)	17 793	26 (29)/38 (33)	0.65	0.39–1.08
Two-County trial: Östergötland County, Sweden Nyström et al. (2002a)	40–49/40–54	17.4	20 744	18 (31)/17 (30)	1.05	0.64–1.71
Two-County trial: Kopparberg County, Sweden Tabár et al. (2000)	40–49/40–54	20	NR	NR	0.76	0.42–1.40
Edinburgh trial, United Kingdom Alexander et al. (1999)	45–49/45–56	14	21 746	34 (47)/42 (53)	0.75	0.48–1.18
CNBSS 1 trial, Canada Miller et al. (2014a)	40–49/40–54	22	50 430	NR	1.09	0.80–1.49
Stockholm trial, Sweden Nyström et al. (2002a)	40–49/40–54	14.9	22 324	17 (34)/11 (13)	1.52	0.80–2.88
Gothenburg trial, Sweden Bjurstam et al. (2003)	39–49/39–55	14	25 941	(25)/(46)	0.65	0.40–1.05
United Kingdom Age trial Moss et al. (2006)	39–41/39–48	10.7	160 921	18 (105)/22 (251)	0.83	0.66–1.04

CI, confidence interval; CNBSS, Canadian National Breast Screening Study; NR, not reported; RR, relative risk.
From IARC (2002).

For the Malmö trials, Andersson & Janzon (1997) combined the data from the Malmö I and Malmö II trials, with a relative risk of death from breast cancer of 0.64 (95% CI, 0.45–0.89). This is the only relative risk presented in Table 4.2 where the upper 95% confidence limit is less than 1.0. In the Malmö I trial, the cumulative mortality curves did not begin to separate until after 5 years of follow-up, but in the Malmö II trial, separation began after the first year. For the Malmö II trial, Nyström et al. (2002a) presented age-adjusted data for women aged 43–49 years.

For the Two-County trial, updated data by age have not been reported for women aged 40–49 years or for women aged 50 years and older, but have been reported by separate segments of the age ranges in different publications. Table 4.2 presents the results from the Swedish overview analysis, where the findings only from Östergötland County were reported

Table 4.3 Age-specific results of randomized trials of the efficacy of mammography screening, with and without clinical breast examination – women aged 50 years and older

Trial, country References	Age (years) at enrolment/ screening	Mean duration of follow-up (years)	No. of women	Breast cancer mortality per 100 000 person-years (no. of breast cancer deaths) in screened/ control group	RR	95% CI
Health Insurance Plan trial, USA Shapiro et al. (1988), IARC (2002)	50–64/50–69	18	NR	(77)/(98)	0.79	0.58–1.08
Malmö I trial, Sweden Andersson et al. (1988)	55–69/55–79	8.8	26 210	(35)/(44)	0.79	0.51–1.24
Two-County trial: Östergötland County, Sweden Nyström et al. (2002a)	50–59/50–64 60–69/60–74	17.4	23 506	27 (53)/29 (54)	0.94 0.72	0.66–1.35 0.52–1.00
Two-County trial: Kopparberg County, Sweden Tabár et al. (2000)	50–59/50–64 60–69/60–74 70–74/70–78	20	22 435	39 (64)/54 (83)	0.46 0.58 0.76	0.30–0.71 0.39–0.87 0.44–1.33
Edinburgh trial, United Kingdom Alexander et al. (1999)	50–54/50–61 55–59/55–66 60–64/60–71	14	11 046 11 858 9 993	56 (44)/52 (35) 55 (43)/76 (55) 67 (42)/76 (44)	0.99 0.65 0.80	0.62–1.58 0.43–0.99 0.51–1.25
CNBSS 2 trial, Canada Miller et al. (2014a)	50–59/50–64	22	39 405		1.02	0.77–1.36
Stockholm trial, Sweden, Nyström et al. (2002a)	50–59/50–64 55–64/55–69	14.9	24 367 26 347	12 (25)/20 (24) 17 (39)/23 (28)	0.56 0.75	0.32–0.97 0.46–1.21
Gothenburg trial, Sweden Bjurstam et al. (2003)	50–59/50–61	14	25 670	(38)/(66)	0.91	0.61–1.36

CI, confidence interval; CNBSS, Canadian National Breast Screening Study; NR, not reported; RR, relative risk.

(Nyström et al., 2002a), with a relative risk of 1.05 (95% CI, 0.64–1.71). In the report by Tabár et al. (2000), the relative risk of death from breast cancer in Kopparberg County was 0.76 (95% CI, 0.42–1.40) for women aged 40–49 years.

Relative risks of less than 1.0 were reported from the Edinburgh trial and the Gothenburg trial for women aged 45–49 years and 39–49 years at entry, respectively; relative risks of more than 1.0 were reported from the CNBSS 1 trial and the Stockholm trial for women aged 40–49 years at entry.

Although analyses are based on women aged 40–49 years at entry into the trials, screening after age 49 years could have influenced the estimated relative risks of breast cancer mortality, so-called "age creep" (de Koning et al., 1995; Smith, 2000). Only the United Kingdom Age trial (Moss, 1999) was designed to overcome this. As stated above, in this trial of women aged 39–41 years at assignment, the ratio of breast cancer deaths in the study group relative to the control group was 0.83 (95% CI, 0.66–1.04) after a mean follow-up of 10.7 years (Moss et al., 2006).

Table 4.3 summarizes the available data on the efficacy of mammography screening for women aged 50 years and older at entry. For the Malmö I trial, data were available only for women aged 55–69 years at entry. For many trials, data are available only for 10-year age groups. Partly because of this age separation, many of the relative risks presented show upper 95% confidence limits of more than 1.0. However, the upper 95% confidence limit was less than 1.0 for women aged 50–59 years and for those aged 60–69 years in Kopparberg County, for women aged 55–59 years in the Edinburgh trial, and for women aged 50–59 years in the Stockholm trial.

In a model-based analysis, Rijnsburger et al. (2004) evaluated whether the lack of benefit from mammography in the CNBSS 2 trial could have been due to a beneficial effect of the CBE performed in both arms for women aged 50–59 years. Using data derived from the CNBSS 2 trial, the Netherlands breast screening programme, and the Two-County trial, it was estimated that a mortality reduction of more than 20% could have been derived from the CBE if compared with a no-screening arm.

The only trial to enrol women aged 70–74 years was the Kopparberg component of the Two-County trial (Tabár et al., 1992). The participation rate of this group was poor, and only two screens were offered. At 15 years after randomization, the relative risk of death from breast cancer in the screened group compared with the control group was 0.79 (95% CI, 0.51–1.22) (Tabár et al., 1995). At 20 years after randomization, the relative risk of death from breast cancer in Kopparberg County was 0.76 (95% CI, 0.44–1.33) (Tabár et al., 2000).

(c) *Meta-analyses of results of randomized trials of mammography screening*

The previous IARC Working Group on breast cancer screening (IARC, 2002) reported the results of its own meta-analysis of the trials, including those using mammography alone compared with no screening as well as all valid trials in women aged 40–49 years. The results are summarized in Table 4.4, together with the results of subsequent meta-analyses. [None of these meta-analyses included the updated results of the Two-County trial or of the CNBSS trials.]

(d) *Reduced incidence of advanced breast cancer*

Most investigators consider that advanced breast cancer should be defined as extensive local involvement or metastatic disease, although the exact definition by stage will vary according to the level of detail recorded. In the randomized screening trials, this level of detail was rarely captured. The available data as reported by the authors of the various trials are presented in Table 4.5.

For the Health Insurance Plan trial, Shapiro (1977) reported that of 299 breast cancers in the study arm detected within 5 years of entry, 102 (34%) were node-positive (for 27, the nodal status was unknown) compared with 121 of 285 (42%) in the control arm (34 of unknown status).

For the Malmö I trial, Andersson et al. (1988) reported that, after an excess of stage II–IV breast cancers ascertained during the first screen, the numbers of breast cancers at these stages gradually became greater in the control group, resulting at 10 years in a cumulative rate per 100 000 person–years of 980 in the study group and 1210 in the control group [relative risk (RR), 0.81]. Most of the excess in the control group was from stage II cancers. There were 26 stage III and 22 stage IV breast cancers ascertained in the study group, and 27 stage III and 32 stage IV breast cancers in the control group (Andersson et al., 1988). No similar data have been reported for the Malmö II trial.

For the Two-County trial, Tabár et al. (1992) estimated the cumulative incidence of breast cancers of stage II or higher during the first 10 years of follow-up. There was an excess incidence in the ASP at year 1, which disappeared by year 3. Subsequently, the rate increased much more slowly in the ASP than in the PSP. At 10 years, the rate per 1000 person–years was just more than 10 in the PSP and less than 8 in the

Table 4.4 Meta-analyses of randomized controlled trials of the efficacy of mammography screening

Reference	Screen[a]	Age at entry (years)	No. of trials[b]	Population (thousands)		Breast cancer deaths		RR	95% CI
				Screened	Control	Screened	Control		
IARC (2002)[c]	M alone	40–49	6	58.6	49.1	166	173	0.81	0.65–1.01
	All	40–49	8					0.88	0.74–1.04
	M alone	50–69	6	188.5	147.8	496	549	0.75	0.67–0.85
Nelson et al. (2009)	All	39–49	8	152.3	195.9	448	625	0.85	0.75–0.96
		50–59	6					0.86	0.75–0.99
		60–69	2					0.68	0.54–0.87
		70–74	1					1.12	0.73–1.72
Canadian Task Force on Preventive Health Care (2011)	All	40–49	8	152.3	195.9	448	625	0.85	0.75–0.96
		50–69	7	135.1	115.2	639	743	0.79	0.68–0.90
		70–74	2	10.3	7.3	49	50	0.68	0.45–1.01
Magnus et al. (2011)[d]	All	39–49	7	144.6	191.6	427	615	0.83	0.72–0.97
Gøtzsche & Jørgensen (2013)	All	39–49	8	142.9	186.6	385	567	0.84	0.73–0.96
		≥ 50	7	146.3	122.6	599	701	0.77	0.69–0.86
Marmot et al. (2013)	All	40–74	9					0.80	0.73–0.89

[a] "All" indicates trials with mammography with or without CBE screening.
[b] The Two-County trial is regarded as two trials: Kopparberg County and Östergötland County.
[c] Excluded the Edinburgh trial.
[d] Included the Edinburgh trial but excluded Kopparberg County and Östergötland County.
CBE, clinical breast examination; CI, confidence interval; M, mammography; RR, relative risk.

ASP [rates approximated from Fig. 4 of Tabár et al. (1992)]. Tabár et al. (1995) reported that the cumulative incidence rate of lymph node-positive breast cancers together with those with distant metastases for women aged 40–49 years at 14 years of follow-up was 28.0 per 100 000 in the ASP and 32.8 per 100 000 in the PSP; the corresponding rates per 100 000 for women aged 50–74 years were 45.1 in the ASP and 64.4 in the PSP.

For the Edinburgh trial, Alexander et al. (1994) reported that of 489 breast cancers ascertained in the study group, 189 (39%) were of stage II (21 mm or larger), III, or IV (10 were of unknown stage), compared with 221 of 400 (55%) in the control group (7 of unknown stage).

For the CNBSS trials, no data have been reported on the incidence of advanced breast cancers, but data were reported on the nodal status of the majority of the breast cancers detected during the screening period, and for an average of 8.5 years of follow-up from enrolment (Miller et al., 1992a, b), and subsequently on tumour size (Miller et al., 2000, 2002). For the CNBSS 1 trial, the total of node-positive breast cancers in the mammography arm was 81 of 245 (33%) with known nodal status (for 33, the nodal status was unknown). The corresponding numbers were 59 of 203 (29%) for the control arm (45 of unknown nodal status) (Miller et al., 1992a). For the CNBSS 2 trial, the corresponding numbers were 83 of 281 (30%) in the mammography arm (47 of unknown nodal status) and 64 of 200 (32%) in the control arm (38 of unknown nodal status) (Miller et al., 1992b).

For the Stockholm trial, data were reported on breast cancers of stage II or higher. There was a cumulative incidence of 4.27 per 1000 in the intervention arm compared with 4.86 per 1000

Table 4.5 Incidence of advanced breast cancer in randomized trials of breast cancer screening

Trial, country[a]	Definition of advanced breast cancer	No. of patients with advanced breast cancer		Cumulative incidence of advanced breast cancer (‰)		RR	95% CI
		Intervention	Control	Intervention	Control		
Health Insurance Plan trial, USA	Stage II or higher	160	188	5.29	6.21	0.85	0.69–1.05
Malmö I trial, Sweden	Stage II or higher	190	231	9.01	10.90	0.83	0.68–1.00
Two-County trial, Sweden	Stage II or higher	524	555	6.80	9.91	0.69	0.61–0.78
CNBSS 1 trial, Canada	Size ≥ 20 mm	111	115	4.40	4.56	0.97	0.74–1.25
CNBSS 2 trial, Canada	Size ≥ 20 mm	114	136	5.78	6.91	0.84	0.65–1.07
Stockholm trial, Sweden	Stage II or higher	172	97	4.27	4.86	0.88	0.68–1.12
Gothenburg trial, Sweden	One or more nodes involved	85	144	3.93	4.81	0.80	0.61–1.05
United Kingdom Age trial	Size ≥ 20 mm	171	386	3.17	3.61	0.88	0.73–1.05

[a] Follow-up periods may differ between trials.
CI, confidence interval; CNBSS, Canadian National Breast Screening Study; RR, relative risk.
Adapted from Autier et al. (2009).

in the control arm, for a relative risk of 0.88 (95% CI, 0.68–1.12) (Table 4.5).

In the Gothenburg trial, the incidence of lymph node-positive breast cancers in the study group was 0.65 per 1000, compared with 0.81 per 1000 in the control group, for a relative risk of 0.80 (95% CI, 0.61–1.05). For women aged 50–59 years, the relative risk was 1.02 (95% CI, 0.70–1.48) (Bjurstam et al., 2003).

In the United Kingdom Age trial, which defined advanced breast cancers as those of 20 mm or larger, the cumulative incidence rate per 1000 was 3.17 in the intervention arm and 3.61 in the control arm, for a relative risk of 0.88 (95% CI, 0.73–1.05) (Moss et al., 2005a) (Table 4.5).

Based on the available data from randomized controlled trials, an association has been observed between the risk of advanced breast cancer and breast cancer mortality (Autier et al., 2009; Tabár et al., 2015a, b; Fig. 4.2).

(e) More-conservative surgery

The extent of use of breast-conserving surgery was reported for the Malmö I trial, although data were missing from some control subjects with stage 0 disease (Andersson et al., 1988). Overall, of 575 women with breast cancer ascertained in the study group, 137 (24%) received breast-conserving surgery, compared with 80 (18%) of 436 in the control group.

Gøtzsche & Jørgensen (2013), in a Cochrane review, reported that the risk ratio for mastectomies in the screened versus unscreened groups based on 5 trials was 1.20 (95% CI, 1.11–1.30) and for lumpectomies and mastectomies combined was 1.35 (95% CI, 1.26–1.44), thus suggesting that screening in the trials did not result in more-conservative surgery. [The Working Group noted that the sources of the data from which these estimates were made are unclear.]

Fig. 4.2 Plot of data from randomized controlled trials, showing the association between the logarithm of relative risk (RR) of advanced breast cancer and of disease-specific mortality, with meta-regression line

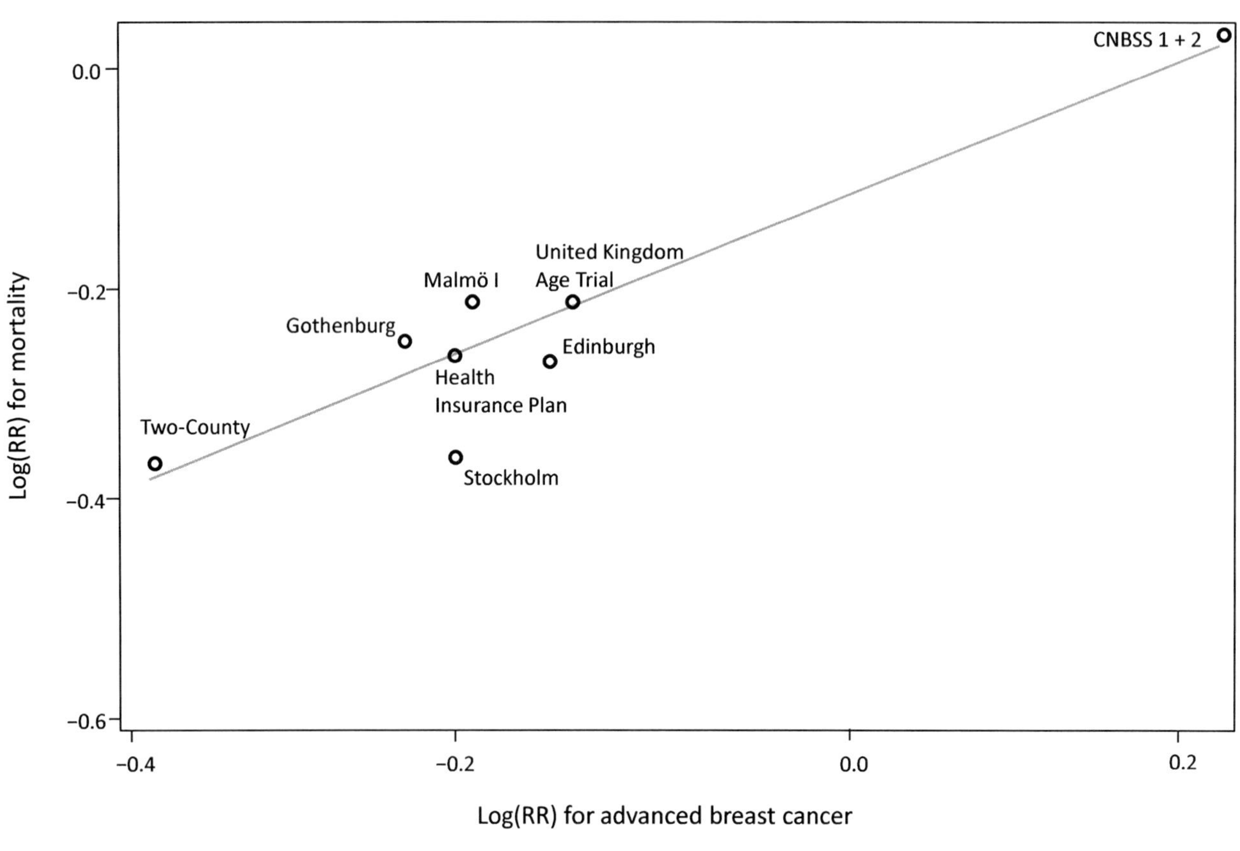

From Tabár et al. (2015a).
CNBSS, Canadian National Breast Screening Study.

4.2.3 Performance indicators

For consistency with Section 5.1 on indicators for monitoring effectiveness of screening, the data available on false-positive mammograms and interval cancers are summarized here, as process indicators of performance in these trials.

(a) False-positive mammograms

For the Malmö trials, Andersson & Janzon (1997) reported that in women younger than 50 years, further examination of false-positives was required in 1260 per 100 000 person–years; the rate of surgery for benign disease was 56 per 100 000 person–years, and the rate of treatment of clinically insignificant cancer was 10 per 100 000 person–years. No data on false-positives were reported for older women.

For the Two-County trial, the rate of recall for assessment for those not found to have breast cancer was 44 per 1000 at the first screen and 22 per 1000 at subsequent screens; the rate of biopsy for benign conditions was 6 per 1000 at the first screen and 1 per 1000 at subsequent screens (Tabár et al., 1992).

In the CNBSS trials, with screening by both mammography and CBE, it is not possible to fully distinguish the contribution of mammography to false-positive detections. As a result of the referrals by the study surgeon, the overall rates of surgical intervention after the first screen were 64 per 1000 in the mammography group and 37 per 1000 in the control group in the CNBSS 1 trial (Miller et al., 1992a) and 58 per 1000 in the mammography group and 25 per 1000 in the control group in the CNBSS 2 trial (Miller et al., 1992b). After subsequent screens, the rates were approximately one half of those after the first screen. These procedures resulted after the first screen in overall rates of biopsy detection of benign lesions of 33.6 per 1000 in the mammography group and 11.5 per 1000 in the control group in the CNBSS 1 trial (Miller et al., 1992a) and 34.8 per 1000 in the mammography group and 8.7 per 1000 in the control group in the CNBSS 2 trial (Miller et al., 1992b). After subsequent screens, the rates of biopsy with detection of benign breast lesions were approximately one third of those after the first screen (Miller et al., 1992a, b).

For the Stockholm trial, Frisell & Lidbrink (1997) reported that the recall rate was 0.8% for all subjects and 1.0% for those in the age group 40–49 years. With only two screening rounds, the rate of false-positives was 242 per 100 000 person–years in women older than 50 years compared with 355 per 100 000 in those younger than 50 years. The rate of benign surgical biopsies in the second round was 21 per 100 000 in women older than 50 years and 49 per 100 000 in those younger than 50 years. In women aged 40–49 years, 1 out of 2.5 surgical biopsies was benign, compared with 1 out of 7 in those older than 50 years.

For the Gothenburg trial, Bjurstam et al. (2003) reported that 5.9% of the participants in the study group were recalled for supplemental mammography at the first screen, and 2.6% at subsequent screens. The percentages of women who had clinical examination and fine-needle aspiration cytology who were not found to have cancer were 1.5% at the first screen and 0.7% at subsequent screens; the corresponding percentages for surgery were 0.3% and 0.1%, respectively.

For the United Kingdom Age trial, Johns et al. (2010a) reported that 14.6% of women in the intervention arm and 18.1% of women attending at least one routine screen experienced one or more false-positive screens during the trial.

(b) Interval cancers

In the Malmö I trial, 100 (17%) breast cancers were detected in the 2-year interval before the next screen was due, out of 581 breast cancers ascertained in the study group (Andersson et al., 1988). Corresponding data have not been reported from the Malmö II trial.

For the Two-County trial, Tabár et al. (1992) reported the incidence of interval cancers as a percentage of the incidence in the control group by age. Over all intervals between screens, the percentage for women aged 40–49 years was 45% in the first year and 62% in the second; the percentages over the 3-year intervals were 17%, 34%, and 63%, respectively, for women aged 50–59 years, 17%, 27%, and 46%, respectively, for those aged 60–69 years, and 8%, 44%, and 48%, respectively, for those aged 70–74 years.

In the CNBSS 1 trial, the rate of interval cancers after the first screen was 0.75 per 1000 in the mammography group and 1.11 per 1000 in the control group. For the second, third, fourth, and fifth screens in the mammography group, the rates were 0.71, 0.36, 0.46, and 0.64 per 1000, respectively (Miller et al., 1992a). In the CNBSS 2 trial, data on interval cancer rates were available for both the mammography group and the control group after all five screens. The rates per 1000 in the mammography group and the control group, respectively, were 0.76 and 0.81 after the first screen, 0.57 and 0.92 after the second screen, 0.46 and 1.52 after the third screen, 0.52 and 0.95 after the fourth screen, and 0.51 and 1.64 after the fifth screen (Miller et al., 1992b).

For the Stockholm trial, Frisell et al. (1986) reported that 60 interval cancers (6 in situ) occurred in the 24 months between the two screens (1.8 per 1000 examinations), and 38 of the cases occurred in the second year. A review of the original mammograms found no indication of an abnormality in 31 cases (2 in situ); 45% of them were in women aged 40–49 years, and only 8 occurred in the first year.

For the Gothenburg trial, Bjurstam et al. (2003) reported that 52 [24%] invasive interval cancers occurred of the total of 220 invasive cancers ascertained in attenders. There were an additional 2 in situ interval cancers of 36 ascertained in attenders. The proportion of invasive interval cancers decreased with increasing age, from 36% at ages 39–44 years to 31% at 45–49 years, 16% at 50–54 years, and 15% at 50–59 years [percentages calculated by the Working Group]. The two in situ interval cancers were ascertained in women younger than 50 years.

In the United Kingdom Age trial, there were 125 (26%) interval cancers and 229 (48%) screen-detected cancers of the total of 482 breast cancers ascertained (Moss et al., 2005b). However, of the total, 9 breast cancers were diagnosed between randomization and invitation, and 61 breast cancers occurred in never-attenders, 44 in lapsed attenders, and 14 in women lost to screening. If these are excluded from the denominator, the percentages become 35% and 65%, respectively.

(c) Overdiagnosis of breast cancer

(i) Definition

Overdiagnosis of breast cancer is detection by screening of a breast cancer (DCIS or invasive carcinoma) that would never have presented clinically during the woman's lifetime if it had not been detected by screening. Overdiagnosis is invariably associated with the use of any method that is able to effectively bring forward the date of diagnosis. The probability that a tumour represents an overdiagnosis versus a timely diagnosis is determined by two components: the speed of growth, which determines the time the tumour would have required to present clinically, and the remaining lifespan of a patient, which depends on the patient's age at diagnosis and other competing causes of death. Overdiagnosis is an important harm caused by screening because of the otherwise unnecessary investigation, treatment, and psychosocial consequences that a diagnosis of cancer entails. Overdiagnosed cases cannot be identified individually, but, based on the above-mentioned components, the majority of overdiagnoses represent slower-growing, lower-grade cancers, both in situ and invasive.

(ii) Counting overdiagnosed cancers

Conceptually, overdiagnosed cancers can be counted as the difference between the numbers of breast cancer cases, including in situ and invasive, accumulated in screened and unscreened cohorts from the beginning of screening in the screened cohort until the end of the compensatory drop in incidence that occurs after screening has ended (i.e. when the lead time of all breast cancer cases diagnosed as a result of screening has elapsed) (Puliti et al., 2011). In principle, randomized screening trials, in which there is a clearly defined end to trial screening and a period of follow-up for new incident cases in both screened and unscreened women beyond the end of the compensatory drop, provide the best estimates of overdiagnosis under the assumption that there is no further screening outside of the trial, or at least that the accrual of diagnosed breast cancers outside of the trial is approximately the same in the two arms (Moss, 2005; Biesheuvel et al., 2007; Independent UK Panel on Breast Cancer Screening, 2012; Marmot et al., 2013). However, this requirement is rarely, if ever, met, or known with any certainty to have been met, by any trial. The time interval that should be allowed for the compensatory drop is uncertain. Information on the timing of the compensatory drop is available from established screening programmes (de Gelder et al., 2011). For a randomized screening trial in which two cohorts of women are recruited, screened or not screened for a period, and followed up for a period, Duffy & Parmar (2013) depicted in Fig. 1 of their article that excess cancers due to lead time accumulate for 10 years, this excess remains constant for as long as screening lasts, and then the excess dissipates over 10 years. Therefore, given the assumptions of Duffy & Parmar (2013) as to median lead time and its distribution, 10 years after screening has ended seems a suitable point at which to attribute any remaining excess to overdiagnosis.

(iii) Estimating the proportion of incident cancers that are overdiagnosed

The Independent United Kingdom Panel on Breast Cancer Screening (Marmot et al., 2013), following earlier work by de Gelder et al. (2011), defined four measures of the overdiagnosis rate based on data from randomized screening trials. In each, the numerator was a count of overdiagnosed cancers. The four denominators were: (A) breast cancers diagnosed over the whole follow-up period in unscreened women (where the follow-up period extends from the beginning of screening in the screened women until the end of follow-up in both screened and unscreened women); (B) breast cancers diagnosed over the whole follow-up period in women invited to screening; (C) breast cancers diagnosed during the screening period in women invited to screening; and (D) breast cancers detected by screening in women invited to screening. The United Kingdom Panel preferred denominators (B), as representing the population perspective, and (C), as representing the perspective of a woman invited to screening.

(iv) Estimates of overdiagnosis rates from the trials

For the Health Insurance Plan trial, cumulative in situ and invasive breast cancer incidence rates at 10 years after the beginning of the trial (~6 years after the end of the trial) were reported as 2.11 per 1000 in women offered screening and 2.09 per 1000 in control women (Table 1 in Shapiro, 1997), from which an overdiagnosis rate of 1% can be estimated, as a proportion of breast cancers diagnosed in unscreened women over the whole follow-up period. The excess number of incident invasive breast cancers at 10 years was 0 (Table 5.1 in Shapiro et al., 1988). However, the year-by-year data on invasive breast cancer do not show a decrease in incident breast cancers in screened women from years 1–4 (screening) to years 5–10 (after screening); the average annual numbers were 62 and 61, respectively. Instead, there was an increase in incident cases in the control group; the corresponding annual average numbers were 55 and 66, respectively. [Therefore, there may have been a period of "catch-up" screening in the control group after trial screening ended, which would bias the estimate of overdiagnosis from the Health Insurance Plan trial downwards.]

In updating results from the Malmö I trial, Zackrisson et al. (2006) reported incidence data separately for women aged 45–54 years and those aged 55–69 years at entry. However, conclusions on overdiagnosis could be drawn only for women aged 55–69 years, whose controls were never screened, in contrast to women aged 45–54 years, whose controls were offered screening after the end of the screening period. In women aged 55–69 years at entry, the relative risk of in situ and invasive breast cancer was 1.10 (95% CI, 0.99–1.22) and the relative risk of invasive breast cancer was only 1.07 (95% CI, 0.96–1.18). Thus, 15 years after the trial ended the rate of overdiagnosis of breast cancer was 10% in women randomized to screening at age 55–69 years compared with an unscreened control group. Njor et al. (2013) questioned the validity of this estimate on several grounds. They argued that older screened women would not have been followed up long enough for the whole of the compensatory drop to have occurred, with resulting upward bias in the overdiagnosis estimate. In addition, since mammography screening was available outside of the screening trial for the whole period, women in the screening arm would have continued to participate in screening after the end of the trial, which would also have biased the overdiagnosis estimate upwards. They presented data [percentages calculated by the Working Group from data in Table 1 in Njor et al. (2013)] showing that 20% of cancers diagnosed in all screened women (34% of cancers in the youngest women) in the 10 years after trial screening ended were asymptomatic, i.e. probably screen-detected. [The Working Group considered both the overdiagnosis estimates of Zackrisson et al. (2006) and the updated estimates of Njor et al. (2013) difficult to interpret.]

At the end of the Two-County trial, in 1985, cumulative in situ and invasive breast cancer incidence rates were 18.50 per 1000 in women offered screening and 18.61 per 1000 in control women, and the excess breast cancer incidence in screened women relative to that in control women was −0.06% (Duffy et al., 2003b). [The numbers of breast cancers contributing to these rates are stated elsewhere to have been those at the end of 1992 (Tabár et al., 1995).] In 2012, cumulative breast cancer incidence numbers every 5 years from the start of the trial until 29 years later were published for the Dalarna (formerly Kopparberg) County component of the trial (Yen et al., 2012). Screening of the control group began after an average of three screens of women in the screened group, 6–8 years after the start. The relative cumulative risk of breast cancer in the screened group was 1.34 (95% CI, 1.13–1.59) at 5 years after the start, 1.03 (95% CI, 0.91–1.16) at 10 years, 1.04 (95% CI, 0.94–1.15) at 15 years, 1.06 (95% CI, 0.97–1.16) at 20 years, 1.02 (95% CI, 0.94–1.11) at 25 years, and 1.00 (95% CI, 0.92–1.08) at 29 years. The authors concluded that "there was no overdiagnosis associated with the additional 3 screens of the [screened group] in the first 8 years of observation." [Because screening of the control group began after the end of scheduled screening in the screened group and continued in that group also, it is not possible to make an estimate of the extent of overdiagnosis caused by the screens in this trial.]

Incidence data from the Edinburgh trial have been reported to 10 years, 3 years beyond the end of the intervention period (Alexander et al., 1994, 1999). Organized service screening began in Scotland in 1988; women in the screening arm of the trial received their first invitation to service screening about 3 years after their last trial screen (year 7). Although it is not stated, it is assumed that women in the control arm could have begun service screening in 1988 if they were then aged 50–64 years, the target age group for service screening. Cumulative in situ and invasive breast cancer incidence rates to 10 years were 22.4 per 10 000 in women randomized to screening and 20.0 per 10 000 in control women (Alexander et al., 1994), from which an overdiagnosis rate of 12% can be estimated, as a proportion of cancers diagnosed in unscreened women over the whole follow-up period. There were 57% fewer incident breast cancers in screened women than in control women during the 3 years of post-screening follow-up, consistent with a substantial compensatory drop (Alexander et al., 1994). [It is doubtful whether 3 years after the end of screening in the trial would have been sufficient for the compensatory drop to have been completed.]

For the CNBSS trials, initiated in 1980, the period of screening was the first 5 years after randomization, and the follow-up period was 20–25 years after randomization (Miller et al., 2014a). Screening was provided in the intervention groups for four or five annual screening rounds. The subsequent history of screening in the intervention and control groups after the end of trial screening was not reported. In the first 5 years, the cumulative incidence of invasive breast cancer in the group offered mammography relative to that in the control group was 1.27 (95% CI, 1.13–1.42), with an excess of cancers in the screened group of 142. After 10 years of follow-up, it was 1.09 (95% CI, 1.01–1.18), and after 25 years it was 1.04 (95% CI, 0.99–1.08) [relative risks and confidence intervals estimated from data in Table 1 in Miller et al. (2014a)]. The excess of breast cancer in the group offered mammography became constant at 106 cancers 15 years after enrolment (i.e. 10 years after the end of screening). This excess was 22% of all screen-detected invasive cancers in the trial (484). Miller (2014) reported that if in situ cancers are included in these estimates, the proportion of screen-detected cancers that were overdiagnosed increases to 35%. [There is a potential contribution of CBE to overdiagnosis in the CNBSS 2 trial, which has not been assessed. Women in both arms of the trial could have joined service mammography screening between 1988 and 1998, when organized screening services were rolled out across Canada, and opportunistic screening could also have occurred. Therefore, the excess cancers in the intervention arm may not be attributable exclusively to the screen-detection in the trials. Correspondingly, accrual of cases in the control arm may also have been inflated by screening. The resulting potential for bias makes the overdiagnosis estimate from the CNBSS trials difficult to interpret.]

The Stockholm trial offered two rounds of mammography screening at an interval of about 2.5 years to 40 318 women, beginning in 1981 and ending in 1985. In 1986, one round of screening was offered to the 19 343 control women, and recording of incident breast cancers in both groups ceased at the end of 1986. At the end of 1985, 371 cancers, both in situ and invasive, had been diagnosed in women randomized to screening, and 257 in control women (adjusted to the size of the population randomized to screening; Frisell et al., 1991), a 44% excess of breast cancer in screened women relative to that in control women. At the end of 1986, 428 cancers had accumulated in women offered screening, and 217 in control women (Frisell et al., 1997) (439 when adjusted as described above; Frisell et al., 1991). [Lack of follow-up for incident breast cancers after the end of the trial period prevents any estimate of overdiagnosis from the Stockholm trial.]

At the end of the Gothenburg trial, both groups were invited to service screening. Incidence of breast cancer (DCIS and invasive) was ascertained until the end of 1996, about 8 years after the end of the trial, and also at the end of the screening phase, which included the first service screening round for control women aged 50–69 years. There was a clear excess of breast cancers 4 years after the start of the trial in women randomized to screening (Fig. 2 in Bjurstam et al., 2003), but there was no excess at the end of the screening phase (excess over control group, −6.0%) or at the end of follow-up, 8 years after the end of the trial (−6.6%, invasive cancer only) [estimates based on data in Table 1 and text in Bjurstam et al. (2003)]. [No explanation has been offered by the authors for this paradoxically lower incidence of breast cancer in the control group than in the screened group.]

(d) Frequency of mammography screening

Only one trial provided informative data about the effects of varying screening frequency. The effect of annual versus 3-yearly mammography screening in increasing the likelihood of an improved outcome was tested in one trial (Breast Screening Frequency Trial Group, 2002). The measured outcomes included tumour size, nodal status, and histological grade of invasive tumours. These data were incorporated into two models to predict breast cancer mortality. Although the tumours diagnosed in women in the study arm were significantly smaller than those in women in the control arm, there was no difference in terms of nodal status or histological grade. The relative risks of predicted deaths from breast cancer for annual versus 3-yearly screening were 0.95 (95% CI, 0.83–1.07) and 0.89 (95% CI, 0.77–1.03) in the two models.

In most of the randomized screening trials, a 1–2-year screening interval was used. In the Two-County trial, a 24-month interval was used for women aged 40–49 years and a 33-month interval for those aged 50–74 years. [Given the different designs of these trials, it is not possible to derive estimates of the comparative efficacy of screening by different intervals by comparing their results.]

(e) Digital mammography

No trials of digital mammography with breast cancer mortality as the end-point have so far been reported. Trials that had breast cancer detection as the end-point are discussed in Section 2.1.3.

4.3 Clinical breast examination

4.3.1 Randomized clinical trials

Comparisons of the efficacy of CBE versus no screening come from three randomized studies (Pisani et al., 2006; Mittra et al., 2010; Sankaranarayanan et al., 2011). One of them closed after the first round of intervention, due to poor compliance (Pisani et al., 2006), and the other two have not yet reported their results on breast cancer mortality (Mittra et al., 2010; Sankaranarayanan et al., 2011).

(a) CBE versus no screening

See Table 4.6.

(i) Mumbai study

The Mumbai study (Mittra et al., 2010) is a cluster RCT that was initiated in 1998 by investigators from the Tata Memorial Hospital, Mumbai, India. Approximately 150 000 women underwent CBE at 24-month intervals, followed by 8 years of active monitoring for breast cancer incidence and mortality in the screening arm and one round of health education at entry, followed by active monitoring for self-reported cases and deaths from breast cancer in the control arm. The screening positivity rates for CBE were 0.46%, 0.77%, and 0.94% for the first, second, and third rounds of screening, respectively. Compliance rates for diagnostic confirmation ranged from 68% for the first round to 78% for the third round. Cancers were confirmed by histology in about 0.04% of women who underwent CBE. The mean age at detection was 49.8 years for both the screen-detected breast cancer cases and women in the control group.

During the corresponding period, in the control arm, there were 18 symptomatic referrals with 3 histologically confirmed cases at the first round, 61 symptomatic referrals with 39 histologically confirmed cases at the second round, and 76 symptomatic referrals with 45 histologically confirmed cases at the third round. Cohen's kappa for the agreement rates for CBE between the expert and the primary health workers was 0.849. In the screening arm, during the first, second, and third screening rounds, respectively, 21, 15, and 12 breast cancers were detected at early stages (stages 0, I, and II), 9, 7, and 9 cases were detected at advanced stages (stages III and IV), and for 2, 2, and 4 cases, staging information was unavailable. In the screening arm overall, [62.4% (78/125)] cancers were diagnosed at early stages and [25.6% (32/125)] at advanced stages, whereas in the control arm, [43.7%] were diagnosed at early stages and [42.5%] at advanced stages. The shift to a lower stage in the screening arm compared with the control arm was statistically significant (P = 0.0082; RR, 1.45; 95% CI, 1.09–1.93) (Table 4.6). The results on breast cancer mortality are awaited.

(ii) Trivandrum study

The Trivandrum cluster randomized study (Sankaranarayanan et al., 2011) began in 2006 in the Trivandrum District of Kerala, India, to evaluate whether three rounds of 3-yearly CBE would reduce advanced disease incidence rates and breast cancer mortality rates. A total of 115 652 healthy women aged 30–69 years in 275 electoral

Table 4.6 Randomized controlled studies of clinical breast examination: performance characteristics and tumour detection

Study Reference	Age range	Performance		Cancers in screening arm[a]		No./% of tumours, by stage[b]	
		Sensitivity	Specificity	Screen-detected cancers	Interval cancers	Screened group	Control group
Mumbai study Mittra et al. (2010)	35–64	57.4%	91.9%	73 (81)	37 (44)	Early lesion, 78 Advanced lesion, 32	Early lesion, 38 Advanced lesion, 37
Trivandrum study Sankaranarayanan et al. (2011)	30–69	51.7%	94.3%	80	28	Early lesion, 43.8% Advanced lesion, 45.0%	Early lesion, 25.4% Advanced lesion, 68.3%
Philippines study Pisani et al. (2006)	35–64	53.2%	100%	68	NA	[17% more advanced lesions in control group]	

[a] Number of tumours with available staging (total number of tumours).

[b] Early lesion included tumour size < 5 cm (T1 and T2), and advanced lesion included T3 and T4.

wards (clusters) were randomly allocated to the intervention group (CBE) or the control group (no screening). An intention-to-treat analysis was performed for comparison of incidence rates between the two groups. Preliminary results for incidence are based on follow-up until 2009, when the first round of screening was completed. Among the 2880 CBE-positive women, 1767 were judged to have a palpable lump and the remaining 1113 to have other abnormalities. The sensitivity was 51.7%, and the specificity was 94.3%. Among the intervention and control groups, 80 and 63 women, respectively, were diagnosed with breast cancer. The percentage of early-stage (stage IIA or lower) breast cancer was 43.8% (95% CI, 32.9–54.6%) in the intervention group versus 25.4% (95% CI, 14.6–36.1%) in the control group ($P = 0.023$), and the percentage of advanced-stage (stage IIB or higher) breast cancer was 45.0% (95% CI, 34.1–55.9%) in the intervention group versus 68.3% (95% CI, 56.8–79.7%) in the control group ($P = 0.005$). This indicates a shift to a lower stage of cancers in the CBE arm.

(iii) Philippines study

The randomized trial in the Philippines (Pisani et al., 2006) began in 1995. Women aged 35–64 years from urban Manila were randomized to five annual CBEs (carried out by trained nurses or midwives) or no screening. The first round of CBE took place in 1996–1997 (over 24 months) and included 151 168 women, who were also instructed in the technique of BSE; 8% of these women refused CBE. Of those examined, 2.5% had palpable lesions and were referred for investigation; of these, 1293 (37.2%) received further investigation. Complete diagnostic follow-up was achieved for only 1220 women (35% of those who were positive on screening); 42.4% refused further investigation, even with a home visit, and 22.6% were lost to follow-up. The sensitivity of annual CBE was 53.2%, and the positive predictive value (PPV) was 1.2%. In the control arm, 17% of the cases presented with advanced disease. Because of the poor compliance with follow-up of screen-positive women, even with home visits, the active intervention was discontinued after the first screening round was completed, in December 1997.

All three studies evaluating CBE versus no screening showed a shift to a lower stage of the tumours detected.

(b) Mammography plus CBE versus no screening

Table 4.7 and Table 4.8 present the study characteristics and the outcome, respectively, of RCTs and other studies evaluating the efficacy of mammography plus CBE compared with no screening or compared with CBE alone.

(i) Health Insurance Plan trial

The Health Insurance Plan trial was the first RCT of breast cancer screening and was designed to assess the role of screening in reducing mortality from breast cancer, using mammography and CBE performed by trained surgeons. Approximately 61 000 women aged 40–64 years were included in the study (Shapiro et al., 1971). The results after 18 years from entry reported a relative risk for death from breast cancer of 0.77 (95% CI, 0.61–0.97). The proportion of cases detected with mammography was low, especially in younger women; also, the benefit appeared to be more due to the earlier detection of advanced rather than early disease (Shapiro, 1994; Miller, 2004). [The individual contribution of each intervention remained ambiguous.] The contribution of CBE in the detection of breast cancer was 67% (Table 4.8).

(ii) Edinburgh trial

The Edinburgh randomized trial of breast cancer screening (Alexander et al., 1994; Alexander, 1997) recruited 44 288 women aged 45–64 years into the initial cohort of the trial during 1978–1981. A total of 22 944 women were randomized into the study group and were offered screening for 7 years; the remaining women constituted the control group. After 10 years, breast cancer mortality was 21% lower in the study group than in the control group (not statistically significant) in women older than 50 years. The relative risk of death from breast cancer in all women was 0.82 (95% CI, 0.61–1.11). The contribution of CBE in the detection of breast cancer was 74% (Table 4.8).

(c) Mammography plus CBE versus CBE alone

The CNBSS 2 trial (Miller et al., 1992a, b; Barton et al., 1999) compared annual CBE plus mammography versus CBE in a randomized setting (Table 4.7 and Table 4.8). Mammography plus CBE detected more node-negative and small breast cancers compared with screening with CBE alone, but there was no impact on breast cancer mortality. Mammography showed no added value to CBE, with a relative risk of 0.97 (95% CI, 0.62–1.52). [The Working Group noted that this study does not allow an evaluation of the efficacy of CBE in reducing breast cancer mortality.]

4.3.2 Nested case–control study

The DOM project, a population-based, non-randomized breast cancer screening programme with physical examination and xeromammography, was started in 1974 in the city of Utrecht, The Netherlands (Table 4.7). A total of 116 cases of breast cancer were detected with screening, of which 55.6% were detected with mammography alone, 9.7% with CBE alone, and 34.6% with combined-modality screening (De Waard et al., 1984). A protective effect of screening against breast cancer mortality was found in a nested case–control study after 8 years of follow-up (odds ratio [OR], 0.30; 95% CI, 0.13–0.70) (Collette et al., 1984), which decreased after 14 years of follow-up (Collette et al., 1992). Analysis within different age subgroups showed the effect to be more pronounced for older women (OR, 0.38; 95% CI, 0.18–0.83) than for younger women (OR, 0.91; 95% CI, 0.39–2.13) (Collette et al., 1992).

Table 4.7 Characteristics of studies evaluating combined mammography and clinical breast examination

Study, country References	Design	Years of recruitment	CBE examiners	Age at entry (years)	No. of women		Screening modality (intervention vs control)
					Intervention	Control	
Randomized controlled trials							
Health Insurance Plan trial, USA Shapiro et al. (1988)	Randomized	1963–1966	Surgeons	40–64	30 131	30 565	CBE annually + mammography annually vs none
Edinburgh trial, United Kingdom Alexander et al. (1994)	Cluster randomized	1979–1988	Physicians, nurses	45–64	22 944	21 344	CBE annually + mammography every 2 years vs none
CNBSS 1 trial, Canada Miller et al. (1992a)	Randomized	1980–1988	Nurses	40–49	25 214	25 216	CBE annually + mammography annually vs CBE at entry
CNBSS 2 trial, Canada Miller et al. (1992b)	Randomized	1980–1985	Nurses	50–59	19 711	19 694	CBE annually + mammography annually vs CBE annually
Nested case–control study							
DOM study, Netherlands Collette (1985), Collette et al. (1992)	Nested case–control	1974–1981	Medical assistants	50–64	14 796 invited: 54 cases, 162 controls	–	CBE annually; mammography annually
Observational studies							
Breast Cancer Detection Demonstration Project Baker (1982), Morrison et al. (1988)	Prospective	1973–1981	Nurses	35–74[a]	283 222[a]	–	CBE + mammography + thermography[b] annually
West London study, United Kingdom Chamberlain et al. (1979)	Prospective	1973–1977	Nurses, then doctors	> 40	2484	–	CBE + mammography at 0, 6, 12, and 24 months
United Kingdom Trial of Early Detection of Breast Cancer Moss et al. (1993), UK Trial of Early Detection of Breast Cancer Group (1993)	Prospective, non-randomized	1979–1988	Physicians, nurses	45–64	45 956	127 109	CBE annually + mammography every 2 years vs none
Data analysis from the National Breast and Cervical Cancer Early Detection Programme Bobo et al. (2000)	Prospective	1995–1998	Doctors	[c]	564 708	–	CBE annually; mammography annually

Table 4.7 (continued)

Study, country References	Design	Years of recruitment	CBE examiners	Age at entry (years)	No. of women		Screening modality (intervention vs control)
					Intervention	Control	
Data analysis of four Canadian breast cancer screening programmes Bancej et al. (2003)	Prospective	1996–1998	Nurses, technologists	50–69	300 303	–	CBE and mammography in alternate years
Breast Cancer Screening Programme at Group Health Cooperative of Puget Sound Oestreicher et al. (2005)	Prospective	1996–2000	Nurses	≥ 40	61 688	–	CBE and mammography every 1–2 years based on breast cancer risk factors
Well Women Clinics, opportunistic breast screening in Hong Kong Special Administrative Region, China Lui et al. (2007)	Prospective	1998–2002	Doctors	≥ 40	29 028	–	CBE + mammography every 2 years (188 women aged 35–39 years also screened based on family history)
Breast care centre, Hong Kong Sanatorium and Hospital, Hong Kong Special Administrative Region, China Kwong et al. (2008)	Prospective	1999–2006	Family physicians	[c]	11 408	–	BSE training; CBE; mammography
Breast screening comparative study in Chengdu, China Huang et al. (2012)	Prospective	2009–2011	Breast surgeon	25–80	3 028	–	CBE, mammography, and ultrasonography annually (2 rounds)

[a] 99.4% of screenees were aged 35–74 years at entry, although any woman seeking screening could participate. At least 283 222 women had been screened as of September 1981.

[b] CBE, mammography, and thermography were used from the start of the project until 1977, when thermography was dropped and mammography was restricted to women aged 50 years and older and women at high risk who were younger than 50 years.

[c] The age range of women who were offered breast screening is not specified. However, some data are presented for women aged ≤ 40 years and for those aged ≥ 65 years.

BSE, breast self-examination; CBE, clinical breast examination; CNBSS, Canadian National Breast Screening Study.

Table 4.8 Outcome of studies of combined mammography and clinical breast examination

Study, country References	No. of rounds	Duration of follow-up (years)	Mortality reduction, RR (95% CI)	No. of cancers detected	
				Total	CBE only No. (%)
Randomized controlled trials					
Health Insurance Plan trial, USA Shapiro et al. (1988), Barton et al. (1999)	4	18	0.77 (0.61–0.97)	132	59 (45%)
Edinburgh trial, United Kingdom Alexander et al. (1994), Barton et al. (1999)	7	10	0.82 (0.61–1.11)	88	3 (3%)[a]
CNBSS 1 trial, Canada[b] Miller et al. (1992a), Barton et al. (1999)	5	7	0.86 (0.73–1.01)	255	61 (24%)
CNBSS 2 trial, Canada[c] Miller et al. (1992b), Barton et al. (1999)	5	7	0.29 (0.14–0.62)	325	39 (12%)
Nested case–control study					
DOM study, Netherlands Collette (1985), Collette et al. (1992)	4	14	0.52 (0.32–0.83)[d]	116[e]	(9.7%)[e]
Observational study					
United Kingdom Trial of Early Detection of Breast Cancer UK Trial of Early Detection of Breast Cancer Group (1993), Barton et al. (1999)	7	10	0.73 (0.63–0.84)	432	24 (6%)

[a] Results based only on data from first round screening.
[b] Mammography + CBE vs CBE at entry.
[c] Mammography + CBE vs CBE annually.
[d] Odds ratio estimated after adjusting for confounding and extending follow-up to 14 years.
[e] Values for the entire cohort.
CBE, clinical breast examination; CI, confidence interval; CNBSS, Canadian National Breast Screening Study; RR, relative risk.

4.3.3 Observational studies

See Table 4.7.

After the success of the Health Insurance Plan trial, several population-based implementation projects and case–control studies evaluated the role of CBE plus mammography for the detection of breast cancer.

In the USA, the Breast Cancer Detection Demonstration Project was initiated by the American Cancer Society and the National Cancer Institute in 1973 (Beahrs & Smart, 1979; Baker, 1982; Morrison et al., 1988). After 5 years of follow-up, 3557 cases of breast cancer had been diagnosed in the screened group, of which 41.6% were detected with mammography alone, 8.7% with CBE alone, and the remainder with both modalities. There was a slight shift to a lower stage; less than 20% of women were diagnosed node-positive, compared with 24% nodal positivity in interval cancers. [Although the Breast Cancer Detection Demonstration Project shows benefit with population-based screening using two modalities and an incremental benefit obtained with CBE, it does not provide effective evidence for the efficacy of CBE in the population.]

The West London study, aiming to screen women older than 40 years in Ealing, London, United Kingdom, began in 1973. Initial screening consisted of two independent CBEs, one by a nurse and one by a doctor, and mammography. Repeat screening was offered after 6, 12, and 24 months to women who had not been diagnosed with breast cancer. Over 3 years, 2484 women were screened, and 83%, 65%, and 53% had repeated screens at 6, 12, and 24 months, respectively. Overall, 34 breast cancers were detected, of which 5 were interval cancers. Of the 29 cases detected by screening, 80% were at an early stage; 10 (29%) of them were detected with mammography alone, 9 with CBE alone (27%), and 10 with both modalities (Chamberlain et al., 1979).

A multicentre project to assess the effect of breast cancer screening with mammography, CBE, and BSE on mortality was started in 1979 by the UK Trial of Early Detection of Breast Cancer Group (1988). The sensitivity of combined-modality screening (mammography plus CBE) was 92% (197/213) and 91% (235/259) for the Edinburgh and Guildford screening centres, respectively, whereas the sensitivity of CBE screening alone was estimated to be 64% (74/115) for both centres; the incremental detection of CBE over mammography was estimated as 8% (Moss et al., 1993). In the 16-year update on mortality (UK Trial of Early Detection of Breast Cancer Group, 1999), in the cohort offered combined-modality breast cancer screening, breast cancer mortality was 27% lower than in the national population (rate ratio, 0.73; 95% CI, 0.63–0.84). [The Working Group noted that this result could be due to a healthy volunteer effect rather than to reduced mortality from screening.]

In the USA, the National Breast and Cervical Cancer Early Detection Program was started to provide screening to poor and uninsured women in a community setting, using combined CBE and mammography (Bobo et al., 2000). Of 752 081 CBEs performed, 6.9% were abnormal. A total of 2852 invasive and 928 in situ cancers were diagnosed; the diagnostic yield was 5 cancers per 1000 CBEs. Across all ages, the sensitivity, specificity, and PPV of CBE were 58.8%, 93.4%, and 4.3% respectively, based on 1-year survival (consistent with results from most RCTs). About 5.1% of cancers were detected with CBE but not with mammography. [The Working Group noted that the CBE practices varied across medical centres (Bobo & Lee, 2000); however, it was felt that this study provides a real-world outcome of implementing CBE as a screening procedure.]

Bancej et al. (2003) analysed the contribution of CBE in four Canadian organized breast cancer screening programmes. CBE detected 45% of cancers in the first screen, and of these, 11% were detected with CBE alone. In rescreening, CBE detected 39% of cancers, and of these, 16% were detected with CBE alone. Without CBE, the programmes would have missed 3 cancers for every 10 000 screens and 3–10 small invasive cancers for every 100 000 screens. The PPV of CBE was 0.9–1.1%.

Oestreicher et al. (2005) prospectively followed 61 688 women aged 40 years and older who were enrolled in the Breast Cancer Screening Program at Group Health Cooperative of Puget Sound, in Seattle, USA, and underwent at least one screening examination with mammography and/or CBE in 1996–2000. The sensitivity of mammography was 78% and that of combined mammography and CBE was 82%, showing an incremental value of CBE in addition to mammography of 4% (Oestreicher et al., 2005). CBE generally added incrementally more to sensitivity among women with dense breasts.

The effect of breast cancer screening using CBE and mammography has also been evaluated more recently in several settings in Asia. The Well Women Clinics in Hong Kong Special Administrative Region, China, offered breast cancer screening with CBE and mammography to women older than 40 years (and to women aged 35–40 years with a family history of breast cancer) in Hong Kong Special Administrative Region every 2 years. In 1998–2002, 29 028 women were screened, and breast cancer was detected in 232 of them; 83 (36%) cancers were detected with CBE, and 15 of them (6.5% of all detected cancers) were not detected with mammography (Lui et al., 2007). Another breast cancer service was set up at the Hong Kong Sanatorium and Hospital in 1999. Over 8 years, 11 408 asymptomatic women were screened with

CBE and mammography and were given instructions on how to perform BSE. A total of 26 breast cancers were diagnosed; 8 of them (31%) were detected with CBE alone (Kwong et al., 2008).

A screening study to compare CBE, mammography, and ultrasonography was carried out in Chengdu, China, in 2009–2011. Among 3028 women aged 25 years and older who were screened with the three techniques, 33 breast cancers were identified after an average follow-up of 1.3 years; 28 (85%) cancers were detected with mammography, 22 (67%) with CBE, and 24 (73%) with ultrasonography. No cases were detected with CBE that were not detected with mammography, whereas three cancers were detected with ultrasonography that were not detected with the other two methods (Huang et al., 2012).

4.4 Breast self-examination

4.4.1 Randomized trials

Two randomized trials of BSE with breast cancer mortality as the primary end-point have been conducted.

(a) St Petersburg trial

The first randomized trial began in Moscow and St Petersburg, Russian Federation, in 1985. Results on deaths from breast cancer have been reported only from the St Petersburg portion of the study (Semiglazov et al., 1999a, b, 2003). In that city, women aged 40–64 years who received medical care at 18 polyclinics and 10 large industrial businesses with health care services were eligible to participate. Nine polyclinics and five businesses were randomly selected as intervention facilities, and the remainder were control facilities. Women who received medical care at the intervention facilities were invited to participate in the trial. Medical personnel in the clinics examined each woman's breasts, and then the women were given detailed BSE instruction in groups of 5–20 women. Each woman was given a calendar to serve as a reminder to practise BSE monthly and to record the dates of her BSEs. All women were also asked to return annually for reinforcement sessions. Women in the control clinics received CBE at entry into the trial and at annual clinic visits, so this was a trial of the additional benefit of BSE in reducing breast cancer mortality in women screened by annual CBE.

The results are summarized in Table 4.9. Approximately 60 000 women were enrolled in each arm of the study (the exact numbers vary in different reports). Significantly more women in the instruction group than in the control group were referred for evaluation of a breast lump ($P < 0.05$), and more were found to have a benign lesion. Somewhat more women in the instruction group than in the control group were also diagnosed with breast cancer, but the difference could be due to chance ($P > 0.05$), and the malignant tumours in the two groups of women did not differ appreciably in size or percentage with axillary node involvement, suggesting that BSE instruction did not result in breast cancer diagnosis at an earlier, less-advanced stage than would be expected in the absence of BSE instruction. Although survival after diagnosis was somewhat more favourable for cases in the instruction group than those in the control group (65% vs 55% at 9 years; relative survival, 0.77 in log-rank test; 53.9% vs 45.3% at 15 years based on 70–75% follow-up), the difference was not statistically significant ($P > 0.05$). After approximately 10 years of follow-up, almost equal percentages of women in the two groups had died of breast cancer.

[In addition to the possibility that BSE would not be efficacious under any circumstances, there are three possible explanations for the results of this study. One is poor compliance with the BSE instruction. Based on a sample of the participants 1 year after BSE training, 82% of the women interviewed reported practising BSE more than 5 times per year, and 53% reported monthly BSE practice. However, by year 4, these percentages

Table 4.9 Results of randomized trials of breast self-examination

Characteristic	St Petersburg trial[a]		Shanghai trial[b]	
	Intervention	Control	Intervention	Control
Age range (years)	40–64	40–64	30–64	30–64
No. of women	57 712	64 759	1 329 769	133 085
No. (%) referred for evaluation/ benign breast lesions[c]	4300 (7.5%)	2438 (3.8%)	2387 (1.8%)	1296 (1.0%)
No. (%) with breast cancer[d]	493 (0.9%)	446 (0.7%)	864 (0.7%)	896 (0.7%)
No. (%) of deaths from breast cancer	157 (0.27%)	167 (0.26%)	135 (0.1%)	131 (0.1%)

[a] From Semiglazov et al. (1999a, b).
[b] From Thomas et al. (2002).
[c] Number referred for further evaluation in the St Petersburg trial, and number of histologically confirmed benign lesions in the Shanghai trial.
[d] After about 10 years in the St Petersburg trial and after 10–11 years in the Shanghai trial.

had dropped to 52% and 18%, respectively. After a re-education programme in 1994, these percentages increased to 76% and 32%, respectively, 8 years after the trial was initiated. Also in 1994, medical personnel observed a random sample of about 400 women practising BSE and recorded their proficiency. Although the reported frequency of correctly practising various aspects of BSE was high, there is no evidence that these observations accurately reflect the routine practice of BSE outside of the clinic setting by all of the women in the instruction group. A second possible reason for the results is that BSE is not effective in reducing mortality from breast cancer in women who are also screened by CBE. A third possible explanation is that women in both groups had easy access to medical care at the polyclinics, and women in the control group tended to present with tumours that were small and at an early stage. Of women in the control group, 17.4% presented with tumours less than 2 cm in diameter, and 46.4% with tumours that had not spread to the axillary lymph nodes.]

(b) Shanghai trial

The second randomized trial was conducted in Shanghai, China (Thomas et al., 1997, 2002). In 1989–1991, more than 266 000 women aged 30–64 years who were current or retired employees of the Shanghai Textile Industry Bureau, working in 519 different factories, were randomized by factory to a BSE instruction group or a control group. Women in the instruction group received initial BSE instruction in groups of about 10 women and two subsequent reinforcement sessions, 1 year and 3 years later, consisting of videos and discussion groups, as well as multiple reminders to practise BSE. Nearly 80% of the women attended all three sessions. In addition, women were asked to attend periodic practice sessions supervised by factory medical workers about every 6 months for 4–5 years. During the first year of the study, 92% of the women attended these sessions; this percentage gradually declined to 74% in the fourth year and 49% in the fifth and last year of the intervention. The women thus practised BSE under supervision on average once every 4–5 months during the first 4–5 years of the trial. The quality of the BSEs at these sessions was high. Women were encouraged to practise BSE monthly, but the frequency and quality of the practice outside of the clinic setting are unknown. No breast cancer screening was offered to women in the control group. A higher level of proficiency in detecting lumps in silicone breast models was demonstrated by randomly selected women in the instruction group compared with the control group.

The results after 10–11 years of follow-up are summarized in Table 4.9. More women were diagnosed with benign breast lesions in the instruction group than in the control group. The numbers of women with breast cancer were similar in the two groups. The breast cancers in the two groups did not differ appreciably in size (44.9% vs 41.6% were ≤ 2 cm in diameter) or stage (47.0% vs 48.3% had no axillary nodal involvement). Also, the numbers of deaths from breast cancer and the cumulative breast cancer mortality rates were nearly identical in the two groups, as were survival rates in women with breast cancer, both from entry into the trial and from date of diagnosis. Evidence was presented that these results cannot be readily explained by the absence of statistical power, insufficient duration or completeness of follow-up, failure of the randomization procedure to select two groups at equal risk of breast cancer, selective exclusions of women after randomization, incomplete or differential ascertainment of breast cancer cases or deaths, screening in the control group, or insufficient breast cancer treatment. The most likely reason for the absence of an effect of BSE instruction on breast cancer mortality in this study is that proficient BSE practice at least once every 5 months for 4–5 years did not result in breast cancer being diagnosed at a sufficiently less advanced stage of progression for appropriate therapy to have altered the course of the disease. There is suggestive evidence that more frequent BSE might have resulted in a more favourable trial result. Among women who attended all of the supervised BSE sessions and those who attended fewer than 70% of the sessions, the percentages with tumours that were less than 2 cm in diameter were 52.3% and 45.3%, respectively, in current workers, and 48.7% and 44.4%, respectively, in retired women.

In summary, the results from both randomized controlled trials provided little evidence that risk of death or of advanced disease is reduced by BSE instruction. In both studies, the women in the control group had easy access to medical care and tended to present with relatively small tumours without regional lymph-node involvement. The efficacy of BSE in populations in which women typically present with more-advanced tumours remains unknown.

4.4.2 Observational studies

(a) Methodological considerations

In evaluating the evidence for the efficacy of BSE from observational studies, several methodological issues must be considered.

BSE must be distinguished from breast awareness. BSE is a screening method used to attempt to detect *asymptomatic* breast cancer before it is clinically apparent (see Section 2.4 for technical details). Breast awareness consists of the education and encouragement of women to seek medical attention for *symptomatic* changes in their breasts that may be due to the presence of breast cancer (see Section 1.5.1 for additional details). These two concepts of breast cancer detection are not always clearly defined or distinguished (Thornton & Pillarisetti, 2008; Mark et al., 2014). Self-reports of BSE practice may include breast awareness, and some cancers that are reported as being detected by BSE may have been symptomatic cancers found by the women themselves through breast awareness.

There are two components to BSE compliance: frequency (typically once a month) and proficiency; these are not consistently considered and reported in observational studies. In addition, there may be underreporting or misclassification of BSE practice. These reporting errors would lead to underestimation of the efficacy of BSE in cohort studies. In case–control studies, if the magnitudes of the reporting errors are different for cases and controls, spurious associations would arise. Finally, the practice of BSE may be related to risk factors for breast cancer, or to other methods of screening, and lead to spurious results if the potential confounding effect of these associations is not taken into account.

There have been a large number of clinical studies of tumour size and stage at diagnosis, and of survival from date of diagnosis, in relation to whether the patient reported that the tumour was detected by BSE, and in relation to reported frequency of BSE practice (IARC, 2002). In most studies, the proportion of women who had early-stage cancer was slightly higher in women who reported detecting their cancer by BSE than in women whose cancer was detected by other means (excluding mammography screening). However, it is not clear whether the women who reported detecting their tumour by BSE were actually practising BSE or whether they were women who simply reported having found their tumour by themselves. Among cases who reported a history of practising BSE, tumour stage was not consistently related to reported BSE frequency. Most studies did show a tendency towards slightly smaller tumour size in women who reported practising BSE monthly than in women who reported practising BSE less frequently, but differential reporting of BSE frequency by women with small and large tumours cannot be ruled out. Survival tended to be somewhat longer in women reporting a history of BSE practice, or who were taught BSE or accepted an invitation to attend a BSE instruction session, than in women not reporting any of these factors, but the magnitude of the differences varied widely among the studies, the differences were not consistently statistically significant, and enhanced lead-time or length bias sampling cannot be ruled out as alternative explanations for the observations. The results of these observational studies of intermediate end-points may thus all be due to bias, confounding, or chance, and the Working Group therefore concluded that they do not contribute meaningful information in formulating an assessment of the efficacy of BSE. These studies will therefore not be considered further in this review. One more-recent study in the USA (Tu et al., 2006) assessed BSE practice before the development of breast cancer, thus avoiding possible reporting bias, and found no association between the quality of BSE practice and either tumour size or stage of disease.

The two randomized trials evaluated the efficacy of BSE instruction, not the actual practice of BSE. The evidence from observational studies that BSE can reduce mortality from breast cancer and detect interval cancers between periodic screenings is reviewed in this section.

(b) Cohort studies

Reports are available from three studies in which breast cancer mortality rates were compared in women who did and did not practise BSE.

Holmberg et al. (1997) calculated breast cancer mortality rates in a cohort of women in the USA who in 1959 were asked a single question: "Many doctors recommend that women examine their breasts monthly. Do you do so?" A "yes" answer presumably indicated that the women practised BSE monthly, and a "no" answer indicated that BSE either was practised less frequently or was not practised. After a 13-year follow-up period, no association was observed between breast cancer mortality and the answer to this question. [The major strengths of this study are its large size, long duration of follow-up, strong statistical power, and control for multiple possible confounders. However, the absence of any detailed information on the frequency or manner of BSE practice by the women in the study reduces the usefulness of the negative findings, since many of the women who reported practising BSE may not have done so adequately.]

In the Mama Program for Breast Screening in Finland (Gastrin et al., 1994), beginning in 1973 women were given detailed BSE instruction in groups of 20–50 women, followed by periodic reminders and annual mailings of calendars for the women to record their BSE practice. Mortality rates in the participants were compared with those in the general population of Finland. The breast cancer mortality rate in the participants was significantly lower than expected (mortality rate ratio, 0.71). This occurred in spite of a higher incidence rate of breast cancer in the participants than expected (incidence rate ratio, 1.19). The reduced rates of death from breast cancer were observed in most age groups of women and were most pronounced in years 3–4 after entry into the study. However, mortality rates from all causes were also significantly lower by the same amount as for breast cancer mortality (standardized mortality ratio, 0.70), suggesting that the participants were healthier than women in the general population, and that their lower breast cancer mortality may have been due to factors related to improved survival, other than early diagnosis resulting from BSE practice, that were not controlled for in the analysis. This contention is supported by the observation that the stage of disease at diagnosis was no different in the women in the study cohort than in other cases in the country. [There is no mention of CBE or mammography screening in the published report, and these screening methods were presumably not taken into account in the data analysis, although the frequency of their use was probably low.] A large majority of the women in the cohort reported on their calendars that they had practised BSE monthly. [This information was not validated and is therefore questionable, and proficiency of BSE practice was not assessed.]

As part of the United Kingdom Trial of Early Detection of Breast Cancer (Ellman et al., 1993; UK Trial of Early Detection of Breast Cancer Group, 1999), women in the cities of Huddersfield and Nottingham were invited to attend BSE education sessions. The sessions included a talk and a film demonstrating BSE. In Huddersfield, calendars were mailed annually, as reminders and as a means to record monthly BSE practice. No further BSE instruction was provided in either city. Breast cancer mortality rates in the women invited to the BSE training session (whether or not they attended) were compared with those in four comparison centres in which women received no breast cancer screening or BSE instruction. No overall difference in breast cancer mortality rates was observed between the women in the two BSE instruction centres combined and the women in the four comparison centres (rate ratio, 0.99; 95% CI, 0.87–1.12). However, the rate ratio in Huddersfield was significantly less than 1 (0.79; 95% CI, 0.65–0.96) and was similar to that observed in the Mama Program for Breast Screening in Finland; at the Huddersfield centre, as in the programme in Finland, calendars were mailed annually, suggesting that the difference could be due to more intensive BSE practice in Huddersfield than in Nottingham (rate ratio, 1.09; 95% CI, 0.95–1.26). In addition, more women in Huddersfield than in Nottingham also received breast-conserving surgery, chemotherapy, and tamoxifen, whereas participation rates in the BSE instruction sessions were higher in Nottingham than in Huddersfield, suggesting that differences in treatment or other factors could explain the discrepant results. No information on compliance was reported.

In summary, although the cohort studies in Finland and the United Kingdom (Huddersfield component) showed that BSE instruction with periodic reminders was associated with a small reduction in breast cancer mortality, it is more likely that these observations are due to factors unrelated to BSE practice. No reliable information on compliance was provided for any of the studies. In the study in the USA, BSE practice was defined by a single question, and in the studies in Finland and the United Kingdom, BSE instruction was given in a single session with no reinforcement sessions. It is therefore reasonable to assume that the frequency and proficiency of BSE practice by the women in these three studies was lower than those in the two randomized trials, which provided more intensive BSE instruction and encouragement to practise, and that the results provide no information on the efficacy of BSE in women who practise BSE regularly and competently.

(c) Case–control studies

Two case–control studies that were nested in prospective studies, and thus did not rely on self-reported BSE practice, have been conducted.

Locker et al. (1989) performed a case–control analysis of data from women invited to enrol in the United Kingdom Trial of Early Detection of Breast Cancer in Nottingham. Of 180 women who died of breast cancer more than 3 months after invitation, 68 (37.8%) had attended the BSE instruction class, compared with 258 (42.8%) of 603 age-matched control women at the Nottingham centre, for an estimated relative risk of 0.70 (95% CI, 0.50–0.97). The comparable relative risk estimate in premenopausal women was 0.85 (95% CI, 0.45–1.60) and in postmenopausal women was 0.66 (95% CI, 0.45–0.97). [These estimates were not controlled for factors other than age that may have been associated with a decision to attend the BSE instruction class, or for treatment or other factors that could influence survival.]

Harvey et al. (1997) conducted a case–control study nested within the CNBSS. Answers to questions about frequency of BSE obtained before enrolment in the trial and during the trial and results of annual assessment of BSE proficiency were compared in 220 cases with fatal or metastatic disease and 2200 age-matched controls selected from trial enrollees. All of the information on BSE was obtained before the development of breast cancer in the cases. Compared with women who practised BSE before enrolment, those who did not had a relative risk of fatal or advanced breast cancer of 1.27 (95% CI, 0.96–1.68), and relative risk estimates decreased with increasing frequency of BSE practice before enrolment. The relative risk of fatal or advanced disease also increased slightly with decreasing frequency of BSE practice during the trial, but none of the estimates or trends were statistically significant ($P > 0.05$). However, there was a significant decrease in estimates of relative risk of fatal or advanced disease with increasing BSE proficiency as observed in clinics by trained examiners 2 years before diagnosis in the cases (Table 4.10). The level of proficiency was defined according to the exclusion of one, two, or three key elements of a proper BSE (visual inspection, use of three middle fingers, and use of finger pads) that were weakly associated with a reduction in risk. Similar but weaker trends in risk were observed in relation to these same levels of proficiency at 1 year and 3 years before diagnosis, but none of the relative risk estimates had 95% confidence limits that excluded 1.0. Also, other elements of BSE practice (systematic search, circular palpation, complete coverage of the breast, and examination of the axilla) were not associated with changes in risk estimates. The relative risk estimates were not found to be confounded by family history of breast cancer, age at menarche or menopause, education level, occupation, or the trial arm to which the woman was allocated.

Two additional case–control studies, which were conducted in the general population and relied on results of interviews with women to obtain information on BSE practice, have been conducted. Both included women with advanced disease (as a surrogate for death from breast cancer) as cases.

In the USA, Newcomb et al. (1991) compared BSE practice in 209 enrollees in a prepaid health plan who developed late-stage (stage III or IV) breast cancer during a defined period of time with BSE practice in 433 age-matched controls selected randomly from enrollees in the same plan. Personal interviews with the women were conducted in which specific questions were asked about various components of the recommended techniques and frequency of practice. Both an open-ended technique and a structured

Table 4.10 Relative risk of death from breast cancer or of advanced disease in relation to proficiency of breast self-examination

Reference, country	Years before diagnosis that assessment was performed	Measure of proficiency	RR (95% CI)
Harvey et al. (1997), Canada	1	All 3 practices included[a]	1.00 (ref)
		1 practice omitted	1.52 (0.93–2.48)
		2 practices omitted	1.53 (0.83–2.84)
		3 practices omitted	1.40 (0.58–3.39)
	2	All 3 practices included[a]	1.00 (ref)
		1 practice omitted	1.82 (1.00–3.29)
		2 practices omitted	2.84 (1.44–5.59)
		3 practices omitted	2.95 (1.19 –7.30)
	3	All 3 practices included[a]	1.00 (ref)
		1 practice omitted	1.21 (0.65–2.28)
		2 practices omitted	0.92 (0.38–2.22)
		3 practices omitted	1.68 (0.59–4.76)
Newcomb et al. (1991), USA	After diagnosis[b]	High proficiency[c]	0.65 (0.33–1.31) [ref][d]
		Moderate proficiency	1.00 (0.56–1.80) [1.53]
		Low proficiency	1.33 (0.83–2.12) [2.05]
		No BSE practice	1.00 (ref) [1.53]

[a] Includes visual inspection, use of three middle fingers, and use of finger pads.
[b] Women were asked about BSE practice 1 year before the date of diagnosis in cases or a comparable reference date in controls.
[c] Proficiency based on a 10-point scoring system of items included in responses to an open-ended questionnaire.
[d] Relative risks in square brackets with high proficiency as the reference category were calculated by the Working Group.
BSE, breast self-examination; ref, reference; RR, relative risk.

interview were used to classify BSE as to level of proficiency. The relative risk of advanced disease in women who ever practised BSE was 1.15 (95% CI, 0.73–1.81), and the relative risk unexpectedly increased with the frequency of BSE practice. However, the women who practised BSE frequently were found to practise it with the lowest level of proficiency, and the relative risk of advanced disease decreased with increasing level of proficiency (Table 4.10). This trend was observed in women with all levels of BSE frequency. [Although the influence of the presence of the disease on responses could have biased this study, it seems unlikely that cases would underreport frequency of BSE practice and overreport proficiency during the same detailed interviews. The relative risk estimates were controlled for age and frequency of CBE. Other risk factors for breast cancer were considered as possible confounders but were found not to alter the values of the estimates.]

Muscat & Huncharek (1991) compared 435 women in Connecticut, USA, with regional or distant breast cancer at diagnosis with 887 control women selected by random-digit dialling. Frequency of BSE practice was ascertained during detailed interviews as part of a larger study on steroid hormones and cancer. No information on proficiency was obtained. BSE practice at least once a month was reported by 27.4% of the cases and 20.5% of the controls. After controlling for family history of breast cancer, age at first birth, race, and frequency of mammograms, a relative risk of 1.27 (95% CI, 0.77–2.07) was estimated, but it is not clear from the report whether this estimate is for women who practised BSE monthly or also less frequently. [As in the study by Newcomb et al. (1991), risk increased with the frequency of

BSE practice, but unlike that study, no information on proficiency was obtained, so it is not known whether this trend is due to confounding by proficiency.]

In summary, the results from case–control studies provided little evidence that risk of death from breast cancer or of advanced disease is reduced by frequent practice of BSE as it is generally practised by women in North America and the United Kingdom. Two of the case–control studies provided evidence to suggest that risk of fatal or advanced disease could be reduced if BSE were practised with a high degree of proficiency. It can be assumed that the documented practice of BSE in the Shanghai trial was performed with a high degree of proficiency, because it was observed by health workers and was the result of intensive instruction over a period of several years; however, such practice about once every 4–5 months for 4–5 years was insufficient to reduce mortality from breast cancer. The efficacy of more frequent, high-proficiency BSE in reducing mortality remains unknown.

(d) Detection of interval cancers

The previous IARC Working Group on breast cancer screening (IARC, 2002) recommended that studies be conducted to assess the efficacy of BSE in detecting interval cancers between periodic mammography screenings. Results of only one such study have been published (Wilke et al., 2009). It involved women who were at high risk of breast cancer (estimated average lifetime risk, > 20%) and therefore probably more highly motivated to practise BSE than other women. A high-risk breast clinic at Duke University, USA, recruited 147 women who had a 5-year Gail-model risk of at least 1.7% and followed them up for an average of 23 months (range, 6–36 months). Risk factors included: a previous histologically confirmed diagnosis of atypical hyperplasia or lobular carcinoma in situ or DCIS; a contralateral invasive breast cancer; a *BRCA1/2* mutation; radiation treatment for Hodgkin lymphoma to the chest, neck, and axilla; or one or more first-degree relatives with premenopausal breast cancer. The women were screened annually with mammography and magnetic resonance imaging (MRI). They also received 6–15 minutes of BSE instruction in conjunction with CBE two or three times a year, and their self-reported home practice of BSE was recorded at each of these sessions. Breast cancer was detected in 12 women, 1 during initial training and 11 during the follow-up period. All 12 women with breast cancer were judged to have complied with the recommendations to practise BSE monthly. Six of the cancers were initially found by BSE (sensitivity, 50%), as were 18 additional masses that were confirmed as not being breast cancer (PPV, 25%). The 5 cases detected by BSE during the follow-up period were detected 6–11 months after the last annual screening.

These results suggest that BSE may be useful in detecting interval cancers in women at high risk of breast cancer who are highly motivated to practise BSE regularly and competently. No information is available to determine whether this would contribute to a reduction in mortality from breast cancer.

References

Alexander F, Roberts MM, Lutz W, Hepburn W (1989). Randomisation by cluster and the problem of social class bias. *J Epidemiol Community Health*, 43(1):29–36. doi:10.1136/jech.43.1.29 PMID:2592888

Alexander FE (1997). The Edinburgh Randomized Trial of Breast Cancer Screening. *J Natl Cancer Inst Monogr*, (22):31–5. PMID:9709272

Alexander FE, Anderson TJ, Brown HK, Forrest AP, Hepburn W, Kirkpatrick AE et al. (1994). The Edinburgh randomised trial of breast cancer screening: results after 10 years of follow-up. *Br J Cancer*, 70(3):542–8. doi:10.1038/bjc.1994.342 PMID:8080744

Alexander FE, Anderson TJ, Brown HK, Forrest AP, Hepburn W, Kirkpatrick AE et al. (1999). 14 years of follow-up from the Edinburgh randomised trial of breast-cancer screening. *Lancet*, 353(9168):1903–8. doi:10.1016/S0140-6736(98)07413-3 PMID:10371567

Allgood PC, Warwick J, Warren RM, Day NE, Duffy SW (2008). A case-control study of the impact of the East Anglian breast screening programme on breast cancer mortality. *Br J Cancer*, 98(1):206–9. doi:10.1038/sj.bjc.6604123 PMID:18059396

Andersson I, Aspegren K, Janzon L, Landberg T, Lindholm K, Linell F et al. (1988). Mammographic screening and mortality from breast cancer: the Malmö mammographic screening trial. *BMJ*, 297(6654):943–8. doi:10.1136/bmj.297.6654.943 PMID:3142562

Andersson I, Janzon L (1997). Reduced breast cancer mortality in women under age 50: updated results from the Malmö Mammographic Screening Program. *J Natl Cancer Inst Monogr*, 22(22):63–7. PMID:9709278

Autier P, Héry C, Haukka J, Boniol M, Byrnes G (2009). Advanced breast cancer and breast cancer mortality in randomized controlled trials on mammography screening. *J Clin Oncol*, 27(35):5919–23. doi:10.1200/JCO.2009.22.7041 PMID:19884547

Bailar JC 3rd, MacMahon B (1997). Randomization in the Canadian National Breast Screening Study: a review for evidence of subversion. *CMAJ*, 156(2):193–9. PMID:9012720

Baines CJ, Christen A, Simard A, Wall C, Dean D, Duncan L et al. (1989). The National Breast Screening Study: pre-recruitment sources of awareness in participants. *Can J Public Health*, 80(3):221–5. PMID:2743247

Baker LH (1982). Breast Cancer Detection Demonstration Project: five-year summary report. *CA Cancer J Clin*, 32(4):194–225. doi:10.3322/canjclin.32.4.194 PMID:6805867

Baker SG, Kramer BS, Prorok PC (2002). Statistical issues in randomized trials of cancer screening. *BMC Med Res Methodol*, 2(1):11. doi:10.1186/1471-2288-2-11 PMID:12238954

Bancej C, Decker K, Chiarelli A, Harrison M, Turner D, Brisson J (2003). Contribution of clinical breast examination to mammography screening in the early detection of breast cancer. *J Med Screen*, 10(1):16–21. doi:10.1258/096914103321610761 PMID:12790311

Barton MB, Harris R, Fletcher SW (1999). The rational clinical examination. Does this patient have breast cancer? The screening clinical breast examination: should it be done? How? *JAMA*, 282(13):1270–80. doi:10.1001/jama.282.13.1270 PMID:10517431

Beahrs OH, Smart CR (1979). Diagnosis of minimal breast cancers in the BCDDP: the 66 questionable cases. *Cancer*, 43(3):848–50. doi:10.1002/1097-0142(197903)43:3<848::AID-CNCR2820430310>3.0.CO;2-1 PMID:427726

Biesheuvel C, Barratt A, Howard K, Houssami N, Irwig L (2007). Effects of study methods and biases on estimates of invasive breast cancer overdetection with mammography screening: a systematic review. *Lancet Oncol*, 8(12):1129–38. doi:10.1016/S1470-2045(07)70380-7 PMID:18054882

Bjurstam N, Björneld L, Duffy SW, Smith TC, Cahlin E, Eriksson O et al. (1997). The Gothenburg breast screening trial: first results on mortality, incidence, and mode of detection for women ages 39–49 years at randomization. *Cancer*, 80(11):2091–9. doi:10.1002/(SICI)1097-0142(19971201)80:11<2091::AID-CNCR8>3.0.CO;2-# PMID:9392331

Bjurstam N, Björneld L, Warwick J, Sala E, Duffy SW, Nyström L et al. (2003). The Gothenburg Breast Screening Trial. *Cancer*, 97(10):2387–96. doi:10.1002/cncr.11361 PMID:12733136

Black WC, Haggstrom DA, Welch HG (2002). All-cause mortality in randomized trials of cancer screening. *J Natl Cancer Inst*, 94(3):167–73. doi:10.1093/jnci/94.3.167 PMID:11830606

Bobo J, Lee N (2000). Factors associated with accurate cancer detection during a clinical breast examination. *Ann Epidemiol*, 10(7):463. doi:10.1016/S1047-2797(00)00099-5 PMID:11018380

Bobo JK, Lee NC, Thames SF (2000). Findings from 752,081 clinical breast examinations reported to a national screening program from 1995 through 1998. *J Natl Cancer Inst*, 92(12):971–6. doi:10.1093/jnci/92.12.971 PMID:10861308

Boyd NF, Jong RA, Yaffe MJ, Tritchler D, Lockwood G, Zylak CJ (1993). A critical appraisal of the Canadian National Breast Cancer Screening Study. *Radiology*, 189(3):661–3. doi:10.1148/radiology.189.3.8234686 PMID:8234686

Breast Screening Frequency Trial Group (2002). The frequency of breast cancer screening: results from the UKCCCR Randomised Trial. *Eur J Cancer*, 38(11):1458–64. doi:10.1016/S0959-8049(01)00397-5 PMID:12110490

Canadian Task Force on Preventive Health Care (2011). Recommendations on screening for breast cancer in average-risk women aged 40–74 years. *CMAJ*, 183(17):1991–2001. doi:10.1503/cmaj.110334 PMID:22106103

Chamberlain J, Clifford RE, Nathan BE, Price JL, Burn I (1979). Error-rates in screening for breast cancer by clinical examination and mammography. *Clin Oncol*, 5(2):135–46. PMID:466892

Cole P, Morrison AS (1980). Basic issues in population screening for cancer. *J Natl Cancer Inst*, 64(5):1263–72. PMID:6767876

Collette HJ, Day NE, Rombach JJ, de Waard F (1984). Evaluation of screening for breast cancer in a non-randomised study (the DOM project) by means of a case-control study. *Lancet*, 1(8388):1224–6. doi:10.1016/S0140-6736(84)91704-5 PMID:6144934

Collette HJ, de Waard F, Rombach JJ, Collette C, Day NE (1992). Further evidence of benefits of a (non-randomised) breast cancer screening programme: the DOM project. *J Epidemiol Community Health*, 46(4):382–6. doi:10.1136/jech.46.4.382 PMID:1431712

Collette HJA (1985). Attempts to evaluate a non-randomized breast cancer screening programme (the 'DOM-project'). *Maturitas*, 7(1):43–50. doi: 10.1016/0378-5122(85)90033-7 PMID:4021828

Cuzick J, Edwards R, Segnan N (1997). Adjusting for non-compliance and contamination in randomized clinical trials. *Stat Med*, 16(9):1017–29. doi:10.1002/(SICI)1097-0258(19970515)16:9<1017::AID-SIM508>3.0.CO;2-V PMID:9160496

de Gelder R, Heijnsdijk EAM, van Ravesteyn NT, Fracheboud J, Draisma G, de Koning HJ (2011). Interpreting overdiagnosis estimates in population-based mammography screening. *Epidemiol Rev*, 33(1):111–21. doi:10.1093/epirev/mxr009 PMID:21709144

de Koning HJ, Boer R, Warmerdam PG, Beemsterboer PM, van der Maas PJ (1995). Quantitative interpretation of age-specific mortality reductions from the Swedish breast cancer-screening trials. *J Natl Cancer Inst*, 87(16):1217–23. doi:10.1093/jnci/87.16.1217 PMID:7563167

de Koning HJ (2009). The mysterious mass(es). [Inaugural address, Professor of Screening Evaluation.] Rotterdam, Netherlands: Erasmus MC. Available from: http://repub.eur.nl/res/pub/30689/oratie.pdf.

De Waard F, Collette HJ, Rombach JJ, Baanders-van Halewijn EA, Honing C (1984). The DOM project for the early detection of breast cancer, Utrecht, The Netherlands. *J Chronic Dis*, 37(1):1–44. doi:10.1016/0021-9681(84)90123-1 PMID:6690457

Dean PB (2007). A withdrawn prepublication. *Lancet*, 369(9565):901. doi:10.1016/S0140-6736(07)60434-6 PMID:17368138

Duffy SW, Parmar D (2013). Overdiagnosis in breast cancer screening: the importance of length of observation period and lead time. *Breast Cancer Res*, 15(3):R41. doi:10.1186/bcr3427 PMID:23680223

Duffy SW, Tabár L, Vitak B, Day NE, Smith RA, Chen HH et al. (2003b). The relative contributions of screen-detected in situ and invasive breast carcinomas in reducing mortality from the disease. *Eur J Cancer*, 39(12):1755–60. PMID:12888371

Duffy SW, Tabár L, Vitak B, Yen MF, Warwick J, Smith RA et al. (2003a). The Swedish Two-County Trial of mammographic screening: cluster randomisation and end point evaluation. *Ann Oncol*, 14(8):1196–8. doi:10.1093/annonc/mdg322 PMID:12881376

Ellman R, Moss SM, Coleman D, Chamberlain J (1993). Breast self-examination programmes in the Trial of Early Detection of Breast Cancer: ten year findings. *Br J Cancer*, 68(1):208–12. doi:10.1038/bjc.1993.315 PMID:8318415

Fagerberg CJG, Tabár L (1988). The results of periodic one-view mammography screening in a randomized, controlled trial in Sweden. In: Day NE, Miller AB, editors. Screening for breast cancer. Toronto, Canada: Hans Huber; pp. 33–8.

Frisell J, Eklund G, Hellström L, Lidbrink E, Rutqvist LE, Somell A (1991). Randomized study of mammography screening – preliminary report on mortality in the Stockholm trial. *Breast Cancer Res Treat*, 18(1):49–56. doi:10.1007/BF01975443 PMID:1854979

Frisell J, Glas U, Hellström L, Somell A (1986). Randomized mammographic screening for breast cancer in Stockholm. Design, first round results and comparisons. *Breast Cancer Res Treat*, 8(1):45–54. doi:10.1007/BF01805924 PMID:3790749

Frisell J, Lidbrink E (1997). The Stockholm Mammographic Screening Trial: risks and benefits in age group 40–49 years. *J Natl Cancer Inst Monogr*, 22(22):49–51. PMID:9709275

Frisell J, Lidbrink E, Hellström L, Rutqvist LE (1997). Followup after 11 years – update of mortality results in the Stockholm mammographic screening trial. *Breast Cancer Res Treat*, 45(3):263–70. doi:10.1023/A:1005872617944 PMID:9386870

Gastrin G, Miller AB, To T, Aronson KJ, Wall C, Hakama M et al. (1994). Incidence and mortality from breast cancer in the Mama Program for Breast Screening in Finland, 1973–1986. *Cancer*, 73(8):2168–74. doi:10.1002/1097-0142(19940415)73:8<2168::AID-CNCR2820730822>3.0.CO;2-V PMID:8156521

Gøtzsche PC, Jørgensen KJ (2013). Screening for breast cancer with mammography. *Cochrane Database Syst Rev*, 6:CD001877. doi:10.1002/14651858.CD001877.pub5 PMID:23737396

Gøtzsche PC, Olsen O (2000). Is screening for breast cancer with mammography justifiable? *Lancet*, 355(9198):129–34. doi:10.1016/S0140-6736(99)06065-1 PMID:10675181

Gulati R, Tsodikov A, Wever EM, Mariotto AB, Heijnsdijk EA, Katcher J et al. (2012). The impact of PLCO control arm contamination on perceived PSA screening efficacy. *Cancer Causes Control*, 23(6):827–35. doi:10.1007/s10552-012-9951-8 PMID:22488488

Hanley JA (2011). Measuring mortality reductions in cancer screening trials. *Epidemiol Rev*, 33(1):36–45. PMID:21624962

Harvey BJ, Miller AB, Baines CJ, Corey PN (1997). Effect of breast self-examination techniques on the risk of death from breast cancer. *CMAJ*, 157(9):1205–12. PMID:9361639

Holmberg L, Duffy SW, Yen AMF, Tabár L, Vitak B, Nyström L et al. (2009). Differences in endpoints between the Swedish W-E (two county) trial of mammographic screening and the Swedish overview: methodological consequences. *J Med Screen*, 16(2):73–80. doi:10.1258/jms.2009.008103 PMID:19564519

Holmberg L, Ekbom A, Calle E, Mokdad A, Byers T (1997). Breast cancer mortality in relation to self-reported use of breast self-examination. A cohort study of 450,000 women. *Breast Cancer Res Treat*, 43(2):137–40. doi:10.1023/A:1005788729145 PMID:9131269

Holmberg LH, Tabár L, Adami HO, Bergström R (1986). Survival in breast cancer diagnosed between mammographic screening examinations. *Lancet*, 328(8497):27–30. doi:10.1016/S0140-6736(86)92569-9 PMID:2873324

Huang Y, Kang M, Li H, Li JY, Zhang JY, Liu LH et al. (2012). Combined performance of physical examination, mammography, and ultrasonography for breast cancer screening among Chinese women: a follow-up study. *Curr Oncol*, 19(Suppl 2):eS22–30. doi:10.3747/co.19.1137 PMID:22876165

IARC (2002). Breast cancer screening. *IARC Handb Cancer Prev*, 7:1–229. Available from: http://www.iarc.fr/en/publications/pdfs-online/prev/handbook7/Handbook7_Breast.pdf.

Independent UK Panel on Breast Cancer Screening (2012). The benefits and harms of breast cancer screening: an independent review. *Lancet*, 380(9855):1778–86. doi:10.1016/S0140-6736(12)61611-0 PMID:23117178

Johns LE, Moss SM, Cuckle H, Bobrow L, Evans A, Kutt E et al.; Age Trial Management Group (2010a). False-positive results in the randomized controlled trial of mammographic screening from age 40 ("Age" trial). *Cancer Epidemiol Biomarkers Prev*, 19(11):2758–64. doi:10.1158/1055-9965.EPI-10-0623 PMID:20837718

Johns LE, Moss SM; Trial Management Group (2010b). Randomized controlled trial of mammographic screening from age 40 ('Age' trial): patterns of screening attendance. *J Med Screen*, 17(1):37–43. doi:10.1258/jms.2010.009091 PMID:20356944

Kerr M (1991). A case-control study of treatment adequacy and mortality from breast cancer for women age 40–49 years at entry into the National Breast Screening Study [dissertation]. Toronto, Canada: University of Toronto.

Kingston N, Thomas I, Johns L, Moss S; Trial Management Group (2010). Assessing the amount of unscheduled screening ("contamination") in the control arm of the UK "Age" Trial. *Cancer Epidemiol Biomarkers Prev*, 19(4):1132–6. doi:10.1158/1055-9965.EPI-09-0996 PMID:20233850

Kopans D (2014). Re: Twenty five year follow-up for breast cancer incidence and mortality of the Canadian National Breast Screening Study: randomised screening trial. http://www.bmj.com/content/348/bmj.g366?tab=responses

Kopans DB (1990). The Canadian screening program: a different perspective. *AJR Am J Roentgenol*, 155(4):748–9. doi:10.2214/ajr.155.4.ajronline_155_4_001

Kopans DB (1993). Mammography. *Lancet*, 341(8850):957 doi:10.1016/0140-6736(93)91246-I PMID:8096288

Kopans DB, Feig SA (1993). The Canadian National Breast Screening Study: a critical review. *AJR Am J Roentgenol*, 161(4):755–60. doi:10.2214/ajr.161.4.8372752 PMID:8372752

Kwong A, Cheung PS, Wong AY, Hung GT, Lo G, Tsao M et al. (2008). The acceptance and feasibility of breast cancer screening in the East. *Breast*, 17(1):42–50. doi:10.1016/j.breast.2007.06.005 PMID:17720500

Locker AP, Caseldine J, Mitchell AK, Blamey RW, Roebuck EJ, Elston CW (1989). Results from a seven-year programme of breast self-examination in 89,010 women. *Br J Cancer*, 60(3):401–5. doi:10.1038/bjc.1989.294 PMID:2789950

Lui CY, Lam HS, Chan LK, Tam KF, Chan CM, Leung TY et al. (2007). Opportunistic breast cancer screening in Hong Kong; a revisit of the Kwong Wah Hospital experience. *Hong Kong Med J*, 13(2):106–13. PMID:17406037

Magnus MC, Ping M, Shen MM, Bourgeois J, Magnus JH (2011). Effectiveness of mammography screening in reducing breast cancer mortality in women aged 39–49 years: a meta-analysis. *J Womens Health (Larchmt)*, 20(6):845–52. doi:10.1089/jwh.2010.2098 PMID:21413892

Mark K, Temkin SM, Terplan M (2014). Breast self-awareness: the evidence behind the euphemism. *Obstet Gynecol*, 123(4):734–6. doi:10.1097/AOG.0000000000000139 PMID:24785598

Marmot MG, Altman DG, Cameron DA, Dewar JA, Thompson SG, Wilcox M (2013). The benefits and harms of breast cancer screening: an independent review. *Br J Cancer*, 108(11):2205–40. doi:10.1038/bjc.2013.177 PMID:23744281

Miller AB (2001). Screening for breast cancer with mammography. *Lancet*, 358(9299):2164, author reply 2167–8. doi:10.1016/S0140-6736(01)07189-6 PMID:11784651

Miller AB (2004). Commentary: a defence of the Health Insurance Plan (HIP) study and the Canadian National Breast Screening Study (CNBSS). *Int J Epidemiol*, 33(1):64–5, discussion 69–73. doi:10.1093/ije/dyh015 PMID:15075146

Miller AB (2014). Implications of the Canadian National Breast Screening Study. *Womens Health (Lond Engl)*, 10(4):345–7. doi:10.2217/whe.14.25 PMID:25259895

Miller AB, Baines CJ, Sickles EA (1990). Canadian National Breast Screening Study. *AJR Am J Roentgenol*, 155(5):1133–4. doi:10.2214/ajr.155.5.2120947 PMID:2120947

Miller AB, Baines CJ, To T, Wall C (1992a). Canadian National Breast Screening Study: 1. Breast cancer detection and death rates among women aged 40 to 49 years. *CMAJ*, 147(10):1459–76. PMID:1423087

Miller AB, Baines CJ, To T, Wall C (1992b). Canadian National Breast Screening Study: 2. Breast cancer detection and death rates among women aged 50 to 59 years. *CMAJ*, 147(10):1477–88. PMID:1423088

Miller AB, Howe GR, Wall C (1981). The National Study of Breast Cancer Screening Protocol for a Canadian randomized controlled trial of screening for breast cancer in women. *Clin Invest Med*, 4(3–4):227–58. PMID:6802546

Miller AB, To T, Baines CJ, Wall C (2000). Canadian National Breast Screening Study-2: 13-year results of a randomized trial in women aged 50–59 years. *J Natl Cancer Inst*, 92(18):1490–9. doi:10.1093/jnci/92.18.1490 PMID:10995804

Miller AB, To T, Baines CJ, Wall C (2002). The Canadian National Breast Screening Study-1: breast cancer mortality after 11 to 16 years of follow-up. A randomized screening trial of mammography in women age 40 to 49 years. *Ann Intern Med*, 137(5 Part 1):305–12. doi:10.7326/0003-4819-137-5_Part_1-200209030-00005 PMID:12204013

Miller AB, Wall C, Baines CJ, Sun P, To T, Narod SA (2014a). Twenty five year follow-up for breast cancer incidence and mortality of the Canadian National Breast Screening Study: randomised screening trial. *BMJ*, 348:g366. doi:10.1136/bmj.g366 PMID:24519768

Miller AB, Wall C, Baines CJ, Sun P, To T, Narod SA (2014b). Re: Twenty five year follow-up for breast cancer incidence and mortality of the Canadian National Breast Screening Study: randomised screening trial. http://www.bmj.com/content/348/bmj.g366?tab=responses

Mittra I, Mishra GA, Singh S, Aranke S, Notani P, Badwe R et al. (2010). A cluster randomized, controlled trial of breast and cervix cancer screening in Mumbai, India: methodology and interim results after three rounds of screening. *Int J Cancer*, 126(4):976–84. doi:10.1002/ijc.24840 PMID:19697326

Morrison AS, Brisson J, Khalid N (1988). Breast cancer incidence and mortality in the Breast Cancer Detection Demonstration Project [published erratum appears in *J Natl Cancer Inst* (1989) Oct 4; 81(19):1513]. *J Natl Cancer Inst*, 80(19):1540–7. doi:10.1093/jnci/80.19.1540 PMID:3193469

Moskowitz M (1992). Guidelines for screening for breast cancer. Is a revision in order? *Radiol Clin North Am*, 30(1):221–33. PMID:1732929

Moss S (1999). A trial to study the effect on breast cancer mortality of annual mammographic screening in women starting at age 40. *J Med Screen*, 6(3):144–8. doi:10.1136/jms.6.3.144 PMID:10572845

Moss S (2005). Overdiagnosis and overtreatment of breast cancer: overdiagnosis in randomised controlled trials of breast cancer screening. *Breast Cancer Res*, 7(5):230–4. doi:10.1186/bcr1314 PMID:16168145

Moss S, Thomas I, Evans A, Thomas B, Johns L; Trial Management Group (2005b). Randomised controlled trial of mammographic screening in women from age 40: results of screening in the first 10 years. *Br J Cancer*, 92(5):949–54. doi:10.1038/sj.bjc.6602396 PMID:15726102

Moss S, Waller M, Anderson TJ, Cuckle H; Trial Management Group (2005a). Randomised controlled trial of mammographic screening in women from age 40: predicted mortality based on surrogate outcome measures. *Br J Cancer*, 92(5):955–60. PMID:15726103

Moss SM, Coleman DA, Ellman R, Chamberlain J, Forrest AP, Kirkpatrick AE et al. (1993). Interval cancers and sensitivity in the screening centres of the UK Trial of Early Detection of Breast Cancer. *Eur J Cancer*, 29A(2):255–8. doi:10.1016/0959-8049(93)90187-K PMID:8422291

Moss SM, Cuckle H, Evans A, Johns L, Waller M, Bobrow L; Trial Management Group (2006). Effect of mammographic screening from age 40 years on breast cancer mortality at 10 years' follow-up: a randomised controlled trial. *Lancet*, 368(9552):2053–60. doi:10.1016/S0140-6736(06)69834-6 PMID:17161727

Muscat JE, Huncharek MS (1991). Breast self-examination and extent of disease: a population-based study. *Cancer Detect Prev*, 15(2):155–9. PMID:2032258

Nelson HD, Tyne K, Naik A, Bougatsos C, Chan BK, Humphrey L; U.S. Preventive Services Task Force (2009). Screening for breast cancer: an update for the U.S. Preventive Services Task Force. *Ann Intern Med*, 151(10):727–37, W237–42. doi:10.7326/0003-4819-151-10-200911170-00009 PMID:19920273

Newcomb PA, Weiss NS, Storer BE, Scholes D, Young BE, Voigt LF (1991). Breast self-examination in relation to the occurrence of advanced breast cancer. *J Natl Cancer Inst*, 83(4):260–5. doi:10.1093/jnci/83.4.260 PMID:1994055

Njor SH, Garne JP, Lynge E (2013). Over-diagnosis estimate from The Independent UK Panel on Breast Cancer Screening is based on unsuitable data. *J Med Screen*, 20(2):104–5. doi:10.1177/0969141313495190 PMID:24065032

Nyström L, Andersson I, Bjurstam N, Frisell J, Nordenskjöld B, Rutqvist LE (2002a). Long-term effects of mammography screening: updated overview of the Swedish randomised trials. *Lancet*, 359(9310):909–19. doi:10.1016/S0140-6736(02)08020-0 PMID:11918907

Nyström L, Andersson I, Bjurstam N, Frisell J, Rutqvist LE (2002b). Update on effects of screening mammography. Authors' reply. *Lancet*, 360(9329):339–40. doi:10.1016/S0140-6736(02)09527-2

Oestreicher N, Lehman CD, Seger DJ, Buist DS, White E (2005). The incremental contribution of clinical breast examination to invasive cancer detection in a mammography screening program. *AJR Am J Roentgenol*, 184(2):428–32. doi:10.2214/ajr.184.2.01840428 PMID:15671358

Olsen O, Gøtzsche PC (2001). Cochrane review on screening for breast cancer with mammography. *Lancet*, 358(9290):1340–2. doi:10.1016/S0140-6736(01)06449-2 PMID:11684218

Paap E, Verbeek A, Puliti D, Broeders M, Paci E (2011). Minor influence of self-selection bias on the effectiveness of breast cancer screening in case-control studies in the Netherlands. *J Med Screen*, 18(3):142–6. doi:10.1258/jms.2011.011027 PMID:22045823

Paap E, Verbeek AL, Botterweck AA, van Doorne-Nagtegaal HJ, Imhof-Tas M, de Koning HJ et al. (2014). Breast cancer screening halves the risk of breast cancer death: a case-referent study. *Breast*, 23(4):439–44. doi:10.1016/j.breast.2014.03.002 PMID:24713277

Pisani P, Parkin DM, Ngelangel C, Esteban D, Gibson L, Munson M et al. (2006). Outcome of screening by clinical examination of the breast in a trial in the Philippines. *Int J Cancer*, 118(1):149–54. doi:10.1002/ijc.21343 PMID:16049976

Porta M, editor (2014). A dictionary of epidemiology, 5th edition. Online version. Oxford University Press. Available from: http://www.oxfordreference.com/view/10.1093/acref/9780195314496.001.0001/acref-9780195314496.

Puliti D, Miccinesi G, Paci E (2011). Overdiagnosis in breast cancer: design and methods of estimation in observational studies. *Prev Med*, 53(3):131–3. doi:10.1016/j.ypmed.2011.05.012 PMID:21658405

Rijnsburger AJ, van Oortmarssen GJ, Boer R, Draisma G, To T, Miller AB et al. (2004). Mammography benefit in the Canadian National Breast Screening Study-2: a model evaluation. *Int J Cancer*, 110(5):756–62. doi:10.1002/ijc.20143 PMID:15146566

Sankaranarayanan R, Ramadas K, Thara S, Muwonge R, Prabhakar J, Augustine P et al. (2011). Clinical breast examination: preliminary results from a cluster randomized controlled trial in India. *J Natl Cancer Inst*, 103(19):1476–80. doi:10.1093/jnci/djr304 PMID:21862730

Semiglazov VF, Manikhas AG, Moiseenko VM, Protsenko SA, Kharikova RS, Seleznev IK et al. (2003). Results of a prospective randomized investigation [Russia (St Petersburg)/WHO] to evaluate the significance of self-examination for the early detection of breast cancer [in Russian]. *Vopr Onkol*, 49(4):434–41. PMID:14569932

Semiglazov VF, Moiseenko VM, Manikhas AG, Protsenko SA, Kharikova RS, Popova RT et al. (1999a). Interim results of a prospective randomized study of self-examination for early detection of breast cancer (Russia (St Petersburg)/WHO) [in Russian]. *Vopr Onkol*, 45(3):265–71. PMID:10443229

Semiglazov VF, Moiseyenko VM, Manikhas AG, Protsenko SA, Kharikova RS, Ivanov VG et al. (1999b). Role of breast self-examination in early detection of breast cancer: Russia/WHO prospective randomized trial in St. Petersburg. *Cancer Strategy*, 1:145–51.

Shapiro S (1977). Evidence on screening for breast cancer from a randomized trial. *Cancer*, 39(6 Suppl): 2772–82. doi:10.1002/1097-0142(197706)39:6<2772::AID-CN-CR2820390665>3.0.CO;2-K PMID:326378

Shapiro S (1994). Screening: assessment of current studies. *Cancer*, 74(Suppl 1):231–8. doi:10.1002/cncr.2820741306 PMID:8004592

Shapiro S (1997). Periodic screening for breast cancer: the HIP randomized controlled trial. Health Insurance Plan. *J Natl Cancer Inst Monogr*, (22):27–30. PMID:9709271

Shapiro S, Strax P, Venet L (1966). Evaluation of periodic breast cancer screening with mammography. Methodology and early observations. *JAMA*, 195(9):731–8. doi:10.1001/jama.1966.03100090065016 PMID:5951878

Shapiro S, Strax P, Venet L (1971). Periodic breast cancer screening in reducing mortality from breast cancer. *JAMA*, 215(11):1777–85. doi:10.1001/jama.1971.03180240027005 PMID:5107709

Shapiro S, Venet W, Strax P, Venet L (1988). Screening for breast cancer: the Health Insurance Plan project and its sequelae, 1963–1986. Baltimore (MD), USA: The Johns Hopkins University Press.

Smith RA (2000). Breast cancer screening among women younger than age 50: a current assessment of the issues. *CA Cancer J Clin*, 50(5):312–36. PMID:11075240

Tabár L (2014). Re: Twenty five year follow-up for breast cancer incidence and mortality of the Canadian National Breast Screening Study: randomised screening trial. http://www.bmj.com/content/348/bmj.g366?tab=responses

Tabár L, Chen H-HT, Duffy SW, Krusemo UB (1999). Primary and adjuvant therapy, prognostic factors and survival in 1053 breast cancers diagnosed in a trial of mammography screening. *Jpn J Clin Oncol*, 29(12):608–16. doi:10.1093/jjco/29.12.608 PMID:10721943

Tabár L, Chen HH, Yen AM, Chen SL, Fann JC, Chiu SY et al. (2015b). Response to Miller et al. *Breast J*, 21(4):459–61. doi:10.1111/tbj.12439 PMID:26010345

Tabár L, Duffy SW, Yen MF, Warwick J, Vitak B, Chen HH et al. (2002). All-cause mortality among breast cancer patients in a screening trial: support for breast cancer mortality as an end point. *J Med Screen*, 9(4):159–62. doi:10.1136/jms.9.4.159 PMID:12518005

Tabár L, Fagerberg CJ, Gad A, Baldetorp L, Holmberg LH, Gröntoft O et al. (1985). Reduction in mortality from breast cancer after mass screening with mammography. Randomised trial from the Breast Cancer Screening Working Group of the Swedish National Board of Health and Welfare. *Lancet*, 1(8433):829–32. doi:10.1016/S0140-6736(85)92204-4 PMID:2858707

Tabár L, Fagerberg G, Chen HH, Duffy SW, Smart CR, Gad A et al. (1995). Efficacy of breast cancer screening by age. New results from the Swedish Two-County Trial. *Cancer*, 75(10):2507–17.

doi:10.1002/1097-0142(19950515)75:10<2507::AID-CNCR2820751017>3.0.CO;2-H PMID:7736395

Tabár L, Fagerberg G, Duffy SW, Day NE, Gad A, Gröntoft O (1992). Update of the Swedish two-county program of mammographic screening for breast cancer. *Radiol Clin North Am*, 30(1):187–210. PMID:1732926

Tabár L, Vitak B, Chen HH, Duffy SW, Yen MF, Chiang CF et al. (2000). The Swedish Two-County Trial twenty years later. Updated mortality results and new insights from long-term follow-up. *Radiol Clin North Am*, 38(4):625–51. doi:10.1016/S0033-8389(05)70191-3 PMID:10943268

Tabár L, Vitak B, Chen TH, Yen AM, Cohen A, Tot T et al. (2011). Swedish two-county trial: impact of mammographic screening on breast cancer mortality during 3 decades. *Radiology*, 260(3):658–63. doi:10.1148/radiol.11110469 PMID:21712474

Tabár L, Yen AM-F, Wu WY-Y, Chen SL-S, Chiu SY-H, Fann JC-Y et al. (2015a). Insights from the breast cancer screening trials: how screening affects the natural history of breast cancer and implications for evaluating service screening programs. *Breast J*, 21(1):13–20. doi:10.1111/tbj.12354 PMID:25413699

Thomas DB, Gao DL, Ray RM, Wang WW, Allison CJ, Chen FL et al. (2002). Randomized trial of breast self-examination in Shanghai: final results. *J Natl Cancer Inst*, 94(19):1445–57. doi:10.1093/jnci/94.19.1445 PMID:12359854

Thomas DB, Gao DL, Self SG, Allison CJ, Tao Y, Mahloch J et al. (1997). Randomized trial of breast self-examination in Shanghai: methodology and preliminary results. *J Natl Cancer Inst*, 89(5):355–65. doi:10.1093/jnci/89.5.355 PMID:9060957

Thornton H, Pillarisetti RR (2008). 'Breast awareness' and 'breast self-examination' are not the same. What do these terms mean? Why are they confused? What can we do? *Eur J Cancer*, 44(15):2118–21. doi:10.1016/j.ejca.2008.08.015 PMID:18805689

Tu SP, Reisch LM, Taplin SH, Kreuter W, Elmore JG, Legge Muilenburg J (2006). Breast self-examination: self-reported frequency, quality, and associated outcomes. *J Cancer Educ*, 21(3):175–81. doi:10.1207/s15430154jce2103_18 PMID:17371185

UK Trial of Early Detection of Breast Cancer Group (1988). First results on mortality reduction in the UK Trial of Early Detection of Breast Cancer. *Lancet*, 2(8608):411–6. PMID:2900351

UK Trial of Early Detection of Breast Cancer Group (1993). Breast cancer mortality after 10 years in the UK Trial of Early Detection of Breast Cancer. *Breast*, 2(1):13–20. doi:10.1016/0960-9776(93)90031-A

UK Trial of Early Detection of Breast Cancer Group (1999). 16-year mortality from breast cancer in the UK Trial of Early Detection of Breast Cancer. *Lancet*, 353(9168):1909–14. doi:10.1016/S0140-6736(98)07412-1 PMID:10371568

van Schoor G, Moss SM, Otten JD, Donders R, Paap E, den Heeten GJ et al. (2011a). Increasingly strong reduction in breast cancer mortality due to screening. *Br J Cancer*, 104(6):910–4. doi:10.1038/bjc.2011.44 PMID:21343930

van Schoor G, Paap E, Broeders MJ, Verbeek AL (2011b). Residual confounding after adjustment for age: a minor issue in breast cancer screening effectiveness. *Eur J Epidemiol*, 26(8):585–8. doi:10.1007/s10654-011-9584-3 PMID:21519892

Weiss NS (2014). All-cause mortality as an outcome in epidemiologic studies: proceed with caution. *Eur J Epidemiol*, 29(3):147–9. PMID:24729152

Wilke LG, Broadwater G, Rabiner S, Owens E, Yoon S, Ghate S et al. (2009). Breast self-examination: defining a cohort still in need. *Am J Surg*, 198(4):575–9. doi:10.1016/j.amjsurg.2009.06.012 PMID:19800471

Yen AM, Duffy SW, Chen TH, Chen LS, Chiu SY, Fann JC et al. (2012). Long-term incidence of breast cancer by trial arm in one county of the Swedish Two-County Trial of mammographic screening. *Cancer*, 118(23):5728–32. doi:10.1002/cncr.27580 PMID:22605639

Yen MF, Tabár L, Vitak B, Smith RA, Chen HH, Duffy SW (2003). Quantifying the potential problem of overdiagnosis of ductal carcinoma in situ in breast cancer screening. *Eur J Cancer*, 39(12):1746–54. doi:10.1016/S0959-8049(03)00260-0 PMID:12888370

Zackrisson S, Andersson I, Janzon L, Manjer J, Garne JP (2006). Rate of over-diagnosis of breast cancer 15 years after end of Malmö mammographic screening trial: follow-up study. *BMJ*, 332(7543):689–92. doi:10.1136/bmj.38764.572569.7C PMID:16517548

Zahl P-H, Gøtzsche PC, Andersen JM, Maehlen J (2006). Results of the Two-County trial of mammography screening are not compatible with contemporaneous official Swedish breast cancer statistics. *Dan Med Bull*, 53(4):438–40. PMID:17150148

5. EFFECTIVENESS OF BREAST CANCER SCREENING

This section considers measures of screening quality and major beneficial and harmful outcomes. Beneficial outcomes include reductions in deaths from breast cancer and in advanced-stage disease, and the main example of a harmful outcome is overdiagnosis of breast cancer. The absolute reduction in breast cancer mortality achieved by a particular screening programme is the most crucial indicator of a programme's effectiveness. This may vary according to the risk of breast cancer death in the target population, the rate of participation in screening programmes, and the time scale observed (Duffy et al., 2013). The technical quality of the screening, in both radiographic and radiological terms, also has an impact on breast cancer mortality. The observational analysis of breast cancer mortality and of a screening programme's performance may be assessed against several process indicators. The major indicators of both the screening process and the clinical outcome, and the associated analytical methodologies, are described below.

5.1 Indicators for monitoring and evaluating effectiveness

5.1.1 Performance indicators

As a general principle, the most important indicator of the effectiveness of a screening programme is its effect on breast cancer mortality. Nevertheless, the performance of a screening programme should be monitored to identify and remedy shortcomings before enough time has elapsed to enable observation of mortality effects.

(a) Screening standards

The randomized trials performed during the past 30 years have enabled the suggestion of several indicators of quality assurance for screening services (Day et al., 1989; Tabár et al., 1992; Feig, 2007; Perry et al., 2008; Wilson & Liston, 2011), including screening participation rates, rates of recall for assessment, rates of percutaneous and surgical biopsy, and breast cancer detection rates. Detection rates are often classified by invasive/in situ status, tumour size, lymph-node status, and histological grade.

Table 5.1 and Table 5.2 show selected quality standards developed in England by the National Health Service (NHS) (Wilson & Liston, 2011; Department of Health, 2013) and in the USA by the Agency for Health Care Policy and Research and endorsed by the American College of Radiology, respectively (Bassett et al., 1994; D'Orsi et al., 2013). Similar sets of standards exist for screening in Australia, Canada, and Europe (National Quality Management Committee of BreastScreen Australia, 2008; Perry et al., 2008; CPAC, 2013) (see Section 3.2). The programmes specify standards – related mainly to the screening process and not directly to technical

Table 5.1 Minimum quality standards and targets considered in the National Health Service breast screening programme in England

Criterion	Standard	Target
Attendance at screening	≥ 70%	80%
Invasive cancers detected, prevalent screen	≥ 3.6/1000	≥ 5.1/1000
Invasive cancers detected, incident screen	≥ 4.1/1000	≥ 5.7/1000
In situ cancers detected, prevalent screen	≥ 0.5/1000	None specified
In situ cancers detected, incident screen	≥ 0.6/1000	None specified
Standardized detection ratio	≥ 1.0	≥ 1.4
Invasive cancers < 15 mm, prevalent screen	≥ 2.0/1000	≥ 2.8/1000
Invasive cancers < 15 mm, incident screen	≥ 2.3/1000	≥ 3.1/1000
Mean glandular radiation dose for standard breast	≤ 2.5 mGy	None specified
Number of repeat examinations (% of total examinations)	< 3%	< 2%
Recall for assessment (% of prevalent screens)	< 10%	< 7%
Recall for assessment (% of incident screens)	< 7%	< 5%
Short-term recall (% of screened women)	< 0.25%	≤ 0.12%
Non-operative diagnosis (% of cancers)	≥ 90%	≥ 95%
Non-operative diagnosis (% of DCIS)	≥ 85%	≥ 90%
Benign biopsies (prevalent screens)	< 1.5/1000	< 1.0/1000
Benign biopsies (incident screens)	< 1.0/1000	< 0.75/1000
Interval cancers within 24 months (screened women)	≤ 1.2/1000	None specified
Interval cancers within 25–36 months	≤ 1.4/1000	None specified
Percentage rescreened within 36 months	≥ 90%	100%
Percentage receiving screening result within 2 weeks	≥ 90%	100%
Assessed within 3 weeks (% of total assessed)	≥ 90%	100%
Percentage non-operative biopsies with result within 1 week	≥ 90%	100%
Percentage referred to surgeon receiving surgical assessment within 1 week	≥ 90%	100%
Percentage admitted for treatment within 2 months of referral	≥ 90%	100%

DCIS, ductal carcinoma in situ.
Adapted from Wilson & Liston (2011) and Department of Health (2013).

aspects of image quality – that all units should attain, as well as achievable targets at which units should aim.

Table 5.1 pertains to a programme that targets women aged 50–70 years with a maximum screening interval of 36 months in high-incidence countries. In the example in England, two-view mammography is used, and the programme changed from film to digital mammography during 2010–2014.

Minimum standards are specified for screening attendance and detection rates, in particular detection rates of small cancers, which are expected to be high in an effective screening programme. Maximum standards are specified for adverse effects of screening, such as radiation dose, and for rates of interval cancers, repeat examinations, and recalls for assessment. In addition, maximum times to events in the screening, diagnostic, and treatment processes are specified; these are important for the patient's experience and quality of life, although they do not necessarily reflect clinical or radiological quality.

Some of the criteria and standards are very specific to the programme. For example, the randomized trials of breast screening observe a higher rate of breast cancer detection at the prevalent (first) screen than at incident (subsequent) screens (see, for example, Tabár et al.,

Table 5.2 Minimum quality standards for mammography in the USA[a]

Criterion	Standard
Recall rate for assessment (% of screened women)	< 10%
Cancer detection rate, prevalent screen (per 1000 screened)	6–10
Cancer detection rate, incident screen (per 1000 screened)	2–4
Positive predictive value of recall for assessment	5–10%
Positive predictive value of biopsy	25–40%
Proportion of screen-detected cancers in situ or TNM stage 0–I	> 50%
Proportion of screen-detected node-positive cancers	< 25%

[a] Values are specified by the United States Agency for Health Care Policy and Research and endorsed by the American College of Radiology.
TNM, tumour–node–metastasis staging system of malignant tumours (see Section 1, Table 1.9).
Adapted from Bassett et al. (1994) and D'Orsi et al. (2013).

1992). However, the detection rate standards are expected to be higher for incident screens because these values are based not on observations of a cohort recruited at the prevalent screen and followed up thereafter but on a programme in which prevalent screens usually take place at about age 50 years and incident screens on average at about age 60 years (when the underlying risk of cancer is higher).

Another measure that is used in the United Kingdom is the standardized detection ratio, obtained by comparing the observed detection rates of invasive cancers by age with those of the Swedish Two-County trial (Tabár et al., 1992), on which the United Kingdom breast screening programme was modelled. At present, the standard is almost invariably exceeded (NHSBSP, 2009), probably at least partly due to the fact that breast cancer incidence in the United Kingdom in the 21st century is higher than that in Sweden in the 1970s and 1980s. This example implies that standards should be revised over time, although it has also been observed that lower standards followed by remedial action have conferred substantial improvements in programme performancc (Blanks et al., 2002). Wallis et al. (2008) gave a demonstration of how careful surveillance of audit standards can lead to changes in practice and improved performance at the local and national levels.

Indicators such as detection rates are typically part of the monitoring system of most screening programmes, but the actual target values will vary according to the screening regimen, the target population, the underlying incidence in the programme's location, and possibly aspects of the health-care delivery systems and the medicolegal environment (Klabunde et al., 2001).

Table 5.2 shows selected standards developed in the USA. These standards include acceptable ranges for positive predictive values (PPVs) of recall for assessment and for recommendation for biopsy. They specify that the proportion of cases recalled for assessment that result in diagnosis of cancer should be 5–10%, and that the proportion of biopsies that result in diagnosis of cancer should be 25–40%. These are powerful measures of the process since they reflect detection rates, recall rates, and biopsy rates.

(b) *Screening sensitivity and interval cancers*

In a screening setting, the prevalence of the disease in screened subjects, expressed as a proportion, is usually very low; a very small number of those screened at each screening round are diagnosed with cancer, whereas thousands of women are screened negative. Typically, in European screening programmes, per 10 000 women screened, about 9500 will have a normal initial result and about 500 will be recalled for further assessment, of whom about 70 will have breast cancer. After the screen, about 10–30 will present with symptomatic interval cancer.

Components of the quality monitoring data listed above can be useful to estimate some important attributes of the screening programme, notably the specificity and sensitivity (the correct classification of negative and positive subjects) and the PPV. Specificity estimates the false-positives, or the complement of the proportion of screened-negative cases that are recalled for further assessment. The classic definition of test sensitivity is the probability that if the screening test is applied to someone with the disease, a positive diagnosis will result. PPV is the proportion of test-positive subjects who are diagnosed as cases at the end of the screening episode and is a function of the prevalence of the lesion. There are costs, both human and economic, to achieving a good balance of these performance parameters.

Other parameters of cancer detection have been defined by Hakama et al. (2007): test sensitivity, programme sensitivity, and episode sensitivity.

(i) Test sensitivity

In a clinical setting, test sensitivity is usually measured by comparison with a "gold standard". This is rarely possible in a screening setting, where the objective of the test is the detection of a lesion in the preclinical detectable phase, and where only those with suspicious initial screening findings receive further investigation. Test sensitivity is the number of cancers detected at a screen divided by the sum of those detected at the screen plus the false-negatives. In principle, the false-negatives can be identified by a radiological audit of the original screening mammograms in those screened negative and subsequently diagnosed with interval breast cancer (Houssami et al., 2006; Perry et al., 2006). This method of estimation involves assumptions about the audit quality, and the audit itself consumes resources, but it is a crucial learning tool and has the potential to improve the programme's ability to detect early-stage cancers.

In the past, a common convention has been to estimate sensitivity as the number of cancers detected at a screen divided by the sum of those detected at the screen plus the interval cancers arising within 1 year. Two main sources of error have been identified: first, the interval cancers arising within 1 year will include true negatives that have entered the preclinical detectable phase during that year, and, second, they will not exclude those cancers missed at the screen but taking longer than 1 year to arise symptomatically (Day, 1985). The reasoning implies that interval cancers are a mixture of missed and newly arising cancers, which tend to be more rapidly developing tumours. This, in turn, suggests that interval cancers will also be a mixture with respect to the aggressive potential of the cancers. In the epoch of film mammography, test sensitivity was reported to range from 83% to 95%, with the higher values observed for screening women older than 50 years (Mushlin et al., 1998). In the epoch of digital mammography, the difference in sensitivity between age groups may be smaller (Vinnicombe et al., 2009).

(ii) Programme sensitivity

Programme sensitivity may be defined as the proportion of cancers diagnosed among women attending a screening programme or as the proportion of cancers diagnosed in the screening-eligible population. The first definition is the number of screen-detected cases divided by the sum of the screen-detected cancers plus the interval cancers. The second definition includes in the denominator cancers diagnosed among those who were invited but did not attend screening. Programme sensitivity is often described as the ability of the programme to detect cancers. It is generally estimated from steady-state screening, from the numbers of cancers diagnosed at several incident screens (not from prevalent screening) and the symptomatic cancers occurring in the same number of intervals between screens.

Programme sensitivity depends on the test sensitivity, the screening interval, and (depending on which measure is used) the attendance rate. It is typically estimated to be 50–60% (Anttila et al., 2002; Zorzi et al., 2010). This means that in organized programmes, about half of the cancers in the target population are detected by screening. Of course, this will depend strongly on the rate of participation in screening.

(iii) Episode sensitivity

Hakama et al. (2007) defined episode sensitivity as the incidence reduction in a specified period after screening compared with the expected incidence in the absence of screening, that is $1 - (P_1/P_0)$, where P_1 is the incidence among the screened subjects in the specified period after screening and P_0 is the expected incidence in the absence of screening (which, in practice, is difficult to estimate).

Taylor et al. (2002, 2004) reviewed estimates of the proportional incidence in the first year of the screening interval, comparing international data published since 1975 and including results from randomized trials and service screening programmes in Australia, Canada, Italy, the Netherlands, Scandinavia, the United Kingdom, and the USA (Health Insurance Plan study). A large variability was reported, with an overall point estimate of the proportional incidence of 18.5% from all randomized trials and 27.3% from service screening programmes, corresponding to episode sensitivity estimates of 91.5% for the randomized trials and 72.7% for service screening.

A pooled analysis in the service screening centres of six European countries (Törnberg et al., 2010) reported a large variation in screening sensitivity and performance, with a proportional incidence of 46% (episode sensitivity, 54%) in the 24 months after screening. The European standards (Perry et al., 2006) were 30% and 50% for the proportional incidence at the prevalent screen and at subsequent screenings, respectively, corresponding to recommended episode sensitivities of 70% and 50%, respectively.

(iv) Interval cancers

Note that all three measures discussed above require an estimation of interval cancer incidence. This illustrates the crucial nature of interval cancers in programme evaluation. Whereas screen detection rates are important, the future cancer risk in those screened negative is at least equally informative about the programme's ability to detect cancer in the preclinical phase.

Bennett et al. (2011) noted the complexity of the evaluation of interval cancers on a large scale. They analysed 26 475 interval cancers in the NHS Breast Screening Programme (England, Wales, and Northern Ireland) and found a large variability in the regional estimates, with an estimate of a higher level than expected on the basis of the randomized trial experience. The conclusion was that comparison of different programmes is possible only if the methodology used is very thorough and guidelines are agreed upon in advance, with accurate follow-up and homogeneous reporting.

Table 5.1 includes standards for maximum interval cancer rates, that is, rates of symptomatic cancers that are diagnosed after a screen with negative findings and before the next scheduled screen (usually a period of 1–3 years). Together with prompt and nearly complete cancer registration, the interval cancer rate can be a powerful indicator of screening quality (Bennett et al., 2011). The observation that interval cancer rates were very high in the early years of the United Kingdom programme in the East of England prompted a radiological audit, which consisted of re-reading previous screening mammograms, both of interval cancers and of non-cancers, without knowledge of the diagnostic result (Day et al., 1995). This identified issues of sensitivity, which were later remedied, and served as a learning resource for quality improvement in other regions of England (Duncan & Wallis, 1995). Interval cancer rates are now considerably lower in the East of England and similar to those in the rest of the United Kingdom (Bennett et al., 2011; Offman & Duffy, 2012). The radiological audit of advanced disease may be suggested in health-care settings where cancer registration systems do not sufficiently identify interval cancers.

Interval cancer rates can also yield inferences about the effect of changes to the screening regimen. The policy of two-view mammography for incident screens was shown first to increase detection rates (Blanks et al., 2005) and subsequently to reduce interval cancer rates by almost exactly the same absolute numbers (Dibden et al., 2014). The concomitant reduction in interval cancer rates gave some assurance that the increased detection capability was not an overdiagnosis phenomenon.

Estimates and characteristics of interval cancers in national and regional screening programmes have been published, confirming the need for surveillance and improvement of service screening (Ganry et al., 2001; Wang et al., 2001; Hofvind et al., 2006; Bucchi et al., 2008; Domingo et al., 2013a; Carbonaro et al., 2014; Dibden et al., 2014; José Bento et al., 2014; Renart-Vicens et al., 2014).

The relationship between detection modality and tumour characteristics of breast cancers has been investigated ever since the first randomized trials (Duffy et al., 1991). Recently, the renewed interest in interval cases and their radiological classification (Houssami et al., 2006) has enabled the analysis of tumour characteristics by detection mode and interval type in terms of new biomolecular classifications and mammographic breast density at screening. Such analyses, along with recent findings with respect to genetic predisposition, have raised interest in personalized screening (Hall & Easton, 2013). Although personalized screening is not simple to incorporate into existing programmes (Paci & Giorgi Rossi, 2010), such interest does indicate that investigation of interval cancers can inform hypotheses to potentially improve screening policy.

(c) Breast cancer mortality

As noted above, the most telling indicator of the effectiveness of a screening programme is its effect on breast cancer mortality. However, estimating this effect is not straightforward (Duffy et al., 2007; Otten et al., 2008; Broeders et al., 2012; Independent UK Panel on Breast Cancer Screening, 2012). Temporal and geographical comparisons are potentially confounded with other parameters that influence breast cancer mortality; simultaneous temporal and geographical control yields more directly interpretable results (Otto et al., 2003; Olsen et al., 2005). The introduction of breast screening as in Finland, with date-of-birth clusters randomized to receive screening first, yields results that may be interpretable directly as estimates of the efficacy of the programme (Hakama et al., 1997). It is worth noting that such designs do not obviate the need for sufficient follow-up. In absolute terms, in the early years of a programme the adverse effects are enumerable, but the benefits in terms of numbers of breast cancer deaths avoided are not.

Arguably the most important issue for observational evaluation of screening and breast cancer mortality is the diagnostic period. Because of the generally good breast cancer survival rates, unrefined mortality (used hereafter to denote breast cancer mortality regardless of the time of diagnosis) in the epoch of screening will be contaminated by a substantial numbers of deaths from cancers diagnosed before screening was initiated (Duffy et al., 2007). This will tend to bias results against screening. The bias can be avoided by using refined or incidence-based mortality (IBM), where mortality is ascertained specific to the diagnostic period (Olsen et al., 2005; Swedish Organised Service Screening Evaluation Group,

2006a, b). Alternatively, the bias can be minimized by estimating the mortality effect in a period beginning some years after the start of screening, albeit with some qualifications on interpretation (Duffy et al., 2010).

Epoch of diagnosis also has implications for treatment and management of breast cancer, so that the before–after comparisons of mortality are almost invariably confounded with changes in treatment, as with the expansion in use of adjuvant systemic therapies in the 1980s and 1990s. This is considered further in Section 5.1.2.

Concerns have been expressed with respect to ascertainment of cause of death (Gøtzsche & Jørgensen, 2013). Results suggest that this is not a serious cause of bias (Goldoni et al., 2009; Holmberg et al., 2009), partly because the number of women with advanced breast cancer who do not die of breast cancer is limited (de Koning et al., 1992). In any case, it can be addressed by estimating the effect of screening on excess mortality in breast cancer cases, which does not require individual determination of cause of death (Jonsson et al., 2007).

Methods and results in terms of breast cancer screening and mortality are dealt with in more detail in Section 5.1.2, and possible surrogate indicators of breast cancer mortality are considered in Section 5.1.3.

5.1.2 Study designs to assess the effectiveness of screening

(a) General principles

Attempts to estimate exact proportions of recent reductions in breast cancer mortality are subject to difficulties in modelling and interpreting the dynamism of incidence, behaviour, screening policy, treatment policy, and the correlations among these. In addition, there are always difficulties in interpreting directions of causality in changes, particularly in breast cancer incidence.

The main observational methods to assess the effect of screening are: (i) analysis of temporal trends in unrefined breast cancer mortality, reporting annual percentage changes in screening and pre-screening periods and change points when trends are estimated to change in magnitude or direction; (ii) comparison of unrefined mortality rates in screening or invited exposed populations with temporal, geographical, or other demographic control; (iii) the same comparison using IBM; and (iv) case–control studies where women who have died of breast cancer are compared with women who have not, with respect to screening histories before diagnosis of the case. In addition, modelling studies can provide information on outcomes beyond the limits of observational studies. This section outlines the principles and practice of each method, illustrating them with published results. First, two commonly occurring biases, and possible methods for their correction, are described.

(i) Self-selection for screening

Any estimate of the effect of being screened might be biased by factors influencing self-selection, such as the risk of death from breast cancer. In the Swedish breast screening trials, women not attending screening had a 36% higher risk of death from breast cancer compared with the uninvited control group (Duffy et al., 2002a). This was a combination of a lower incidence of breast cancer and a considerably higher case fatality rate (Duffy et al., 1991). A difference of this nature would induce a bias in favour of screening if not addressed by design or analysis.

Cuzick et al. (1997) developed a method to correct for this bias in randomized controlled trials (RCTs), assuming a latent non-attender population in the control group. Duffy et al. (2002a) adapted this for case–control studies and later for other designs of observational studies (Swedish Organised Service Screening Evaluation Group, 2006a). The correction depends crucially

Table 5.3 Odds ratios, with and without correction for self-selection bias, for breast cancer mortality associated with screening in five regions of the Netherlands

Region[a]	Uncorrected OR (95% CI)	RR, non-participants/uninvited (95% CI)[b]	OR corrected for self-selection bias (95% CI)
1	0.67 (0.42–1.08)	0.64 (0.46–0.90)	0.40 (0.22–0.74)
2	0.52 (0.38–0.73)	0.77 (0.63–0.93)	0.38 (0.25–0.57)
3	0.27 (0.12–0.62)	0.92 (0.65–1.30)	0.24 (0.10–0.62)
4	0.44 (0.32–0.60)	1.08 (0.82–1.43)	0.49 (0.30–0.78)
5	0.46 (0.30–0.72)	1.08 (0.85–1.37)	0.51 (0.30–0.87)

[a] Region 1: Bevolkingsonderzoek Noord-Nederland; region 2: IKA; region 3: Limburg; region 4: Bevolkingsonderzoek Borstkanker Zuidwest Nederland; region 5: Vroege Opsporing Kanker Oost-Nederland.

[b] Region-specific estimates of the relative risk of breast cancer death in non-participants compared with uninvited women.

CI, confidence interval; OR, odds ratio; RR, relative risk.

Adapted from *Breast*, Volume 23, issue 4, Paap et al. (2014), Breast cancer screening halves the risk of breast cancer death: a case-referent study, pages 439–444, Copyright (2014), with permission from Elsevier.

on an estimate of the relative risk of breast cancer death in non-attenders compared with an uninvited population. Although this can be readily estimated within a given trial, in observational studies this is not generally the case. In the past, observational studies have relied on a relative risk estimate of 1.36 from the Swedish trials (e.g. Allgood et al., 2008) and, more recently, on estimates from the target population (Paap et al., 2011). Paap et al. (2011) noted that in the Netherlands, the non-participant population had, if anything, a lower a priori risk of breast cancer death compared with the participant population. Table 5.3 shows the odds ratios (with and without correction for self-selection bias) for breast cancer mortality associated with screening, and the relative risks for non-participants in screening, in five regions of the Netherlands. Those regions with a non-participant relative risk greater than 1 had a corrected odds ratio that was less extreme than the uncorrected one, whereas those regions with a non-participant relative risk less than 1 had a more extreme corrected odds ratio. This leads to the observation that in the organized screening in the Netherlands, self-selection bias appeared to have only a minor effect (Otto et al., 2012a).

Differences in prognosis between attenders and non-attenders could be explained by: a different underlying risk of disease; different help-seeking habits for symptoms, which lead, in turn, to differences in stage at presentation; varying compliance with treatment; or different comorbidities, which have a bearing on outcome (Aarts et al., 2011). Socioeconomic status has been suggested as the major confounder of both outcome and participation in screening (Palli et al., 1986; Aarts et al., 2011), although adjustment for it made almost no difference to the estimated effect of attending screening (Palli et al., 1986).

There is greater uncertainty about the appropriate correction in observational studies with respect to randomized trials when estimating the effect of actually being screened. However, Duffy et al. (2002a) illustrated that the relative risk of breast cancer death may differ a priori between attenders and non-attenders, in ways that are not related to screening and thus completely annul the benefit observed among the screened population. The authors first considered a Swedish case–control study with an uncorrected relative risk of 0.50 for being screened, and then calculated that the a priori risk of breast cancer death among non-attenders would have to be 1.53 to be entirely due to self-selection bias, in a programme with 70% attendance. For a true (i.e. often suggested by trials' meta-analyses) relative risk of 0.80 associated with invitation to screening, the relative risk would have to be 1.23. Such reverse calculation of the required size of the bias to annul the result, or to give a result consistent with the trials, may provide some assistance in interpreting the results of observational estimates of the effect of actually being screened.

(ii) Screening opportunity bias

Screening opportunity bias pertains particularly to case–control studies, where controls can only be exposed to screening if they attended their last screen, whereas cases can be exposed to screening if they attended their last screen or were screen-detected (Walter, 2003). This means that if the screens at which any screen-detected cases were detected are included as exposure, there is a bias against screening, and if they are excluded, there is a bias in favour of screening. Duffy et al. (2008) developed a method that estimates the additional opportunity for screening exposure among the cases and yields a correction to the odds ratio for this, obtaining an estimate that lies between the odds ratios including and excluding the detection screen.

(b) Prospective or retrospective cohort analysis of unrefined mortality

A common evaluation technique consists of comparing rates of unrefined mortality (i.e. regardless of time of diagnosis) in a screened versus an unscreened population (whether historical or contemporaneous or both). An early but very clear example of this approach is the estimation of the effect of the NHS Breast Screening Programme in England and Wales by Blanks et al. (2000). The authors fitted age-cohort models to breast cancer mortality data recorded over the period 1971–1989, before the advent of substantial screening coverage, and projected these to estimate the expected mortality in the absence of screening for the period 1990–1998, in which the screening programme was achieving high coverage. The authors compared the observed reductions in mortality with expected rates for the age groups 55–69, 50–54, and 75–79 years. The observed reductions in breast cancer mortality were 21.3% in the age group 55–69 years and 14.9% in the age groups 50–54 years and 75–79 years, age groups that might reasonably be expected to be unaffected by breast screening. The estimated reduction in breast cancer mortality associated with the NHS Breast Screening Programme was 6.4%. The authors noted that the inclusion of deaths from cancers diagnosed before the screening started would dilute the observed benefit of screening. Duffy et al. (2002b) subsequently showed that more than half of the breast cancer deaths in a given 10-year period are from cancers diagnosed before screening started, and consequently that the effect on mortality from cancers diagnosed in the screening epoch is likely to be twice as high as the 6.4% mortality reduction estimated. For this and other reasons, the full effect of the screening programme was unlikely to be seen until between 2005 and 2010.

As with any temporal comparison, the issue of confounding with treatment arises. Although the age groups above the screening range might not have benefited fully from the therapeutic changes, it is reasonable to suppose that the age groups below the screening range would have done so. The greater mortality reduction in 1998 in the age group 50–54 years compared with the age group 75–79 years (17.0% vs 12.8%) appears to bear this out.

(c) Prospective or retrospective cohort analysis of incidence-based mortality

Incidence-based mortality studies are cohort studies in which the incidence-based mortality from breast cancer diagnosed after the first invitation to screening is compared with an estimate of expected breast cancer mortality in the absence of screening. The breast cancer mortality expected in a situation without screening can be estimated using breast cancer mortality rates in a cohort not (yet) invited to screening, or using historical data on breast cancer mortality patterns from the same region. Ideally, historical and current data on breast cancer mortality from a region in which screening is absent are included, to account for possible temporal changes that affect breast cancer mortality (e.g. improvements in breast cancer treatment). Incidence-based mortality studies have several methodological advantages, including avoidance of lead-time bias and achieving appropriate correspondence in time of the breast cancer incidence and mortality between the study and control cohorts.

Suppose a screening programme started in 1990, in a stable target population of 100 000 women aged 50–69 years. One might have available data to compare breast cancer mortality in the 1 000 000 person–years of eligible follow-up in 1990–1999 with the same mortality in the corresponding 1 000 000 person–years of observation in 1980–1989, before the screening was initiated. However, such a comparison of deaths from breast cancer regardless of time of diagnosis would include in 1990–1999 deaths from breast cancers diagnosed before 1990 and so with no potential for exposure to screening. The IBM approach would include only deaths from cancers diagnosed at ages 50–69 years during either 1990–1999 or 1980–1989. Although this approach may incur some conservative bias due to lead time, this would be outweighed by the correct classification of exposure to invitation to screening (Swedish Organised Service Screening Evaluation Group, 2006a). Since the risk of breast cancer death may change with time since diagnosis, it is desirable that the observation periods with and without screening be of equal duration.

A real instance of this approach is now considered. The study of Olsen et al. (2005) compared changes in incidence-based breast cancer mortality in the period 1991–2001 in the Copenhagen screening programme with changes in the rest of Denmark (which was without a screening programme and was consequently taken as the national control group). Incidence-based breast cancer mortality rates declined from 69 per 100 000 in the pre-screening period to 52 per 100 000 in the screening period in the Copenhagen area, and almost no change (from 52 to 53 per 100 000) was observed in the national control group. This observation led to an estimated relative risk of breast cancer death of 0.75 (95% confidence interval [CI], 0.63–0.89). Any changes in therapy in the Copenhagen area over the period would also have been seen in the national control group, given the standardization of treatment performed in accordance with the Danish Breast Cancer Cooperative Group (Fischerman & Mouridsen, 1988). Since the only deaths included were those from cancers diagnosed during the relevant periods, there was no dilution of the effect of the screening due to deaths from cancers diagnosed before screening started.

(d) Case–control studies

In a case–control study, exposure to screening (history of breast cancer screening attendance) is compared between women who died of breast cancer (cases) and women who did not die of breast cancer (controls). Potentially important biases associated with case–control studies include selection bias and information bias related to the time at which exposure is defined. Because screening attendance is used as the exposure measure, selection bias plays an important role, as women attending screening might be more health-conscious than women not attending screening. Selection bias influences the estimated effect of the study in favour of screening but may be corrected, at least partially, using statistical methods (adaptation by Duffy et al., 2002a of the correction of Cuzick et al., 1997 for RCTs). For a correct estimate of selection bias, it is crucial to have data available on the variables that influence breast cancer mortality, or on breast cancer mortality between attenders and non-attenders (Paap et al., 2014).

Generally speaking, the definition of exposure to screening can lead to bias both in favour of screening and against screening. If exposure is defined as “ever screened” versus “never screened”, bias will occur in favour of screening. Because all cases have died of breast cancer and were therefore very likely to have been diagnosed with breast cancer some time before death, most will have stopped being invited to screening some time before death. In contrast, controls (most of whom were not diagnosed with breast cancer) would have continued to be invited to screening up to near the time of their death, and would thus have been more likely to be exposed to screening. This difference in the probability of having been screened would lead to bias in favour of screening. This bias in favour of screening is eliminated if exposure is defined as screening attendance to the time of the case’s breast cancer diagnosis, so that exposure stops simultaneously for cases and controls. Although in this design the bias in favour of screening is eliminated, bias against screening is likely to occur because a case is eligible to be screened until cancer is detected either clinically or by screening, whereas controls matched to a case with a cancer detected by screening are eligible to be screened only until the cancer of their matched case is detected by screening. This bias can be corrected by defining exposure for controls matched to cases with a screen-detected cancer to the time at which cases with a screen-detected cancer would have been clinically diagnosed (in the absence of screening), but this requires an estimate of the screening lead time for each case (Connor et al., 2000). Exposure of controls matched to cases with a clinical diagnosis remains unchanged.

Essential elements in performing case–control studies are: (i) sampling cases and controls from the same population (i.e. controls that would have had the same probability of becoming cases); (ii) qualitatively equal information on the primary outcome measure; and (iii) correct definition of (population-based) mammography screening exposure. In countries with complete population registries and full coverage of cancer registries and vital statistics, such case–control studies approximate nested case–control studies. Examples of this type of study are the case–control studies done in the Netherlands (e.g. Paap et al., 2014).

Case–control studies consistently report a greater breast cancer mortality reduction associated with screening (up to 50%) compared with the RCTs (Walter, 2003; Broeders et al., 2012). Only a small part of this difference in breast cancer mortality reduction can be explained by differences in study design. RCTs compare breast cancer mortality in women offered screening with that in women not offered screening. The estimated effect is influenced by the participation rate (women who decline the invitation to screening are included in the screened group) and by contamination of the control group. In contrast, most case–control studies estimate breast cancer mortality reduction in women who are screened compared with women who are not screened, thereby excluding women who decline the invitation to screening from the case group and avoiding contamination of the control group. Therefore, the effect estimate assessed in case–control studies can be expected to be stronger, even if adjusted for selection effects.

The independent United Kingdom panel on breast cancer screening reviewed the usefulness of case–control studies in estimating breast cancer mortality reduction associated with screening and considered that bias could inflate the estimate of benefit and that the RCTs provide more reliable evidence for mortality reduction (Marmot et al., 2013). However, the number of screens performed in current screening programmes outnumbers the women screened in the RCTs by hundreds of millions. Therefore, studies conducted in high-quality organized invitation systems, which have almost complete follow-up data and high acceptance rates, can best estimate whether currently implemented programmes are of benefit to women invited (effectiveness).

The case–control approach is a relatively quick and inexpensive one, based on the principle that if the screening is reducing mortality, women who have died of breast cancer will be characterized by lesser screening histories than those who have not. It does have specific complexities and risks of bias (Walter, 2003; Duffy, 2007; Verbeek & Broeders, 2010). However, these can to some extent be addressed by design and analytical tactics. Within opportunistic, rather than organized, screening, the case–control approach is one of the few evaluation options available. In some health-care environments, it may not be possible to link screening and mortality records, in which case the advanced disease status might be used to define cases (with the possibility to be interviewed with respect to screening status in the absence of screening records).

A notable feature of the case–control evaluation is that its primary comparison is made between participants and non-participants in the screening programme, and this option thus introduces the possibility of self-selection bias. Duffy et al. (2002a) developed a correction for this bias that requires a reliable estimate of the relative risk of breast cancer death in non-attenders versus those not invited to screening. This may be difficult to estimate; however, the method also provides an estimate of how large this relative risk would have to be for the observed benefit to be entirely due to self-selection bias.

An example of a case–control evaluation is the study of the effect of participation in the BreastScreen Australia programme, which has been inviting women aged 50–69 years to 2-yearly mammography since the mid-1990s (Nickson et al., 2012). The 427 breast cancer deaths occurring at some time during 1995–2006 were compared with 3650 controls who were alive. A variable number of controls, selected by incidence density sampling, were matched by month and year of birth to cases (Greenland & Thomas, 1982). In each case–control matched set, a date of first diagnosis of breast cancer (in the majority, the date of diagnosis of the case) was defined as the reference date. The primary definition of exposure to screening was having had a mammogram between the woman's 50th birthday and the case–control set reference date. Exposure to screening was less common in cases than in controls (39% vs 56%). The odds ratio associated with screening, adjusted for remoteness of residence and socioeconomic status, was 0.48 (95% CI, 0.38–0.59). A series of sensitivity analyses yielded a range of 0.44 to 0.52.

This result may be affected by self-selection bias, despite the adjustment for socioeconomic status and the various sensitivity analyses performed. However, to be entirely due to self-selection bias, the a priori risk of breast cancer death in non-participants compared with uninvited women would have to be at least 1.80, which seems unlikely given the evidence that participants are at a higher risk of breast cancer than non-participants (Thompson et al., 1994; van Schoor et al., 2010; Beckmann et al., 2013). Clearly, the self-selection bias can act in either direction. However, the results do indicate that case–control evaluations appear to be less conservative compared with prospective evaluation approaches.

(e) Ecological studies

An ecological study makes use of aggregated data for exposure or outcome identification, or both, rather than individual-level assessment of the association of the exposure with the outcome.

Ecological studies are generally accorded a lower status than randomized trials or studies using individual data, such as case–control and cohort studies. However, there may be cases where a well-conducted ecological study is more pertinent than a poorly conducted cohort or case–control study. In fact, for population interventions such as mammography breast cancer screening, the distinctions between these study types may be blurred, making it more important to consider the studies on a case-by-case basis, or at least according to a finer subdivision of types.

Two factors limit the ability to interpret findings in ecological studies. First, the ecological fallacy relates to the uncertain relationship between the mean and the median of characteristics of individuals in cells of aggregated data. Thus, the average use of screening in region A may be higher than that in region B, but if this average is due to very intensive use by a small number of women, one would not expect to see an overall mortality advantage for the women in region A. Second, differences in outcomes may be explained by other risk factors that differ between two regions. These may not be adjusted for, because they are unknown, are unmeasured, or are measured only on average (which returns one to the ecological fallacy). Adequate treatment of these two issues is a necessary condition for considering an ecological study as informative with respect to the effectiveness of mammography screening.

Ecological studies for breast cancer mortality compare data in countries or areas before and after the introduction of screening (interrupted time series), or concurrently between areas with and without screening (geographical comparisons). In the first type of study, extrapolation of time trends means that decisions must be made, for example about the linearity or otherwise of the trend, the choice of time periods considered as "before" and "after" screening, and the age groups included. In the second type of study, choices must be made about the areas to include, the time period considered, and the age groups included. Such decisions, which can appear to have been made rather arbitrarily, can have a profound impact on the estimates obtained. Lack of comparability and different time trends in the groups being contrasted could lead to substantial bias.

Ecological studies that use temporal trends fit regression models to national or regional published mortality data, commonly to estimate annual rates of change in mortality over time and to assess whether and to what extent breast cancer screening affects them. The change points are either dictated by the date of introduction of screening programmes or estimated from the data using joinpoint regression models (Mukhtar et al., 2013). Studies comparing the *levels* of mortality rates between screening and non-screening periods are not included in this definition (please refer to Sections 5.1.2b and c).

Mukhtar et al. (2013) analysed unrefined breast cancer mortality data (i.e. regardless of epoch of diagnosis) from 1971 or 1979 to 2009 in England, using log-linear models with joinpoint regression. They estimated similar contemporaneous downward trends in mortality during the screening epoch for women younger than 50 years and for those older than 50 years, the lower age limit for screening in Oxford. The joinpoint regression estimated no changes in trends for women aged 64 years or younger but significant changes in the late 1980s in older women. In England as a whole, the authors estimated the largest decreasing relative trend in women younger than 40 years. Years of peak mortality were observed in the mid- to late 1980s, before an effect of screening would be expected.

The authors concluded that screening was unlikely to have affected breast cancer mortality. Problems with this interpretation include the following. (i) The greatest mortality reduction in the most recent period was observed for the youngest age group. Rates were rising in the screening age group until the mid-1980s and falling thereafter. (ii) Because of the methodology's choice of discontinuities at different ages, the calendar periods comparing the screening and non-screening age groups are not the same. (iii) Screening was mostly confined to ages 50–64 years, and the effect on mortality would be quite substantial in the late sixties and early seventies rather than in the early fifties. (iv) The emphasis on individual years of peak mortality and year-to-year trends loses sight of the more stable mortality estimates as a whole. The level of mortality was considerably lower in the screening epoch than in the pre-screening epoch, and this difference was most pronounced in the screening age group. (v) The maximum number of change points allowed should be specified. This will also affect their estimated occurrence.

Usually, it is most difficult to anticipate the occurrence of a change point, or its magnitude, based on year-to-year trends in unrefined mortality. This may influence the subjective decision about the number of joinpoints and about whether trends of decreasing mortality would have continued unabated in the absence of screening. Nevertheless, despite the significant complexities of analysis and interpretations, trend studies can be informative, such as the Otto et al. (2003) study.

(f) Modelling studies

Formally, RCTs answer one specific outcome question, namely whether mammography screening reduces breast cancer mortality, given the exact design features, like fixed interval, starting age, and stopping age, and given the background situation of the control group to compare with. Modelling studies are generally intended to predict outcomes beyond the (limited) end of the trial follow-up, and for different schedules of screening. They seek to avoid possible overestimation of the effect of screening on breast cancer mortality, due to lead-time and length bias, by modelling the breast cancer process more directly. The essence of modelling is simulating the natural history of disease, based on the best available data. This is realized by incorporating variables associated with the disease process and with detection and treatment of breast cancer, including the mean duration of the preclinical detectable phase, the probability of transition to the next tumour stage, age- and stage-specific sensitivity of mammography, and stage-specific response to treatment (Berry et al., 2005; Groenewoud et al., 2007). As an example, the number and the time frame of interval cancers being diagnosed give estimates of sensitivity, whereas the detection rates (by stage, age, calendar year, etc.) and interval cancers together give information on the sojourn times of disease (duration of period when cases are screen-detectable). Modelling produces estimates of these unobservable phenomena, and thus there is sometimes scepticism about the evidence coming from modelling studies. Modelling tries to incorporate all available screen and non-screen data and to give the best estimate of the natural history of disease and of what would have happened if no screening had been implemented. In the evaluation of screening, when it is already being introduced, such model predictions are valuable to evaluate and steer the programme, and they are also advisable before implementation for estimating the optimal programme of screening with its benefits and harms as well as its cost–effectiveness. With good estimates, especially of the screen-detectable period, overdiagnosis can be estimated (van Ravesteyn et al., 2015).

However, all good modelling analyses that predict the consequences of treating earlier in the natural history of disease are dependent on efficacy measures, from RCTs or high-quality observational studies, to estimate such results. Therefore, high-quality models are calibrated to such high-quality data (de Koning et al., 1995). The advantage is that differences in protocol, for example attendance and referral rates, and in follow-up period can specifically be taken into account.

In such modelling, the natural history of breast cancer in the absence of screening is first modelled. Some women in the simulated population may develop breast cancer, which develops from a small preclinical lesion to a symptomatic cancer, possibly leading to breast cancer death. In each stage, a lesion may grow to the next stage, regress, or be clinically diagnosed because of symptoms. The natural course of the disease may be interrupted by screening, at which a preclinical lesion can become screen-detected. Screen detection can result in the detection of smaller tumours, which may entail a survival benefit. Each screen-detected or clinically diagnosed tumour may be treated with adjuvant systemic therapy, which may also improve survival. Critical components of such models are the assumed natural history component, the effects of interrupting by screening or treatment, and extrapolating lifetime harms and benefits (Heijnsdijk et al., 2012). In principle, such elements are calibrated and validated against data from trials and observational studies, and criteria to evaluate models have been proposed (Habbema et al., 2014).

5.1.3 Surrogate indicators of effect on mortality

As noted above, although in principle the main indicator of the effectiveness of a screening programme is its impact on breast cancer mortality, to estimate this impact in practice can be complicated. The population incidence of advanced-stage disease (Smith et al., 2004; Autier et al., 2011) or predicted mortality from the stage of disease diagnosed have been suggested as surrogates for mortality. Randomized trials show that screening that results in a reduction in the incidence of node-positive breast cancer is also accompanied by a reduction in mortality (Smith et al., 2004). A review confirmed this strong inverse association of exposure to screening and of screen detection with nodal status and tumour size (Nagtegaal & Duffy, 2013). To consider potential confounding, the incidence of disease should be compared before and after the introduction of screening, to account for changes in treatment as well as more complete pathological staging and reporting (e.g. the implementation of sentinel node biopsy) in the screening epoch. This gives rise to further complexities of analysis and interpretation of data (Swedish Organised Service Screening Evaluation Group, 2007).

Another possible confounder is the increase in breast cancer incidence recorded in almost all parts of the world in the second half of the 20th century, which is related to mortality and incidence of advanced disease as well as to the introduction of screening. Thus, there are methodological problems when trying to estimate the expected incidence of disease by stage in the absence of screening.

Despite these problems, the rates of advanced-stage disease are still a very direct measure of the impact of early detection by screening, as several studies have reported. To estimate the potential beneficial effect, not simply the proportion of cases with advanced-stage disease but also the reduction in the absolute rate of advanced-stage disease should be reported.

Thus, the incidence of advanced-stage disease might be used as a surrogate for the effect of screening on mortality, but the above-mentioned limitations should be considered. Other indicators include the detection rate of interval cancers and of small tumours, which are necessary but not sufficient indicators of the success of screening (Day et al., 1989, 1995; Tabár et al., 1992). Although they are less direct, these indicators are often more generally observable than the absolute population incidence of advanced-stage disease.

5.2 Preventive effects of mammography

5.2.1 Incidence-based cohort mortality studies

IBM studies are the most methodologically robust studies for evaluating the effectiveness of service mammography in reducing breast cancer mortality (see Section 5.1.1). They are cohort studies usually conducted in association with a population-based mammography screening programme. Their defining feature is the observation of deaths from breast cancer in women diagnosed after their first invitation to (or attendance to) mammography screening, that is, at a time when their risk of breast cancer death could have been affected by screening. The expected number of breast cancer deaths is estimated in women diagnosed with breast cancer but not invited to screening compared with a matching cohort of women over a similar period of time.

The screening and non-screening cohorts can be fixed or dynamic, most commonly dynamic. For those invited to screening, the date of first invitation is taken from screening records or is estimated from the cohort member's residence location and the history of the roll-out of screening in the study area and period. For those not invited to screening, the date of first invitation may be allocated to correspond in age and time to those invited, or at about the midpoint of the first screening round for those invited. The two cohorts' age distributions are usually matched, as are the periods over which their breast cancer experience is recorded. In most cases, incident breast cancers during the accrual period for the study (which begins at the date of first invitation to screening for each woman) and the associated breast cancer deaths are identified in a population-based cancer registry, and deaths from other causes in a regional or national death register. In some studies, one or both cohorts have also been identified in national registers and individual women tracked into and out of the cohorts for accurate estimation of person–years of experience; otherwise, the person–years are estimated using aggregated population data.

This description of the results of IBM studies is based on studies correctly characterized as IBM studies, mostly covered by two recent systematic reviews. The first of these, the Euroscreen review, systematically searched for relevant studies published up to February 2011 in women aged 50–69 years covered by European population-based screening mammography programmes (Broeders et al., 2012; Njor et al., 2012). The second had a similar search strategy to the Euroscreen review but without age restriction or limitation to European populations, and included studies published up to January 2013 (Irvin & Kaplan, 2014). Additional IBM studies were found in an unrestricted systematic search that covered literature published between March 2011 and 22 July 2014. One study published after July 2014 (Coldman et al., 2014) and two early studies not identified in the searches (Morrison et al., 1988 and Thompson et al., 1994) were also known to the Working Group.

Four analyses that were excluded from the Njor et al. (2012) review report were also excluded by the Working Group, on the grounds that they were based exclusively on some or all of the data used for previous reports. However, there remains significant overlap among several studies, which is detailed below.

In almost all instances, the studies reviewed were conducted in areas where population-based service mammography screening had been implemented. There is, in principle, no reason for not conducting such studies within a population exposed only to opportunistic screening, but they are more readily conducted in areas of population-based screening and the Working Group knew of no IBM studies that had been conducted in an area with exclusively opportunistic screening.

The following summary of results of IBM studies is organized into two broad sections: studies that report on breast cancer mortality reduction after mammography screening of women in age groups that include most or all of the age range 50–69 years, and studies that report on mortality reduction from screening in an age group that lies mainly below or above that age range (i.e. women younger than 50 years or older than 69 years).

(a) Women aged 50–69 years invited to screening

The results of studies of mammography screening mainly in women aged 50–69 years are summarized in Table 5.4 and Table 5.5. Table 5.4 covers estimates of relative risk of breast cancer death in women invited to mammography screening relative to women not invited. Table 5.5 does the same for women who were invited and attended screening relative to women who were invited but did not attend. Studies are ordered in the table by the country in which they were conducted (with countries in the order in which their mammography screening programmes were first introduced) and within each country by the earliest date of mammography screening that was included in the analysis.

All analyses reviewed here included women in the age group 50–69 years, with the exception of four analyses in which the women invited or otherwise targeted for screening were aged up to 59 or 64 years and one in which only women from age 55 years were invited. Eight analyses included women invited to screening before age 50 years, and five analyses included women invited to screening beyond age 69 years.

(i) Sweden

The six reports based on population-based mammography screening in Sweden have multiple overlaps in space and time; that is, they drew on geographical mammography experience for more than a year that overlapped with that drawn on by at least one other study. The experiences in the reports of Duffy et al. (2002a, b) are almost completely a subset within that of the Swedish Organised Service Screening Evaluation Group (2006a, b) reports; however, the reports of Duffy et al. (2002a, b) provide valuable additional results and so are included separately in Table 5.4 and below. The whole mammography experience of Jonsson et al. (2007) is also included in that of Swedish Organised Service Screening Evaluation Group (2006a, b), but it does provide some independent information since it uses contemporary and not historical control areas. Most of the screening experience in two of the seven screening areas of Jonsson et al. (2001) overlaps with that in Swedish Organised Service Screening Evaluation Group (2006a, b), and two of the control counties overlap more than 50% of the time with the control counties in Jonsson et al. (2007). The screening experience of the one screening county in Jonsson et al. (2003a) overlaps by 2 years that of Duffy et al. (2002a, b) and by 1 year that of Swedish Organised Service Screening Evaluation Group (2006a, b). The screening experience of one of the two counties included in Tabár et al. (2001) is also included in Duffy et al. (2002a, b) and Swedish Organised Service Screening Evaluation Group (2006a, b).

Sweden's first population-based mammography screening programme was introduced in 1974 to cover women aged 40–64 years in Gävleborg County. Jonsson et al. (2003a) primarily compared IBM in Gävleborg County with an age-matched control population from four neighbouring counties without mammography screening programmes. Cohorts of women were defined in Gävleborg County according to the date at which invitation to screening began in their district, and corresponding cohorts were created in the control counties. Incident breast cancers and their dates of diagnosis were identified, and their date and cause of death obtained from the Swedish Cancer Registry; aggregated population data were used to estimate person–years at risk. The study also included a reference period (1964–1973), in which any pre-existing difference in breast cancer mortality between Gävleborg County and the control counties could be estimated and adjusted for in the analysis. Incident breast cancers were accrued for 10 years, and the follow-up period for breast cancer mortality was 22 years; cases were accrued only in the age group 40–64 years, and follow-up extended to age 79 years. [These differences in accrual and follow-up periods and age

Table 5.4 Incidence-based mortality studies of the effectiveness of invitation to mammography screening[a] mainly in women aged 50–69 years, by country and follow-up period

Reference	Areas, earliest year of programme screening, screening age, screening interval	Person-years[b]	Duration of screening	Accrual and follow-up periods	Diagnosis and death age ranges	Individual or aggregate data	Temporal and geographical similarity of comparison group	Time-balanced follow-up periods?	Adjustments	Breast cancer mortality RR (95% CI)[c]	Comments
Sweden											
Jonsson et al. (2003a)	Gävleborg County and 4 other counties 1974 40–64 yr average, 38 mo (earlier) and 23 mo (later)	Invited 885 000 Not invited 2 581 000	10 yr	1974–1986 (max 10 yr) Same + 12 yr	40–64 yr Same + 15 yr	Individual for breast cancer cases; aggregate, all other women	Same period; different counties	Yes	Age, follow-up time, county, period (study or reference)	0.86 (0.71–1.05)	RR, 0.82 adjusted for lead-time bias; adjustment for inclusion bias[d] did not change RR
Tabár et al. (2001)	2 counties 1978 40–69 yr 1.5–2 yr	Invited 1 100 931 Not invited 1 213 136	≤ 9 yr	1988–1996 Same	40–69 yr Not stated	Individual for breast cancer cases; aggregate, all other women	Different periods; same areas	No (screening period was 1 yr shorter than non-screening period)	Selection bias	0.52 (0.43–0.63) 0.64 (0.30–1.36)[e]	It is uncertain whether there is lead-time bias

Table 5.4 (continued)

Reference	Areas, earliest year of programme screening, screening age, screening interval	Person-years[b]	Duration of screening	Accrual and follow-up periods	Diagnosis and death age ranges	Individual or aggregate data	Temporal and geographical similarity of comparison group	Time-balanced follow-up periods?	Adjustments	Breast cancer mortality RR (95% CI)[c]	Comments
Duffy et al. (2002b)	7 counties 1978–1994 40 or 50 yr to 69 or 74 yr 1.5–2.75 yr	Invited 3 815 330 Not invited 3 693 064	5–20 yr	1978–1997 to 1994–1998 Same	40–69 yr (6 counties), 50–59 yr (1 county) Same	Individual for breast cancer cases; aggregate, all other women	Different periods; same areas	Yes	Lead-time bias, time trend in breast cancer mortality	0.74 (0.68–0.81)[f] ≤ 10 yr of screening: 0.82 (0.72–0.94) > 10 yr of screening: 0.68 (0.60–0.77)	Analyses in 5 counties based on ≤ 10 yr of screening, in 2 counties based on > 10 yr. Substantial overlap with Swedish Organised Service Screening Evaluation Group (2006a)
Swedish Organised Service Screening Evaluation Group (2006a)	13 areas 1980–1990, depending on area 40 or 50 yr to 69 yr, depending on area probably mostly 2 yr	Invited 7 542 833 Not invited 7 265 841	11–22 yr, depending on area	1980–2001 to 1990–2001 Same	40–69 yr (8 areas) or 50–69 yr (5 areas) Maximum follow-up age not stated	Individual for breast cancer cases; aggregate, all other women	Different periods; same areas	Yes	Time trend in breast cancer mortality	0.73 (0.69–0.77)	Updated and expanded analysis incorporating almost all data used for Duffy et al. (2002b)
Jonsson et al. (2001)	12 counties 1986 50–69 yr 2 yr	Invited 2 036 000 Not invited 1 265 000	7 yr	1986–1994 Same + 3 yr	50–69 yr Same + 10 yr	Individual for breast cancer cases; aggregate, all other women	Same period; different counties	Yes	Age, year of follow-up, area, period	0.90 (0.74–1.10)	RR, 0.87 adjusted for inclusion bias.[d] Lead-time bias estimated to be −0.4%

Table 5.4 (continued)

Reference	Areas, earliest year of programme screening, screening age, screening interval	Person-years[b]	Duration of screening	Accrual and follow-up periods	Diagnosis and death age ranges	Individual or aggregate data	Temporal and geographical similarity of comparison group	Time-balanced follow-up periods?	Adjustments	Breast cancer mortality RR (95% CI)[c]	Comments
Jonsson et al. (2007)	4 counties 1989 40–74 yr average, 20–22 mo	Invited 1 223 346 Not invited 915 948	7 yr	1989–1996 Same + 5 yr	50–69 yr Same + 10 yr	Individual for breast cancer cases; aggregate, all other women	Different period (accrual 1989–1996 for study group, 1988–1994 for control group); different areas	No (study group follow-up to 2001, control group to 1998)	Age	50–69 yr: 0.86 (0.86–1.17) 40–74 yr: 0.74 (0.58–0.94)[g]	Lead-time bias estimated to be −2% at ages 50–69 yr and 40–74 yr ~85% of invited women screened
The Netherlands											
Peer et al. (1995)	2 cities 1975 35–64 yr 2 yr	Invited 166 307 Not invited 154 103	15 yr	1975–1990 Same	35–64 yr Same	Individual for breast cancer cases; aggregate, all other women	Same period; different cities	Yes	None stated	0.94 (0.68–1.29)	Study followed for 15 yr a cohort aged 35–49 yr at first invitation. Cities may differ in underlying breast cancer mortality trends
United Kingdom											
UK Trial of Early Detection of Breast Cancer Group (1999)[a]	England and Scotland, 6 health service areas 1979 45–64 yr 2 yr	Invited 793 288 Not invited 2 346 328	7 yr	1979–1995 Same	45–80 yr Same	Individual	Same period; different health service areas	Yes	Age, pre-trial breast cancer mortality	0.73 (0.63–0.84)	Screening included annual CBE 65% of invited women screened

Table 5.4 (continued)

Reference	Areas, earliest year of programme screening, screening age, screening interval	Person-years[b]	Duration of screening	Accrual and follow-up periods	Diagnosis and death age ranges	Individual or aggregate data	Temporal and geographical similarity of comparison group	Time-balanced follow-up periods?	Adjustments	Breast cancer mortality RR (95% CI)[c]	Comments
Finland											
Hakama et al. (1997)	84% of munici-palities 1987 50–64 yr 2 yr	Invited 400 804 Not invited 299 228	≤ 6 yr	1987–1992 Same	50–64 yr Same	Individual for all women	Same period; same areas	Yes	Age	0.76 (0.53–1.09)	Approximately 1/6 of women invited to 1 screening round, 1/3 to 2 rounds, and 1/2 to 3 rounds 85% of invited women screened
Anttila et al. (2002)	Helsinki 1986 50–59 yr 2 yr	Invited 161 400 Uninvited 155 400	0.5–10.5 yr; 1–5 screening rounds	1986–1997 Uncertain	50–59 yr Uncertain	Individual for breast cancer cases; aggregate, all other women	Different period; same area	Yes	Age at death, time trend in breast cancer mortality at age 40–49 yr in screened and unscreened cohorts	0.81 (0.62–1.05)	Possible difference in age of case accrual and follow-up, and therefore lead-time bias
Parvinen et al. (2006)	Turku 1987 55–74 yr 2 yr	Invited 204 896 Not invited 199 329	11 yr	1987–1997 Same + 4 yr	55–74 yr Same + 10 yr	Individual for invited women; aggregate for not invited women	Different periods; same area	Yes	Age, time trend in mortality extrapolated from 1970 to 1986	55–74 yr: 0.58 (0.41–0.83) 65–69 yr: 0.42 (0.21–0.84)	Some lead-time bias

Table 5.4 (continued)

Reference	Areas, earliest year of programme screening, screening age, screening interval	Person–years[b]	Duration of screening	Accrual and follow-up periods	Diagnosis and death age ranges	Individual or aggregate data	Temporal and geographical similarity of comparison group	Time-balanced follow-up periods?	Adjustments	Breast cancer mortality RR (95% CI)[c]	Comments
Anttila et al. (2008)	410 munici-palities 1987 50–69 yr 2 yr	Invited 1 822 900 Not invited no estimate provided	≤ 5 yr	1992–1996 Same + 3 yr	50–69 yr Same + 10 yr	Individual for breast cancer cases; aggregate, all other women	Different period; same area	No	Age at diagnosis, cohort, year	0.89 (0.81–98)	Some lead-time bias. Breast cancer mortality in the absence of screening was extrapolated from statistical models of breast cancer mortality from 1971 to 1986 and in age groups 40–49 yr and 65–69 yr up to 1991

Table 5.4 (continued)

Reference	Areas, earliest year of programme screening, screening age, screening interval	Person–years[b]	Duration of screening	Accrual and follow-up periods	Diagnosis and death age ranges	Individual or aggregate data	Temporal and geographical similarity of comparison group	Time-balanced follow-up periods?	Adjustments	Breast cancer mortality RR (95% CI)[c]	Comments
Sarkeala et al. (2008a, b)	260 munici-palities 1987 50–69 yr (up to 74 yr in some munici-palities) 2 yr	Invited 2 330 266 Not invited 401 002	≤ 12 yr	1992–2003 Same	50–69 yr Same	Individual for invited women; aggregate for not invited women	Different period; same area	Yes	Age at death, centre recall categories, period, calendar year within period, interaction between calendar year and age	0.78 (0.70–0.87) 50–59 yr: 1.04 (0.81–1.31) 50–59 yr (up to 69 yr): 0.84 (0.75–0.92) 50–69 yr (up to 74 yr): 0.72 (0.51–0.97)	Time trend in breast cancer mortality taken account of by modelled adjustment for calendar period. 87% of invited women screened. The material was grouped by screening policy of the municipality
Italy											
Paci et al. (2002)	Florence 1990 50–69 yr 2 yr	Invited 254 890 Not invited not stated	≤ 7 yr	1990–1996 Same + 3 yr	50–76 yr Same + 3 yr	Individual for breast cancer cases; aggregate, all other women	Different period; same area	Yes	None stated	0.81 (0.64–1.01)	Some lead-time bias

Table 5.4 (continued)

Reference	Areas, earliest year of programme screening, screening age, screening interval	Person-years[b]	Duration of screening	Accrual and follow-up periods	Diagnosis and death age ranges	Individual or aggregate data	Temporal and geographical similarity of comparison group	Time-balanced follow-up periods?	Adjustments	Breast cancer mortality RR (95% CI)[c]	Comments
Spain											
Ascunce et al. (2007)	Navarre 1990 50–69 yr 2 yr	Invited 293 000 Not invited 289 000[h]	5 yr	1997–2001 Same	50–69 yr Uncertain	Individual for breast cancer cases; aggregate, all other women	Different period; same area	Yes	Age	0.58 (0.44–0.75)	Lead-time bias is possible. RR not adjusted for trend in breast cancer mortality; RR for age 30–44 yr was 1.07, for age ≥ 75 yr was 1.03
Denmark											
Olsen et al. (2005)	Copenhagen 1991 50–69 yr 2 yr	Invited 430 823 Not invited 634 224	≤ 10 yr	1991–2001 Same	50–69 yr, mainly 50–79 yr	Individual for all women	Different period; same city	Yes	Age, exposure, period, region, period*region	0.75 (0.63–0.89)	Some lead-time bias. Adjusted for underlying mortality trend and difference between regions by including period*region term in model

Table 5.4 (continued)

Reference	Areas, earliest year of programme screening, screening age, screening interval	Person–years[b]	Duration of screening	Accrual and follow-up periods	Diagnosis and death age ranges	Individual or aggregate data	Temporal and geographical similarity of comparison group	Time-balanced follow-up periods?	Adjustments	Breast cancer mortality RR (95% CI)[c]	Comments
Norway											
Kalager et al. (2010)	1996–2005, depending on area 50–69 yr 2 yr	Invited 2 337 323 Not invited 2 197 469	10 yr in 1 region; 2–6 yr in 5 regions	1996–2005 Same	50–69 yr Same + 9 yr	Individual for breast cancer cases; aggregate, all other women	Different period; same area	No	Age	[0.88[g] (0.73–1.05)]	Some lead-time bias. Widespread opportunistic screening before programme began
Olsen et al. (2013)	1996–2005, depending on area 50–69 yr 2 yr	Invited 1 182 747 Not invited 1 152 755	≤ 6 yr	1996–2001 or 2002 1996–2001 or 2008[i]	50–69 50–69 or 50–81[i]	Individual for all women	Different period; same counties	Yes	Age at death, breast cancer mortality trend in reference region[j]	0.89 (0.71–1.12) from the “evaluation” model	Some lead-time bias. Study group screened 1–3 times in the population-based programme. Widespread opportunistic screening before programme began

Table 5.4 (continued)

Reference	Areas, earliest year of programme screening, screening age, screening interval	Person–years[b]	Duration of screening	Accrual and follow-up periods	Diagnosis and death age ranges	Individual or aggregate data	Temporal and geographical similarity of comparison group	Time-balanced follow-up periods?	Adjustments	Breast cancer mortality RR (95% CI)[c]	Comments
Weedon-Fekjær et al. (2014)	1996–2005, depending on area 50–69 yr 2 yr	Invited 2 407 709 Not invited 12 785 325	1–15 yr median, 4.5 yr	1986–2009 Same	50–79 yr Same	Individual for all women	Partly different period (1986–2009 for all women, 1995–2009 for invited women); whole country	No	Age, period, cohort, county, lead-time bias	0.72 (0.64–0.79)	Bulk of "not invited" follow-up was in 1986–1995. Widespread opportunistic screening before programme began

[a] One study evaluated invitation to mammography plus CBE.

[b] Person–years: number of women or number of breast cancer deaths.

[c] All RRs are for breast cancer as the underlying cause of death.

[d] Bias from inclusion of deaths from breast cancers that were diagnosed in the period between becoming eligible for screening (either by start of screening or by reaching a certain age) and being invited to be screened.

[e] Estimated trend-adjusted, obtained by the Working Group by dividing the authors' estimate by the incidence-based mortality RR comparing women aged 40–69 years not invited to screening in 1988–1996 with women aged 40–69 years in 1968–1977.

[f] Estimated by combining RRs for ≤ 10 yr screening and > 10 yr screening using a fixed effects meta-analytic method.

[g] RR and 95% CI adjusted for trend or geographical difference in underlying mortality were calculated as ratio of the authors' estimated RRs comparing screening area with control period or area; 95% CI of ratio estimated using method in Altman & Bland (2003) as implemented in http://www.hutchon.net/CompareRR.htm.

[h] Estimated from number of breast cancer deaths and breast cancer mortality rate in Table 4 of the article.

[i] Alternative dates applied to two different birth cohorts.

[j] RR and 95% CI adjusted for time trend in mortality calculated as ratio of the authors' estimated RR comparing women aged 40–69 years invited to screening in 1988–1996 with women aged 40–69 years in 1968–1977, before screening, and their estimated RR comparing women aged 20–39 years not invited to screening in 1988–1996 with women aged 20–39 years in 1968–1977; 95% CI of ratio estimated using method in Altman & Bland (2003) as implemented in http://www.hutchon.net/CompareRR.htm.

CBE, clinical breast examination; CI, confidence interval; mo, month or months; RR, relative risk; yr, year or years.

Table 5.5 Incidence-based mortality studies of the effectiveness of participation in mammography screening[a] mainly in women aged 50–69 years, by country and follow-up period

Reference	Areas, earliest year of programme screening, screening age, screening interval	Person-years[b]	Duration of screening	Accrual and follow-up periods	Diagnosis and death age ranges	Individual or aggregate data	Temporal and geographical similarity of comparison group	Time-balanced follow-up periods?	Adjustments	Breast cancer mortality RR (95% CI)[c]	Comments
Sweden											
Tabár et al. (2001)	2 counties 1978 40–69 yr 1.5–2 yr	Screened 932 229 Not screened 168 702	≤ 9 yr	1988–1996 Same	40–69 yr Not stated	Individual for breast cancer cases; aggregate, all other women (including participation in screening)	Different periods; same areas	No (screening period was 1 yr shorter than non-screening period)	None Time trend	0.37 (0.30–0.46) [0.46 (0.21–0.97)]	Uncertain whether there is lead-time bias. Not adjusted for self-selection bias
Duffy et al. (2002b)	7 counties 1978–1994 40 or 50 yr to 69 or 74 yr 1.5–2.75 yr	Screened 2 687 855 Not screened 628 681	5–20 yr	1978–1997 to 1994–1998 Same	40–69 yr (6 counties), 50–59 yr (1 county) Same	Individual for breast cancer cases; aggregate, all other women (including participation in screening)	Different periods; same areas	Yes	Lead-time bias, self-selection bias	0.61 (0.55–0.68)	See also Swedish Organised Service Screening Evaluation Group (2006a). Adjusted for self-selection bias using method of Duffy et al. (2002b)

Table 5.5 (continued)

Reference	Areas, earliest year of programme screening, screening age, screening interval	Person-years[b]	Duration of screening	Accrual and follow-up periods	Diagnosis and death age ranges	Individual or aggregate data	Temporal and geographical similarity of comparison group	Time-balanced follow-up periods?	Adjustments	Breast cancer mortality RR (95% CI)[c]	Comments
Swedish Organised Service Screening Evaluation Group (2006a)	13 areas 1980–1990, depending on area 40 or 50 yr to 69 yr, depending on area probably mostly 2 yr	Screened 5 612 312 Not screened 1 930 521	11–22 yr, depending on area	1980–2001 to 1990–2001 Same	40–69 yr (8 areas) or 50–69 yr (5 areas) Maximum follow-up age not stated	Individual for breast cancer cases; aggregate, all other women (including participation in screening)	Different periods; same areas	Yes	Lead-time bias, self-selection bias using method of Duffy et al. (2002b)	0.57 (0.53–0.62)	Updated and expanded analysis based on analysis in Duffy et al. (2002b)
Jonsson et al. (2007)	4 counties 1989 40–74 yr average, 20–22 mo	Invited 1 223 346 Not invited 915 948 (Only 9% of breast cancer cases were in women who did not attend screening)	7 yr	1989–1997 Same + 4 yr	50–69 yr 50–79 yr	Individual for breast cancer cases; aggregate, all other women	Different period (accrual 1989–1997 for study group, 1988–1994 for control group); different counties	No (study group follow-up to 2001, control group to 1998)	Age, difference in breast cancer mortality between study group and control group in preceding 7 yr, self-selection for screening	0.70 (0.57–0.86)	Lead-time adjustment was estimated to be –2% ~85% of invited women screened Adjusted for self-selection bias using method of Cuzick et al. (1997)

Table 5.5 (continued)

Reference	Areas, earliest year of programme screening, screening age, screening interval	Person–years[b]	Duration of screening	Accrual and follow-up periods	Diagnosis and death age ranges	Individual or aggregate data	Temporal and geographical similarity of comparison group	Time-balanced follow-up periods?	Adjustments	Breast cancer mortality RR (95% CI)[c]	Comments
Finland											
Sarkeala et al. (2008b)	260 munici-palities 1987 50–59 yr (invited); 60–69 yr (optional) 2 yr	Screened 1 023 598 Not screened 1 365 177 ("screened" = screened after first invitation; "not screened" includes not invited and invited but not screened)	≤ 12 yr	1992–2003 Same	50–79 yr 60–79 yr	Individual for screened women; aggregate for unscreened women	Different period; same area	Yes	Age at death, screening policy category, calendar period. Adjusted for self-selection bias using method of Cuzick et al. (1997)	0.63 (0.53–0.75)[d]	Time trend in breast cancer mortality taken account of by modelled adjustment for calendar period
Italy											
Puliti & Zappa (2012)	Florence 1991 50–69 yr 2 yr	Screened 466 205 Not screened 248 182	1–16 yr	1992–2007 Same + 1 yr	50–85 yr 50–86 yr	Individual for all women	Same period; same population	Yes	Age at entry, marital status, deprivation index. No additional adjustment for self-selection bias	0.51 (0.40–0.66)	Some lead-time bias

Table 5.5 (continued)

Reference	Areas, earliest year of programme screening, screening age, screening interval	Person–years[b]	Duration of screening	Accrual and follow-up periods	Diagnosis and death age ranges	Individual or aggregate data	Temporal and geographical similarity of comparison group	Time-balanced follow-up periods?	Adjustments	Breast cancer mortality RR (95% CI)[c]	Comments
Canada											
Coldman et al. (2014)	7 provinces 1990 Most ≥ 40 yr Most 40–49 yr 1 yr ≥ 50 yr 2 yr	Screened and not screened 20 200 000	1–20 yr	1990–2009 Same	40–99 yr Same	Individual for screened women; aggregate for unscreened women	Same period; same population	Yes	Age	0.60 (0.52–0.67)	Self-selection bias estimated for British Columbia women aged 40–49 yr at entry using an ad hoc approach: unadjusted RR, [0.43 (0.28–0.61)]; adjusted RR, [0.39 (0.19–0.91)]

Table 5.5 (continued)

Reference	Areas, earliest year of programme screening, screening age, screening interval	Person–years[b]	Duration of screening	Accrual and follow-up periods	Diagnosis and death age ranges	Individual or aggregate data	Temporal and geographical similarity of comparison group	Time-balanced follow-up periods?	Adjustments	Breast cancer mortality RR (95% CI)[c]	Comments
Denmark											
Olsen et al. (2005)	Copenhagen 1991 50–69 yr 2 yr	Invited 430 823 Not invited 634 224 (Not separately estimated for screened and not screened women)	≤ 10 yr	1991–2001 Same	50–69 yr, mainly 50–79 yr	Individual for all women	Different period; same city	Yes	Age, exposure, period, region, period*region. Adjusted for underlying mortality trend by including period*region term in model	0.60 (0.49–0.74)	0.63 adjusted for self-selection bias using an ad hoc approach. ~71% participation; widespread opportunistic screening before programme began
Norway											
Hofvind et al. (2013)	Norway 1996–2005, depending on area 50–69 yr 2 yr	Screened 4 814 060 Not screened 988 641	1–15 yr median, 4.5 yr	1996–2009 Same + 1 yr	50–84 yr 50–85 yr	Individual for all women	Same period; same population	Yes	Age, calendar period, time in screened or unscreened cohort, self-selection bias using method of Cuzick et al. (1997)	0.57 (0.51–0.64)	Some lead-time bias. Estimated RR in those invited, 0.64. Widespread opportunistic screening before programme began

Table 5.5 (continued)

Reference	Areas, earliest year of programme screening, screening age, screening interval	Person-years[b]	Duration of screening	Accrual and follow-up periods	Diagnosis and death age ranges	Individual or aggregate data	Temporal and geographical similarity of comparison group	Time-balanced follow-up periods?	Adjustments	Breast cancer mortality RR (95% CI)[c]	Comments
USA											
Morrison et al. (1988)[a]	BCDDP (29 centres) 1973–1977 35–74 yr 1 yr	Screened 55 053 White women	5 yr	1–9 yr after first screen [1973–1986]	35–83 yr 35–83 yr	Individual for screened women; aggregate for unscreened women	Same period; comparison derives from SEER	Yes	Age, calendar period, lead-time bias	0.80 Age at entry: 35–49 yr: 0.89 50–59 yr: 0.76 60–74 yr: 0.74	Expected deaths accounts for exclusion of prevalent cases, which would otherwise have contributed to observed deaths. Some self-selection bias. Screening included CBE

Table 5.5 (continued)

Reference	Areas, earliest year of programme screening, screening age, screening interval	Person–years[b]	Duration of screening	Accrual and follow-up periods	Diagnosis and death age ranges	Individual or aggregate data	Temporal and geographical similarity of comparison group	Time-balanced follow-up periods?	Adjustments	Breast cancer mortality RR (95% CI)[c]	Comments
Thompson et al. (1994)[a]	Western Washington State 1985 ≥ 40 yr 1–3 yr	Whole cohort: 94 656 women Subcohort: 2242, including 5 breast cancer deaths	≤ 3.5 yr in programme < 5 yr including opportu-nistic	1982–1988 Same	≥ 40 yr Same	Individual for all women	Same period; same area	Yes	Age, mother's history of breast cancer, nulliparity, history of breast biopsy	≥ 40 yr: 0.80 (0.34–1.85) ≥ 50 yr: 0.61 (0.23–1.62)	Screening included CBE. Unadjusted RR, 1.09 (0.58–2.07)

[a] Two studies evaluated invitation to mammography plus CBE.

[b] Person–years: number of women or number of breast cancer deaths.

[c] RRs are for breast cancer as the underlying cause of death when alternative estimates (e.g. excess mortality) are also provided.

[d] Estimated by combining RRs and 95% CIs, using a fixed effects model, across the three screening policy categories in Table 3 of the article. In an earlier analysis of similar data (Sarkeala et al., 2008a), the authors reported an RR for screening of 0.66 (95% CI, 0.58–0.75) in women aged 50–69 years in follow-up, which, when adjusted for self-selection, became 0.72 (95% CI, 0.56–0.88).

BCDDP, Breast Cancer Detection Demonstration Project; CI, confidence interval; mo, month or months; RR, relative risk; SEER, Surveillance, Epidemiology, and End Results; yr, year or years.

groups created the possibility of lead-time bias in the results. Also, bias due to inclusion of some cases of breast cancer that occurred early in the roll-out of screening and before the first invitation to screening (inclusion bias) was possible.] The estimated IBM relative risk for death from breast cancer was 0.86 (95% CI, 0.71–1.05) based on breast cancer deaths ascertained as the underlying cause of death from the death certificate and adjusted for age, follow-up time, county, and period (study or reference). Corresponding relative risks were 0.82 (no CI stated) after adjustment for lead-time and inclusion biases, 0.82 (95% CI, 0.65–1.03) when based on an estimate of excess mortality due to breast cancer, which does not require use of the certified underlying cause of death, and 0.93 (95% CI, 0.77–1.11) when based on the "rest of Sweden" as the control group.

The relative risk of 0.86 (95% CI, 0.71–1.05) was chosen from the alternatives listed above to be reported in the table. This choice was made a priori on the grounds that: (i) the relative risk was based on the underlying cause of death (the excess mortality measure is not consistently reported in the studies reviewed); (ii) it was the most fully adjusted relative risk that also included its 95% confidence interval; (iii) the Working Group considered four neighbouring counties to be a more nearly similar control group for the study group than the whole of the rest of Sweden; and (iv) this study overlapped the least with other Swedish studies.

Jonsson et al. (2001) and Jonsson et al. (2007) had fundamentally the same design as Jonsson et al. (2003a), except that Jonsson et al. (2007) made historical rather than geographical comparisons of breast cancer mortality in women invited to screening in a later period with that in women in the same population not invited to screening in an earlier period. [Jonsson et al. (2007) is the weakest of the three, because of its overlaps with Jonsson et al. (2001) and Swedish Organised Service Screening Evaluation Group (2006a, b) and because of the difference in the length of the follow-up periods in women invited and not invited to screening.] The IBM relative risk in invited women aged 50–69 years was 0.90 (95% CI, 0.74–1.10) (0.87 adjusted for inclusion bias, and with lead-time bias estimated to be −0.4%) in Jonsson et al. (2001) and 0.86 (95% CI, 0.86–1.17) (lead-time bias estimated to be −2%) in Jonsson et al. (2007).

Tabár et al. (2001) estimated post-RCT effectiveness of mammography screening in the Swedish Two-County study by comparing post-RCT experience with a balanced period of pre-RCT experience. [The reporting of this analysis is limited; there is uncertainty as to whether the result may be affected by lead-time bias and whether there is any statistical adjustment of the relative risks.] To obtain the IBM relative risk for breast cancer mortality in women invited to screening, the authors first estimated the IBM relative risk for attendance to screening (by comparing breast cancer mortality in women aged 40–69 years who attended screening in 1988–1996 with that in women aged 40–69 years in 1968–1977, before any screening) and then adjusted this for self-selection bias to obtain an adjusted relative risk for invitation to screening of 0.52 (95% CI, 0.43–0.63). [However, this estimate was not adjusted for the underlying trend in breast cancer mortality between 1968–1977 and 1988–1996.]

In a similar historical control-design IBM study based in seven Swedish counties, Duffy et al. (2002a, b) estimated an IBM relative risk of 0.74 (95% CI, 0.68–0.81) for screening in women aged 40–69 years based on 5–20 years of screening and follow-up until 1997 or 1998, and adjusted for lead-time bias and the underlying time trend in breast cancer mortality. For counties with 10 years or less of screening, the estimated relative risk was 0.82 (95% CI, 0.72–0.94), and for counties with more than 10 years of screening, it was 0.68 (95% CI, 0.60–0.77).

The Swedish Organised Service Screening Evaluation Group (2006a, b) analysis was of a similar design but expanded to 13 areas of Sweden and had 11–22 years of screening experience of women aged 40–69 years or 50–69 years and followed up until 2001. The IBM relative risk for screening at age 40–69 years was 0.73 (95% CI, 0.69–0.77) after adjustment for the underlying trend in breast cancer mortality.

(ii) The Netherlands

Peer et al. (1995) compared breast cancer mortality in women born in 1925–1939 who were resident in Nijmegen and were offered mammography screening every 2 years from 1975 until the end of 1990 with that of age-matched women resident in Arnhem and not offered screening. Cause of death was ascertained from clinical records and was considered to be breast cancer if metastases had been diagnosed and other causes of death could be ruled out. The IBM relative risk for breast cancer mortality in Nijmegen women relative to Arnhem women was 0.94 (95% CI, 0.68–1.29). [Breast cancer mortality in women aged 35–64 years had been reported to be lower in Nijmegen than that in Arnhem in 1970–1974. This difference was observed not to persist in the period 1975–1979. No adjustment was made for possible differences or trends in underlying breast cancer mortality rates.]

(iii) United Kingdom

The United Kingdom Trial of Early Detection of Breast Cancer (UK Trial of Early Detection of Breast Cancer Group, 1999) was a non-randomized trial that began in 1979 and preceded population-based mammography screening in the United Kingdom by 10 years. IBM to 16 years of follow-up was compared between two health service areas in which women aged 45–64 years were invited to be screened by mammography and clinical breast examination (CBE) every 2 years for four rounds, with CBE only in the intervening years, and two areas in which women received the usual care. The relative risk was 0.73 (95% CI, 0.63–0.84).

(iv) Finland

Five studies have reported IBM analyses of mammography screening in Finland. [Overlaps are not accurately identifiable from published reports but seem likely.] The study of Hakama et al. (1997) overlaps minimally with the studies of Anttila et al. (2008) and Sarkeala et al. (2008a, b) because Hakama et al. (1997) covered screening in 1987–1992 and the other three covered screening from 1992 to 2002 or 2003. Anttila et al. (2008) and Sarkeala et al. (2008a, b), which cover 410 and 260 municipalities, respectively, appear to overlap substantially; each of these two studies also overlaps with that of Parvinen et al. (2006), in which the intervention group primarily covered the "entry" cohort in the city of Turku in 1987. The study of Anttila et al. (2002), which included screening in Helsinki in the period 1986–1997, does not overlap with that of Hakama et al. (1997) or with that of Sarkeala et al. (2008a, b) but is assumed to overlap with that of Anttila et al. (2008) in the period 1992–1997. On these bases, it appears that Hakama et al. (1997), Anttila et al. (2002), and Sarkeala et al. (2008a, b) give nearly complete coverage of screening in Finland from 1986 to 2003 with minimal overlap.

Hakama et al. (1997) compared IBM in women aged 50–64 years invited and not invited to mammography screening in 84% of municipalities in 1987–1992, the first 6 years of nationwide screening in Finland. Individual year-of-birth cohorts of women were progressively invited for the first time during this period and experienced up to three screening rounds. The estimated relative risk of breast cancer death was 0.76 (95% CI, 0.53–1.09). The analysis of Anttila et al. (2002) of screening of women in Helsinki over the period 1986–1997 compared IBM in women born in 1935–1939, who had been invited to screening, with that in women born in 1930–1934, who had not. The estimated relative risk of breast cancer death was 0.81 (95% CI, 0.62–1.05) after adjustment for age at death and the estimated trend in breast cancer mortality from the trend across the two cohorts at age 40–49 years. [There may be lead-time bias in this result.] Using data from 260 Finnish municipalities and modelling the time trend in breast cancer mortality in the absence of screening, with mortality data from 1974–1985 providing estimated pre-screening mortality, Sarkeala et al. (2008a) estimated an IBM relative risk for invitation to screening in 1992–2003 of 0.78 (95% CI, 0.70–0.87) at age 50–69 years. All municipalities regularly invited only women aged 50–59 years. In those municipalities that had regularly invited women aged 50–69 years (and up to 74 years in some of these) throughout the study period, the corresponding IBM relative risk was 0.72 (95% CI, 0.51–0.97). Incidence and death were measured at age 60–79 years, whereas no impact was observed in municipalities that had stopped screening at age 59 years (Sarkeala et al., 2008b). Studies with variable screening policies provided no clear evidence for a difference in the relative risk for screening between the first 5 years (Hakama et al., 1997) and the next 10 years (Anttila et al., 2002; Sarkeala et al., 2008a, b). In addition, the results of Parvinen et al. (2006) demonstrated a significant effect in women screened regularly at age 55–74 years since 1987 in the "entry" cohort of the screening programme in the municipality of Turku (Table 5.4).

(v) Italy

Paci et al. (2002) estimated the IBM relative risk for women aged 50–69 years invited to screening in the first 7 years of population-based mammography screening in Florence over the period 1990–1999. The expected number of deaths in the absence of invitation to screening was estimated from the expected number of incident breast cancers in women not yet invited to screening in each half-year of the period 1990–1996 and the estimated number of breast cancer deaths to 1999 (from estimated case fatality rates for up to 9.5 years after diagnosis) in women expected to be diagnosed with breast cancer in each of these half-year cohorts. The estimated relative risk was 0.81 (95% CI, 0.64–1.01). [The nature of 13 breast cancer deaths classified as "other" (neither invited nor not invited, and treated as not invited in the analysis) is unclear. If they had been treated as invited, the relative risk would have been 0.83.]

(vi) Spain

Based on a population-based mammography screening programme targeting women aged 45–64 years in Navarre, Ascunce et al. (2007) reported an IBM relative risk of 0.58 (95% CI, 0.44–0.75) for invitation to screening of women aged 50–69 years in 1997–2001. There was no adjustment for the overall trend in breast cancer mortality; the corresponding relative risk was 1.07 (95% CI, 0.66–1.74) in women aged 30–44 years and 1.03 (95% CI, 0.77–1.37) in those aged 75 years and older (outside the target age group). The relative risk adjusted for the average of these two trends was 0.56 (95% CI, 0.39–0.80).

(vii) Denmark

Based on linked screening registry, cancer registry, cause of death registry, and population register data for individual women, Olsen et al. (2005) analysed IBM for invitation to screening in the first 10 years (1991–2001) of population-based mammography screening offered every 2 years to women aged 50–69 years in Copenhagen. Three comparison groups, Copenhagen in 1981–1991 and Denmark (except Copenhagen and two other areas with population-based screening before 2001) in 1991–2001 and 1981–1991 (secondary control groups to provide data on the underlying trend in breast cancer mortality), were constructed from women's individual records in the population register, and the women were allocated pseudo-dates of first invitation. In all cases, women with prevalent breast cancer before their real date or pseudo-date of invitation were excluded. Analysis was done by way of a Poisson regression model of breast cancer mortality with age, whether invited or not, period, region, and interaction between period and region as covariates, thus adjusting the estimate of effect of invitation for differences in age, place, and time between invited and not invited women. The estimated IBM relative risk for invitation to screening was 0.75 (95% CI, 0.63–0.89).

(viii) Norway

A population-based programme that offers mammography screening every 2 years to women aged 50–69 years began as a pilot programme in four of the 19 Norwegian counties in 1996; roll-out to the rest of the country began 2 years later and was completed in 2005 (Hofvind et al., 2013). Population-based screening was preceded by widespread opportunistic screening, to the extent that 38% of women who had their first mammogram within the programme in 1996–2006 had received a mammogram within the preceding 3 years, and 64% had ever had a mammogram (Hofvind et al., 2013). Also, importantly, the roll-out of population-based screening in Norway was accompanied by or preceded by the establishment of multidisciplinary breast cancer care units in each county, in which all women being investigated or treated for breast cancer (whether screen-detected or not) were managed (Kalager, 2011).

Three studies have reported on IBM in women invited to screening in the Norwegian population-based programme. One included population-based screening experience accumulated to 2001–2002 in women in the four pilot study counties (Olsen et al., 2013). The second included the experience in the whole country to the end of 2005 (Kalager et al., 2010), thus fully with overlapping the first. The third included the experience in the whole country to the end of 2009 (Weedon-Fekjær et al., 2014), thus fully overlapping with both of the others.

Olsen et al. (2013) compared mortality from breast cancer diagnosed after screening began in women in the four pilot screening counties with the corresponding mortality in women in these counties over the 6 years before screening began. They adjusted their comparison for the underlying trend in breast cancer mortality by estimating it in five non-screening counties in similar periods before and after the beginning of 1996. The authors linked individual data obtained from the central population register, cancer registry, and cause of death registry for all women within the scope of their analysis; aggregated data were not required. However, they did not have individual screening data, so women in the screening counties during the screening period were allocated the date of first invitation to screening in their municipality as their first invitation date. Women included in the 6-year control period for the screening counties were allocated pseudo-dates of invitation 6 years before those in the screening period. The maximum period of screening was 6 years. The authors estimated the IBM relative risk for invitation to screening to be 0.89 (95% CI, 0.71–1.12). [This relative risk includes lead-time bias. Also, the underlying downtrend may have been greater in screening counties than in non-screening counties, due to the introduction of multidisciplinary breast cancer care units along with screening.]

The analysis of Kalager et al. (2010) used a similar approach to that of Olsen et al. (2013) except that it covered mammography screening in the period 1996–2005 and had individual data only for women who had been diagnosed with breast cancer. To address effects of the underlying trends in breast cancer mortality, comparisons were made between women invited to screening in 1996–2005 and corresponding women not invited to screening in 1986–1995, and vice versa. The comparisons were made primarily in women aged 50–69 years at diagnosis of breast cancer. [Balanced breast cancer accrual and follow-up periods and age groups avoided lead-time bias. However, as a consequence of the manner of roll-out of population-based screening in

Norway, the group invited to screening and its historical comparison were concentrated in the second halves of the compared periods and the group not invited to screening and its historical comparison were concentrated in the first halves, making the latter a potentially inaccurate estimate of the underlying trend in breast cancer mortality in the group offered screening.] The authors estimated the relative risk comparing IBM for the group invited to screening relative to its historical comparison group to be 0.72 (95% CI, 0.63–0.81) and the corresponding relative risk in the group not invited to screening to be 0.82 (95% CI, 0.71–0.93). [From these relative risks, the Working Group estimated the IBM for invitation to screening adjusted for the underlying mortality trend to be 0.88 (95% CI, 0.73–1.05). The Working Group noted, in agreement with Olsen et al. (2013), that the mortality trend in areas without screening may not accurately indicate the trend in areas with screening.]

Weedon-Fekjær et al. (2014) obtained individually linked data for all women, as Olsen et al. (2013) had, and in addition obtained individual dates of screening invitations. Unusually, however, they based their analysis of invitation to screening over the period 1996–2009 on the complete, dynamic population of Norwegian women aged 50–79 years in 1986–2009. Thus, their population of women unexposed to screening included women from 10 years before the implementation of population-based screening; as a result, they drew on nearly 13 million person–years of experience before invitation to screening and only 2.4 million after. The IBM relative risk for invitation to screening was estimated to be 0.72 (95% CI, 0.64–0.79) using a complex Poisson regression modelling approach. [The authors noted that they could not exclude possible effects of the establishment of multidisciplinary breast cancer care centres in parallel with the roll-out of the screening programme.]

[The relative risks for invitation to screening of these three, overlapping studies of the Norwegian experience are compatible to the extent that their 95% confidence intervals overlap, although the upper limit for the Weedon-Fekjær et al. (2014) study is less than the point estimates for the other two studies, suggesting that it could be lower. In principle, a lower relative risk in Weedon-Fekjær et al. (2014) would be expected because: it includes a later 4 years of the population-based programme's experience than the other two studies; it would be based, on average, on longer periods of individual women's experience in the programme; and it would be less affected by the previous high level of opportunistic screening. It might also, perhaps, be affected by the inclusion of a large volume of pre-screening breast cancer mortality experience, which, in the event of a falling trend in underlying breast cancer mortality, might produce an artificially lower relative risk. There is evidence of such a trend (Kalager et al., 2010), and it could be sufficient to explain the difference between the estimate of Weedon-Fekjær et al. (2014) and those of the other two studies. Although the adjustment for period should have addressed this issue, the statistical dominance of person–years before 1996 may have compromised the effectiveness of this adjustment.]

Summary

The IBM relative risks for invitation to screening ranged overall from 0.58 to 0.94, with a median value of 0.78. Lead-time bias was the most common residual bias and would be expected to be conservative. If the Swedish, Finnish, and Norwegian studies that are overlapped substantially or fully by other studies (Duffy et al., 2002b; Jonsson et al., 2007; Anttila et al., 2008; Kalager et al., 2010; Olsen et al., 2013) are removed, the range of the remaining 14 studies is the same as for all 19 studies and the median is little changed, at 0.77. Furthermore, if all Norwegian studies are removed because of the introduction of multidisciplinary breast care centres in parallel with screening, the range remains the same and the median is 0.76. The United Kingdom Trial of Early Detection of Breast Cancer (relative risk [RR], 0.73; 95% CI, 0.63–0.84) included annual CBE in the intervention.

(b) Women aged 50–69 years who attended screening

The design and results of studies reviewed are summarized in Table 5.5. Studies are ordered in the table by the country in which they were conducted (with countries in the order in which their mammography screening programmes were first introduced) and within each country by the earliest date of mammography screening that was included in the analysis.

Most of the studies in Table 5.5 were based on the same mammography experience as was used for analyses of the outcomes of invitation to screening. Self-selection for attendance is an important issue in these analyses because the numerator for the IBM relative risk for breast cancer mortality is based on the experience of women attending screening while the denominator is based on all women in a different era or area who were not invited to screening or on women in the same area and era who chose not to attend screening. Self-selection may bias the IBM relative risk estimate if it creates a difference in the underlying risk of breast cancer death between women attending screening and all women, or women not attending screening.

(i) Sweden

Tabár et al. (2001) reported an estimate of the IBM relative risk for women aged 40–64 years attending screening of 0.37 (95% CI, 0.30–0.46). [The estimate appears not to have been adjusted either for self-selection or for the underlying time trend in breast cancer mortality. However, data on this trend in women aged 20–39 years in 1968–1977 or 1988–1996 were reported, and the Working Group used this trend to obtain an adjusted IBM relative risk of 0.46 (95% CI, 0.21–0.97). This relative risk may still be affected by self-selection bias.]

The other three Swedish studies that estimated IBM relative risk for attendance to screening (Duffy et al., 2002a, b; Swedish Organised Service Screening Evaluation Group, 2006a, b; Jonsson et al., 2007) overlapped substantially with one another in their coverage of the screening experience, and Swedish Organised Service Screening Evaluation Group (2006a, b) included the experience of one of the counties analysed in Tabár et al. (2001). These three studies variously covered screening of women aged 40–74 years, but mostly aged 50–69 years, and screening during various parts of the period 1978-2001. The results, each adjusted for self-selection bias, were reasonably similar (Table 5.5): the IBM relative risks were 0.61 (95% CI, 0.55–0.68) for Duffy et al. (2002a, b), 0.57 (95% CI, 0.53–0.62) for Swedish Organised Service Screening Evaluation Group (2006a, b), and 0.70 (95% CI, 0.57–0.86) for Jonsson et al. (2007). The methods of adjustment for self-selection bias were, respectively, that of Duffy et al. (2002a, b), a refinement of that method as reported in Swedish Organised Service Screening Evaluation Group (2006a, b), and the method of Cuzick et al. (1997).

(ii) Finland

One Finnish study has estimated the IBM relative risk for attendance to screening (Sarkeala et al., 2008b). Based on the same data set as used for Sarkeala et al. (2008a), this study was designed primarily to assess the effect of different screening centre policies on screening effectiveness. Screened women attended between 1992 and 2003; unscreened women included those residing in the same areas in 1974–1985 and women who were invited in 1992–2003 but did not attend. The IBM relative risk for attendance to screening was 0.63 (95% CI, 0.53–0.75), adjusted for self-selection bias using the method of Cuzick et al. (1997).

(iii) Italy

Based on a similar population of women invited to the first screening round (1991–1993) in Florence described in Paci et al. (2002) (Table 5.4), Puliti & Zappa (2012) followed up women invited to mammography screening every 2 years at age 50–69 years for incidence of breast cancer to 2007 and mortality from breast cancer and other causes to 2008 (Table 5.5). The estimated IBM relative risk for women who had ever been screened relative to those who had never been screened was 0.51 (95% CI, 0.40–0.66). This estimate was adjusted for marital status and small-area deprivation index in the hope of reducing self-selection bias. [There would also have been some lead-time bias because the mortality follow-up period was 1 year longer than the period of incident breast cancer accrual.]

(iv) Canada

Based on data obtained from seven of the 12 provincial mammography screening programmes established in or after 1988 under the Canadian Breast Cancer Screening Initiative, Coldman et al. (2014) reported an IBM relative risk of 0.60 (95% CI, 0.52–0.67) for women who were screened at least once in the period 1990–2009 (Table 5.5). For the seven individual provinces, the relative risk ranged from 0.41 (95% CI, 0.33–0.48) in New Brunswick to 0.73 (95% CI, 0.68–0.78) in Ontario. The analysis was based on 20.2 million person–years of experience. Population data from Statistics Canada indicated that 32.4% (Ontario) to 53.0% (New Brunswick) of women aged 50–69 years attended screening in 2005–2006 and that 56.1% (Manitoba) to 64.3% (Quebec) reported undergoing bilateral mammography during the same period. An ad hoc method (described fully in the authors' online supplementary methods) was used to adjust the relative risk in British Columbia for self-selection.

(v) Denmark

Olsen et al. (2005), who estimated the IBM relative risk for women invited to screening in the Copenhagen population-based mammography programme (Table 5.4), also estimated the IBM relative risk for women screened relative to those not screened, which was 0.60 (95% CI, 0.52–0.67) unadjusted for self-selection for screening. The relative risk adjusted for self-selection using an ad hoc approach was estimated to be 0.63 (95% CI not reported).

(vi) Norway

In a study of women invited to attend the Norwegian Breast Cancer Screening Program, Hofvind et al. (2013) compared breast cancer mortality in women who accepted the invitation with that in women who did not (Table 5.5). This study is based entirely on linked unit record data of individual women invited to attend a population-based mammography screening programme, which included screening history, cancer registrations, and death records. Women could contribute person–years of experience to both the unscreened and the screened group. Overall, 84% of women attended screening for 1–15 years, with a median of 4.5 years. Accrual of incident breast cancers ended in 2009, and emigration and mortality follow-up continued until the end of 2010. The relative risk of death from breast cancer in screened relative to unscreened women was estimated to be 0.57 (95% CI, 0.51–0.64) adjusted for age at breast cancer diagnosis, calendar year, time since inclusion in the unscreened or screened group, and self-selection bias estimated using the average estimate of the breast cancer mortality relative risk for non-attenders relative to uninvited women (1.36; 95% CI, 1.11–1.67, from Duffy et al. 2002a, b) and the study estimate of attendance in response to a screening invitation. The authors noted that 38% of women first attending the Norwegian Breast Cancer Screening Program in 1996–2006 reported having had a mammogram within the preceding 3 years, which could have biased the estimate of programme effectiveness. They also noted that the contemporaneous introduction of multidisciplinary breast care centres should not have biased their relative risk estimates because only women who were invited to the programme were included in the analysis. [No adjustment was made for lead-time bias.]

(vii) USA

Morrison et al. (1988) examined breast cancer mortality within the Breast Cancer Detection Demonstration Project, which was initiated in 1973 by the American Cancer Society and the National Cancer Institute to demonstrate the feasibility of large-scale screening for breast cancer (Beahrs et al., 1979; Baker, 1982). Screening was initially with two-view mammography, CBE, and thermography, but in later years thermography was dropped and mammography use was reduced, particularly in women younger than 50 years. Morrison et al. (1988) estimated the ratios (observed to expected) for death from breast cancer to be 0.80 overall and 0.89, 0.76, and 0.74, respectively, for women aged 35–49, 50–59, and 60–74 years at entry. [No confidence intervals or *P* values were reported.]

A case–cohort study approach was used by Thompson et al. (1994) to evaluate the effect of a mammography screening programme offered from 1985 to eligible members of a health maintenance organization in Washington State. Women aged 40–49 years were offered screening in the programme only if they had a risk factor for breast cancer, and women aged 50 years and older were invited every 1–3 years, depending on their risk factors; all were recommended to have annual CBE. A randomly selected age-stratified sample representing 2.4% of women was selected as a subcohort to represent the experience of all women in the cohort in the analysis. The formal screening programme began in 1985 and included mammography every 1–3 years depending on risk and annual CBE. About 10% of the women had been screened before implementation of the programme. By 1988 (3.5 years after implementation of the programme), about 34–56% of women (depending on age) had been screened. The IBM relative risk adjusted for mother's history of breast cancer, nulliparity, and history of previous breast biopsy was 0.61 (95% CI, 0.23–1.62) for women aged 50 years and older.

Summary

The IBM relative risks for attendance to screening ranged from 0.51 to 0.80 after adjustment for self-selection. The lower value of 0.46 of Tabár et al. (2001) was not adjusted for selection bias, and it is likely that the value of 0.51 of Puliti & Zappa (2012) was incompletely adjusted for self-selection bias. The relative risks for the remaining studies ranged from 0.57 to 0.80 (median, 0.60) when including only the largest of the substantially overlapping Swedish studies (Swedish Organised Service Screening Evaluation Group, 2006a, b). The two studies in the USA (RR, 0.80 for each) included CBE in the intervention.

(c) Women younger than 50 years or older than 69 years

Only studies designed to separate the effect of screening on breast cancer mortality in a specified age group were considered to be informative. To study effectiveness of screening in women younger than 50 years, the analysis of breast cancer mortality should be limited to deaths in women whose breast cancer was diagnosed when they were younger than 50 years, unless screening was offered only to women while they were younger than 50 years (see Section 4.2.1 for discussion of age creep). Similarly, to study effectiveness of screening in women older than 69 years, the analysis should be limited to women first offered screening when they were older than 69 years and to breast cancer deaths that followed a diagnosis of breast cancer when the women were older than 69 years. Only results of studies that meet these criteria are included in this section. Studies are not included that presented age-specific results for women younger than 50 years but included deaths from breast cancers diagnosed at later ages (UK Trial of Early Detection of Breast Cancer Group, 1999; Coldman et al., 2014) or for women older than 69 years at death from breast cancer who had not been offered screening (Ascunce et al., 2007; Sarkeala et al., 2008b; Kalager et al., 2010; Weedon-Fekjær et al., 2014) or had not been first offered screening in this age group (Jonsson et al., 2007).

The design and results of studies reviewed for this section are summarized in Table 5.6, by age (younger than 50 years or older than 69 years) and by country (in the order in which their mammography screening programmes were first introduced), and within each country by the earliest date of mammography screening that was included in the analysis.

(i) Women younger than 50 years

Sweden

Jonsson et al. (2000) compared IBM in women with breast cancer diagnosed at age 40–49 years in 14 Swedish study-group areas in which population-based mammography screening was offered from age 40 years and 15 control-group areas in which it was offered from age 50 years. These areas excluded five in which RCTs of screening had been conducted, one in which screening had been introduced very early, and one that offered screening from age 45 years. Women in the study group entered the study when screening started in their area. In both groups, mortality follow-up was to age 59 years, creating the possibility of lead-time bias in the result. A geographically identical, historical reference period (1976–1986) was defined for the study group and for the control group. The estimated IBM relative risk for women invited to screening at age 40 years was 0.91 (95% CI, 0.72–1.15), compared with the geographical areas that started screening at age 50 years, and adjusting for year of follow-up, geographical area, and time period. [Geographical area, as included in the model, was not defined but is likely to have been highly correlated with invitation to screening; therefore, the reported relative risk may be unreliable.]

The mammography screening experience of Jonsson et al. (2007) overlaps almost completely with that analysed by Jonsson et al. (2000), and also compares IBM in women invited and not invited to screening over unbalanced time periods. The IBM relative risk for invitation to screening in women aged 40–49 years was 0.64 (95% CI, 0.43–0.97). [The Working Group estimated the IBM relative risk to be 0.51 (95% CI, 0.29–0.90) after adjustment for the difference in underlying breast cancer mortality with reference to results in the authors' Table 3. Lead-time bias was estimated to be −5%.]

Hellquist et al. (2011) updated the analysis of Jonsson et al. (2000) and extended the period of accrual of breast cancer cases from 1997 to 2005. Women in 34 Swedish counties or screening areas were considered invited to screening if they resided when aged 40–49 years in an area that invited women of this age to screening (the same logic was applied for uninvited women in control areas during 1986–2005, with the same average follow-up time and mid-calendar year of follow-up). Such areas were required to have offered screening to women aged 40–49 years for at least 6 years from 1986 to 2005 (mean, 15.8 years). Only breast cancers incident at age 40–49 years were included. The IBM relative risk adjusted for misclassification of breast cancer cases in women invited to screening was 0.74 (95% CI, 0.66–0.83). Assuming 1 month and 1 year of lead time produced estimates of lead-time bias of −0.01% and −0.05%, respectively. Adjusted relative risks for breast cancer deaths in women diagnosed at ages 40–44 years and 45–49 years were estimated to be 0.83 (95% CI, 0.70–1.00) and 0.68 (95% CI, 0.59–0.78), respectively. Adjusted relative risks in women who

Table 5.6 Incidence-based mortality studies of the effectiveness of invitation to mammography screening[a] mainly in women younger than 50 years or older than 69 years

Reference Country	Areas, earliest year of programme screening, screening age, screening interval	Person–years[b]	Duration of screening	Accrual and follow-up periods	Diagnosis and death age ranges	Individual or aggregate data	Temporal and geographical similarity of comparison group	Time-balanced follow-up periods?	Adjustments	Breast cancer mortality RR (95% CI)[c]	Comments
Women younger than 50 years											
Jonsson et al. (2000) Sweden	29 areas 1986–1997, depending on area 40–49 yr 18–22 mo; average, 20 mo	Invited 2 229 000 Not invited 3 383 000	3–10 yr average, 8.0 yr	1986–1996 Same	40–49 yr Same + 10 yr	Individual for breast cancer cases; aggregate, all other women	Same period; different areas	No (follow-up in study population was from start of screening in each area; in control population, it was from 1987)	Year of follow-up, area, time period	0.91 (0.72–1.15)	Lead-time bias estimated to be −0.4%, and inclusion bias −3% RR was 0.97 after excluding > 8 yr of follow-up from control group
Jonsson et al. (2007) Sweden	4 counties 1989 40–49 yr average, 20–22 mo	Invited 485 468 Not invited 387 173	7 yr	1989–1996 Same + 5 yr	40–49 yr Same + 10 yr	Individual for breast cancer cases; aggregate, all other women	Different period (accrual 1989–1996 for study group, 1988–1996 for control group); different areas	No (study group follow-up to 2001, control group to 1998)	Not stated	[0.51 (0.29–0.90)[d]]	RR adjusted by the Working Group for difference in underlying breast cancer mortality. Lead-time bias estimated to be −5%

Table 5.6 (continued)

Reference Country	Areas, earliest year of programme screening, screening age, screening interval	Person–years[b]	Duration of screening	Accrual and follow-up periods	Diagnosis and death age ranges	Individual or aggregate data	Temporal and geographical similarity of comparison group	Time-balanced follow-up periods?	Adjustments	Breast cancer mortality RR (95% CI)[c]	Comments
Hellquist et al. (2011) Sweden	34 areas 1986–1997, depending on area 40–49 yr 18 mo	Invited 6 994 421 Not invited 8 843 852	6–20 yr	1986–2005 Same	40–49 yr 40–68 yr	Individual for women who died of breast cancer; aggregate, all other women	Same period; different areas (3 of 34 areas changed status)	Yes	Breast cancer cases in study-group women known not to have been invited to screening; contamination in control group	Invited to screening: [0.79 (0.67–0.92)] Ever screened: [0.76 (0.64–0.89)[d]]	RR adjusted for pre-screening differences in breast cancer mortality. Lead-time bias estimated to be −0.01% to −0.05%
Hakama et al. (1995) Finland	City of Kotka 1982 40–51 yr 2 yr	Invited to screening 38 220 Attended screening 32 910 Not screened 56 233	8–9 yr	1982–1990 Same + 1 yr	40–54 yr 40–55 yr	Yes	Same period; same area	Yes	Age	Invited to screening: 0.11 (0.00–0.71) Attended screening: 0.10 (0.00–0.53)	Screening included CBE. Lead-time bias possible. RR based on 1 breast cancer death. Programme sensitivity estimated to be 25%

Table 5.6 (continued)

Reference Country	Areas, earliest year of programme screening, screening age, screening interval	Person–years[b]	Duration of screening	Accrual and follow-up periods	Diagnosis and death age ranges	Individual or aggregate data	Temporal and geographical similarity of comparison group	Time-balanced follow-up periods?	Adjustments	Breast cancer mortality RR (95% CI)[c]	Comments
Women older than 69 years											
Jonsson et al. (2003b) Sweden	23 areas 1986–1990, depending on area 70–74 yr 22.8 mo	Invited 1 251 000 Not invited 580 000	8–12 yr average, 8.1 yr	1986–1998 Same	70–74 yr; Same + 12 yr	Individual for breast cancer cases; aggregate, all other women	Same period; different areas	Yes	Age during follow-up, area, time period	Underlying cause of death: 0.96 (0.73–1.25) Excess mortality estimate: 0.84 (0.59–1.19)	RR adjusted for both inclusion bias and lead-time bias was estimated to be 0.93 for underlying cause of death and 0.78 for excess mortality (95% CIs not reported)
Van Dijck et al. (1997) The Netherlands	2 cities 1977 68–83 yr 2 yr	Invited 60 313 Not invited 61 832	13 yr	1977–1990 Same	68–95 yr 68–95 yr	Individual for breast cancer cases; aggregate, all other women	Same period; different cities	Yes	Difference in underlying risk of breast cancer in the 2 cities	[0.89 (0.56–1.40)]	Women first invited to screening at age 68 yr or older; 46% of invited women screened once or more

Table 5.6 (continued)

Reference Country	Areas, earliest year of programme screening, screening age, screening interval	Person–years[b]	Duration of screening	Accrual and follow-up periods	Diagnosis and death age ranges	Individual or aggregate data	Temporal and geographical similarity of comparison group	Time-balanced follow-up periods?	Adjustments	Breast cancer mortality RR (95% CI)[c]	Comments
Coldman et al. (2014) Canada	7 provinces 1990 70–79 yr No recall after 69 yr	Screened and not screened at all ages 20 200 000 (Analysis for screening 70–79 yr based on 4 of 7 provinces)	1–20 yr, all women not known, women 70–79 yr	1990–2009 Same	70–99 yr Same	Individual for screened women; aggregate for unscreened women	Same period; same population	Yes	Age	0.65 (0.56–0.74)	Not adjusted for self-selection bias (see Table 5.5). Analysis based on age at first participation in organized screening; previous opportunistic screening cannot be excluded

[a] Two studies evaluated invitation to mammography plus CBE.
[b] Person–years: number of women or number of breast cancer deaths.
[c] RRs are for breast cancer as the underlying cause of death when alternative estimates (e.g. excess mortality) are also provided.
[d] RRs and 95% CIs adjusted for trend or geographical difference in underlying mortality were calculated as ratio of the authors' estimated RRs comparing screening area with control period or area; 95% CI of ratio estimated using the method in Altman & Bland (2003) as implemented in http://www.hutchon.net/CompareRR.htm. With reference to Hellquist et al. (2011), see also Weedon-Fekjær et al. (2014).
CI, confidence interval; mo, month or months; RR, relative risk; yr, year or years.

attended screening were 0.71 (95% CI, 0.62–0.80), 0.82 (95% CI, 0.67–1.00), and 0.63 (95% CI, 0.54–0.75) for the age groups 40–49, 40–44, and 45–49 years, respectively. These estimates were made by adjusting the estimates for invitation to screening using the method of Cuzick et al. (1997). The above estimates were not adjusted for a pre-screening difference in breast cancer mortality (RR, 0.94; 95% CI, 0.85–1.05) between screening and non-screening areas; taking this into account, the Working Group calculated an IBM relative risk of [0.79 (95% CI, 0.67–0.92)] for invited women and [0.76 (95% CI, 0.64–0.89)] for women who were ever screened using a method developed by Altman & Bland (2003).

Finland

Mammography was initiated on a pilot basis in Finland in the early 1980s. Women born in 1940 or 1942 were invited to attend screening with mammography and CBE in 1982; women born in 1936 or 1938 were invited in 1983, and thus they were aged 40–47 years at entry. They were re-invited every 2 years until 1990 (a total of four or five invitations), and women were considered to be non-attenders if they did not attend the first round. Women born in alternate years from 1935 to 1943 were used as a control cohort. The IBM relative risk was 0.11 (95% CI, 0.00–0.71) for invitation to screening and 0.10 (95% CI, 0.00–0.53) for attendance to screening (Hakama et al., 1995). [The Working Group agreed with the authors' opinion that an estimated programme sensitivity of 25% was too low for programme effectiveness to be the sole explanation for the very low relative risk.]

Summary

The Swedish study of Hellquist et al. (2011) encompassed the whole screening experience covered by Jonsson et al. (2000) and Jonsson et al. (2007) and provided IBM relative risks of 0.74 (95% CI, 0.66–0.83) for being invited to screening and 0.71 (0.62–0.80) for being ever screened. No weight was given to the very low relative risk that Hakama et al. (1995) observed, because it was based on only one death and appears incompatible with the estimated screening programme sensitivity of 25%.

(ii) Women older than 69 years

Sweden

The results of Jonsson et al. (2003b) are similar to those of Jonsson et al. (2000), except that the analysis was based on first invitation to screening of women aged 65–74 years and covered 23 areas (16 study-group areas and 7 control-group areas) and not 29; the additional exclusions were principally counties in which screening did not begin until after 1990. The mean follow-up time was 10.1 years in the study group (8.1 years if estimated individual date of first screening was used, and not date of start of the screening programme in each area) and 9.3 years in the control group. Breast cancer deaths included in the analysis were only those that followed a diagnosis of breast cancer at age 70–74 years. The IBM relative risk for invitation to screening was 0.96 (95% CI, 0.73–1.25) when breast cancer mortality was based on underlying cause of death and adjusted for the difference in underlying mortality between the study-group and control-group areas. With further adjustment for inclusion bias and lead-time bias, the relative risk was 0.93 (95% CI not reported). The authors argued that the underlying cause of death may have been a particularly inaccurate classifier of mortality due to breast cancer in older women and that an excess mortality estimate would be more accurate. The corresponding excess mortality estimate of the relative risk was 0.84 (95% CI, 0.59–1.19) adjusted for the difference in underlying mortality between the study-group and control-group areas; with further adjustment for inclusion bias and lead-time bias, the relative risk was 0.78.

Jonsson et al. (2007) also reported on IBM associated with invitation to screening at age 70–74 years. However, the two screening counties in this study were also study-group (screening) counties in the Jonsson et al. (2003b) study, and the periods covered by the two studies were nearly the same. Therefore, Jonsson et al. (2007) was not considered to provide independent evidence.

The Netherlands

Van Dijck et al. (1997) reported on IBM in women first invited to mammography screening at age 68–83 years in the city of Nijmegen compared with that in the city of Arnhem over an accrual and follow-up period of 1977–1990. Attendance rates in Nijmegen fell sharply with age, from approximately 70% in women in their late sixties to about 40% in those in their seventies and to less than 20% for the first round and less than 10% for the second and later rounds in women in their eighties and nineties. Screening began in Arnhem in 1989. The IBM relative risk for invitation to screening over the whole study period was estimated to be 0.80 (95% CI, 0.53–1.22), which became [0.89 (95% CI, 0.56–1.40)] when adjusted for the estimated difference in underlying breast cancer mortality between Nijmegen and Arnhem (see Table 5.6). For the period 9–13 years after the start of screening, the IBM relative risk estimate was 0.53 (95% CI, 0.27–1.04), and 0.59 (95% CI, 0.30–1.16) after adjusting for the difference in underlying breast cancer mortality.

Canada

In the Canadian provincial mammography screening programmes (Coldman et al., 2014), the relative risk for women first screened at age 70–79 years was 0.65 (95% CI, 0.56–0.74) in the four provinces that offered screening to women in this age group. The province-specific relative risks varied from 0.63 (95% CI, 0.49–0.76) to 0.84 (95% CI, 0.36–1.31). The authors estimated that self-selection bias was conservative (–9% in an analysis limited to women aged 40–49 years in British Columbia). [This estimate may not be applicable to screening of women aged 70–79 years. Also, opportunistic breast screening before first screening in the provincial programmes could have affected the reported results, particularly in the age group 70–79 years.]

Summary

Three studies reported potentially valid estimates of IBM relative risks for breast cancer mortality in women older than 69 years: one for the age group 68–83 years (Van Dijck et al., 1997), one for 65–74 years (Jonsson et al., 2003b), and one for 70–79 years (Coldman et al., 2014). The reported relative risks, of 0.89 (95% CI, 0.56–1.40) by Van Dijck et al. (1997), 0.96 (95% CI, 0.73–1.25) by Jonsson et al. (2003b), and 0.65 (95% CI, 0.56–0.74) by Coldman et al. (2014), are heterogeneous. However, the heterogeneity is reduced if the excess mortality estimate of the relative risk, 0.84 (95% CI, 0.59–1.19), of Jonsson et al. (2003b) is accepted as the more accurate estimate from that study. Lack of adjustment for self-selection bias and lack of consideration of possible effects of previous opportunistic screening limit the weight that can be given to the result of Coldman et al. (2014).

5.2.2 Case–control studies

The reported case–control studies are presented by country in the text and tables. All case–control studies are based on defined populations, but some of these are specific cohorts, with the methods of analysis being a case–control study nested within the cohort. In many case–control studies, the risk estimates are calculated for women who participated in screening compared with women who had been invited (or to whom screening was otherwise offered) but who did not participate. The non-participating women may have a different risk of death from breast cancer compared with the average population (Cuzick et al., 1997; Duffy et al., 2002a;

Swedish Organised Service Screening Evaluation Group, 2006a; Sarkeala et al., 2008a, b), so this may result in selection bias. If the case–control study is based on systematic historical databases on screening, information bias can be considered minimal. However, in other case–control studies, information bias may be a problem. Rather few case–control studies have assessed screening impact compared with expectation in the absence of screening (or invitation) in the average population, as is usually done in cohort mortality studies. There are further limitations in the reported case–control studies in taking into account full screening histories in the risk estimates, and consequently there is wide variation in the follow-up windows for incidence and mortality after index screening. This potentially affects the magnitude of the estimates, even though these follow-up details are not always reported in connection with the individual studies. Some studies used only age at death in matching, whereas most studies also matched on residence at the time of diagnosis of the case. In addition, since the risk of breast cancer could be different among women who attend screening after receiving an invitation compared with those who are invited but do not attend, selection factors may confound the estimates of efficacy. A potential asset in case–control studies is that an adjustment for sociodemographic factors can also be attempted.

(a) Case–control studies within service screening programmes

See Table 5.7.

(i) United Kingdom

Allgood et al. (2008) performed a case–control study in the East Anglia region. The cases were deaths from breast cancer in women diagnosed between the ages of 50 years and 70 years, after the initiation of the East Anglia Breast Screening Programme in 1989. The controls were women (two per case) who had not died of breast cancer, from the same area, matched by date of birth to the cases. Each control was known to be alive at the date of death of her matched case. All women were known to the breast screening programme and had been invited, at least once, to be screened. The unadjusted odds ratio for risk of death from breast cancer in women who attended at least one routine screen compared with those who did not attend was 0.35 (95% CI, 0.24–0.50), and 0.65 (95% CI, 0.48–0.88) after adjusting for self-selection bias using the more conservative intention-to-treat analysis (Duffy et al., 2002a).

Fielder et al. (2004) conducted a case–control study to estimate the effect of service screening, as provided by the NHS Breast Screening Programme, on breast cancer mortality in Wales. The 419 cases were deaths from breast cancer in women aged 50–75 years at diagnosis who were diagnosed after the start of screening in 1991 and who died after 1998. The 717 controls were women who had not died of breast cancer or any other condition during the study period. The aim was to select one control from the same general practitioner's practice and another from a different general practitioner's practice within the same district, matched by year of birth. The unadjusted odds ratio for risk of death from breast cancer in women who attended at least one routine screen compared with those who had never been screened was 0.62 (95% CI, 0.47–0.82), and 0.75 (95% CI, 0.49–1.14) after excluding cases diagnosed before 1995 and adjusting for self-selection bias.

(ii) Iceland

Gabe et al. (2007) conducted a case–control study to evaluate the impact of the Icelandic breast screening programme, which was initiated in November 1987 in Reykjavik and covered the whole country from December 1989, comprising biennial invitation to mammography screening for women aged 40–69 years. The cases were deaths from breast cancer matched by age and

Table 5.7 Case–control studies of the effectiveness of mammography screening within service screening programmes, by country

Reference	Area, year programme began, screening age and interval, women included	No. of breast cancer deaths, source, time period for breast cancer deaths, years of diagnoses; proportion of eligible women included	Screening exposure; age of included women	No. of controls, source, whether same source population as cases, matching variables, alive at date of death or diagnosis of case	Linkage or use of screening, cancer registry, death databases; data items available	Issues or items related to screening history; whether prevalent cases were excluded	Adjustments	Breast cancer mortality OR (95% CI)
United Kingdom								
Allgood et al. (2008)	East Anglia 1989 50–70 yr active, ≥ 70 yr allowed 3-yearly Women registered with GP	284 East Anglia cancer registry database 1995–2004 from 1995 16 deaths excluded	At least 1 invitation to breast screening 50–70 yr	568 NHS Exeter system database Same source as cases DOB; most were from same health authority as case Alive at DOD of case	All 3 DOB, date of diagnosis, DOD, screening history (time since last screen, number of screens)	Prevalent cases were minimized by restricting to deaths and diagnoses from 1995, 6 yr after start of programme	SES, self-selection bias using method of Duffy et al. (2002a)	0.65 (0.48–0.88) for at least 1 screen
Fielder et al. (2004)	Wales 1989 50–75 yr 3-yearly Women registered with GP and identified in health authority registers	419 Breast Test Wales database and "standard death registration" 1998–2001 from 1991 84%	At least 1 invitation before date of diagnosis or pseudo-diagnosis 50–75 yr	717 Database of those eligible for screening in Breast Test Wales Year of birth; 1 control from same GP and 1 from other GP Alive at time of diagnosis of case	Breast Test Wales for screening history and breast cancer diagnoses Year of birth, date of diagnosis, screening history (time since last screen, number of screens)	All cancers diagnosed early in the programme in 1991–1994 excluded; controls with breast cancer diagnosis were eligible	Self-selection bias using method of Duffy et al. (2002a)	0.75 (0.49–1.14) for at least 1 screen

Table 5.7 (continued)

Reference	Area, year programme began, screening age and interval, women included	No. of breast cancer deaths, source, time period for breast cancer deaths, years of diagnoses; proportion of eligible women included	Screening exposure; age of included women	No. of controls, source, whether same source population as cases, matching variables, alive at date of death or diagnosis of case	Linkage or use of screening, cancer registry, death databases; data items available	Issues or items related to screening history; whether prevalent cases were excluded	Adjustments	Breast cancer mortality OR (95% CI)
Iceland								
Gabe et al. (2007)	1987 40–69 yr 2-yearly All women in age group	226 Source not stated 1990–2002 from start of service screening 7 deaths before 1990 excluded	Ever screened before date of diagnosis or pseudo-diagnosis 40–70+ yr	902 National registry Same source as cases DOB, screening area Alive at DOD of case	Probably the national cancer and screening registries DOB, date of diagnosis, DOD, urban/rural residence, screening history (time since last screen, number of screens)	Excluded 7 deaths before 1990; screening history excluded after diagnosis for controls diagnosed with cancer	Self-selection bias using method of Duffy et al. (2002a), and screening opportunity bias	0.65 (0.39–1.09)
The Netherlands								
Broeders et al. (2002)	Nijmegen 1975 50–69 yr until 1997; 50–74 yr thereafter 2-yearly All women	157 Screening registry 1987–1997 Last 10 yr of the programme NR	At least 1 invitation 50–74 yr	785 Same source population as cases Alive and residing in Nijmegen at DOD of case, invited to participate in the index screening round, free of breast cancer at their index invitation	Data on invitation and participation were kept in the screening registry	Analysis includes only women who attended screening	Age at screening	0.68 (0.33–1.41) By age: 40–49 yr: 0.90 (0.38–2.14) 50–59 yr: 0.71 (0.35–1.46) 60–69 yr: 0.80 (0.42–1.54) 70–79 yr: 1.13 (0.50–2.58) > 79 yr: 2.92 (0.55–15.4)

Table 5.7 (continued)

Reference	Area, year programme began, screening age and interval, women included	No. of breast cancer deaths, source, time period for breast cancer deaths, years of diagnoses; proportion of eligible women included	Screening exposure; age of included women	No. of controls, source, whether same source population as cases, matching variables, alive at date of death or diagnosis of case	Linkage or use of screening, cancer registry, death databases; data items available	Issues or items related to screening history; whether prevalent cases were excluded	Adjustments	Breast cancer mortality OR (95% CI)
van Schoor et al. (2011)	Nijmegen 1975 Invitations sent to women aged ≥ 35 yr	282 Women invited to the screening programme in Nijmegen NR 1975–2008 191 cases were screened and 91 not screened	Screening invitation during a 4-yr period before breast cancer diagnosis of the case (biennial screening schedule including 2 consecutive invitations) 50–69 yr	1410 Same source as cases Eligible for screening, not having breast cancer at the time of invitation, and living in Nijmegen at DOD of case; 5 per case randomly sampled	Separate registry on all breast cancer patients in Nijmegen diagnosed within and outside the screening programme Vital status from the Municipal Personal Records Database Assessments of causes of death by a committee of physicians unaware of the screening history		Including an interaction term, the combination of screening and calendar year, in the logistic regression model; corrected for the confounding influence of age at index invitation by stratification into 5-yr age groups	By calendar period: 1975–2008: 0.65 (0.49–0.87) 1975–1991: 0.72 (0.47–1.09) 1992–2008: 0.35 (0.19–0.64)

Table 5.7 (continued)

Reference	Area, year programme began, screening age and interval, women included	No. of breast cancer deaths, source, time period for breast cancer deaths, years of diagnoses; proportion of eligible women included	Screening exposure; age of included women	No. of controls, source, whether same source population as cases, matching variables, alive at date of death or diagnosis of case	Linkage or use of screening, cancer registry, death databases; data items available	Issues or items related to screening history; whether prevalent cases were excluded	Adjustments	Breast cancer mortality OR (95% CI)
Paap et al. (2010)	Limburg Province 1989 50–75 yr every 2 yr Women aged 50–75 yr who received at least 1 invitation to screening in the region	118 Women invited to screening in IKL region Deaths between 2004 and 2005 Years of diagnosis NR Proportion of eligible cases included NR	Received at least 1 invitation to the service screening programme 50–75 yr	118 Same source population as cases Matched for year of birth and area of residence Alive at DOD of case	IKL includes a screening registry and a cancer registry Cause of death was determined by linkage to Statistics Netherlands For cases, DOD, DOB, date of diagnosis	For cases and controls, complete screening history was obtained from the screening registry. Controls with breast cancer diagnosis at time of invitation to screening were excluded	Self-selection bias	0.24 (0.10–0.58)

Table 5.7 (continued)

Reference	Area, year programme began, screening age and interval, women included	No. of breast cancer deaths, source, time period for breast cancer deaths, years of diagnoses; proportion of eligible women included	Screening exposure; age of included women	No. of controls, source, whether same source population as cases, matching variables, alive at date of death or diagnosis of case	Linkage or use of screening, cancer registry, death databases; data items available	Issues or items related to screening history; whether prevalent cases were excluded	Adjustments	Breast cancer mortality OR (95% CI)
Paap et al. (2014)	(5 of 9 screening regions) 1990 50–74 yr 2-yearly All women	1233 Netherlands Cancer Registry 2004 or 2005 from start of service screening Proportion NR	Screened at index invitation (most recent before diagnosis of case) or the preceding screening round 50–75 yr	2090 Women in 5 regions with at least 1 screening invitation Same source as cases Year of birth, area of residence, screening invitation in same round as case index invitation Alive at DOD of case	All 3 DOB, date of diagnosis, DOD, screening history (time since last screen, number of screens)	Screening participation restricted to maximum 2 rounds	Self-selection bias using correction factor for each region based on IBM method (Paap et al., 2011), and for screening opportunity bias (control matched to screening round of index invitation of case)	0.42 (0.33–0.53)

Table 5.7 (continued)

Reference	Area, year programme began, screening age and interval, women included	No. of breast cancer deaths, source, time period for breast cancer deaths, years of diagnoses; proportion of eligible women included	Screening exposure; age of included women	No. of controls, source, whether same source population as cases, matching variables, alive at date of death or diagnosis of case	Linkage or use of screening, cancer registry, death databases; data items available	Issues or items related to screening history; whether prevalent cases were excluded	Adjustments	Breast cancer mortality OR (95% CI)
Otto et al. (2012b)	South-western region 1990 50–69 yr (extended to 75 yr in 1998) 24.5 mo All female residents	755 Cohort of women invited by the screening organization in south-western Netherlands 1995–2003 1990–2003 98.6%	Index period: time period from index invitation backward to a maximum of 2 invitations before the index invitation; total number of invitations varied from 1 to 3 per case–control set 50–75 yr	3739 Same source as cases 5 controls per case, matched on year of birth, year of first invitation, and number of invitations before diagnosis of case	Linkage with cause of death registry and cancer registry, Comprehensive Cancer Centre Rotterdam, and Statistics Netherlands	Screening histories for all women ever invited to a mammography screening examination were systematically retrieved from the same database	Self-selection bias	49–75 yr: 0.51 (0.40–0.66) 50–69 yr: 0.61 (0.47–0.79) 50–75 yr: 0.52 (0.41–0.67) 70–75 yr: 0.16 (0.09–0.29)
Italy								
Puliti et al. (2008)	Northern and central Italy, 5 regions 1990 50–69 yr 2-yearly	1750 Regional mortality registers 1988–2002 from year before start of service screening to end of 2001 Proportion NR	Any service screen before date of diagnosis or pseudo-diagnosis 50–74 yr	7000 All women 50–69 yr resident in the selected areas for any period of time Same source as cases DOB and resident in the municipality in year of death of subject	IMPACT database used cancer, screening, and mortality registers DOB, screening history (screening in 3 yr before diagnosis of case, number of screens)	Not-yet-invited women included in unscreened; free of breast cancer diagnosis before diagnosis date of case	Self-selection bias using method of Duffy et al. (2002a) and own correction factor	0.55 (0.36–0.85)

Table 5.7 (continued)

Reference	Area, year programme began, screening age and interval, women included	No. of breast cancer deaths, source, time period for breast cancer deaths, years of diagnoses; proportion of eligible women included	Screening exposure; age of included women	No. of controls, source, whether same source population as cases, matching variables, alive at date of death or diagnosis of case	Linkage or use of screening, cancer registry, death databases; data items available	Issues or items related to screening history; whether prevalent cases were excluded	Adjustments	Breast cancer mortality OR (95% CI)
Australia								
Roder et al. (2008)	South Australia 1989 50–69 yr active; 40–49 yr and ≥ 70 yr allowed 2-yearly	491 South Australia Cancer Registry 2002–2005 from 1994 94%	BreastScreen attendance before date of diagnosis or pseudo-diagnosis 45–80 yr	1473 Electoral roll Same source as cases	All 3 DOB, screening history (number of screens)	Date of breast cancer diagnosis for case; only if date of diagnosis in controls later than in case	SES, remoteness, access (ARIA)	0.59 (0.47–0.74) 0.70 (NR) adjusted for self-selection bias
Nickson et al. (2012)	Western Australia mid-1990s 50–69 yr active; 40–49 yr allowed 2-yearly	427 Western Australia Cancer Registry 1995–2006 from 1995 Proportion NR	Receiving a screening mammogram between age 50 yr and reference date 50–69 yr	Average 8.5 controls per case Electoral roll 1995–2006 Same source population as cases Month and year of birth of case; Western Australia resident at time of diagnosis of cases Alive at DOD of case	All 3 DOB, date of any cancer diagnosis, DOD, screening history (year of first screen)	Earliest breast cancer diagnosis in case–control set; women were excluded if they had a screen before age 50 yr	SES, remoteness, HRT use, family history of breast cancer	0.48 (0.38–0.59)

ARIA, Accessibility/Remoteness Index of Australia; CI, confidence interval; DOB, date of birth; DOD, date of death; GP, general practitioner; HRT, hormone replacement therapy; IBM, incidence-based mortality; IKL, Comprehensive Cancer Centre Limburg; mo, month or months; NHS, National Health System; NR, not reported; OR, odds ratio; SES, socioeconomic status; yr, year or years.

screening area to population-based controls. The unadjusted odds ratio for risk of death from breast cancer in women who attended at least one screen compared with those who had never been screened was 0.59 (95% CI, 0.41–0.84), and 0.65 (95% CI, 0.39–1.09) after correction for both self-selection bias and screening opportunity bias.

(iii) The Netherlands

Broeders et al. (2002) conducted a case–control study to describe the effect of population-based mammography screening in Nijmegen on breast cancer mortality, based on a 20-year follow-up period. The risk of death from breast cancer was calculated per 10-year moving age group for women who had attended the index screening (the screening immediately before diagnosis of breast cancer) versus those who had not. Odds ratios were presented by age group for both participation in index screening (see Table 5.7) and participation in either the index screening or the previous screening, or both; none showed a statistically significant effect. The youngest 10-year age group that showed an effect was women aged 45–54 years at their index screening; the odds ratio in women aged 45–49 years was 0.56 (95% CI, 0.20–1.61). The odds ratios for women aged 40–49 years were 0.90 (95% CI, 0.38–2.14) for participation in the index screening and 0.84 (95% CI, 0.30–2.29) for participation in the index screening and the previous screening. The corresponding odds ratios for women aged 70–79 years were 1.13 (95% CI, 0.50–2.58) and 0.70 (95% CI, 0.32–1.54). There was no limitation in these analyses as to age at first attendance to screening. [This analysis overlaps partly with that of van Schoor et al. (2010) (see Section 5.2.2b).]

By 2008, 55 529 women had received an invitation to screening in Nijmegen, and another case–control study was performed (van Schoor et al., 2011). The odds ratio for breast cancer death in the screened group over the complete period was 0.65 (95% CI, 0.49–0.87). Analyses were also performed by calendar period of index invitation to screening (see Table 5.7). [It is unclear why the numbers analysed for the two screening periods are so much less than the overall total of cases and controls included in this study.]

Paap et al. (2010) designed a case–control study to investigate the effect of mammography screening at the individual level. The study population included all women aged 50–75 years in Limburg Province who had been invited to the screening programme in 1989–2006. The unadjusted odds ratio for the screened versus the unscreened women was 0.30 (95% CI, 0.14–0.63), and 0.24 (95% CI, 0.10–0.58) after adjustment for self-selection. [This analysis includes only deaths in the most recent screening years. Deaths in the period from inception of the programme in 1989 until 2003 were not included.]

Paap et al. (2014) estimated the effect of the Dutch screening programme on breast cancer mortality by means of a large multiregion case–control study. They identified all breast cancer deaths in 2004 and 2005 in women aged 50–75 years who had received at least one invitation to the service screening programme in five participating screening regions. Cases were individually matched to controls from the population invited to screening. Conditional logistic regression was used to estimate the odds ratio of breast cancer death according to individual screening history. The unadjusted odds ratio for breast cancer death in screened versus unscreened women was 0.48 (95% CI, 0.40–0.58), and 0.42 (95% CI, 0.33–0.53) after adjustment for self-selection bias using regional correction factors for the difference in the baseline risk of breast cancer death between screened and unscreened women.

Otto et al. (2012b) conducted a case–control study in the south-western region of the Netherlands for the period 1995–2003, including women aged 49–75 years. There was no restriction with respect to age at first invitation. The all-age odds ratio for the association between attending screening at the index invitation and risk of breast cancer death was 0.56 (95% CI, 0.44–0.71), and 0.51 (95% CI, 0.40–0.66) for women attending any of the three screening examinations (for analyses by age at the index invitation, see Table 5.7).

(iv) Italy

Puliti et al. (2008) conducted a case–control study to evaluate the impact of service screening programmes on breast cancer mortality in five regions of Italy. The odds ratio for invited women compared with not-yet-invited women was 0.75 (95% CI, 0.62–0.92). When the analyses were restricted to invited women, the odds ratio for screened women compared with never-respondent women, corrected for self-selection bias, was 0.55 (95% CI, 0.36–0.85).

(v) Australia

Roder et al. (2008) conducted a case–control study of women in South Australia aged 45–80 years during 2002–2005 (diagnosed after the start of BreastScreen Australia) and live controls (three per death) randomly selected from the state electoral roll after date-of-birth matching. The programme has provided biennial screening, with two-view mammography and double reading, since its inception. It actively targets women aged 50–69 years and allows access to women aged 40–49 years and those aged 70 years and older. The odds ratio for breast cancer death in all BreastScreen participants compared with non-participants was 0.59 (95% CI, 0.47–0.74). The corresponding odds ratio in women younger than 50 years at diagnosis was 1.18 (95% CI, 0.70–1.98) and in those aged 70 years and older at diagnosis was 0.43 (95% CI, 0.25–0.72). Compared with non-participants, the odds ratio was 0.70 (95% CI, 0.47–1.05) for women last screened through BreastScreen more than 3 years before diagnosis of the index case, and 0.57 (95% CI, 0.44–0.72) for women screened more recently.

Nickson et al. (2012) conducted another case–control study within BreastScreen Australia, in which women aged 50–69 years on the electoral roll (98.9% of the eligible population) are invited to attend screening. Eligible women were those aged 50 years and older on the Western Australian electoral roll between 1995 and 2006. The cases were women from this population who died of breast cancer between 1995 and 2006. Controls (10 per case) were selected by incidence density sampling from the source population (those with a breast cancer diagnosis were not excluded). Exposure to screening was defined as receipt of a screening mammogram from BreastScreen at any point between the woman's 50th birthday and the case–control set reference date (the date of earliest breast cancer diagnosis for that set; for 89%, this was the date of diagnosis of the case); 56% of controls and 39% of cases attended screening. The odds ratio from the primary analyses (adjusted for remoteness and relative socioeconomic disadvantage) was 0.48 (95% CI, 0.38–0.59). The odds ratio was found to vary little by reference age group or year of death and was robust to sensitivity analyses.

(b) Other case–control studies

See Table 5.8.

(i) The Netherlands

In 1974, de Waard et al. (1984a) set up a population-based study of periodic screening by xeromammography of women aged 50–64 years in Utrecht; 72% of invited women attended the first of four rounds. The effect of the programme on breast cancer mortality was evaluated in a nested case–control study, which showed an odds ratio for breast cancer mortality in women who had ever been screened of 0.30 (95% CI, 0.13–0.70) compared with those who had never been screened (Collette et al., 1984). The odds ratios for women aged 50–54, 55–59, 60–64, and 65–69 years at diagnosis were 1.13, 0.31, 0, and 0.10, respectively. [These estimates were based on

Table 5.8 Other case–control studies of the effectiveness of mammography screening

Reference	Area, year programme began, screening age and interval, women included	No. of breast cancer deaths, source, time period for breast cancer deaths, years of diagnoses; proportion of eligible women included	Screening exposure; age of included women	No. of controls, source, whether same source population as cases, matching variables, alive at date of death or diagnosis of case	Linkage or use of screening, cancer registry, death databases; data items available	Issues or items related to screening history; whether prevalent cases were excluded	Adjustments	Breast cancer mortality OR (95% CI)
The Netherlands								
Collette et al. (1984)	Utrecht 1974 50–64 yr at the start of the project All women born in 1911–1925 (72% attended screening)	46 Birth cohort under study 1974–1981 Screening at the first visit and after 12, 18, and 24 mo 20% screened	Screening at first visit and after 12, 18, and 24 mo 50–64 yr 50–54 yr	138 Birth cohort under study, same source 3 controls for each case, lived in Utrecht when the case died and same year of birth as case 43% screened	All breast cancer patients included in breast cancer registry; dates of diagnosis checked with general practitioners' registries	Screening histories of cases and controls for the time up to and including date of diagnosis of case	Stratification by birth cohort or age	0.30 (0.13–0.70)
Miltenburg et al. (1998)	Utrecht 1974–1975 ≤ 2 yr All women born in 1911–1925	177 Birth cohort under study 1975–1992 NR	At 1, 1.5, 2, and 4 yr 50–64 yr	531 Birth cohort under study, same source 3 per case, same birth year, living in Utrecht in 1974, selected from the screening intervention file	Linkage to DOM project breast cancer registry; causes of death provided by general practitioners or hospitals	Screening history for the time up to and including date of diagnosis; 17 yr of follow-up of screening programme; for both cases and controls, participation was low; exclusion of cases with follow-up of < 1 yr	Stratification by birth cohort	0.54 (0.37–0.79) By birth cohort: 1911–1915: 0.40 (0.21–0.75) 1916–1920: 0.57 (0.31–1.04) 1921–1925: 0.71 (0.34–1.48)

Table 5.8 (continued)

Reference	Area, year programme began, screening age and interval, women included	No. of breast cancer deaths, source, time period for breast cancer deaths, years of diagnoses; proportion of eligible women included	Screening exposure; age of included women	No. of controls, source, whether same source population as cases, matching variables, alive at date of death or diagnosis of case	Linkage or use of screening, cancer registry, death databases; data items available	Issues or items related to screening history; whether prevalent cases were excluded	Adjustments	Breast cancer mortality OR (95% CI)
Verbeek et al. (1985)	Nijmegen Reference to Verbeek et al. (1984)	62 residents 1975–1982 NR	Diagnosed after first screening invitation; stratification by age at first invitation	310 Birth cohort under study, same source 5 per case, same year of birth as case, and same invitation history	NR	NR	Residential district and marital status	0.51 (0.26–0.99) By age: 35–49 yr: 1.2 (0.31–4.8) 50–64 yr: 0.26 (0.10–0.67) ≥ 65 yr: 0.81 (0.23–2.8)
Van Dijck et al. (1996)	Nijmegen 1975 35–64 yr (since 1977, also older women) 2-yearly Women invited to participate at age ≥ 65 yr and free of breast cancer at first screening invitation	82 Nijmegen population of invited women, before 1 January 1994 NR	Index round: most recent invitation before diagnosis of primary breast cancer 65–92 yr	410 Age-matched population in Nijmegen, invited to screening at same index round as the case	Cause of death classified by a panel of physicians unaware of the screening history	Patients with advanced breast cancer who died of other, unrelated causes not included as cases	NR	By age: ≥ 65 yr: 0.56 (0.28–1.13) 65–74 yr: 0.45 (0.20–1.02) ≥ 75 yr: 1.05 (0.27–4.14)

Table 5.8 (continued)

Reference	Area, year programme began, screening age and interval, women included	No. of breast cancer deaths, source, time period for breast cancer deaths, years of diagnoses; proportion of eligible women included	Screening exposure; age of included women	No. of controls, source, whether same source population as cases, matching variables, alive at date of death or diagnosis of case	Linkage or use of screening, cancer registry, death databases; data items available	Issues or items related to screening history; whether prevalent cases were excluded	Adjustments	Breast cancer mortality OR (95% CI)
van Schoor et al. (2010)	Nijmegen 1975 40–69 yr 2-yearly Women invited to the screening	272 Women invited to screening programme in Nijmegen NR 1975–1990 NR	1975–1990 40–69 yr at invitation	1360 Same source Risk sets of controls from which 5 controls were randomly sampled for each case, eligible for screening, and living in Nijmegen at date of death of case	Linkage to vital status from the Municipal Personal Records Database Assessments of causes of death made by a committee of physicians	NR	For differences in age at index invitation between the comparison groups by stratification; thereafter, combination of screening and age as an interaction term to the logistic model Sensitivity analysis for obesity, socioeconomic group, nulliparity, late age at menopause, early age at menarche, and family history	By age: 40–49 yr: 0.50 (0.30–0.82) 50–59 yr: 0.54 (0.35–0.85) 60–69 yr: 0.65 (0.38–1.13)
Italy								
Palli et al. (1989)	Florence 1970 40–70 yr Invitation every 30 mo All residents	103 death certificates 1977–1987 After at least a first invitation to the programme and within 3 yr of the last invitation NR	After at least a first invitation to the programme 40–70 yr	515 Same source Selected for year of birth and town of residence 5 per case	Form completed for each woman, with clinical and demographic information	Screening history until date of diagnosis from the Centre for the Study and Prevention of Oncological Diseases	Number of children, age at first birth, civil status, years of education, occupation, place of birth, family history, screening history for cervical cancer, self-referred to breast clinic for mammography	By age at diagnosis: 40–49 yr: 0.63 (0.24–1.6) ≥ 50 yr: 0.51 (0.29–0.89)

Table 5.8 (continued)

Reference	Area, year programme began, screening age and interval, women included	No. of breast cancer deaths, source, time period for breast cancer deaths, years of diagnoses; proportion of eligible women included	Screening exposure; age of included women	No. of controls, source, whether same source population as cases, matching variables, alive at date of death or diagnosis of case	Linkage or use of screening, cancer registry, death databases; data items available	Issues or items related to screening history; whether prevalent cases were excluded	Adjustments	Breast cancer mortality OR (95% CI)
USA								
Elmore et al. (2005)	California, Massachusetts, Minnesota, Oregon, and Washington	1351 deaths from breast cancer or causes possibly related to breast cancer 1983–1998 1983–1993 100% from 4 of 6 sites, 25% from 1 site, 33% from 1 site	3 yr up to and including the index date: the date of first symptom or suspicion of cancer (in the breast where the cancer was later identified); same date allocated to matched controls 40–49 yr 50–69 yr	2501 Same source as cases Matched on health plan, age, and level of risk for breast cancer, who were alive on the date that the matched case subject had died, and were active health plan members at the time of the matched case subject's breast cancer diagnosis	Health plan information linked to SEER cancer registries or other cancer registries, and medical chart review	Screening history for 3 yr before index date (mammography and CBE) extracted from medical record review; diagnosis of breast cancer before 1983 was excluded	Race, comorbidity, and age at first birth	By age at screening by CBE or mammography: 40–65 yr: 0.91 (0.78–1.07) 40–49 yr: 0.92 (0.76–1.13) 50–65 yr: 0.87 (0.68–1.12) By age at screening by mammography: 40–65 yr: 0.92 (0.79–1.08) 40–49 yr: 0.85 (0.69–1.05) 50–65 yr: 1.04 (0.82–1.33)

Table 5.8 (continued)

Reference	Area, year programme began, screening age and interval, women included	No. of breast cancer deaths, source, time period for breast cancer deaths, years of diagnoses; proportion of eligible women included	Screening exposure; age of included women	No. of controls, source, whether same source population as cases, matching variables, alive at date of death or diagnosis of case	Linkage or use of screening, cancer registry, death databases; data items available	Issues or items related to screening history; whether prevalent cases were excluded	Adjustments	Breast cancer mortality OR (95% CI)
Norman et al. (2007)	CARE multicentre study NR 40–64 yr White women and Black women in metropolitan Atlanta, Georgia; Detroit, Michigan; Los Angeles, California; Philadelphia, Pennsylvania; and Seattle, Washington	553 Women with a new diagnosis of invasive breast cancer in 1994–1998 who died NR 1994–1998 NR	At least 1 screening mammogram in the 2 yr before the reference date (month and year of initial diagnosis for cases) 40–64 yr	4016 Women identified by random-digit dialling who had never been diagnosed with cancer	Standard SEER follow-up procedures used, primarily passive linkage with state death records; for the Pennsylvania site, state death records used	Screening histories from population screening registries or medical records	BMI, family history, education, marital status, parity, alcohol consumption in year before reference date, smoking status, number of pre-existing medical conditions, use of oral contraceptive, use of combined estrogen–progestin hormone replacement therapy, use of estrogen therapy, and less than twice the federal poverty threshold for household income. Model with stratification by age was further adjusted for menopausal status	By age group: 40–49 yr: 0.89 (0.65–1.23) 50–64 yr: 0.47 (0.35–0.63)

BMI, body mass index; CARE, Contraceptive and Reproductive Experiences; CBE, clinical breast examination; CI, confidence interval; mo, month or months; NR, not reported; OR, odds ratio; RR, relative risk; SEER, Surveillance, Epidemiology, and End Results; yr, year or years.

small numbers, and no confidence intervals were given.]

An updated case–control analysis 17 years after the initiation of this project was reported by Miltenburg et al. (1998). Controls (three for each case) were defined as women with the same year of birth as the case, living in the city of Utrecht at the time the case died, and having had the opportunity to be screened in the DOM project. The odds ratio for breast cancer mortality for screening in the period 1975–1992 was 0.54 (95% CI, 0.37–0.79). Stratification by birth cohort is given in Table 5.8.

In 1975, a population-based screening programme was set up in Nijmegen, a city with about 150 000 inhabitants (Peeters et al., 1989a). The first screening round, in 1975–1976, involved 23 000 women born in 1910–1939, who were thus aged 35–64 years. In the subsequent screening rounds, the same birth cohort was invited, as well as 7700 women born before 1910. The odds ratio for death from breast cancer estimated in a case–control analysis was 1.2 (95% CI, 0.31–4.8) for women aged 35–49 years, 0.26 (95% CI, 0.10–0.67) for those aged 50–64 years, and 0.81 (95% CI, 0.23–2.8) for those aged 65 years and older (Verbeek et al., 1985).

In a further case–control study based on the Nijmegen population, Van Dijck et al. (1996) selected women who were 65 years or older when first invited to screening. The rate ratio of breast cancer mortality in women who had participated regularly (i.e. in the two most recent screening rounds before diagnosis) compared with those who had not participated in screening was 0.56 (95% CI, 0.28–1.13). The rate ratio for women aged 65–74 years at the most recent invitation was 0.45 (95% CI, 0.20–1.02), and for women aged 75 years and older it was 1.05 (95% CI, 0.27–4.14). [The Working Group estimated rate ratios for women who had ever been screened by combining, using fixed effects meta-analysis, reported relative risks for women who had been screened regularly and women who had been screened "otherwise" relative to women who had not been screened. The estimates rate ratios were 0.68 (95% CI, 0.44–1.05) for all ages, 0.54 (95% CI, 0.31–0.95) for ages 65–74 years, and 0.94 (95% CI, 0.45–1.88) for ages 75 years and older. Forty of the 82 deaths from breast cancer included in this study were included in a separate IBM analysis of effectiveness of screening in women aged 68–83 years at entry into the Nijmegen screening programme (Van Dijck et al., 1997).]

van Schoor et al. (2010) designed a case–control study to investigate the effect of biennial mammography screening on breast cancer mortality in women aged 40–69 years between 1975 and 1990 in Nijmegen. In women aged 40–49 years at their index screening (in cases, the last screening before diagnosis of breast cancer), the odds ratio for screening was 0.50 (95% CI, 0.30–0.82). Similarly, an odds ratio of 0.54 (95% CI, 0.35–0.85) was reported for women aged 50–59 years, and an odds ratio of 0.65 (95% CI, 0.38–1.13) for those aged 60–69 years.

(ii) Italy

Between 1970 and 1980, women aged 40–70 years living in 24 municipalities in Florence were invited to mammography screening with craniocaudal and mediolateral oblique views every 2.5 years. In 1989, the screening area was extended to include the city of Florence. Palli et al. (1986, 1989) conducted a case–control study within this population to estimate the impact on breast cancer mortality. The odds ratios for women aged 40–49 years and for those aged 50 years and older at diagnosis of breast cancer were estimated to be 0.63 (95% CI, 0.24–1.6) and 0.51 (95% CI, 0.29–0.89), respectively.

(iii) USA

Elmore et al. (2005) conducted a matched case–control study among women enrolled in six health plans in the states of California, Massachusetts, Minnesota, Oregon, and Washington and examined the efficacy of screening by mammography and/or CBE among women in two age cohorts (40–49 years and 50–65 years) and in two levels of breast cancer risk (in women at average risk and women with a family history and/or previous breast biopsy) until 1983–1998. The effect of screening with mammography, or of screening with mammography and CBE, during the 3 years before the index date (defined as the date of first suspicion of breast abnormalities in case subjects, with the same date used for matched control subjects) was evaluated. For women aged 40–49 years at diagnosis of breast cancer, the odds ratio was 0.85 (95% CI, 0.65–1.23), and for women aged 50–65 years, the odds ratio was 0.47 (95% CI, 0.35–0.63) for screening with mammography alone. The odds ratio for women at an increased risk was 0.74 (95% CI, 0.50–1.03) and for women at average risk was 0.96 (95% CI, 0.80–1.14); however, the difference was not statistically significant ($P = 0.17$).

Norman et al. (2007) used data from a subset of the Women's Contraceptive and Reproductive Experiences (CARE) Study, a population-based multicentre case–control study of risk factors for breast cancer among White and Black women conducted in metropolitan Atlanta, Georgia; Detroit, Michigan; Los Angeles, California; Philadelphia, Pennsylvania; and Seattle, Washington, to estimate the relative mortality rates from invasive breast cancer among women with at least one screening mammogram in the 2 years before a baseline reference date compared with unscreened women, adjusting for potential confounding. The odds ratio for breast cancer death within 5 years after diagnosis was 0.89 (95% CI, 0.65–1.23) for ages 40–49 years at diagnosis and 0.47 (95% CI, 0.35–0.63) for ages 50–64 years at diagnosis.

A meta-analysis was performed of some of the earlier case–control studies (Demissie et al., 1998), and Broeders et al. (2012) conducted a meta-analysis of seven more recent case–control studies. The combined unadjusted odds ratio in women who were screened versus those who were not screened was 0.46 (95% CI, 0.40–0.54), and 0.52 (95% CI, 0.42–0.65) when adjusted for self-selection using the method of Duffy et al. (2002a). The crude odds ratio for breast cancer mortality reduction, translated to intention-to-treat estimates for women who were invited versus those who were not invited was 0.69 (95% CI, 0.57–0.83).

(c) *Specific age groups*

Several of the case–control studies summarized above reported results in several age groups, including those that lie below or above the age range 50–69 years. Such results can be validly used to infer the effectiveness, or otherwise, of screening women younger than 50 years, provided they are based only on deaths from breast cancer of women whose breast cancer was diagnosed when they were younger than 50 years. The results that permit this inference are those of Palli et al. (1989), Broeders et al. (2002), Elmore et al. (2005), Norman et al. (2007), and Roder et al. (2008) (see Table 5.8).

The use of results from case–control studies to infer effectiveness at ages older than 69 years is less straightforward because, even if they are based only on deaths from breast cancer of women whose breast cancer was diagnosed when they were older than 69 years, the relative risk of death calculated will have been influenced by screening at age 69 years and younger, assuming screening effectiveness (Otto et al., 2012b). This influence can only be removed by limiting the analysis to women *first* offered screening after age 69 years. No case–control study has been done in a context in which this limitation could be applied; however, that of Van Dijck et al. (1996) was limited to women first offered screening from age 65 years.

5.2.3 Ecological studies

In assessing the effectiveness of breast cancer screening, the Working Group considered that accurate information on standards of breast cancer treatment in different regions analysed and careful matching of regions by treatment standards or adjustment for differences between regions in treatment standards are minimum criteria for validity of ecological studies. Therefore, simple comparisons of trends between unmatched regions or without potentially effective statistical adjustment, or in a single region over time, were excluded.

Correcting for differences in underlying incidence is a challenge. Differences in incidence between regions, or across time, may indicate an important difference in baseline risk that must be adjusted for, or they may indicate overdiagnosis and should not be adjusted for. These studies were therefore excluded, as were any that measured differences in survival, due to the well-recognized issue of lead time.

Studies of population-based screening in Europe were reviewed to assess the value of trend analyses in population breast cancer mortality (Moss et al., 2012). A literature review identified 17 reports, of which 12 provided quantitative estimates of the impact of screening. Due to differences in comparisons and outcome measures, no pooled estimate of effectiveness was calculated. Overall, this approach proved to be of limited value for assessment of screening impact.

For the purpose of selecting studies to review, the Working Group defined the following subcategories:

Category 1: Single-country or single-region studies that consider time trends in total incidence or total mortality, or that use, at best, different age groups to standardize treatment effects. These studies were excluded because of the impossibility of disentangling temporal changes in incidence, overdiagnosis, lead-time effect, and changes in treatment.

Category 2: Studies that measure proportional distribution of breast cancers by stage, proportional or relative survival, or post-diagnosis survival time over time or between countries with different screening protocols. These studies were excluded because of the potential bias due to overdiagnosis or the clear bias due to earlier diagnosis in screened women (lead-time bias).

Category 3: Studies of incidence of advanced-stage breast cancers over time between matched regions. These studies were included, subject to appropriate care having been taken to match or otherwise account for differences in risk factors or treatment. It is also necessary to account for differing completeness or reliability of staging. The advantage of such studies is that they should minimize the effects of overdiagnosis (which would generate mostly early-stage cancers) and differences in treatment. Correction is still required for a changing underlying rate of breast cancer incidence. This correction is generally based on the assumption that this change is driven by lifestyle changes, which change progressively, and in a similar manner in matched regions. Hence, smooth temporal trends are used to model the underlying rate, whereas effects of screening should manifest both by more rapid changes and by contrasts between regions that introduced screening on different dates.

Category 4: Studies of breast cancer mortality over time in matched regions. These studies raise the same issues as those of advanced-stage breast cancers, with the further complication of potential or real differences in treatment. This may include the availability of systemic hormone treatments or the organization of health-care systems.

A total of 87 studies were identified by the Working Group through literature searches and were reviewed for initial categorization according to the above criteria. After the initial exclusion of studies in categories 1 (n = 25) or 2 (n = 20), studies of other designs (9 case–control studies, 4 cohort studies, and 3 studies based on RCTs), and studies with other limitations (n = 12), 14 studies were further considered. Eight of these were then identified as IBM studies (Tabár et al., 2001; Duffy et al., 2002b; Jonsson et al., 2003a, b; Parvinen et al., 2006; Anttila et al., 2008; Sarkeala et al., 2008b; Kalager et al., 2010) and were therefore excluded. Of the remaining six ecological studies, two were judged to be uninformative: Das et al. (2005) used correlation as the measure of association, and Autier et al. (2011) may have been biased by the evolution of staging data over the study period; the remaining four studies were found to be informative. One additional informative study was identified separately (Otto et al., 2003) and was included in the review.

Otto et al. (2003) reviewed mortality trends in the Netherlands from 1980 to 1998, using clustered municipality-level data in 1-month bands, including the progressive introduction of screening from 1989 until 1997. Four age bands were compared to detect changes in treatment effectiveness: 45–54, 55–64, 65–74, and 75–84 years. Rates of change and cumulative changes were estimated in both the pre-screening and screening eras. Analysis was via linear splines (i.e. a single joinpoint). There was a downturn in mortality for the middle two age bands (55–64 years and 65–74 years) coincident with the introduction of screening, with an accumulated mortality reduction by 1999 estimated to be 19.1%. The annual rate of decline (annual percentage change) was 1.7% (95% CI, 1–2.4%) in these two age groups combined and 1.2% (95% CI, 0.1–2.4%) in the younger age group (45–54 ycars). There was no significant change in the older age group (75–84 years). Before screening, the trend was upward at 0.3% per year.

Törnberg et al. (2006) compared time trends in breast cancer incidence and mortality after the introduction of mammography screening in Copenhagen, Helsinki, Stockholm, and Oslo. In Helsinki, screening was offered to women aged 50–59 years, starting in 1986, and in the other three capitals, screening was offered to women aged 50–69 years, starting between 1989 and 1996. Peaks in breast cancer incidence depended on the age groups covered by the screening, the length of the implementation of screening, and the extent of background opportunistic screening. No mortality reduction after the introduction of screening was visible after 7–12 years of screening in any of the capitals. [No visible effect on mortality reduction was expected in Oslo, due to too short an observation period.]

Jørgensen et al. (2010) compared breast cancer mortality trends in Denmark, between Copenhagen (where screening was introduced in 1991) and Funen County (where screening started in 1993) and the rest of Denmark (which served as an unscreened control group). Unscreened age groups were used to further control for effects of changing treatment. Screening was offered to women aged 55–74 years, and mortality was evaluated in three age bands: 35–54, 55–74, and 75–84 years. The pre-screening period was 1982–1991, and the post-screening period was restricted to 1997–2006, to allow for a lag in benefit. The annual percentage change in breast cancer mortality was evaluated by Poisson regression. For the likely-to-benefit age band (55–74 years), the annual percentage change changed from +1 to −1% in the screening areas and from +2 to −2% in the non-screening areas. For the younger age band (35–54 years), the annual percentage change changed from +2% to −5% in the screening areas and from 0% to −6% in the non-screening areas. No significant changes were observed in the older age band.

The mortality benefit of attending screening was estimated using a Markov model of disease progression based on three regions in France (Uhry et al., 2011). Attempts were made to correct for opportunistic screening, and overdiagnosis was included as an explicit assumption, at either

10% or 20%. The corresponding estimates of mortality reduction were 23% (95% CI, 4% to 38%) and 19% (95% CI, −3% to 35%). [Problems of model fit were reported.]

Poisson regression was used in a study reanalysing population data from the era of Swedish screening trials (Haukka et al., 2011). [The data used were from NORDCAN (Engholm et al., 2010), which had variable levels of agreement with trial data where it could be compared.] The model assumed a delayed step change due to screening after the staggered introduction by region, with different lead times tested for best fit. Using the 3-year lead time estimate, breast cancer mortality decreased by 16% (RR, 0.84; 95% CI, 0.78–0.91) in the screening age group 40–69 years and by 11% (RR, 0.89; 95% CI, 0.80–0.98) in the age group 70–79 years.

5.2.4 Other measures of screening performance

See Table 5.9.

(a) Studies reporting on tumour size and nodal status in women aged 50–69 years

Hofvind et al. (2012c) compared incidence of advanced breast cancer cases diagnosed among screened and unscreened women aged 50–69 years in Norway. A total of 11 569 breast tumours (1670 ductal carcinoma in situ [DCIS] and 9899 invasive cancer) were diagnosed among 640 347 women who were invited to the screening programme during the study period. Participants in the screening programme accounted for 9726 breast tumours (1517 DCIS and 8209 invasive cancer) and non-participants accounted for 1843 breast tumours (153 DCIS and 1690 invasive cancer). When cases were compared between participants and non-participants, a significant reduction was observed in stage III (RR, 0.5; 95% CI, 0.4–0.7) and stage IV (RR, 0.3; 95% CI, 0.2–0.4) cancers, in tumours larger than 50 mm (RR, 0.4; 95% CI, 0.4–0.6), and in distant metastasis (RR, 0.3; 95% CI, 0.2–0.4). Distributions by stage, size, and nodal status were similar in women who did not attend screening and those who were not invited.

Domingo et al. (2013b) analysed data on invitation to organized screening programmes in Copenhagen (first eight invitations rounds, 1991–2008) and in Funen (first six invitation rounds, 1993–2005) (Table 5.10). Both programmes offered biennial screening to women aged 50–69 years. The Working Group calculated the rate ratios and 95% confidence intervals for tumour size and nodal status of screen-detected breast cancers versus those diagnosed in women who were not screened, for Copenhagen and Funen together. Among screen-detected cancers, a significant increase in detection of tumours of size 0–10 mm [RR, 2.91; 95% CI, 2.47–3.44] and 11–20 mm [RR, 1.27; 95% CI, 1.14–1.41] and a reduction in detection of tumours of size 21–30 mm [RR, 0.47; 95% CI, 0.40–0.55] and larger than 30 mm [RR, 0.26; 95% CI, 0.21–0.33] and in node–positive cancers [RR, 0.61; 95% CI, 0.54–0.67] were estimated. The rates of large screen-detected cancers were significantly lower, and screen-detected cancers were significantly less frequently lymph node-positive.

(b) Studies reporting incidence rates since the beginning of the screening period

Foca et al. (2013) analysed data from 700 municipalities in Italy, with a total population of 692 824 women aged 55–74 years targeted by organized mammography screening from 1991 to 2005. The effect of the screening was evaluated from year 1 (the year screening started at the municipal level) to year 8 (based on the decreasing number of available municipalities). The study was based on a total of 14 447 incident breast cancers. The observed 2-year, age-standardized (Europe) incidence rate ratio (ratio of the incidence rate to the expected rate) was calculated. Expected rates were estimated assuming that the incidence of breast cancer was stable and

Table 5.9 Studies using stage or indicators of stage at diagnosis of breast cancer as measures of screening performance

Reference	Areas, earliest year of programme screening, age, interval	Duration of screening Individual or aggregate data	Compared groups: contemporary or historical, period(s) covered, nature of groups	Denominators for rate/proportions calculations	Period of observation for screened and not screened	Adjustments	RR (95% CI) unless otherwise stated[a]	Comments
Hofvind et al. (2012c)	Norway 1996 50–69 yr 2 yr	1–12 yr Individual	Contemporary 1996–2007 Invited and screened, invited but not screened	Invitations to screening Screened: 1 475 978 (9726) Not screened: 449 747 (1843)	2 yr after each invitation to screening	None	*Stage:*[b] 0: 3.0 (2.6–3.6) I: 2.0 (1.8–2.2) II: 1.2 (1.1–1.3) III: 0.5 (0.4–0.7) IV: 0.3 (0.2–0.4) *Tumour size:* > 50 mm: 0.4 (0.4–0.6) *Node-positive:* No: 2.0 (1.8–2.1) Yes: 1.1 (1.0–1.2) *Distant metastasis:* No: 1.8 (1.7–1.9) Yes: 0.3 (0.2–0.4)	Distributions by stage, size, and nodal status were similar between not attending and not invited women
Domingo et al. (2013b)	Denmark (Copenhagen and Funen) 50–69 yr 2 yr	Copenhagen: 8 biennial screening rounds Funen: 6 biennial screening rounds Individual	Same years of observation	Copenhagen: Participants: 214 088 Not screened: 139 461 Funen: Participants: 486 722 Not screened: 230 153	Copenhagen: 1991–2008 Funen: 1993–2005		Rate ratios[c] *Tumour size:* ≤ 10 mm: [2.91 (2.47–3.44)] 11–20 mm: [1.27 (1.14–1.41)] 21–30 mm: [0.47 (0.40–0.55)] > 30 mm: [0.26 (0.21–0.33)] *Node-positive:* No: [1.61 (1.47–1.77)] Yes: [0.61 (0.54–0.67)] See Table 5.10 for original data	

Table 5.9 (continued)

Reference	Areas, earliest year of programme screening, age, interval	Duration of screening Individual or aggregate data	Compared groups: contemporary or historical, period(s) covered, nature of groups	Denominators for rate/ proportions calculations	Period of observation for screened and not screened	Adjustments	RR (95% CI) unless otherwise stated[a]	Comments
Foca et al. (2013)	Italy (700 munici-palities) 1991–2005 55–74 yr	1991–2005 Individual	(Analysis from year 1 to year 8) year 1: 692 824 women year 8: 300 859 women Total number of eligible cancer cases: 14 447 Advanced cancers analysed: 4036 (28%) pT2–pT4 cancers	Study end-points: total incidence of breast cancer incidence of pT2–pT4 breast cancer	1991–2005 (analysis from year 1 to year 8)		*1–2 yr after introduction of screening:* Total breast cancer: 1.35 (1.03–1.41) pT2–pT4: 0.97 (0.90–1.04) *5–6 yr after introduction of screening:* Total breast cancer: 1.14 (1.08–1.20) pT2–pT4: 0.79 (0.73–0.87) *7–8 yr after the introduction of screening:* Total breast cancer: 1.14 (1.08–1.21) pT2–pT4: 0.71 (0.64–0.79)	Excluded women aged 50–54 yr Restricted to municipalities in which the proportion of total incident cancers detected by screening reached 30% within year 2 Annual incidence expected in the absence of screening assumed stable and equivalent to that observed in the past 3 yr before year 1 Effect evaluated based on the decreasing number of available municipalities Supplementary analysis of the subgroup of municipalities that had a complete 8-yr period of observation

Table 5.9 (continued)

Reference	Areas, earliest year of programme screening, age, interval	Duration of screening Individual or aggregate data	Compared groups: contemporary or historical, period(s) covered, nature of groups	Denominators for rate/ proportions calculations	Period of observation for screened and not screened	Adjustments	RR (95% CI) unless otherwise stated[a]	Comments
Nederend et al. (2012)	Netherlands 50–75 yr 2 yr Women aged 50–69 yr (75 yr in 1998)	1997–2008	351 009 consecutive screens of 85 274 women			Age, family history of breast cancer, previous breast surgery, use of HRT, initial screen, interval between 2 latest screens, breast density at latest screening mammogram, mammographic abnormality, tumour histology of invasive cancers	Rate per 1000 (95% CI) *Advanced cancers:* 1997–1998: 1.5 (1.2–1.9) 1999–2000: 1.6 (1.3–2.0) 2001–2002: 1.6 (1.3–2.0) 2003–2004: 1.6 (1.3–1.9) 2005–2006: 1.5 (1.2–1.8) 2007–2008: 1.9 (1.5–2.2) Total: 1.6 (1.5–1.8) *Non-advanced cancers:* 1997–1998: 3.0 (2.5–3.5) 1999–2000: 3.3 (2.8–3.8) 2001–2002: 3.0 (2.5–3.5) 2003–2004: 3.9 (3.4–4.4) 2005–2006: 3.3 (2.9–3.7) 2007–2008: 3.3 (2.9–3.7) Total: 3.3 (3.1–3.5)	At multivariate analysis, women with a ≥ 30-mo interval between the latest two screens had an increased risk of screen-detected advanced breast cancer (OR, 1.63; 95% CI, 1.07–2.48)

Table 5.9 (continued)

Reference	Areas, earliest year of programme screening, age, interval	Duration of screening Individual or aggregate data	Compared groups: contemporary or historical, period(s) covered, nature of groups	Denominators for rate/ proportions calculations	Period of observation for screened and not screened	Adjustments	RR (95% CI) unless otherwise stated[a]	Comments
Autier & Boniol (2012)	West Midlands, United Kingdom 1988 50–64 yr	1988–2004 Aggregate	No comparison APC of the incidence rates of lymph node-positive/ negative and of tumours > 50 mm reported for the screening period	First procedure based on CI5*plus* (Ferlay et al., 2014) and on proportions derived from Nagtegaal et al. (2011), for distinguishing cancers found in women attending and not attending screening	Data reported for the screening period 1989–2004 only		APC See Fig. 5.1	The > 50 mm cut-off is not appropriate to study changes in incidence rates of advanced cancers in a country with a high level of awareness, as United Kingdom Sources for estimation of incidence trends of advanced breast cancer NR
Eisemann et al. (2013)	Germany First screening units in 2005 50–69 yr 2 yr	2005– Aggregate		Breast cancer epidemiology in Germany in 2008–2009 (data sources: German Centre for Cancer Registry Data, Society of Epidemiolo-gical Cancer Registries in Germany, and German Federal Office of Statistics)			*Stage:* T1: ~40% T2: ~30% T3: ~4% T4: 5% Not known: ~13% Carcinoma in situ: 9%	Of the newly diagnosed patients in 2007–2008

Table 5.9 (continued)

Reference	Areas, earliest year of programme screening, age, interval	Duration of screening Individual or aggregate data	Compared groups: contemporary or historical, period(s) covered, nature of groups	Denominators for rate/ proportions calculations	Period of observation for screened and not screened	Adjustments	RR (95% CI) unless otherwise stated[a]	Comments
Elting et al. (2009)	Texas, USA > 40 yr	2002–2004 Individual	Incident breast cancer cases diagnosed among women aged > 40 yr in 2004 Total of 12 469 women	Risk of invasive breast cancer and DCIS in Texas Counties with facility compared with counties without facilities	2004	Age, race, ethnicity, higher probabilities of advanced disease among African-American and Hispanic women	*Stage at diagnosis:* DCIS: 1.27 (1.07–1.5) Regional nodes: 1.12 (0.98–1.27) Locally advanced or distant disease: 0.81 (0.66–0.98) Factors associated with diagnosis of DCIS compared with local disease: In-county facility 1.32 (0.98–1.77) Factors associated with diagnosis of locally advanced or disseminated disease compared with local disease: In-county facility 0.36 (0.26–0.51) ($P < 0.001$)	Significant associations between the absence of in-county mammography facilities and both low odds of screening and high odds of diagnosis at a late stage of breast cancer

Table 5.9 (continued)

Reference	Areas, earliest year of programme screening, age, interval	Duration of screening Individual or aggregate data	Compared groups: contemporary or historical, period(s) covered, nature of groups	Denominators for rate/ proportions calculations	Period of observation for screened and not screened	Adjustments	RR (95% CI) unless otherwise stated[a]	Comments
Bleyer & Welch (2012)	USA, SEER data ≥ 40 yr	NR Aggregate	Historical Before mammography (1976–1978) Three decades later (2006–2008)	Trend data from the National Health Interview Survey Trend data on incidence and survival rates obtained from the 9 long-standing SEER areas Annual estimates of population of women aged ≥ 40 yr obtained from United States Census	Before mammography (1976–1978) Three decades later (2006–2008)	Excluded excess cases associated with use of HRT	Number of cases per 100 000 women in 1976–1978 (2006–2008): DCIS: 7 (56) localized disease: 105 (178) regional disease: 85 (78) distant disease: 17 (17)	
Helvie et al. (2014)	USA, 18 SEER geographical areas, which captured cancer data from 27.8% of the United States population > 40 yr	2007–2009	Trend		Before mammography (1977–1979) Mammography screening period (2007–2009)	Underlying temporal trends	Late-stage breast cancer incidence decreased by 37%, with a reciprocal increase in early-stage rates Late-stage breast cancer incidence decreased by from 21% to 48% Total invasive breast cancer incidence decreased by 9%	Projected incidence stage-specific values were compared with actual observed values in 2007–2009. Used different APC estimates

Table 5.9 (continued)

Reference	Areas, earliest year of programme screening, age, interval	Duration of screening Individual or aggregate data	Compared groups: contemporary or historical, period(s) covered, nature of groups	Denominators for rate/ proportions calculations	Period of observation for screened and not screened	Adjustments	RR (95% CI) unless otherwise stated[a]	Comments
Hou & Huo (2013)	USA, 18 SEER registries No data on screening	2000–2009	Trend Breast cancer incidence rates from 2000 to 2009	Incidence rates of in situ, localized, regional, distant (per 100 000)		None	*DCIS* (all racial groups): APC, 2.3–3.0% ($P < 0.005$) *Localized breast cancer:* non-Hispanic Black women: APC, 1.3% ($P = 0.004$) Asian women: APC, 1.2% ($P = 0.03$) *Regional and distant cancers:* non-Hispanic White women: APC, −2.5% ($P = 0.02$) Hispanic women: APC, −1.1% ($P = 0.006$)	It is unlikely that the overall trends of incidence rates are due to changes in mammography screening rate, since mammography use did not change substantially from 2000 to 2010

Table 5.9 (continued)

Reference	Areas, earliest year of programme screening, age, interval	Duration of screening Individual or aggregate data	Compared groups: contemporary or historical, period(s) covered, nature of groups	Denominators for rate/ proportions calculations	Period of observation for screened and not screened	Adjustments	RR (95% CI) unless otherwise stated[a]	Comments
DeSantis et al. (2014)	USA, SEER Program, SEER 9 registries	NR Aggregate	Historical	Data about incidence, probabilities of developing cancer, and cause-specific survival obtained from the SEER Program Prevalence data on mammography by age and state obtained from the 2010 and 2012 Behavioral Risk Factor Surveillance System	1975–2010	Rates age-adjusted to the 2000 United States standard population within each age group	*Correlation between mammography screening prevalence in 2010 and breast cancer stage at diagnosis (2006–2010):* Non-Hispanic White women: in situ stage, $r = 0.62$ ($P < 0.001$) late stage, $r = -0.51$ ($P < 0.001$) African-American women: in situ stage, $r = 0.47$ ($P < 0.006$) late stage, NS	

[a] Comparing screened and unscreened.
[b] Calculated using COMPARE2 in WinPepi V11.39 (http://www.brixtonhealth.com/pepi4windows.html).
[c] Calculated using Stata/SE 13.1.
APC, annual percentage change; CI, confidence interval; DCIS, ductal carcinoma in situ; HRT, hormone replacement therapy; IRR, incidence rate ratio; NR, not reported; NS, not significant; OR, odds ratio; RR, relative risk; SEER, Surveillance, Epidemiology, and End Results; yr, year or years.

Table 5.10 Number of breast cancers (invasive and carcinoma in situ) detected at screening in participants, diagnosed as interval cancers in participants, or diagnosed in unscreened women (Copenhagen and Funen screening programmes, Denmark)

Invitation round	Screened women								Unscreened women				
	Participants	Screen-detected cancers (of which CIS)	Proportion[a]	Rate[a,b]	Interval cancers (of which CIS)	Proportion[a]	Rate[a,c]	False-positive rate (%)	Unscreened women	Diagnosed cancers (of which CIS)	Proportion[a]	Rate[a,d]	Total rate[a,e]
Copenhagen screening programme													
1	30 388	361 (44)	11.88	5.79	58 (2)	1.93	0.79	5.6%	14 763	128 (8)	8.67	4.23	5.91
2	26 109	164 (17)	6.28	3.13	65 (6)	2.51	1.25	4.0%	15 960	62 (0)	3.95	1.96	3.45
3	25 153	156 (18)	6.20	3.41	59 (3)	2.36	1.18	2.5%	15 968	70 (3)	4.38	2.41	3.81
4	25 427	147 (18)	5.78	2.79	73 (1)	2.89	1.44	2.4%	16 260	108 (4)	6.64	3.21	3.80
5	25 059	145 (22)	5.79	2.97	66 (3)	2.65	1.32	1.8%	17 281	94 (6)	5.44	2.79	3.69
6	25 271	180 (42)	7.12	3.28	62 (1)	2.47	1.24	1.5%	18 149	109 (4)	6.01	2.77	3.73
7	26 205	227 (40)	8.66	3.36	83 (2)	3.20	1.60	1.4%	18 846	163 (5)	8.65	3.35	4.07
8	30 476	242 (47)	7.94	3.48	89 (2)	2.94	1.47	1.4%	22 234	162 (5)	7.29	3.20	4.10
Total (1–8)	214 088	1622 (248)	7.48	3.57	555 (20)	2.61	1.31	2.6%	139 461	896 (35)	6.43	3.02	4.09
Funen screening programme													
1	41 519	401 (59)	9.66	4.47	89 (4)	2.16	1.08	1.7%	14 593	187 (11)	12.81	5.93	5.58
2	44 117	236 (35)	5.35	2.67	124 (6)	2.83	1.41	1.1%	13 892	89 (7)	6.41	3.20	3.87
3	44 892	216 (21)	4.81	2.41	140 (4)	3.13	1.57	1.1%	14 805	90 (8)	6.08	3.04	3.74
4	45 817	273 (35)	5.96	2.98	128 (4)	2.81	1.41	1.0%	15 430	90 (1)	5.83	2.92	4.01
5	47 458	257 (19)	5.42	2.71	112 (3)	2.37	1.19	0.8%	15 591	94 (7)	6.03	3.01	3.67
6	48 831	285 (31)	5.84	2.92	109 (4)	2.25	1.12	0.8%	16 381	101 (5)	6.17	3.08	3.80
Total (1–6)	272 634	1668 (200)	6.12	3.02	702 (25)	2.59	1.30	1.1%	90 692	651 (39)	7.18	3.54	4.10
Total	486 722	3290 (448)	6.76	3.27	1257 (45)	2.60	1.30	1.8%	230 153	1548 (74)	6.73	3.22	4.10

[a] Proportion per 1000 women, and rate per 1000 person–years.

[b] Person–years at risk to develop a screen-detected cancer were estimated as number of participants multiplied by length of invitation round.

[c] Person–years at risk to develop an interval cancer were estimated as number of participants, minus participants with screen-detected cancers, multiplied by 2.

[d] Person–years at risk to develop a cancer outside screening were estimated as number of unscreened women multiplied by length of invitation round.

[e] For simplicity, for each invitation round based on the total of screen-detected cancers, interval cancers, and cancers in unscreened women, although part of the interval cancers were diagnosed during the next invitation round.

CIS, carcinoma in situ.

From Domingo et al. (2013a). Aggressiveness features and outcomes of true interval cancers: comparison between screen-detected and symptom-detected cancers, *European Journal of Cancer Prevention*, volume 22, issue 1, pages 21–28, Copyright (2013), with permission from the publisher, Wolters Kluwer Health.

Fig. 5.1 Annual incidence rates from 1989 to 2004 of advanced breast cancer in women aged 50–64 years in the West Midlands, United Kingdom

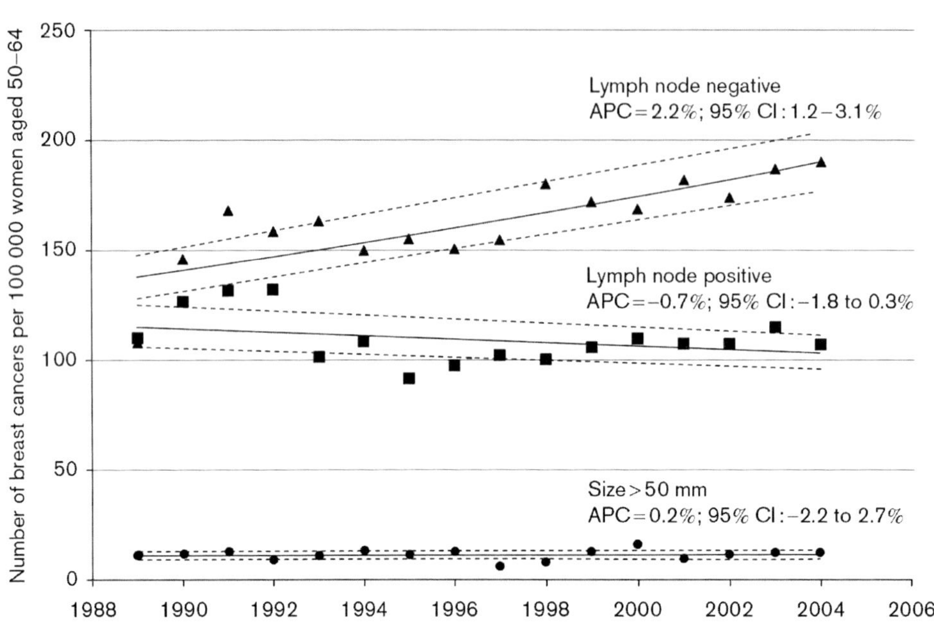

APC, annual percentage change; CI, confidence interval.
From Autier & Boniol (2012). The incidence of advanced breast cancer in the West Midlands, United Kingdom, *European Journal of Cancer Prevention*, volume 21, issue 3, pages 217–221, Copyright (2012), with permission from the publisher, Wolters Kluwer Health.

equivalent to that in the 3 years before year 1. The incidence rate ratio for pT2–pT4 breast cancers was 0.97 (95% CI, 0.90–1.04) in years 1 and 2, 0.81 (95% CI, 0.75–0.88) in years 3 and 4, 0.79 (95% CI, 0.73–0.87) in years 5 and 6, and 0.71 (95% CI, 0.64–0.79) in years 7 and 8. A significant and stable decrease in the incidence of late-stage breast cancer was observed from the third year of screening onward.

Nederend et al. (2012) analysed a consecutive series of 351 009 screening mammograms of 85 274 women aged 50–75 years, who underwent biennial screening in a breast screening region in the Netherlands in 1997–2008. A total of 1771 screen-detected cancers and 669 interval cancers were diagnosed in 2440 women. The authors observed, as expected, no decline in detection rates of advanced breast cancer during each round of 12 years of biennial screening mammography in the screened population. In the source population (data from a cancer registry), no decline in advanced breast cancer has been reported.

Autier & Boniol (2012) estimated incidence trends in advanced breast cancer from 1989 to 2004 in the West Midlands (United Kingdom), where breast screening started in 1988 for women aged 50–64 years (Fig. 5.1). The authors extracted numbers of breast cancer cases from the *Cancer Incidence in Five Continents* database (Ferlay et al., 2014). They used published data (Lawrence et al., 2009; Nagtegaal et al., 2011) for the annual percentage change (APC) in the incidence rates of lymph node-positive/node-negative breast cancer and of tumours larger than 50 mm for the screening period. According to their analysis, the incidence rates of node-positive breast cancer increased from 1989 to 1992 and then decreased below the pre-screening level in 1993–1995 but returned to pre-screening levels in 1996–2000 and then stabilized. From 1989 to 2004, the APC was 2.2% (95% CI, 1.2% to 3.1%) for node-negative cancers and −0.7% (95% CI, −1.8% to 0.3%) for node-positive cancers. The incidence of tumours larger than 50 mm remained stable from 1989 to 2004 (APC, 0.2%; 95% CI, −2.2% to 2.7%).

Eisemann et al. (2013) reported data from 2008–2009 in Germany, where breast cancer screening started in 2005, biennially, for women aged 50–69 years. From 2002 to 2007, the absolute number of breast cancer diagnoses (including in situ cases) increased markedly, by 15%: for in situ tumours, by +94%; for T1 tumours, by +18%; for T2 tumours, by +11%; for T3 tumours, by +14%; and for tumours of unknown stage, by +24%. A decrease of about −10% was observed for T4 tumours. [No comparison of rates of advanced cancers was reported in the screened or invited population versus the population not screened or not invited.]

Elting et al. (2009) assessed the association between in-county mammography facilities (in 2002–2004) and mammography screening and breast cancer diagnosis at a late stage among women in Texas older than 40 years. Half of the 254 counties had no mammography facility. In 2004, a total of 12 469 of the 4 639 842 women in Texas older than 40 years were diagnosed with either invasive breast cancer or DCIS (risk per 10 000 women aged > 40 years, 26.87; 95% CI, 26.4–27.3). The risk of diagnosis at early and late stages varied significantly between counties with and without mammography facilities. After accounting for confounding by age, race, and ethnicity, multivariate analysis showed that women who lived in counties with facilities were more likely to be diagnosed with DCIS (odds ratio [OR], 1.32; 95% CI, 0.98–1.77; $P = 0.06$) and significantly less likely to be diagnosed at an advanced stage (OR, 0.36; 95% CI, 0.26–0.51; $P < 0.001$) than their counterparts who lived in counties without a facility. These differences were observed despite adjustment for higher probabilities of advanced disease among African-American and Hispanic women.

(c) Studies reporting incidence rates using SEER data

Bleyer & Welch (2012) used data from the Surveillance, Epidemiology, and End Results (SEER) Program of the United States National Cancer Institute to examine trends from 1976 to 2008 in the incidence of early-stage and late-stage breast cancer among women aged 40 years and older. The 3-year period 1976–1978 was chosen to obtain the estimate of the baseline incidence of breast cancer detected without mammography. During this period, the incidence of breast cancer was stable and few cases of DCIS were detected (findings compatible with the very limited use of screening mammography). The estimate of the current incidence of breast cancer was based on the 3-year period 2006–2008. To eliminate the effect of use of hormone replacement therapy, the observed incidence was truncated if it was higher than the estimate of the current incidence (the annual incidence per 100 000 women of DCIS was not allowed to exceed 56.5 cases, of localized disease to exceed 177.5 cases, of regional disease to exceed 77.6 cases, and of distant disease to exceed 16.6 cases, during the period 1990–2005). A substantial increase in the use of screening mammography during the 1980s and early 1990s among women aged 40 years and older in the USA, a substantial concomitant increase in the incidence of early-stage breast cancer among these women, and a small decrease in the incidence of late-stage breast cancer were observed. A large increase in cases of early-stage cancer (absolute increase of 122 cases per 100 000 women) and a small decrease in cases of late-stage cancer (absolute decrease of 8 cases per 100 000 women) were observed. The trends in regional and distant late-stage breast cancer showed that the variable pattern in late-stage cancer (which includes the excess diagnoses associated with use of hormone replacement therapy in the late 1990s and early 2000s) was almost entirely attributable to changes in the incidence of regional (largely node-positive) disease. However, the incidence of distant (metastatic) disease remained unchanged (95% CI for the APC, −0.19% to 0.14%). The SEER data did not distinguish between women who were screened and those who were not screened.

Helvie et al. (2014), similarly to Bleyer & Welch (2012), compared the SEER breast cancer incidence and stage for the pre-mammography period (1977–1979) and the mammography screening period (2007–2009) in women older than 40 years. The authors estimated pre-screening temporal trends using several measures of APC. Stage-specific incidence values for 1977–1979 (baseline) were adjusted using APC values of 0.5%, 1.0%, 1.3%, and 2.0% and then compared with observed stage-specific incidence in 2007–2009. Pre-screening APC temporal trend estimates ranged from 0.8% to 2.3%. The joinpoint estimate of 1.3% for women older than 40 years approximated the four-decade-long APC trend of 1.2% noted in the Connecticut Tumor Registry. At an APC of 1.3%, late-stage breast cancer incidence decreased by 37% (56 cases per 100 000 women), with a reciprocal increase in early-stage rates noted from 1977–1979 to 2007–2009. The resulting late-stage breast cancer incidence decreased by 21% at an APC of 0.5% and by 48% at an APC of 2.0%. Total invasive breast cancer incidence decreased by 9% (27 cases per 100 000 women) at an APC of 1.3%. [According to the authors, a substantial reduction in late-stage breast cancer has occurred in the mammography era when appropriate adjustments are made for pre-screening temporal trends.]

Hou & Huo (2013) analysed the SEER age-standardized breast cancer incidence rates from 2000 to 2009, for 677 774 women aged 20 years and older. This study represents a descriptive analysis of population-based cancer incidence rates from 18 SEER registries with high-quality data, representing 28% of the United States population. Since 2004, incidence rates in women aged 40–49 years increased significantly for most racial/ethnic groups (overall APC, 1.1%; $P = 0.001$). The incidence rate of DCIS increased significantly in all racial/ethnic groups, with an APC range from 2.3% to 3.0% ($P < 0.005$). The incidence rate of localized breast cancer increased significantly in non-Hispanic Black women (APC, 1.3%; $P = 0.004$) and Asian women (APC, 1.2%; $P = 0.03$). The incidence rates of regional and distant cancers decreased significantly in non-Hispanic White women from 2000 to 2004 (APC, −2.5%; $P = 0.02$) and in Hispanic women from 2000 to 2009 (APC, −1.1%; $P = 0.006$). [It is possible that the changes in incidence rates are due in part to improvements in cancer screening methods and, therefore, advances in early detection. It is unlikely that the overall trends of incidence rates are due to changes in the mammography screening rate, since mammography use did not change substantially from 2000 to 2010, although it increased by large magnitudes in small groups with growing populations, such as new immigrants and Asian-Americans.]

DeSantis et al. (2014) obtained data on incidence, probability of developing cancer, and cause-specific survival from SEER, and data on the prevalence of mammography by age from the 2010 and 2012 Behavioral Risk Factor Surveillance System, to assess the relationship between mammography screening rates in 2010 and breast cancer stage at diagnosis in 2006–2010. Among non-Hispanic White women, state-level mammography screening prevalence was positively correlated with the percentage of breast cancers diagnosed at the in situ stage (correlation coefficient, $r = 0.62$; $P < 0.001$) and negatively correlated with the percentage of breast cancers diagnosed at late stages ($r = -0.51$; $P < 0.001$).

(d) Modifying effects of breast density

Given that increased mammographic breast density is associated with lower sensitivity and higher interval cancer rates (Mandelson et al., 2000), its potential role as an effect modifier of mammography screening effectiveness is of interest. The effect of breast density on case fatality rate, or breast density as a modifier, has been investigated in several studies. Only one of these has examined differences in survival of women with interval cancers in those with dense versus non-dense breasts. This study in Sweden found that women with interval cancers had worse survival than women with screen-detected cancers (hazard ratio [HR], 1.69; 95% CI, 1.03–2.76, overall) and that interval-cancer survival was poorer in those with non-dense breasts (HR, 1.76; 95% CI, 1.01–3.09) than in those with dense breasts (HR, 1.26; 95% CI, 0.47–3.38) (Eriksson et al., 2013). These effects were observed after adjustment for tumour size and lymph-node metastasis at diagnosis. [Before adjustment, hazard ratios were stronger.]

The remaining studies examined the impact of breast density on survival or mortality rates within populations where screening is available, but they did not differentiate between interval and screen-detected cancers. In a cohort in Denmark participating in biennial mammography at ages 50–69 years, during 1991–2001, the case fatality rate was lower in women with mixed/dense breasts than in those with fatty breasts (HR, 0.60; 95% CI, 0.43–0.84) (Olsen et al., 2009). [Although the case fatality rate is lower for women with dense breasts, it should be noted that because more women with dense breasts develop breast cancer, more women with dense breasts die from breast cancer overall.] In the USA, a study using the Carolina Mammography Registry (22 597 breast cancers) showed no difference in breast cancer mortality between women with dense breasts and those with fatty breasts, after adjusting for incidence differences (HR, 0.908; $P = 0.12$) (stage-adjusted) (Zhang et al., 2013). Similarly, the American College of Radiology Breast Imaging Reporting and Data System (BI-RADS) density score was not associated with breast cancer survival (HR for breast cancer death, 0.92; 95% CI, 0.71–1.19) in the United States Breast Cancer Surveillance Consortium (Gierach et al., 2012), except for an increased risk of breast cancer death among women with low breast density (BI-RADS 1) who were obese or had tumours larger than 20 mm. The Kopparberg RCT, in Sweden, suggested that women with dense breasts have higher breast cancer incidence rates (multivariate RR, 1.57; 95% CI, 1.23–2.01) and breast cancer mortality (RR, 1.91; 95% CI, 1.26–2.91), but that there was no clear difference in survival between women with dense breasts and those with non-dense breasts (HR, 1.41; 95% CI, 0.92–2.14) (not adjusted for tumour characteristics) (Chiu et al., 2010). One study found poor survival in women with dense breasts compared with those with fatty breasts in women diagnosed at the first screening round but not in those diagnosed at later rounds (rounds 5–10) (van Gils et al., 1998).

[The Working Group noted that although breast cancers occurring in dense breasts are more likely to be interval cancers, there is no indication that breast cancer survival rates are poorer for these cancers (despite a shorter lead-time bias). In addition, the studies were performed with screen-film mammography, so it is difficult to extrapolate the results to digital methods.]

(e) Effects of population-based mammography screening in the presence of adjuvant systemic therapy

RCTs of mammography screening, mostly performed in the 1980s or earlier, have reported reductions in breast cancer mortality in women aged 50–69 years. However, the present-day relevance of these trials has been debated because the management and treatment of breast cancer has changed considerably in the past decades (Gøtzsche & Nielsen, 2009; Kalager et al., 2010; Paci & EUROSCREEN Working Group, 2012; Marmot et al., 2013). Adjuvant systemic therapy has been increasingly used since the late 1980s, and its dissemination and effectiveness have progressed since then (van de Velde et al., 2010).

Such developments have probably affected the impact of screening, also in service screening programmes (Berry et al., 2005). This section discusses studies of the effects of adjuvant systemic therapy and mammography screening in current health-care systems.

The effects of adjuvant treatment and mammography screening were calculated for the Netherlands using the Microsimulation Screening Analysis (MISCAN) model (de Gelder et al., 2015). [Models can extrapolate findings from screening and adjuvant treatment trials to actual populations, can allow for comparison of intervention strategies, and can separate effects on the natural history of disease, for example screening effects and adjuvant treatment effects (Berry et al., 2005; Mandelblatt et al., 2009) (see Section 5.1.2f).] In the MISCAN model, the progression was modelled as a semi-Markov process through the successive preclinical invasive stages T1a, T1b, T1c, and T2+. The mean duration of the preclinical detectable phase, the probability of a transition between the stages, and the mammography sensitivity were then estimated, using detailed data from screening registries. Data on adjuvant systemic therapy were derived from comprehensive cancer centres. Cure and survival rates after screen detection were based on RCTs (de Koning et al., 1995; Tabár et al., 2000; Nyström et al., 2002; Bjurstam et al., 2003). The risk of death from breast cancer after adjuvant treatment was modelled using the rate ratios from the meta-analysis of the Early Breast Cancer Trialists' Collaborative Group (2005). In 2008, adjuvant treatment was estimated to have reduced the breast cancer mortality rate in the simulated population by 13.9%, compared with a situation without treatment. Biennial screening between age 50 years and age 74 years further reduced the mortality rate by 15.7%. Extending screening to age 48 years would lower the mortality rate by 1.0% compared with screening from age 50 years; 10 additional screening rounds between age 40 years and age 49 years would reduce this rate by 5.1%. Adjuvant systemic therapy and screening reduced breast cancer mortality by similar amounts.

A previous modelling study, which included six natural history models for the population in the USA, had estimated an approximately equal contribution of adjuvant therapy and screening to the observed mortality reduction in the USA (Berry et al., 2005), using very similar techniques to those described above.

These analyses have recently been updated, taking into account the receptor-specific heterogeneity of breast cancer (Munoz et al., 2014), by using six established population models with ER-specific input parameters on age-specific incidence, disease natural history, mammography characteristics, and treatment effects to quantify the impact of screening and adjuvant therapy on age-adjusted breast cancer mortality in the USA by ER status from 1975 to 2000. In 2000, actual screening and adjuvant treatment were estimated to have reduced breast cancer mortality by 34.8%, compared with the situation if no screening or adjuvant treatment had been present; a reduction by 15.9% was estimated to have been a result of screening, and 23.4% as a result of treatment. For ER-positive cases, adjuvant treatment made a higher relative contribution to breast cancer mortality reduction than screening, whereas for ER-negative cases the relative contributions were similar for screening and adjuvant treatment. Although ER-negative cases were less likely to be screen-detected than ER-positive cases (35.1% vs 51.2%), when they were screen-detected, the survival gain was greater for ER-negative cases than for ER-positive cases (5-year breast cancer survival, 35.6% vs 30.7%).

5.3 Adverse effects of mammography

5.3.1 False-positive rates

A screening test is not diagnostic but should identify asymptomatic women who are at risk of harbouring an undiagnosed cancer. The screening episode in organized screening should end with an unequivocal diagnostic report: there is or there is not cancer (Perry et al., 2006). A woman in whom an abnormality is detected by screening and whose investigations end with a negative result has a false-positive result. This result closes the screening episode.

In a recent survey of 20 population-based screening programmes in 17 European countries, the Euroscreen and EUNICE Working Group (Hofvind et al., 2012a) reported average recall rates varying from 9.3% at the initial screening episode (range, 2.2–15.6%) to 4.0% at subsequent screening episodes (range, 1.2–10.5%). The average rates of needle biopsy were 2.2% at the initial screening and 1.1% at subsequent screenings. The variation depends on differences between national protocols and a variety of local conditions. Over the whole diagnostic phase, the benign-to-malignant ratio ranged from 0.09 in the United Kingdom to 0.21 in Luxembourg, with an average of 0.11.

The difference in the performance of the assessment phase between opportunistic screening and service screening has been estimated by comparing screening in the USA and population-based programmes in Europe. Smith-Bindman et al. (2005) compared the performance of screening in the United Kingdom and the USA. The outcomes included (per 1000 women screened for 20 years) a detection rate of carcinoma in situ of 12.3 in the USA compared with 8.3 in the United Kingdom, a rate of non-invasive diagnostic tests for assessment of recalled women of 553 in the USA compared with 183 in the United Kingdom, and a biopsy rate of 142 in the USA compared with 85 in the United Kingdom, of which 54 and 25, respectively, were open surgical biopsies.

Hofvind et al. (2012b) compared the Norwegian mammography screening programme with screening practice in Vermont, USA (Vermont is a member of the Breast Cancer Surveillance Consortium, an initiative of the United States National Cancer Institute), showing that higher recall rates and lower specificity in the USA were not associated with higher sensitivity. These differences may be explained by professional practices, since screening centres in the USA usually have small volumes of mammography readings, and double reading is not a quality requirement in the USA as it is in Europe (Burnside et al., 2014).

The cumulative risk of a false-positive recall is one of the most important harms of screening. The false-positive rate is estimated from the recall rate by subtracting the cancer detection rate in the same screening episode. The cumulative risk of a false-positive result is defined as the cumulative risk of recall for further assessment at least once during the screening period (usually 10 biennial screening episodes in organized programmes) minus the cumulative risk of cancer detection over the same period. There is a similar definition for the cumulative risk of having an invasive procedure (needle biopsy or surgical biopsy) with a benign outcome.

A systematic review has been made of publications estimating the cumulative risk of a false-positive result in European population-based mammography screening programmes (Hofvind et al., 2012a). Four studies were included, based on data from the 1990s and conducted in Denmark, Italy, Norway, and Spain. Results updated with a further 9 years of experience in Norway have since been published (Román et al., 2013). The cumulative risk of any further assessment without cancer diagnosis varied from 8.1% to 20.4% in the most recent period (ending variously in 2001 to 2010), and the cumulative risk of assessment with an invasive procedure without cancer diagnosis varied from 1.8% to 4.1%.

The cumulative risk of false-positives is higher in opportunistic mammography screening, which is the usual modality in the USA. Elmore et al. (1998) estimated that 41% of screened women had at least one false-positive result over 10 screening episodes. Hubbard et al. (2010) applied statistical models to more recent data from the Breast Cancer Surveillance Consortium for women aged 40–59 years at entry and followed up over their screening history. The risk of a false-positive over 10 screening mammograms varied between 58% and 77%.

Román et al. (2012) assessed factors affecting the false-positive rate after any assessment, and after assessment with an invasive procedure, in a retrospective cohort in Spain. The authors reported that the false-positive risk after assessment with an invasive procedure was less for digital mammography (RR, 0.83) than for non-digital mammography, and they estimated a total cumulative risk of 20.4%, ranging from 51.4% for the highest risk profile to 7.5% for the lowest risk profile. The risk after assessment with all procedures and with invasive procedures was estimated to be higher for younger women (OR, 1.30 for age 40–44 years; OR, 1.26 for age 40–54 years; reference category, age 65–69 years).

In the USA, Kerlikowske et al. (2013) assessed the cumulative risk by breast density and risk profile. The cumulative probability of a false-positive mammography result was higher among women with extremely dense breasts who underwent annual mammography and either were aged 40–49 years (65.5%) or used combined estrogen–progestogen hormone therapy (65.8%), and was lower among women aged 50–74 years who underwent biennial or 3-yearly mammography and had scattered fibroglandular densities (30.7% and 21.9%, respectively) or fatty breasts (17.4% and 12.1%, respectively).

Indicators of the cumulative risk of false-positives are included as possible harms of screening in the balance sheet of benefits and harms. The Euroscreen mammography screening balance sheet considered 1000 women who were aged 50 or 51 years at the start of their screening regimen. The cumulative risk of false-positives was estimated to be 200 over the 10 screening rounds from age 50 years to age 69 years; 170 women were recalled for further assessment without invasive procedures, and 30 women had further assessment with invasive procedures (Paci & EUROSCREEN Working Group, 2012).

5.3.2 Overdiagnosis

The definition of overdiagnosis and estimates of overdiagnosis in randomized trials of mammography screening have been presented in Section 4.2.3c. The quantification of overdiagnosis is important in observational studies because this harm was not a primary end-point of the RCTs and estimates are influenced by local screening practice and technological innovation. Other approaches, such as radiological doubling time, have been suggested as useful indicators for the study of overdiagnosis, but in this section overdiagnosis is considered as an epidemiological construct, based on a retrospective analysis of breast cancer diagnosis in the population.

Several approaches have been proposed for estimating overdiagnosis in observational studies.

The *cumulative incidence method* estimates overdiagnosis by following up a cohort of women, invited and not invited to screening or screened and not screened. The ideal study would require the follow-up of pairs of birth or enrolment age cohorts in which one cohort is invited to screening and the other is not invited (Møller et al., 2005; Biesheuvel et al., 2007). The attribution of an individual time zero to each invited woman allows for estimation of changes in incidence over the screening period in the population and monitoring of the compensatory drop phase after the end of screening (Fig. 5.2).

Fig. 5.2 Observed and modelled breast cancer incidence per 100 000 person-years in the presence and absence of screening in 1990–2006

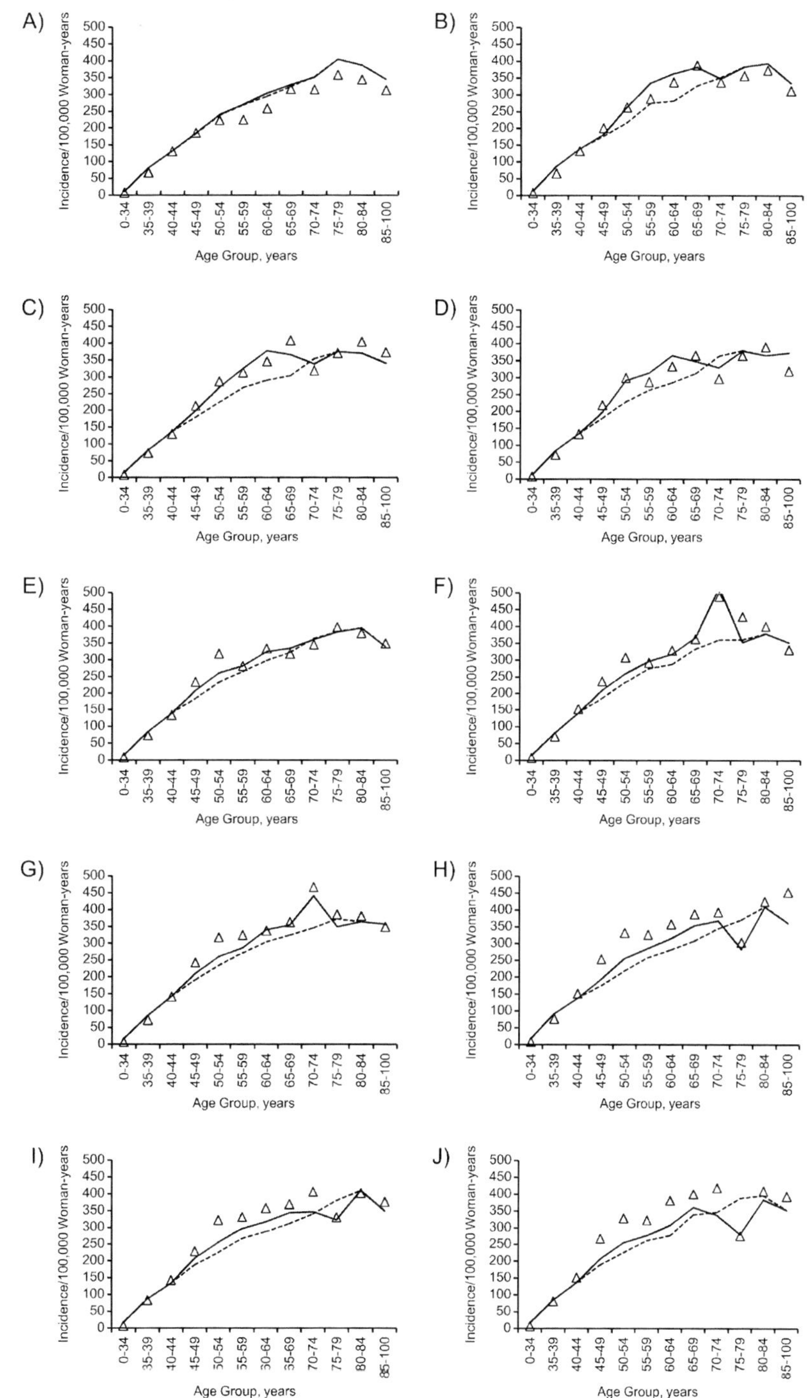

Values after years indicate: percentage of the target population aged 49–69 years invited, fraction of prevalent screenings. (A) 1990: 9.2%, 74%; (B) 1992: 47.4%, 77%; (C) 1994: 74.3%, 49%; (D) 1996: 92.0%, 39%; (E) 1998: 80.8%, 20%; (F) 1999: 91.8%, 19%; (G) 2000: 94.4%, 18%; (H) 2002: 96.1%, 14%; (I) 2004: 95.8%, 14%; (J) 2006: 92.2%, 13%. Solid lines, modelled with screening; dashed lines, modelled without screening; triangles, observed.

From de Gelder et al. (2011a). Interpreting overdiagnosis estimates in population-based mammography screening, *Epidemiologic Reviews*, 2011, volume 33, issue 1, pages 111–121, by permission of Oxford University Press.

The *incidence-rate method* compares the average annual incidence of breast cancer over a defined period of follow-up in a specified age group of women who were offered or accepted screening with an estimate of the average annual incidence of breast cancer during the same period in women who were not offered screening or were not screened. Overdiagnosis is taken to be any excess in incidence in the former over the latter once the screening lead time has been accounted for. Several methods have been suggested for the adjustment for lead time, with the aim of overcoming the frequent difficulty of too short a follow-up period for the lead time to have passed in all women under observation who had been invited to screening or were screened.

In a methodological study, Etzioni et al. (2013) contrasted an incidence excess approach with a lead-time approach. The *lead-time approach* uses the disease incidence under screening to make inferences about the lead time or the natural history of the disease. Using the *incidence excess approach*, the authors suggested that the estimate should consider the time needed for screening dissemination and the compensatory drop, as expressed by incidence rates at older ages. In the presence of a shorter follow-up time and/or unequal screening periods in the age cohorts of women, statistical adjustment for lead time is required. This can be based on estimates of lead time derived from clinical cancers (such as estimates derived from experience before the introduction of population screening programmes) or estimates from modelling studies.

Simulation, using statistical modelling, of lifetime individual histories with or without screening is often used to overcome the complexity of screening evaluation, in particular to account for lead time and to give understandable outcomes (see Section 5.1.2f). Complex models such as these need a set of assumptions about natural history of the disease and screening performance (Tan et al., 2006), which would ideally be clearly stated in reports based on the models' use but generally are not. Importantly, too, a paucity of relevant empirical evidence means that assumptions about the proportion of preclinical cancers that are non-progressive and the range and distribution of lead time, which are critical to modelled estimates of overdiagnosis, are very uncertain.

Duffy & Parmar (2013), using estimates of the incidence rate in the United Kingdom and an exponential distribution of the lead time, simulated the time course of incidence rates during and after the screening period in the absence of overdiagnosis. With a 20-year period of screening (from age 50 years to age 69 years), a period of at least 10 years must elapse after the screening period (to when women are aged 79 years) for the *excess incidence rate* to be close to the rate observed in the absence of screening (to within 1% of excess with 30 years of follow-up from the start of screening). It is important to note that in the same simulation, 10 years of observation of a population of women screened from age 50–69 years at the start of screening will give an incidence excess of 50%. This model assumed an average lead time of 40 months. However, some estimates are much lower (see, for example, Feinleib & Zelen, 1969). Although there is disagreement over the average and distribution of lead time for breast cancer, the main conclusion is that an adequate correction for lead time is needed in the absence of a sufficient follow-up period to distinguish *excess of incidence* due to lead time from *overdiagnosis*.

An important factor determining the observational estimate of overdiagnosis is the estimate of the underlying incidence. In descriptive epidemiological studies, an estimate of incidence in the absence of screening is needed. In comparative studies, the reference population should be comparable to the invited population so far as is possible in terms of the background incidence rate, breast cancer risk factors, socioeconomic status, and use of health services other than for mammography. If rates from the same or another historical (pre-screening) population are used, the time trend in the underlying incidence must be estimated, a projection made to the screened population, and sensitivity analyses of the estimates made that take account of variation in the trend due to unpredicted changes in population composition or the prevalence of risk factors. Self-selection bias should also be considered and adjusted for if attenders only are evaluated.

Adjustment for lead time and estimation of the underlying incidence of breast cancer in the absence of screening (control of confounding due to differences in breast cancer risk factors between screened and unscreened women) were considered as the main problems in estimating overdiagnosis in observational studies (Njor et al., 2013a), but these are not the only factors to be considered. Others include (Njor et al., 2013a): the nature and quality of the observational data used; what estimate was actually reported as a measure of overdiagnosis (ideally classified in the terms outlined by the Independent UK Panel on Breast Cancer Screening, 2012), which is sometimes not clearly described, and, for the Independent United Kingdom Panel's measure A or B, how long the period of follow-up was after screening stopped (periods beyond about 10 years from the end of screening will cause progressive "dilution" of the overdiagnosis estimate; de Gelder et al., 2011a); whether the estimate was based on women invited to screening or women who attended screening; what the screening policies were during the period of screening to which the overdiagnosis estimate related (e.g. age at starting and at stopping screening, and screening interval); and whether the estimate is based on steady-state screening or screening that includes all or a proportion of the period after initiation of screening during which women across the whole screening age range are receiving their first invitations to screening (inclusion of this period will produce higher estimates due to greater inclusion of prevalent screens, in which the probability of overdiagnosis is higher than it is for incident screens).

Observational studies of overdiagnosis for women aged 50–69 years are summarized in Table 5.11 and Table 5.12. Table 5.11 covers studies reviewed by the Euroscreen Working Group (Puliti et al., 2012), which included all 13 observational studies conducted in Europe that were published up to February 2011. Table 5.12 covers 17 studies conducted in Europe and published from February 2011 to November 2014, when the Handbook Working Group met, or conducted outside Europe and published up to November 2014.

Estimates of the overdiagnosis risk, principally the Independent United Kingdom Panel's measure A (the excess cancers expressed as a proportion of cancers diagnosed over the whole follow-up period in unscreened women), ranged from −0.7% to 76% for invasive cancer only and from 1% to 57% for invasive and in situ cancers together.

The Euroscreen Working Group characterized overdiagnosis estimates as made with or without correction for lead time and underlying incidence trend. The reported estimates that were considered as adequately adjusted for both biases (from 6 of the 13 studies) ranged from 1% to 10% excess over the expected incidence for all breast cancers (measure A) (1% to 10% for invasive cancer only, from 4 studies, and 1% to 7% for invasive and in situ cancers, from 4 studies). The majority of the studies used temporal trends or geographical differences in dynamic populations to adjust for the underlying incidence. Only two studies used the cohort population approach, and a few studies used statistical modelling for the estimate. The Euroscreen Working Group derived a summary estimate of overdiagnosis of 6.5% of the incidence in the absence of screening. This is the estimate of the overdiagnosis in women screened between the ages of 50 years and 69 years and followed up for 10 years after the last screening, and included carcinoma in

Table 5.11 Studies of the estimates of overdiagnosis in Europe[a]

Reference	Population		Intervention	Comparison				Outcomes[b]	
	Country (area) Calendar period of screening[c]	Type of population and study design	Age and interval of screening Start year of screening[d]	Reference population	Adjustment for breast cancer risk	Adjustment for lead time	Mean follow-up after end of screening (range)	Estimate of overdiagnosis (only invasive)	Estimate of overdiagnosis (in situ and invasive)
Peeters et al. (1989a, b)	Netherlands (Nijmegen) 1975–1986	Dynamic population Ecological	35–65+ yr 2 yr 1975	Incidence in county not invited to screening (1970–1975)	Birth year	No adjustment	Not applicable	NR	11%
Paci et al. (2004)	Italy (Florence) 1990–1999	Dynamic population Cohort	50–69 yr 2 yr 1990	Pre-screening incidence (1985–1990)	Age	Statistical adjustment	Not applicable	0–1%	5%
Zahl et al. (2004)	Norway (AORH counties) 1996–2000	Dynamic population Ecological	50–69 yr 2 yr 1996	(i) Pre-screening incidence (1991–1995, projected to 2000) (ii) Contemporary incidence in unscreened counties (1991–2000)	Age, temporal trend	No adjustment[e]	2.5 yr (1–4 yr)	54%	NR
Zahl et al. (2004)	Sweden 1986–2000	Dynamic population Ecological	40–74 yr; 50–74 yr 2 yr 40–49 yr 18 mo 1986	Pre-screening incidence (1971–1985, projected to 2000)	Age, temporal trend	No adjustment[e]	Compensatory drop not considered in analysis	45%	NR
Jonsson et al. (2005)	Sweden (11 counties) 1986–2000	Dynamic population Ecological	40–74 yr; 50–74 yr 2 yr 40–49 yr 18 mo 1986	Pre-screening incidence (1971–1985)	Age, temporal trend, and area	Statistical adjustment	12.8 yr	0–54%, depending on age	NR
Olsen et al. (2006)	Denmark (Copenhagen) 1991–1995	Fixed population Cohort	50–69 yr 2 yr 1991	Incidence among screened women	Not needed	Statistical adjustment	Not applicable	NR	7%[f]

Table 5.11 (continued)

Reference	Population		Intervention		Comparison			Outcomes[b]	
	Country (area) Calendar period of screening[c]	Type of population and study design	Age and interval of screening Start year of screening[d]	Reference population	Adjustment for breast cancer risk	Adjustment for lead time	Mean follow-up after end of screening (range)	Estimate of overdiagnosis (only invasive)	Estimate of overdiagnosis (in situ and invasive)
Paci et al. (2006)	Italy (6 northern and central areas) 1991–2001	Dynamic population Cohort	50–74 yr 2 yr 1991	Pre-screening incidence (1986–1990, in women aged 40–79 yr)	Age, temporal trend, and area	Statistical adjustment	Not applicable	3.2%	4.6%
Waller et al. (2007)	England and Wales 1987–2001	Dynamic population Ecological	50–64 yr (extended to age 70 yr in 2001) 3 yr 1988	Pre- and post-screening incidence (1971–2001)	Age, period, birth cohort, use of HRT	Compensatory drop	1–3 yr	10%[e]	NR
Jørgensen& Gøtzsche (2009)	England and Wales 1987–1999	Dynamic population Ecological	50–64 yr 3 yr 1987	Pre-screening incidence (1971–1984)	Age and temporal trend	Compensatory drop	2.3 yr (0–15 yr)	41%	57% (assuming 10% CIS)
Jørgensen & Gøtzsche (2009)	Sweden 1986–2006	Dynamic population Ecological	Different age ranges: the broadest, 40–74 yr; the most common, 50–74 yr 2 yr 40–49 yr 18 mo 1986	Pre-screening incidence (1971–1985)	Age and temporal trend	Compensatory drop	3.9 yr (1–10 yr)	31%	46% (assuming 10% CIS)
Jørgensen& Gøtzsche (2009)	Norway (AORH counties) 1995–2006	Dynamic population Ecological	50–69 yr (and 50% of the population aged 70–74 yr) 2 yr 1995	Pre-screening incidence (1980–1994)	Age and temporal trend	Compensatory drop	4.7 (1–10 yr)	37%	52% (assuming 10% CIS)

Table 5.11 (continued)

Reference	Population		Intervention		Comparison			Outcomes[b]	
	Country (area) Calendar period of screening[c]	Type of population and study design	Age and interval of screening Start year of screening[d]	Reference population	Adjustment for breast cancer risk	Adjustment for lead time	Mean follow-up after end of screening (range)	Estimate of overdiagnosis (only invasive)	Estimate of overdiagnosis (in situ and invasive)
Puliti et al. (2009)	Italy (Florence) 1990–2004	Birth cohort	50–69 yr 2 yr 1990	Pre-screening incidence (1986–1990)	Age and temporal trend	Compensatory drop	4.7 yr (1–14 yr)	0.99%	1.0%
Jørgensen et al. (2009)	Denmark (Copenhagen and Funen) 1991–2003	Dynamic population Ecological	50–69 yr 2 yr Copenhagen: 1991 Funen: 1993	Incidence in neighbouring unscreened area (1971–1990)	Age	Compensatory drop	4.6 yr (1–10 yr)	NR	33%
Duffy et al. (2010)	England 1988–2004	Dynamic population Cohort and ecological	50–64 yr (extended to 70 yr in 2001) 3 yr 1988	Pre-screening incidence (1974–1988)	Age and temporal trend	Compensatory drop	5 yr (1–15 yr)	3.3%[e]	NR
Martinez-Alonso et al. (2010)	Spain (Catalonia) 1990–2004	Dynamic population Statistical model	50–64 yr (extended to 65–69 yr) 2 yr 1990	Pre- and post-screening incidence (women aged 20–84 yr from 1980–2004)	Age, year of birth, fertility rate, and use of mammography	Statistical adjustment	Not applicable	0.4%–46.6%, depending on birth cohort	NR
de Gelder et al. (2011b)	Netherlands 1989–2006	Dynamic population MISCAN model	49–69 yr (extended to 74 yr) 2 yr 1990	Predicted incidence without screening	Not needed	Compensatory drop	6.1 yr (1–16 yr)	NR	3.6%

[a] Studies published up to February 2011 and included in the review by Euroscreen.
[b] Measures of overdiagnosis are equivalent to measure A of the Independent UK Panel on Breast Cancer Screening (2012).
[c] Period of screening that contributed to the estimate of overdiagnosis.
[d] First year of the screening programme or intervention to which the overdiagnosis estimate relates.
[e] A compensatory drop was observed by Zahl et al. (2004) (11% in Norway and 12% in Sweden) but was not taken into account in the estimation of overdiagnosis because it was not statistically significant.
[f] Recalculated as measure A by Puliti et al. (2012).
AORH, Akershus, Oslo, Rogaland, Hordaland; CIS, carcinoma in situ; HRT, hormone replacement therapy; MISCAN, Microsimulation Screening Analysis; NR, not reported; yr, year or years.
Modified from Puliti et al. (2012).

Table 5.12 Studies of estimates of overdiagnosis in Europe (published from February 2011 to November 2014) and in other countries (published up to November 2014)

Reference	Population	Intervention		Comparison			Outcomes		
	Country (area) Calendar period of screening[a]	Type of population and study design	Age and interval of screening Start year of screening[b]	Reference population	Adjustment for breast cancer risk	Adjustment for lead time	Measure of overdiagnosis[c]	Estimate of overdiagnosis (only invasive)	Estimate of overdiagnosis (in situ and invasive)
Jørgensen & Gøtzsche (2009)	Australia (New South Wales) 1996–2002	Dynamic population Ecological	50–69 yr 2 yr 1988	Pre-screening incidence (1972–1987)	Age and temporal trend	Compensatory drop: no drop was observed in women aged 70–79 yr	Measure A	38%	53%
Jørgensen & Gøtzsche (2009)	Canada (Manitoba) 1995–2005	Dynamic population Ecological	50–69 yr (extended to 70–84 yr) 2 yr 1995 (Opportunistic screening began in 1979)	Pre-screening incidence (1970–1978)	Age and temporal trend	Compensatory drop: allowed for a decrease in incidence in women aged 70–84 yr	Measure A	35%[d]	44%
Morrell et al. (2010)	Australia (New South Wales) 1999–2001	Dynamic population Ecological	50–69 yr 2 yr 1988	(i) Incidence trend in women aged < 40 yr and ≥ 80 yr (1972–2001) (ii) Pre-screening incidence trend in women aged 50–69 yr (1972–1983)	Age, use of HRT, obesity, nulliparity, and temporal trend	Statistical adjustment assuming 5 yr lead time	Measure A	(i) 42% (ii) 30%	NR

Table 5.12 (continued)

Reference	Population	Intervention			Comparison		Outcomes		
	Country (area) Calendar period of screening[a]	Type of population and study design	Age and interval of screening Start year of screening[b]	Reference population	Adjustment for breast cancer risk	Adjustment for lead time	Measure of overdiagnosis[c]	Estimate of overdiagnosis (only invasive)	Estimate of overdiagnosis (in situ and invasive)
Junod et al. (2011)	France 1988–2005	Dynamic population Ecological	50–69 yr (1988–1998) 50–74 yr (1999–present) 3 yr (1988–1998) 2 yr (1999–present) 1988	(i) For women aged 50–64 yr, incidence in the same age cohort born 15 yr earlier (1926–1930) (ii) For women aged 65–79 yr, incidence in the same age cohort born 15 yr earlier (1911–1915)	Age, use of HRT, alcohol, and obesity	None	Measure A	(i) 76% (ii) 23%	NR
Seigneurin et al. (2011)	France (Isère) 1991–2006	Statistical model of birth cohorts 1922–1956	50–69 yr 2 yr and opportunistic 1991	Predicted pre-screening incidence (birth cohorts 1900–1950)	Age, temporal trend, and opportunistic screening	Simulation of sojourn times with various distributions of unknown parameters	Excess cancers as a proportion of: (i) those detected by screening (ii) those diagnosed in the whole population	(i) 3.3% (ii) 1.5%	Only in situ: (i) 31.9% (ii) 28.0% 31.9%
Zahl & Mæhlen (2012)	Norway 1996–2009	Dynamic population Ecological	50–69 yr 2 yr 1996	Pre-screening incidence (1991–1995)	Age, area, population growth, introduction of screening mammography, and temporal trend	Compensatory drop: 1–14 yr since last screen	Measure A	NR	50%
Puliti et al. (2012)	Italy (Florence) 1991–2008	Dynamic population Cohort	60–69 yr 2 yr 1991	Incidence in screening non-attenders	Age, marital status, and SES	Compensatory drop: 5–14 yr since last screen	Measure A	5%	10%

Table 5.12 (continued)

Reference	Population	Intervention		Comparison			Outcomes		
	Country (area) Calendar period of screening[a]	Type of population and study design	Age and interval of screening Start year of screening[b]	Reference population	Adjustment for breast cancer risk	Adjustment for lead time	Measure of overdiagnosis[c]	Estimate of overdiagnosis (only invasive)	Estimate of overdiagnosis (in situ and invasive)
Kalager et al. (2012)	Norway 1996–2005	Dynamic population Ecological	50–69 yr 2 yr 1996	(i) Contemporary incidence in county not invited to screening (1996–2005) (ii) Historical county pre-screening incidence (1986–1995)	Age, temporal trend, and area	Compensatory drop: included women up to age 79 yr in incidence and up to 10 yr since last screen	Measure A	(i) 18% (ii) 25%[e]	NR
Bleyer &Welch (2012)	USA 1979–2008	Dynamic population Ecological	≥ 40 yr 1 yr 1971	Incidence before widespread screening (1976–1978)	Age, use of HRT, and temporal trend	No explicit adjustment for lead time. Overdiagnosis estimated from difference between increase in incidence of early breast cancer and fall in incidence of advanced breast cancer when screening steady state reached	Overdiagnosed cancers as a percentage of all cancers diagnosed in the population	20%	31%

Table 5.12 (continued)

Reference	Population	Intervention		Comparison			Outcomes		
	Country (area) Calendar period of screening[a]	Type of population and study design	Age and interval of screening Start year of screening[b]	Reference population	Adjustment for breast cancer risk	Adjustment for lead time	Measure of overdiagnosis[c]	Estimate of overdiagnosis (only invasive)	Estimate of overdiagnosis (in situ and invasive)
Falk et al. (2013)	Norway 1995–2009	Dynamic population Cohort	48–71 yr 2 yr 1995	Incidence in women who had never attended screening in three groups: (1) pre-screening modelled incidence based on women aged 40 yr in 1993–1995 (2) pre-screening incidence in women of screening age in 1980–1984 (3) pre-screening incidence in women in birth cohort 1903–1907	Age, area, calendar year, and temporal trend	Compensatory drop: up to 10 yr since last screen	Measure A	Attenders: 11.4–13.4% Invited: 9.6–11.3%	Attenders: 16.5–19.6% Invited: 13.9–16.5%
Lund et al. (2013)	Norway 2002–2010	Dynamic population Cohort	52–69 yr 2 yr 2002	Incidence in unscreened women	Age, parity, use of HRT, family history, and BMI	Compensatory drop: included women up to age 79 yr in incidence	Measure A	7.5%	22.0%

Table 5.12 (continued)

Reference	Population	Intervention		Comparison			Outcomes		
	Country (area) Calendar period of screening[a]	**Type of population and study design**	**Age and interval of screening Start year of screening**[b]	**Reference population**	**Adjustment for breast cancer risk**	**Adjustment for lead time**	**Measure of overdiagnosis**[c]	**Estimate of overdiagnosis (only invasive)**	**Estimate of overdiagnosis (in situ and invasive)**
Njor et al. (2013b)	Denmark (Copenhagen and Funen) (i) Copenhagen: 1991–2005 (ii) Funen: 1993–2004	Dynamic population Birth cohorts: (i) 1921–1935 (ii) 1923–1934	56–69 yr 2 yr (i) 1991 (ii) 1993	Incidence in: (1) historical pre-screening birth cohorts from same regions (2) contemporary regions not invited to screening (3) national pre-screening historical birth cohort	Temporal trend and area	Compensatory drop: ≥ 8 yr since last screen	Measure A	(i) 5% (ii) 1%	(i) 6% (ii) 1% Pooled: 2.3%
Coldman & Phillips (2013)	Canada (British Columbia) 2000–2009	Dynamic population Cohort	40–49 yr 1 yr ≥ 50 yr 2 yr 1988	Incidence in women who did not attend screening	Age	Compensatory drop: included women up to age 89 yr (screening ceased at age 79 yr)	Measure A	5.4%	17.3%
Coldman & Phillips (2013)	Canada (British Columbia) 1988–2009	Dynamic population Ecological	40–49 yr 1 yr ≥ 50 yr 2 yr 1988	Pre-screening incidence (1970–1979) projected to 2005–2009	Age and temporal trend	Compensatory drop: included women up to age 89 yr (screening ceased at age 79 yr)	Measure A	−0.7%	6.7%

Table 5.12 (continued)

Reference	Population	Intervention			Comparison		Outcomes		
	Country (area) Calendar period of screening[a]	Type of population and study design	Age and interval of screening Start year of screening[b]	Reference population	Adjustment for breast cancer risk	Adjustment for lead time	Measure of overdiagnosis[c]	Estimate of overdiagnosis (only invasive)	Estimate of overdiagnosis (in situ and invasive)
Heinävaara et al. (2014)	Finland (Helsinki) 1986–1997	Dynamic population Ecological	50–59 yr 2 yr 1986	Incidence in: (i) last unscreened birth cohort (1930–1934) (ii) 5-yr birth cohorts from 1920–1924 to 1930–1934 (from statistical model)	Age and cohort	(i) Compensatory drop to 13–14 yr since last screen (ii) Removal of modelled screening effect at age 50–59 yr and 60–64 yr from observed incidence in 1935–1939 cohort	Measure A	NR	(i) 7% (ii) 5%
Gunsoy et al. (2014)	United Kingdom 1975–2013	Dynamic population Markov model	47–73 yr 3 yr 1988	Model calibrated against United Kingdom incidence rates for 1971–2010 and cancer detection rates for screening from 1994–2009	Not required	Compensatory drop: minimum of 12 yr of follow-up since last screen	Measure A	NR	5.6%

Table 5.12 (continued)

Reference	Population	Intervention			Comparison		Outcomes		
	Country (area) Calendar period of screening[a]	Type of population and study design	Age and interval of screening Start year of screening[b]	Reference population	Adjustment for breast cancer risk	Adjustment for lead time	Measure of overdiagnosis[c]	Estimate of overdiagnosis (only invasive)	Estimate of overdiagnosis (in situ and invasive)
Beckmann et al. (2015)	Australia (South Australia) 1989–2010	Dynamic population Case–control study nested within a cohort	40–69 yr 1 yr (increased risk) or 2 yr 1989	Women who did not attend screening in 1989–2010	Age, temporal trend (1977–1988), SES, and area	Compensatory drop: included women up to age 85 yr in incidence and ≥ 10 yr since last screen	Measure A[f]	[8.3%]	[16.0%]

[a] Period of screening that contributed to the estimate of overdiagnosis.
[b] First year of the screening programme or intervention to which the overdiagnosis estimate relates.
[c] Measures are equivalent to measure A of the Independent UK Panel on Breast Cancer Screening (2012) unless otherwise indicated.
[d] This estimate was not adjusted for lead time.
[e] Results are those from the authors' Approach 1, which the Working Group considered to be the preferred of the two approaches the authors took to adjustment for lead time.
[f] The estimate of the percentage risk of overdiagnosis reported in Beckmann et al. (2015) is measure B, with women exposed to screening as the denominator. The Working Group recalculated this as measure A using data provided in Beckmann et al. (2015).
BMI, body mass index; HRT, hormone replacement therapy; NR, not reported; OD, overdiagnosis; SES, socioeconomic status; yr, year or years.

situ (Paci & EUROSCREEN Working Group, 2012), measure A as defined by the Independent UK Panel on Breast Cancer Screening (2012).

The IARC Working Group also sought to distinguish analyses that adequately adjusted for lead time and for the underlying breast cancer incidence trend: these were the analyses of Puliti et al. (2012), Kalager et al. (2012), Falk et al. (2013), Lund et al. (2013), Njor et al. (2013a), Heinävaara et al. (2014) (estimate A1 only), and Beckmann et al. (2015). The range of estimates from these studies was 2% to 25% for invasive cancer only and 2% to 22% for invasive and in situ cancers together.

5.3.3 Overtreatment

Over the past 50 years, breast cancer care has moved from aggressive, mutilating surgery to breast-conserving treatment (Fisher et al., 2002; Veronesi et al., 2002). This change was the starting point for improvements in other treatment and assessment areas, such as, for example, the sentinel lymph node procedure, which has been well established in clinical practice since the early 2000s (Veronesi et al., 2003). Detection of early, indolent lesions, such as carcinoma in situ (Ernster et al., 2002), is a major area of concern. In a recent international survey, Lynge et al. (2014) documented the wide variability in the occurrence of in situ breast cancer across countries. In a comparison with European programmes, higher probabilities for the occurrence of carcinoma in situ were reported in the USA. This finding is associated with higher false-positive rates and biopsy rates in the diagnostic assessment phase (Smith-Bindman et al., 2005).

Carcinomas in situ have high survival rates after treatment, but studies have shown that only a proportion of them, depending mainly on the pathological grade, would have progressed to invasiveness over the lifetime of the woman in the absence of early diagnosis. Overdiagnosed breast cancer cases are all overtreated. Carcinoma in situ is considered a major area of overtreatment. However, overtreatment is a harm not limited to screen-detected cases. Clinicians follow shared guidelines, primarily based on the stage at presentation of the disease. Screen-detected cases, when treated in the same cancer unit, will receive treatment by tumour characteristics. Chemotherapy and hormone therapy for breast cancer are progressively being extended to very early and less-progressive cancers (Peto et al., 2012), with important implications when there is a growing proportion of early, high-survival-rate breast cancers.

An example of the relationship between overdiagnosis and overtreatment is the comparison of mastectomy rates in the screening and pre-screening epochs. In a Cochrane systematic review (Gøtzsche & Jørgensen, 2013), a 31% increase in mastectomy and lumpectomy rates (20% excess of mastectomies) was estimated in the intervention group compared with the control group. This estimate considered all breast cancer cases detected in the screening period (i.e. the excess of incidence observed in the screening arm).

Zorzi et al. (2006) evaluated the use of mastectomy in Italy in the period 1997–2001, during which a large number of screening programmes were implemented, using individual data classified by stage and modality of diagnosis in relation to screening. The probability of a mastectomy increased with age and primary tumour size, and screen-detected cases were half as likely to be treated with mastectomy as non-screen-detected cases. The increasing rates of early-stage cancers (< 30 mm) and the use of breast-conserving treatment paralleled a decline in the mastectomy rate and in the incidence of advanced-stage cancers (> 30 mm), showing an appropriate use of the surgical approach.

Suhrke et al. (2011), using population-based data in the epoch of change to a service screening programme, showed an increase in rates of breast surgery and also an increase in mastectomy rates immediately after the start of the screening programme. They described a recent decline in mastectomy rates and suggested that the change affected all age groups and that it is likely to have resulted from changes in surgical policy.

5.3.4 *Risk of breast cancer induced by radiation*

Exposure of the breast to ionizing radiation may induce breast cancers (see Section 1.3.4). The low dose of X-ray photon radiation received during mammography is thus considered as a potential adverse effect of breast cancer screening. The number of cancers caused by screening with mammography must be estimated to evaluate the balance between benefits and risks. However, due to the small number of expected cases, it is not possible to estimate such a number from epidemiological data. Thus, numerous studies have used a quantitative risk assessment approach. This approach is based on a large number of hypotheses arising from current scientific knowledge and on hypotheses about screening modalities.

(a) Hypotheses for quantitative risk assessment

(i) Hypotheses about risk models

Hypotheses about risk models come from the selection of the most reliable studies on the relationship between radiation exposure and breast cancer risk (see Section 1.3.4). Hypotheses are made about the form of this relationship, the modifying effect of time and age at exposure, the latency time between exposure and risk, and transposition from high to low dose and low exposure rate.

The most recent models for such an exercise in the general population arise from the BEIR VII models of the United States National Academy of Sciences (National Research Council, 2006), with recommendations of the use of an excess absolute risk model for breast cancer risk (National Research Council, 2006; ICRP, 2007; Wrixon, 2008). This model assumes no threshold, even at a very low dose, and a decreasing effect with increasing age at exposure. Coefficients are estimated from atomic bomb survivors and women medically exposed to radiation (see Section 1.3.4). Because these studies are based on a higher dose and a higher dose rate than those typically involved in mammography screening, an effort was made by some authors to produce results taking into account transposition factors from high to low dose and dose rate (dose and dose rate effectiveness factor). Values of this factor in the context of mammography generally vary between 1 and 2 (National Research Council, 2006; Law et al., 2007; Heyes et al., 2009).

A hypothesis about the latency time for the induction of a breast cancer by radiation is also needed for risk assessment. A latency time of 10 years is generally used, with values varying from 5 years to 15 years.

(ii) Hypotheses about doses received during mammography

The estimation of doses received by the glandular tissue of the breast depends on breast thickness and density. Based on an extensive literature review, a historical reconstruction of doses received during mammography shows a strong decrease over time, with an estimated mean glandular dose to the breast of 2 mGy per view since 2000 (Thierry-Chef et al., 2012) (see Section 1, Fig. 1.16). Moreover, recent use of digital mammography (instead of screen-film mammography) has led to new estimates of doses received (Hendrick et al., 2010; Hauge et al., 2014).

(iii) Hypotheses about the target population and screening modalities

To fully develop the risk assessment, scenarios for the target population and screening modalities (age range, frequency, number of examinations at each screening, additional views, etc.) have been developed.

(b) Outcomes from risk assessment

Risk assessment studies provide estimated numbers of radiation-induced breast cancer cases and/or deaths, with a range of estimates according to variations in hypotheses. Estimation of prevented deaths based on assumptions about mortality reduction by screening modalities is performed in most studies, and calculation of benefit–risk is provided. Because the risk of radiation-induced cancer applies only to women who underwent mammography, hypotheses about mortality reduction should apply only to attendees; this is not always made explicit in publications. Thus, benefit–risk estimates provided by studies should be interpreted with caution.

(i) Risk assessment studies in the general population

Risk assessment studies performed in the early 2000s or earlier used risk models that are no longer recommended by international committees (Howe et al., 1981; Feig & Hendrick, 1997; Beemsterboer et al., 1998a; Mattsson et al., 2000; Law & Faulkner, 2001, 2002, 2006; León et al., 2001; Berrington de González & Reeves, 2005; Ramos et al., 2005). Since 2010, all studies have used the excess absolute risk model recommended by BEIR VII and contemporary estimates of mean glandular dose to the breast from either screen-film or digital mammography (Hendrick, 2010; O'Connor et al., 2010; de Gelder et al., 2011b; HPA, 2011; Yaffe & Mainprize, 2011; Hauge et al., 2014). These recent studies are now considered to be the most relevant and are summarized below (Table 5.13). In addition, one study used a biological model (Bijwaard et al., 2010, 2011).

(ii) Estimates for screening starting at about age 50 years

The Health Protection Agency estimated the number of cancer cases and cancer deaths after radiation exposure from a large number of sources, including screening mammography, in the United Kingdom population (HPA, 2011). The number of radiation-induced breast cancer cases after a single two-view screen every 3 years at age 47–73 years was estimated to be 28 per 100 000 women screened, and the number of breast cancer deaths under the same conditions was estimated to be 10 per 100 000 women screened. Assuming 500 prevented deaths from screenings, the authors estimated the net benefit (deaths prevented minus deaths induced) to be 490 [ratio of prevented to induced deaths of 50].

O'Connor et al. (2010) estimated the number of breast cancer cases induced by screen-film mammography, digital mammography, and other imaging techniques in a United States setting. They estimated that 21 cancer cases would be induced by digital mammography and 27 by screen-film mammography for annual screening per 100 000 women screened at age 50–80 years, and that there would be 6 or 7 induced deaths. Using different mortality reduction hypotheses, they estimated ratios of prevented to induced deaths of 116 and 135 for screen-film and digital mammography, respectively.

In Norway, Hauge et al. (2014) estimated the number of radiation-induced breast cancer cases after a single two-view digital mammography screening every 2 years from age 50 years to age 69 years to be 10 (range, 1.4–36) per 100 000 women screened, and the number of induced deaths per 100 000 women screened to be 1 (range, 0.1–3). Assuming a 40% mortality reduction among attendees, the authors estimated that 350 lives would be saved compared with 3 or fewer deaths induced [ratio of prevented to induced deaths of at least 117].

In the Netherlands, calculations were performed for a biennial digital mammography screening between the ages of 50 years and 74 years [12 screening sessions] (de Gelder et al., 2011b). The authors estimated 7.7 radiation-induced breast cancer cases (range, 5.9–29.6) and 1.6 radiation-induced breast cancer deaths

Table 5.13 Risk assessment studies of breast cancer induced by mammography screening[a]

Reference Country	Mean glandular dose to the breast	Risk model	Target population, screening modalities	Lifetime calculation	Radiation-induced cases	Radiation-induced deaths	Benefit–risk: ratio of prevented to induced deaths
Hendrick (2010) USA	3.7 mGy for 2-view DM 4.7 mGy for two-view SFM	EAR model from BEIR VII Modifying effect of age	Annual screening for 40–80 yr	NA	NA	20 (DM) and 25 (SFM) deaths	NA
O'Connor et al. (2010) USA	3.9 mGy for 2-view DM 4.9 mGy for 2-view SFM: inclusion of extra views	EAR model from BEIR VII Modifying effect of age Latency, 5 yr DDREF, 1.5	Annual screening for 40–80 yr and for 50–80 yr	Until 80 yr	Screening 40–80 yr: 56 (DM) and 71 (SFM) cases Screening 50–80 yr: 21 (DM) and 27 (SFM) cases Screening 40–49 yr: 35 (DM) and 44 (SFM) cases	Screening 40–80 yr: 15 (DM) and 19 (SFM) deaths Screening 50–80 yr: 6 (DM) and 7 (SFM) deaths Screening 40–49 yr: 9 (DM) and 11 (SFM) deaths	Assuming a mortality reduction of 15% from screening before age 60 yr and 32% after age 60 yr, ratio of prevented to induced deaths: Screening 40–80 yr: 44 (SFM) and 56 (DM) Screening 50–80 yr: 116 (SFM) and 135 (DM) Screening 40–49 yr: 3 (SFM and DM)
de Gelder et al. (2011b) Netherlands	1.3 mGy per view (range, 1–5 mGy)	EAR model from BEIR VII Modifying effect of age No latency DDREF, 1.5	Screening for 40–74 yr or 50–74 yr Every 2 yr 2 views at first round 1 view at subsequent rounds	Until 100 yr	Screening 40–74 yr: 17.1 cases (range, 13.1–65.6) Screening 50–74 yr: 7.7 cases (range, 5.9–29.6)	Screening 40–74 yr: 3.7 deaths (range, 2.9–14.4) Screening 50–74 yr: 1.6 deaths (range, 1.3–6.3)	Assuming 26% mortality reduction, ratio of prevented to induced deaths: Screening 40–74 yr: 349 Screening 50–74 yr: 684 (range, 178–889)
HPA (2011) United Kingdom	4.5 mGy for 2-view screening	EAR model from Preston et al. (2007) (see Section 1.3.4) Modifying effect of age Latency, 10 yr	Screening for 40–73 yr Annually before 50 yr Every 3 yr after 50 yr	Until 85+ yr	Screening 40–47 yr: 61 cases Screening 47–73 yr: 28 cases	Screening 40–47 yr: 20 deaths Screening 47–73 yr: 10 deaths	Net benefit (deaths prevented minus deaths induced): 80 for age 40–47 yr; 490 for age 47–73 yr [ratio of prevented to induced deaths, 50]

Table 5.13 (continued)

Reference Country	Mean glandular dose to the breast	Risk model	Target population, screening modalities	Lifetime calculation	Radiation-induced cases	Radiation-induced deaths	Benefit–risk: ratio of prevented to induced deaths
Yaffe & Mainprize (2011) Canada	3.7 mGy for 2-view DM	EAR model from BEIR VII Modifying effect of age Latency, 10 yr	Annual screening for 40–55 yr Every 2 yr for 55–74 yr	Until 109 yr	Screening 40–49 yr: 59 cases Screening 40–74 yr: 86 cases	Screening 40–49 yr: 7.6 deaths Screening 40–74 yr: 11 deaths	Assuming 24% mortality reduction, ratio of prevented to induced deaths: Screening 40–49 yr: 11.4 Screening 40–74 yr: 46
Hauge et al. (2014) Norway	2.5 mGy for 2-view DM (range, 0.7–5.7 mGy)	EAR model from BEIR VII Modifying effect of age Latency, 5 or 10 yr DDREF, 1 or 2	Screening for 50–69 yr Every 2 yr	Until 85 or 105 yr	10 cases (range, 1.4–36)	1 death (range, 0.1–3.1)	Assuming 40% mortality reduction among attendees, 350 lives saved compared with 3 or fewer deaths induced [ratio of prevented to induced deaths, at least 117]

[a] Calculated values are per 100 000 women screened.

BEIR VII, Biologic Effects of Ionizing Radiation, Report VII (National Research Council, 2006); DDREF, dose and dose rate effectiveness factor; DM, digital mammography; EAR, excess absolute risk; NA, not available; SFM, screen-film mammography.

(range, 1.3–6.3) per 100 000 women screened, assuming a glandular dose of 1.3 mGy per view. Using a simulation model (MISCAN) to estimate deaths prevented due to screening, they estimated a ratio of prevented to induced deaths of 684. When a glandular dose of 5 mGy per view was assumed, the ratio decreased to 178 and the number of radiation-induced deaths increased to 6.3.

Bijwaard et al. (2010, 2011) performed a risk assessment using a mechanistic, biologically based model that assumes a two-stage mutation for carcinogenesis. With this approach, the authors estimated that for five mammography screenings of 2 mGy starting at age 50 years [biennial screening until age 60 years], 1.3 breast cancer cases would be induced per 100 000 women screened (Bijwaard et al., 2010), and 200 cases for 15 screenings of 4 mGy.

(iii) Estimates for screening starting at age 40 years

In the United Kingdom calculation (HPA, 2011), the number of radiation-induced breast cancer cases after annual two-view screening at ages 40–47 years was estimated to be 61 per 100 000 women screened. Using a hypothesis about survival, the authors estimated the number of radiation-induced breast cancer deaths after annual two-view screening at ages 40–47 years to be 20 per 100 000 women screened. Assuming 100 prevented deaths from screening, they estimated the net benefit (deaths prevented minus deaths induced) to be 80 [ratio of prevented to induced deaths of 5].

In the USA, Hendrick (2010) estimated the number of deaths induced by annual mammography per 100 000 women screened at age 40–80 years to be 20 for digital mammography and 25 for screen-film mammography. In the study of O'Connor et al. (2010), the authors estimated the number of breast cancers induced by annual mammography per 100 000 women screened at age 40–49 years to be 35 for digital mammography and 44 for screen-film mammography, and the number of radiation-induced breast cancer deaths to be 9 for digital mammography and 11 for screen-film mammography. According to a hypothesis about mortality reduction, they estimated a ratio of prevented to induced deaths of about 3 for both modalities.

In Canada, Yaffe & Mainprize (2011) estimated that mammography screening annually from age 40 years to age 55 years and biennially until age 74 years would induce 86 breast cancers cases (59 for the screening period 40–49 years) and 11 breast cancers deaths (7.6 for the screening period 40–49 years) per 100 000 women screened. Assuming a 24% reduction in mortality, they estimated a ratio of prevented to induced deaths of 46 for age 40–74 years (11.4 for age 40–49 years). The ratio of lives saved to lives lost is 78 for age 40–74 years (27 for age 40–49 years).

In the Netherlands, calculations were performed for biennial mammography screening between age 40 years and age 74 years; the authors estimated the number of breast cancer cases per 100 000 women screened to be 17.1 (range, 13.1–65.6) and the number of radiation-induced breast cancer deaths to be 3.7 (range, 2.9–14.4) (de Gelder et al., 2011a). Using a simulation model (MISCAN) to estimate deaths prevented due to screening, they estimated a ratio of prevented to induced deaths of 349. The study using a mechanistic model estimated 1.5 cases per 100 000 women screened for five mammography screenings of 2 mGy starting at age 40 years (Bijwaard et al., 2010).

(iv) Women at an increased risk

Among women at an increased risk of breast cancer, screening procedures are recommended earlier in life and at a higher frequency than in the general population (see Section 5.6). Due to the increased risk of radiation-induced breast cancer when exposure occurs at a younger age and because of the higher radiosensitivity of women with a familial predisposition (see Section 1.3.6), separate risk assessment must be performed for women at an increased risk.

An excess relative risk model was used to estimate the lifetime risk of radiation-induced breast cancer mortality from five annual mammography screenings in young women harbouring a *BRCA* mutation (Berrington de González et al., 2009). They estimated the lifetime risk of radiation-induced breast cancer mortality per 10 000 women screened annually to be 26 (95% CI, 14–49) for screening at age 25–29 years, 20 (95% CI, 11–39) for screening at age 30–34 years, and 13 (95% CI, 7–23) for screening at age 35–39 years. [This calculation was based on model risk and coefficients estimated from the general population, and the higher sensitivity to radiation of these women was not taken into account.] A large European study among carriers of *BRCA1/2* mutations suggested that exposure to diagnostic radiation before age 30 years for these women was associated with an increased risk of breast cancer at dose levels considerably lower than those at which increases had previously been found (Pijpe et al., 2012).

Benefit–risk estimates for women at an increased risk need to consider: the age-dependent higher risk of radiation in younger women and in women with specific gene mutations; their age-dependent overall measured breast cancer risk; and the contribution of mammography to early detection, which itself may depend on patient age, the type of genetic mutation (*BRCA1* vs *BRCA2*), and the availability of magnetic resonance imaging (MRI).

5.3.5 *Psychological consequences of mammography screening*

Participation in breast cancer screening can have psychological or psychosocial consequences for women. Section 3.1.4 summarizes the psychological impacts of an invitation to screening, of a negative result, of a diagnosis of breast cancer, and of interval cancer, as well as the impact of a false-positive result on further participation. This section presents the studies reviewed for the evaluation of the psychological consequences of a false-positive result and of DCIS.

Several reviews have focused on the long-term psychological implications of a false-positive result (Rimer & Bluman, 1997; Steggles et al., 1998; Brodersen et al., 2004; Brett et al., 2005; Brewer et al., 2007; Hafslund & Nortvedt, 2009; Salz et al., 2010; Bond et al., 2013a, b). The two reviews by Bond et al. (2013a, b) evaluate the same set of studies, so one has been excluded. The review by Rimer & Bluman (1997) has also been excluded, due to its lack of relevance. In this section, the outcomes of the informative reviews (Table 5.14) and results from more recent individual studies are presented.

(a) Outcomes from reviews

Negative outcomes were reported from studies using validated measures during the period between receiving a recall letter and the recall appointment (Sutton et al., 1995; Chen et al., 1996; Lowe et al., 1999; Lampic et al., 2001; Sandin et al., 2002), at the recall appointment (Ellman et al., 1989; Cockburn et al., 1992; Swanson et al., 1996; Lowe et al., 1999; Ekeberg et al., 2001; Meystre-Agustoni et al., 2001), or immediately after receiving a recall letter (Cockburn et al., 1994; Lidbrink et al., 1995; Olsson et al., 1999; Lindfors et al., 2001).

The main psychological consequences of a false-positive result were psychological distress, somatization, depression, fear, anxiety, worry, an increase in women's perceived likelihood of developing breast cancer, a decrease in the perceived benefits of mammography, and an increase in the frequency of breast self-examination (BSE) (Salz et al., 2010). [These outcomes may be contextualized as symptoms, but it is unclear how they would affect women in their everyday lives.]

Salz et al. (2010) performed a meta-analysis of the effect of false-positive mammograms on generic and specific psychosocial outcomes. From 17 studies presented in 21 articles, they found that across six generic outcomes, the only consistent effect was generalized anxiety (Ellman et al., 1989; Gram et al., 1990; Bull & Campbell, 1991; Lerman et al., 1991a, 1993; Cockburn et al., 1994; Ong et al., 1997; Scaf-Klomp et al., 1997; Brett et al., 1998; Pisano et al., 1998; Olsson et al., 1999; Aro et al., 2000; Lipkus et al., 2000; Brett & Austoker, 2001; Lampic et al., 2001, 2003; Meystre-Agustoni et al., 2001; Sandin et al., 2002; Barton et al., 2004; Jatoi et al., 2006; Tyndel et al., 2007).

(i) Short-term effects

All reviews concluded that there are short-term psychological consequences (up to 3 months) from having a recall. In one review (Brodersen et al., 2004), all 22 studies that investigated short-term consequences reported adverse short-term consequences. In a review based on 54 articles, Brett et al. (2005) concluded that the negative psychological impact was significantly higher for women who had a recall than for women who received a clear negative result after participation in mammography screening, although three studies reported no difference in the psychological impact of mammography screening between women who received a clear negative result and those who had a false-positive result (Bull & Campbell, 1991; Lightfoot et al., 1994; Aro et al., 2000). Other negative consequences reported in women who had a false-positive result were more intrusive thoughts, worry about breast cancer, greater requirements for social support, being more busy than usual to keep their thoughts away from the clinical visit, or difficulties sleeping (Bull & Campbell, 1991; Lightfoot et al., 1994; Scaf-Klomp et al., 1997; Gilbert et al., 1998; Aro et al., 2000). Two studies reported that 30% (Austoker & Ong, 1994) and 40% (Scaf-Klomp et al., 1997) of women felt very anxious when they received a recall letter. One study that looked at how having a false-positive result influences quality of life found a marked decrease in quality of life for recalled women (Lowe et al., 1999).

(ii) Long-term effects

Based on the available reviews, results about long-term consequences are more ambiguous and inconsistent (Brodersen et al., 2004; Brett et al., 2005; Brewer et al., 2007). Several studies did not find increases in long-term levels of anxiety among women who had a false-positive result (Gram et al., 1990; Cockburn et al., 1994; Lidbrink et al., 1995; Gilbert et al., 1998; Lowe et al., 1999; Ekeberg et al., 2001; Lampic et al., 2001; Sandin et al., 2002), and two studies were inconclusive (Scaf-Klomp et al., 1997; Aro et al., 2000). Other studies reported that the anxiety experienced was greater among women who had a false-positive result than among women who received a clear negative result, at 4–6 months after recall (Ellman et al., 1989; Brett et al., 1998; Olsson et al., 1999; Lampic et al., 2001), 6–12 months after recall (Lampic et al., 2001; Hislop et al., 2002), and 24 months after recall (Lipkus et al., 2000). One review found no long-term symptoms of depression among women who received a false-positive result (Brewer et al., 2007).

(iii) Breast cancer-specific measures

One review investigated the effects on health-care use and symptoms (Brewer et al., 2007). The findings suggested that having a false-positive result increases anxiety related to breast cancer-specific measures (Brewer et al., 2007). Three studies found that women who received a false-positive result reported conducting BSE statistically significantly more frequently (Bull & Campbell, 1991; Aro et al., 2000; Lampic et al., 2001). Women who had a false-positive result also reported higher levels of worry and increased concern about breast cancer (Lerman et al., 1991a, b; Scaf-Klomp et al., 1997; Brett et al., 1998; Aro et al., 2000; Lipkus et al., 2000; Sandin et al., 2002; Absetz et al., 2003). In their meta-analysis, Salz et al. (2010) found statistically significant effects on all eight breast cancer-specific outcomes: distress about breast cancer, somatization or symptoms in the breast, fear of developing breast cancer, anxiety about breast cancer, worry about breast cancer, perceived likelihood of breast cancer, perceived benefits of mammography, and frequency of BSE. The largest effect was for anxiety about breast cancer ($r = 0.22$) and the smallest was for fear ($r = 0.08$); all eight pooled effect sizes were statistically significant.

(iv) Screening factors

Screening factors associated with greater adverse psychological effects were: previous false-positive results (Brett & Austoker, 2001; Haas et al., 2001; Lampic et al., 2001), pain at previous mammography screening (Ong & Austoker, 1997; Drossaert et al., 2002), dissatisfaction with information and communication during screening (Austoker & Ong, 1994; Brett et al., 1998; Brett & Austoker, 2001; Dolan et al., 2001), and waiting time between recall letter and assessment appointment (Gram et al., 1990; Thorne et al., 1999; Brett & Austoker, 2001; Lindfors et al., 2001).

Elements of the structure of the screening programme were also found to be important. The extent of further investigation seemed to determine the extent of negative psychological outcomes. Women who underwent a surgical biopsy before receiving a clear result experienced the greatest anxiety (Ellman et al., 1989; Lerman et al., 1991b; Ong & Austoker, 1997; Brett et al., 1998; Lampic et al., 2001), as did those asked to come back for further tests after 6 months or 1 year (Ong et al., 1997; Brett et al., 1998; Brett & Austoker, 2001). On-site evaluation was shown to reduce the stress of having a false-positive result (Lindfors et al., 2001). Biopsy-specific events appeared to be more distressing than follow-up mammography, and distress risk factors included younger age, less education, and no family history of breast cancer (Steffens et al., 2011).

Reported sociodemographic factors often associated with greater adverse psychological outcomes were younger age, less education, living in an urban area, having one child or no children, and manual occupation (Brett et al., 2005). Other studies found no impact of age (Brett et al., 1998; Brett & Austoker, 2001; Lampic et al., 2001) or employment (Olsson et al., 1999). One study with 910 participants in California, USA, found that Asian ethnicity, annual income greater than US$ 10 000, and weekly attendance of religious services were significantly associated with decreased depressive symptoms (Alderete et al., 2006).

(b) Recent individual studies

More recent studies, not included in the reviews, have used the Hospital Anxiety and Depression Scale, the Psychological Consequences Questionnaire, and the Consequences of Screening in Breast Cancer questionnaire to study psychological consequences of mammography screening (Table 5.14). Consistent with findings from a study conducted in 1996–1997 (Ekeberg et al., 2001), Schou Bredal et al. (2013) found that recall after mammography among women with a false-positive result was associated with transiently increased anxiety and a slight increase in depression. At 4 weeks after screening, the level of anxiety was the same and depression was lower compared with the general female Norwegian population (Schou Bredal et al., 2013).

In a study in Spain, participants were found to worry little until they underwent mammography, but levels of worry increased when the women were notified by telephone call of the need for further testing (Espasa et al., 2012). A substantial proportion of women requiring further assessment reported that they were at least somewhat worried about having breast cancer throughout the screening process, but

Table 5.14 Measures used in 70 studies of psychological consequences of a false-positive result of mammography screening

Questionnaire used	Reference for method	No. of studies in which scale was used
Psychological Consequences Questionnaire	Cockburn et al. (1992)	13
Hospital Anxiety and Depression Scale	Zigmond & Snaith (1983)	7
General Health Questionnaire	Goldberg (1978)	4
State Trait Anxiety Inventory	Spielberger et al. (1970)	5
Hopkins Symptom Checklist	Rickels et al. (1976)	3
Other scales (Beck Depression Inventory, K6)	Beck et al. (1961), Derogatis et al. (1983), Brewer et al. (2004)	40

Compiled by the Working Group, based on the reviews by Steggles et al. (1998), Brodersen et al. (2004), Brett et al. (2005), Brewer et al. (2007), Hafslund & Nortvedt (2009), Salz et al. (2010), and Bond et al. (2013b).

levels of anxiety and depression, measured by the Hospital Anxiety and Depression Scale, showed no statistically significant differences among women who had invasive complementary tests, non-invasive tests, and negative screening results (Espasa et al., 2012).

In a longitudinal study in Denmark, psychological effects of false-positive results were assessed with the Consequences of Screening in Breast Cancer questionnaire. At 6 months after the final diagnosis, women with a false-positive finding reported changes in existential values and inner calmness as great as those reported by women with a diagnosis of breast cancer; 3 years after the final diagnosis, women who had a false-positive result consistently reported greater negative psychosocial consequences in all 12 psychosocial outcomes compared with women who had a normal finding (Brodersen & Siersma, 2013). However, after 5 years, there was no statistically significant difference between the two groups in reported psychosocial aspects (Osterø et al., 2014).

When women who were first-time participants in mammography screening were compared with women with repeated screening experience, women in both groups reported experiencing high levels of anxiety before the diagnosis was known, and no differences were found in anxiety, depressive symptoms, or quality of life (Keyzer-Dekker et al., 2012).

In a study in 98 women, women reported a significant increase in anxiety after being notified of the need to return for follow-up testing, and significant positive associations were found between anxiety and behavioural approach, behavioural avoidance, cognitive approach, and cognitive avoidance coping in cross-sectional analyses (Heckman et al., 2004). Moreover, cognitive avoidance coping was a strong predictor of final levels of state anxiety in these women (Heckman et al., 2004).

These findings are consistent with qualitative studies in Scandinavia and North America. Norwegian women expressed mixed emotions over being recalled; information about recall rates and breast cancer risk was seen as alarming, and the short time between recall and examination was seen as reassuring but was also perceived as an indication of malignancy (Solbjør et al., 2011). Swedish women who were recalled described the recall process as "a roller coaster of emotions" (Bolejko et al., 2013). Qualitative studies from North America have described the psychological effects of the waiting process experienced by women, their unmet informational and psychosocial needs (Doré et al., 2013), anxieties generated by waiting and wondering, and fears of iatrogenic effects of follow-up tests such as biopsies and repeat mammograms (Padgett et al., 2001).

(c) Diagnosis of ductal carcinoma in situ

Psychological consequences of DCIS are included in this section because increasing participation in mammography screening means an increasing number of DCIS detections among women, but the effect of DCIS on psychological issues has been little explored. Women may not be aware of having DCIS, because surgeons might differ in how they inform women about this condition. Potentially, some women with DCIS are informed that they have breast cancer while others are informed that they do not have breast cancer. A study with semi-structured interviews of women previously diagnosed with and treated for DCIS identified six key themes: (i) invisibility of DCIS, (ii) uncertainty, (iii) perceptions of DCIS, (iv) acceptance of treatment, (v) social support, and (vi) moving on, which highlight the substantial challenges faced by women diagnosed with DCIS (Kennedy et al., 2008).

No articles focused on non-invasive breast cancer or DCIS before 1997 (Webb & Koch, 1997). A review of quality-of-life issues among patients with DCIS (Ganz, 2010) found that women with DCIS experience psychological consequences to a lesser extent than women with breast cancer, but few studies have compared these women with healthy women. Of greater concern, women with DCIS demonstrate severe misconceptions about their risk of invasive breast cancer (Ganz, 2010).

One study of 10 women with DCIS found that they would have liked to have received more information about DCIS when they were invited to routine screening (Prinjha et al., 2006). In another study, 45 women took part in an initial interview after a diagnosis of DCIS, and 27 took part in a follow-up interview 9–13 months later (Kennedy et al., 2012). Women's early perceptions of DCIS merged with and sometimes conflicted with their beliefs about breast cancer, and their perceptions and experiences of the condition shifted over time.

A study in Australia also found misunderstanding and confusion among women diagnosed with DCIS and a desire for more information about their breast disease (De Morgan et al., 2011). Approximately half of the participants worried about their breast disease metastasizing, approximately half expressed high decisional conflict, 12% were anxious, and 2% were depressed. Logistic regression analysis demonstrated that worry about dying from the breast disease was significantly associated with not knowing that DCIS could not metastasize (De Morgan et al., 2011). In five focus group interviews involving 26 women diagnosed with DCIS, women were confused about whether or not they had cancer that could result in death, and this confusion was compounded by the use of the term "carcinoma" and by the recommendation of treatments such as mastectomy (De Morgan et al., 2002).

In a study of 487 women who were newly diagnosed with DCIS, financial status was inversely associated with anxiety and depression at the 9-month follow-up, and women with medium or low socioeconomic status were vulnerable to escalating anxiety and depression after a DCIS diagnosis (de Moor et al., 2010). A study in the USA of approximately 800 Latina and Euro-American women with DCIS found that younger age, not having a partner, and lower income were related to lower quality of life in various domains (Bloom et al., 2013).

5.4 Cost–effectiveness and balance of harms and benefits

Decisions about implementation of health-care interventions are based primarily on benefits and a favourable harm–benefit ratio, but – to use limited resources efficiently – are also often based on cost–effectiveness analyses. A cost–effectiveness analysis compares different policies, including the current one, with no intervention (average cost–effectiveness) or compares a more-intensive programme with a less-intensive one (incremental cost–effectiveness). Often, the incremental cost–effectiveness ratio (ICER) is estimated for each policy, expressed as the ratio of the change in costs to the change in effects compared with a less-intensive alternative or the current policy. In a cost–effectiveness analysis, future costs and effects are taken into account and both are discounted at a chosen annual discount rate, to account for time preference. A new strategy is considered cost-effective if it results in an additional effect (compared with a baseline) at acceptable additional costs (or even savings). One should stress the fact that the change in effects is as important as, and in the practice of policy-making even more important than, the change in costs: how much will the population benefit from the resources invested? Effects are often defined as disease-specific deaths prevented and life years gained but are ideally adjusted for quality of life, resulting in quality-adjusted life years (QALYs) (Weinstein & Stason, 1977). For breast cancer screening, factors that could negatively affect quality of life are, among others, the screening examination, false-positive referrals, earlier and often more intensive treatment, overdiagnosis, and simply the earlier knowledge of cancer (Korfage et al., 2006). All such harms are included when adjusting the life years gained for negative quality-of-life effects. Positive side-effects, such as a reduced need for expensive palliative treatments because fewer women are dying of breast cancer, can and should also be incorporated into such cost–effectiveness analyses.

To determine whether an intervention produces reasonable amounts of benefits and limited harms for the resources invested, the cost–effectiveness ratios are usually compared with cost–effectiveness thresholds. A frequently used cost–effectiveness threshold is £30 000 per QALY gained (NICE, 2014). In the USA, interventions below the threshold of US$ 50 000 per QALY are generally considered cost-effective, interventions between US$ 50 000 per QALY and US$ 100 000 per QALY are considered moderately or borderline cost-effective, and those that exceed US$ 100 000 per QALY are generally not considered cost-effective (Grosse, 2008). It has recently been recommended that a threshold of US$ 200 000 per QALY should be used for the USA (Neumann et al., 2014). The relatively high threshold of US$ 200 000 per QALY relates to the fact that health-care costs in the USA are generally considerably higher than those in Europe. Looking more globally, the World Health Organization (WHO) has suggested a cost–effectiveness threshold of 3 times the national gross domestic product per capita (WHO, 2014). Practically, for low-income regions the maximal values for being cost-effective are about US$ 5000 (WHO, 2001). [A clear distinction has to be made for cost-efficacy estimates of trials, which often relate to the limited time frame of an RCT, in which not all benefits have accrued yet but where it is likely that cost and harms have already been prominent.]

Costs that should be considered in a cost–effectiveness analysis of breast cancer screening are costs associated with the organization of the programme (e.g. cost of invitations, screening costs), costs related to the diagnostic workup of both true-positives and false-positives, and additional treatment costs (e.g. due to more and earlier treatments). A few years after implementation, screening will lead to cost savings in treatment due to a decrease in the number of cases of advanced disease needing treatment (de Koning et al., 1992). The cost savings depend mostly on the cost for advanced disease and the magnitude of the effectiveness of the screening programme. In a full cost–effectiveness analysis, direct medical costs, direct non-medical costs (travel and time), and indirect costs (e.g. due to sick leave) must be considered.

Ideally, all possible screening policies that are relevant are compared in a cost–effectiveness analysis. However, it is not feasible to compare all scenarios of interest in an RCT or an observational study. In addition, trials deliver (at best) costs per case detected. This is not an appropriate measure for cost–effectiveness because it lacks information about the effectiveness of screening (in terms of life years gained or breast cancer deaths averted). Furthermore, the aim of a cost–effectiveness analysis on breast cancer screening is to assess the effectiveness of a screening programme in an actual population rather than in a controlled setting. By the use of mathematical models, findings from RCTs and observational studies can be extrapolated to simulated populations (Berry et al., 2005). Models are especially suitable for a cost–effectiveness analysis because the key elements of screening, including the screening strategy (starting age, stopping age, and screening interval), the target population (e.g. at average or increased risk), and the time point of the analysis, can be altered and/or compared. Furthermore, long-term lifetime effects can be predicted, and life years gained or QALYs can be calculated (Groenewoud et al., 2007) (see Section 5.1.2f for further details).

5.4.1 Mammography screening programmes in developed countries

Under the assumption that mammography screening programmes are effective in reducing breast cancer mortality in women at average risk of breast cancer, numerous cost–effectiveness analyses have shown that organized mammography screening can be cost-effective (van Ineveld et al., 1993; Leivo et al., 1999; Stout et al., 2006; Groenewoud et al., 2007; Carles et al., 2011; Pataky et al., 2014).

Most population-based screening programmes screen women at biennial intervals (Giordano et al., 2012). Annual screening strategies may improve the detection of rapidly growing tumours. However, despite the greater effectiveness, screening strategies that consist of annual screening are often found to be less efficient and less cost-effective, due to a disproportionate increase in costs or due to diminishing returns; about 80% of the effect of annual screening is retained when screening is performed every 2 years (Mandelblatt et al., 2009; Stout et al., 2014). Schousboe et al. (2011) demonstrated that, in the United States setting, even if annual mammography is restricted to certain risk groups, based on age or breast density, the costs exceed US$ 100 000 per QALY gained. In contrast, Carles et al. (2011) reported several cost-effective annual screening strategies in Spain. However, ICERs increased markedly when comparing annual screening with biennial screening, as reported in other studies.

Organized mammography screening has been shown to be more cost-effective than opportunistic mammography screening (Bulliard et al., 2009; de Gelder et al., 2009). In Switzerland, the costs per life year gained of opportunistic screening were twice those of organized screening (de Gelder et al., 2009). This difference was caused predominantly by the higher costs of mammography for opportunistic screening and the more frequent use of additional imaging in combination with opportunistic screening.

Cost–effectiveness ratios obtained from studies of screening programmes in different countries are not easily comparable, due to differences in assumptions about effects and costs, time horizon, discount rate, and calculation methods (Brown & Fintor, 1993; de Koning, 2000). Furthermore, epidemiological factors (background risk of breast cancer), the performance of the screening test, and the organization of the national screening programme and the health-care system all influence cost–effectiveness. The cost–effectiveness of a screening programme also depends on its characteristics, including attendance rate, screening interval, and age group targeted for screening.

5.4.2 Screening in low- and middle-income countries

A detailed cost–effectiveness analysis on breast cancer screening in India has been reported, in which the natural history of breast cancer was calibrated against available data on breast cancer incidence, stage distribution, and mortality in India (Okonkwo et al., 2008). The model was used to estimate the costs of breast cancer screening in India, its effects on mortality, and its cost–effectiveness (i.e. costs of screening per life year gained or per life saved). Screening using CBE or mammography among different age groups and at various frequencies was analysed. Stage-dependent sensitivities of CBE in this study were based on data from the Canadian National Breast Screening Study (CNBSS) (Rijnsburger et al., 2004). Alternative (lower) estimates of stage-dependent sensitivities of CBE were based on data from 752 000 CBEs delivered to low-income women in the USA in 1995–1998 through the National Breast and Cervical Cancer Early Detection Program of the United States Centers for Disease Control and Prevention (Bobo et al., 2000).

Okonkwo et al. (2008) expressed costs in international dollars (Int.$), the currency used by WHO; an international dollar has the same purchasing power in a particular country as a United States dollar has in the USA. Under the assumption that such screening programmes are as effective as is seen in mammography trials, the estimated mortality reduction was the greatest for programmes targeting women between age 40 years and age 60 years. Using a 3% discount rate, a single CBE at age 50 years had an estimated cost–effectiveness ratio of Int.$ 793 per life year gained and resulted in a reduction in breast cancer mortality of 2%. The cost–effectiveness ratio increased to Int.$ 1135 per life year gained for every 5-yearly CBE (age 40–60 years) and to Int.$ 1341 for biennial CBE (age 40–60 years); the corresponding reductions in breast cancer mortality were 8.2% and 16.3%, respectively. CBE performed annually from age 40 years to age 60 years was predicted to be nearly as efficacious as biennial mammography screening for reducing breast cancer mortality, while incurring only half the net costs.

The main factors affecting cost–effectiveness were breast cancer incidence, stage distribution, and cost savings on palliative care averted (Okonkwo et al., 2008). The estimated cost–effectiveness of CBE screening for breast cancer in India compares favourably with that of mammography in developed countries. [The study relied on an assumption about the efficacy of CBE in reducing breast cancer mortality in India, which has not been verified in randomized trials comparing CBE with no screening but was based on the CNBSS 2 trial, assuming that the effect of stage shift from mammography trials can be extrapolated.]

More recently, several studies have investigated the expected cost–effectiveness of different strategies in Costa Rica and Mexico (Niëns et al., 2014), Ghana (Zelle et al., 2012), and Peru (Zelle et al., 2013). In Costa Rica, the current strategy of treating breast cancer at stages I to IV at a geographical coverage level of 80% seems to be the most cost-effective, with an ICER of US$ 4739 per disability-adjusted life year (DALY) averted. At a coverage level of 95%, biennial CBE screening could double life years gained and can still be considered very cost-effective (ICER, US$ 5964 per DALY averted). For Mexico, the results indicate that at a coverage level of 95%, a mass media awareness-raising programme could be the most cost-effective (ICER, US$ 5021 per DALY averted). If more resources are available in Mexico, biennial mammography screening for women aged 50–70 years (ICER, US$ 12 718 per DALY averted), adding trastuzumab (ICER, US$ 13 994 per DALY averted), or screening women aged 40–70 years biennially plus trastuzumab (ICER, US$ 17 115 per DALY averted) are less cost-effective options (Niëns et al., 2014).

Breast cancer in Ghana is characterized by low awareness, late-stage treatment, and poor survival. Biennial screening with CBE of women aged 40–69 years, in combination with treatment of all stages, seems the most cost-effective intervention (ICER, US$ 1299 per DALY averted). Mass media awareness-raising is the second-best option (ICER, US$ 1364 per DALY averted) (Zelle et al., 2013). The current breast cancer programme in Peru (US$ 8426 per DALY averted) could be improved by implementing 3-yearly or biennial screening strategies. These strategies seem the most cost-effective in Peru, particularly when mobile mammography is applied (from US$ 4125 per DALY averted) or when CBE screening and mammography screening are combined (from US$ 4239 per DALY averted).

The impact of the various screening interventions on stage distribution was estimated on the basis of a model using proportional detection rates (Duffy & Gabe, 2005). The authors applied a stage shift from developing countries to the Dutch screening programme and corrected this shift for locally relevant attendance rates and the epidemiology and demography. The age-specific sensitivity of tests and the sojourn times (CBE sojourn times are two thirds those of mammography) were based on the literature (Duffy & Gabe, 2005; NETB, 2014). The effectiveness of the awareness-raising interventions is based on a study in Malaysia (Devi et al., 2007), where a 2-fold reduction in advanced breast cancer was observed when a mass media campaign was applied. However, evidence on the effectiveness of awareness-raising, CBE, and mammography screening is absent in many countries. Also, these programmes require substantial organizational, budgetary, and human resources, and the accessibility of diagnostic, referral, treatment, and palliative care facilities for breast cancer should simultaneously be improved.

5.4.3 Harm–benefit ratio and generalizability

As already pointed out, the expected effects – both benefits and harms – and the cost of an intervention are context-specific. In public health, medicine, and any other field, inferences and extrapolations to other populations and individuals are needed. The average estimates for relative benefits, observed in IBM, nested case–control cohort, and case–control studies, in which biases have been minimized as much as possible, need to be extrapolated, as well as the estimates for overdiagnosis, false-positives, and radiation risk. To incorporate all of these and to estimate values as specifically as possible for different populations with different age structures, life expectancies, incidence, mortality, and treatment levels, statistical models are used.

The harm–benefit ratio has been calculated for different settings. The Independent United Kingdom Panel estimated that the United Kingdom screening programmes currently prevent 1300 deaths from breast cancer per year, equivalent to about 22 000 years of life being saved. Per 10 000 women invited to screening, it is estimated that 43 deaths from breast cancer are prevented and 129 cases of breast cancer represent overdiagnosis (Marmot et al., 2013). The Euroscreen Working Group estimated that for every 10 000 women screened biennially from age 50 or 51 years until age 68 or 69 years, about 80 deaths from breast cancer are prevented, versus about 40 cases overdiagnosed (Paci & EUROSCREEN Working Group, 2012). In the Netherlands, it has been estimated that each year 775 breast cancer deaths are prevented, versus 300 overdiagnosed cases (1 million invitations per year) (NETB, 2014).

5.4.4 Lower age limit for screening

Women younger than 50 years may benefit less from mammography screening, due to a lower breast cancer incidence, a lower sensitivity of mammography due to denser breast tissue, a lower PPV, higher false-positive rates, and possibly more aggressive tumour growth (Carney et al., 2003; Buist et al., 2004). Therefore, the cost–effectiveness ratio is less favourable for younger women than for older women. For instance, a recent analysis showed that for Canada the most cost-effective strategies were biennial screening from age 50 years to age 69 years (ICER, US$ 28 921 per QALY), followed by biennial screening from age 40 years to age 69 years (ICER, US$ 86 029 per QALY) (Pataky et al., 2014).

In addition, the efficacy or effectiveness of screening, in terms of breast cancer mortality reduction, in women screened from age 40 years (Alexander et al., 1999; Smith et al., 2004; Moss et al., 2006; Hellquist et al., 2011) is less precisely estimated, due to small numbers of breast cancer deaths, than that in women screened from age 50 years, and may therefore be underestimated or overestimated in cost–effectiveness analyses. It could even be more cost-effective to screen women aged 50–69 years more frequently than to include women younger than 50 years (de Koning et al., 1991).

A study in which the Dutch MISCAN model was used to assess the cost–effectiveness of different policies for breast cancer screening in Catalonia, Spain (using Dutch data on costs) demonstrated that it is comparably cost-effective to extend screening from age 50 years to age 45 years and to extend screening from age 64 years to age 69 years (Beemsterboer et al., 1998b). The researchers emphasized that extending the upper age limit would result in a greater reduction in breast cancer mortality, whereas extending screening to younger women could lead to more life years gained. A more recently performed cost–effectiveness analysis, also focusing on screening in Catalonia, showed that biennial screening from age 45 years (to age 69 years or 74 years), annual screening from age 40 years (to age 69 years or 74 years), and annual screening from age 45 years (to age 69 years) (ranked in order of effectiveness) are all cost-effective strategies, with incremental costs per QALY gained of less than €30 000 (Carles et al., 2011).

A study based on data from the USA demonstrated that biennial mammography screening from age 40 years to age 49 years is cost-effective only for women with BI-RADS 3 or 4 breast density, women with both a previous breast biopsy and a family history of breast cancer, and women with BI-RADS 3 or 4 breast density and either a previous breast biopsy or a family history of breast cancer, assuming a cost–effectiveness threshold of US$ 100 000 per QALY gained (Schousboe et al., 2011). In contrast, another study, using five independent models of digital mammography screening in the USA, found that extending biennial screening from women aged 50–74 years to those aged 40–49 years would lead to incremental costs of US$ 55 100 per QALY gained, which was considered to be cost-effective (Stout et al., 2014). Annual mammography, which may improve detection of rapidly growing tumours that may be more common among younger women, was considered not cost-effective in both studies. As mentioned previously, age considerations may be different for developing countries.

5.4.5 Upper age limit for screening

Breast cancer incidence and breast cancer detection rates are higher in women aged 70 years and older, which may increase the effect of screening. However, compared with younger women, older women are more subject to numerous illnesses and conditions that negatively affect life expectancy, thereby limiting the beneficial effect of screening on life expectancy and potentially increasing costs of screening. Furthermore, attendance rates may be lower among older women, which would also negatively affect the cost–effectiveness ratio.

Women older than 74 years were not included in any breast cancer screening trial (see Section 4.2). Model simulations demonstrated that screening women aged 50–75 years and screening women with high bone mineral density up to age 79 years are both cost-effective strategies (Boer et al., 1995; Kerlikowske et al., 1999). Correspondingly, two systematic reviews showed that ceasing screening at age 75 years or 79 years instead of at age 65 years or 69 years is cost-effective, even for women who are not screened regularly before age 65 years (Barratt et al., 2002; Mandelblatt et al., 2003).

5.4.6 Digital mammography

In several countries, digital mammography has practically replaced film mammography (NHS, 2005; NETB, 2014). The sensitivity of digital mammography may be higher than that of film mammography for women younger than 50 years and for women with dense breasts (Pisano et al., 2008). However, the specificity of digital mammography may be slightly lower than that of film mammography (Skaane, 2009; Kerlikowske et al., 2011). Referral rates are likely to increase with digital mammography, depending on the baseline situation of referrals, but this is especially pertinent in the implementation phase. Because of the differences in test characteristics and in costs of mammography, cost–effectiveness ratios are likely to differ as well. A modelling study that used data from the DMIST trial found that, compared with film mammography, digital mammography is not cost-effective (US$ 331 000 per QALY gained), except when limited to women aged 40–49 years (Tosteson et al., 2008). However, digital mammography targeted to younger ages combined with film mammography from age 50 years is usually not a feasible strategy because film mammography has practically been replaced by digital mammography. Another study showed that digital mammography increases the number of false-positive findings by 220 per 1000 women compared with film mammography, leading to additional costs of US$ 350 000 per 1000 women, whereas the gain in benefits relative to film mammography is small (Stout et al., 2014).

5.4.7 Impact of individual risk factors

In most countries, organized mammography screening applies to all women in a targeted age group (usually 50–69 years or 50–74 years) with a relatively low (average) risk of breast cancer. Because breast cancer risk is associated with risk factors including age, reproductive history, a previous breast biopsy, and a family history of breast cancer (see Section 1.3), costs and benefits of screening may be affected by a woman's individual risk of breast cancer. More personalized mammography screening, by selecting the starting and stopping ages and the screening interval based on a woman's breast cancer risk profile, is therefore being considered in several research projects.

A cost–effectiveness study based on data from women in the USA showed that biennial mammography from age 40 years is cost-effective for women with high breast density (BI-RADS 3 or 4) and either a family history of breast cancer or a previous breast biopsy (< US$ 50 000 per QALY gained), and moderately cost-effective for women with high breast density only or both a previous breast biopsy and a family history of breast cancer (< US$ 100 000 per QALY gained) (Schousboe et al., 2011). Annual mammography was estimated to cost more than US$ 100 000 per QALY gained for any group at an increased risk, and was therefore not considered cost-effective.

Another study based on population data from the USA, using five independent models, showed that annual digital mammography screening for women aged 40–74 years with high breast density (BI-RADS 3 or 4) resulted in 3-fold higher incremental costs per additional QALY gained relative to biennial screening for all women aged 40–74 years (Stout et al., 2014). The incremental benefits of annually screening women aged 40–49 years with (extremely) dense breasts were small, predominantly accounting for the increase in ICERs.

Women with heterogeneously or extremely dense breasts and a negative screening mammogram may be considered for supplemental screening. The most readily available supplemental screening modality is ultrasonography, but little is known about its effectiveness when performed after negative screening mammography (see Section 5.5.1a). Sprague et al. (2015) used three independent simulation models to assess the lifetime benefits, harms, and cost–effectiveness from the payer perspective of supplemental ultrasonography screening for women with dense breasts compared with screening with digital mammography alone. They found that supplemental ultrasonography screening for women with dense breasts undergoing routine digital mammography screening would substantially increase costs while producing relatively small benefits in breast cancer deaths averted and QALYs gained. The cost–effectiveness ratio was US$ 325 000 per QALY gained (range, US$ 112 000–766 000). Restricting supplemental ultrasonography screening to women with extremely dense breasts would cost US$ 246 000 per QALY gained (range, US$ 74 000–535 000) relative to biennial mammography alone for women aged 50–74 years.

5.4.8 Quality of life

A Dutch analysis of cost–effectiveness and quality of life conducted in 1991 included estimates on 15 phases induced and/or prevented by the screening programme (de Koning et al., 1991). It appeared that 85% of the decrements in quality of life due to screening were due to the additional years in follow-up after diagnosis (of which about half were due to earlier detection and about half due to life years gained). False-positives comprised only a small component, as did the initial years of overdiagnosed cases. However, about 66% of the decrements were counterbalanced by gains; 70% of these gains imply reductions in palliative treatments for women with advanced disease. It was estimated that correcting the life years gained for quality of life would imply a 3% difference, that is, 3% fewer life years gained when adjusted for quality of life. The most unfavourable sensitivity analysis estimated a 19.7% decrease.

Vilaprinyo et al. (2014) estimated QALYs for the different breast cancer disease states. They used the health-related quality of life measures obtained from the EuroQol EQ-5D self-classifier in the study of Lidgren et al. (2007), which provided health-related quality of life measures for the first year after primary breast cancer (EQ-5D = 0.696), the second and following years after primary breast cancer or recurrence (EQ-5D = 0.779), and the metastatic breast cancer state (EQ-5D = 0.685). For false-positive mammograms, the authors assumed an average annualized loss of quality of life of 0.013. To obtain the value of 0.013, they assumed that 50% of women with a false-positive result would experience anxiety sufficient to increase the mood subscale of the EuroQol instrument from 0 to 1, lasting a total of 2 months. According to the United States EQ-5D tariffs, such a change for an entire year represents a decrease in the QALY value of 0.156. In the sensitivity analysis, the authors assessed the impact of changing the disutility by false-positives to 0 and to 0.026.

5.5 Other imaging techniques

This section reports evidence on the efficacy or effectiveness of imaging modalities other than screen-film mammography or standard digital mammography, where applied for population screening of asymptomatic women of about average (population) risk. Studies that included women at above average risk were considered, but not those in which study subjects were restricted to classifications of increased risk. Studies of cohorts of women defined by dense breast tissue on mammography (but not restricted to women at an increased risk) were also reviewed.

The following imaging technologies were reviewed: breast ultrasonography, digital breast tomosynthesis, MRI (other than screening of women at increased risk), electrical impedance technology for breast imaging, scintimammography, and positron emission mammography. No RCTs examining the efficacy of these imaging technologies for population breast screening were available to the Working Group.

For two imaging technologies (ultrasonography in dense breasts and digital breast tomosynthesis in population screening), there was evidence from non-randomized studies of incremental (additional) cancer detection when applied as adjunct screening to mammography. The evidence for the preventive effects, adverse effects, and cost–effectiveness of these two technologies is presented in Sections 5.5.1, 5.5.2, and 5.5.3, respectively. Other imaging technologies, for which there was very little or no data on efficacy or effectiveness, or for which population screening studies have not been conducted, are briefly outlined in Section 5.5.4.

5.5.1 Preventive effects

(a) Breast ultrasonography

Ultrasonography has had a role in diagnosis of breast disease for approximately 30 years and has been used for the workup of screen-detected abnormalities and for image-guided needle biopsy (see Section 2.2.1 for technical details). Because dense breast tissue is a risk factor for breast cancer (McCormack & dos Santos Silva, 2006) and reduces the sensitivity of mammography, and hence is associated with a greater likelihood of an interval cancer in mammography screening (Ciatto et al., 2004a), evaluations of breast ultrasonography screening have often focused on populations defined by mammographic density (Buchberger et al., 2000; Houssami et al., 2009; Corsetti et al., 2011; Houssami & Ciatto, 2011; Venturini et al., 2013).

No RCTs examining the efficacy of screening by ultrasonography or of adjunct ultrasonography in women with dense breast tissue on mammography (i.e. mammography alone vs mammography plus ultrasonography) were identified by the Working Group. A recent Cochrane systematic review (Gartlehner et al., 2013) evaluated the literature to assess the effectiveness of ultrasonography screening as adjunct to mammography in women *at average risk* of breast cancer. None of the studies identified (no randomized, prospective, or controlled studies) reported sound evidence supporting ultrasonography as adjunct to mammography in population breast screening. An RCT on the efficacy of adjunct ultrasonography for breast cancer screening, called the Japan Strategic Anti-Cancer Randomized Trial, was noted (Ishida et al., 2014). This trial aimed to recruit 100 000 women aged 40–49 years and has recently closed to recruitment; its results have not yet been reported.

Several studies of breast ultrasonography screening, all non-randomized and without a comparison or control group, have examined the *incremental* cancer detection of breast ultrasonography in women with *dense breast tissue and negative mammography*. Table 5.15 presents the studies that have reported data for both true-positive detection and false-positives (or additional recall) attributed to ultrasonography screening. Studies that recruited women with dense breast tissue conditional to also being classified as at an increased risk were not considered (e.g. Berg et al., 2008). However, studies that defined subjects on the basis of dense breast tissue but also included some women or subgroups with additional risk factors were included and reviewed.

The majority of the studies were retrospective, and all were designed to assess incremental

Table 5.15 Studies of adjunct ultrasonography in screening asymptomatic women with mammography-negative dense breast tissue

Reference Country	Study characteristics; no. screened with US[a]; age	Breast density[b]	Preventive or screening effect			Adverse effect	
			Additional detection: no. of *US-only* detected cancers (% of screens *or* subjects)	Characteristics of US-only detected cancers (vs cancers detected by M, where reported): by tumour stage or pathological tumour size; axillary node status[c]	Interval cancers	No. of false-positives attributed to adjunct US (% of screens *or* subjects)	
						Surgical biopsy	Additional testing
Buchberger et al. (2000) Austria	Non-randomized, retrospective, no comparison group n = 8103 asymptomatic women who had negative M and CBE (included some with PHBC) 35–78 yr (mean, 49 yr)	2–4	32 (0.39%)	Mean invasive cancer size, 9.1 mm (not significantly different from M-detected cancers) NR	NR	229 (2.8%) (includes CNB)	136 (1.7%): FNB or aspiration of complex lesions
Kaplan (2001) USA	Non-randomized, retrospective, no comparison group; most had negative M/CBE n = 1862 35–87 yr	3, 4	6 (0.32%)	All 6 cancers early stage: 1 in situ, 5 stage I all node-negative[c]	NR	51 (2.7%)	117 (6.3%): 45 needle biopsy, 72 imaging review/follow-up
Kolb et al. (2002) USA	Non-randomized, retrospective, no comparison group n = 12 193 screens (4897 women) who had negative M and CBE (included some with PHBC or FHBC) mean, 54.7 yr	2–4	33 cancers in 31 women (0.27%)	89% in situ or stage I cancers; mean size, 9.9 mm (stage and size not different from M-detected) 89% node-negative	NR	287 (2.4%)	5.3% had biopsy or follow-up imaging
Corsetti et al. (2008, 2011) Italy	Non-randomized, retrospective, no comparison group n = 9157 screens in self-referring women with negative M mean, 52 yr	3, 4	37 (0.40%)	Early-stage (in situ or small invasive) cancers: 64.8% vs 35.5%, $P = 0.001$ positive nodes: 13.5% vs 31.3%, $P = 0.047$	8 interval cancers from 7172 negative screens at 1 yr: 1.1/1000	83 (0.9%)	399 (4.4%) had FNB and/or CNB

Table 5.15 (continued)

Reference Country	Study characteristics; no. screened with US[a]; age	Breast density[b]	Preventive or screening effect			Adverse effect	
			Additional detection: no. of *US-only* detected cancers (% of screens *or* subjects)	Characteristics of US-only detected cancers (vs cancers detected by M, where reported): by tumour stage or pathological tumour size; axillary node status[c]	Interval cancers	No. of false-positives attributed to adjunct US (% of screens *or* subjects): Surgical biopsy	No. of false-positives attributed to adjunct US (% of screens *or* subjects): Additional testing
Kelly et al. (2010) USA	Non-randomized, retrospective *n* = 6425 screens in 4419 asymptomatic women (included some with PHBC or FHBC) ≥ 35 yr	3, 4 with or without additional risk factor	23 (0.52%) M detection: 3.6/1000 US detection: 7.2/1000	US detected more invasive cancers ≤ 10 mm (14 of 21) than mammography ($P < 0.01$) NR	11 interval cancers at 1 yr: 1.7/1000	NR	False-positives NR recall 7.2% for US vs 4.2% for M ($P < 0.01$); 9.6% for combined M + US
Hooley et al. (2012) USA	Non-randomized, retrospective, no comparison group *n* = 935 women with recent negative M who also had US (included some at intermediate or high risk) 29–89 yr (mean, 52 yr)	3, 4	[3 (0.32%)] reported as 3.2; 95% CI, 0.8–10/1000 screens	All 3 cancers < 10 mm (includes 1 DCIS) all node-negative	NR	NR	51 (5.5%) needle biopsy 187 (20%) short-interval follow-up
Weigert & Steenbergen, (2012) USA	Non-randomized, retrospective chart review from radiology services, no comparison group *n* = 8647 women with recent negative M who also had US screen age of cancer patients, 42–78 yr	3, 4 (> 50% of breast dense)	28 (0.32%) including 2 ADH and 1 LCIS; re-calculated as [25 (0.29%)]	Average size, 19 mm (for 17 invasive cancers) 1 node-positive	1 interval cancer at 6 mo	NR	429 (4.96%) recommended to have biopsy
Venturini et al. (2013) Italy	Non-randomized, prospective screening study tailored to breast density and (intermediate) risk: women with negative M and dense breasts *n* = 835 women 40–49 yr	3, 4	2 (0.24%)	Both cancers < 15 mm 1 node-positive	NR	10 (1.2%) (mostly needle biopsy)	False-positive invasive tests: 0.9% for US vs 0.1% for M Short-interval follow-up: 7.5% for US vs 0.3% for M

Table 5.15 (continued)

Reference Country	Study characteristics; no. screened with US[a]; age	Breast density[b]	Preventive or screening effect			Adverse effect	
			Additional detection: no. of *US-only* detected cancers (% of screens *or* subjects)	Characteristics of US-only detected cancers (vs cancers detected by M, where reported): by tumour stage or pathological tumour size; axillary node status[c]	Interval cancers	No. of false-positives attributed to adjunct US (% of screens *or* subjects)	
						Surgical biopsy	Additional testing
Brem et al. (2014) USA	Non-randomized, prospective screening study tailored to breast density (included some intermediate risk groups) *n* = 15 318 women ≥ 25 yr	3, 4	30 (0.19% of all screened women)	Similar mean cancer size for M-detected (13 mm) and US-detected (12.9 mm) US-only detected cancers were more frequently invasive than M-detected cancers ($P < 0.05$)	NR	3.6% increase in biopsy rate	Recall rate (not restricted to false-positive recalls): 15% for M vs 28.5% for M with adjunct US ($P < 0.001$)

[a] The study of Kelly et al. (2010) used *automated* whole-breast ultrasonography, and the study of Brem et al. (2014) used *3D automated* breast ultrasonography. All other studies used handheld ultrasonography.

[b] Based on BI-RADS (Breast Imaging Reporting and Data System; D'Orsi et al., 2013) density categories: 1, almost entirely fatty (< 25% fibroglandular); 2, scattered fibroglandular densities (25–50% fibroglandular); 3, heterogeneously dense (51–75% fibroglandular); 4, extremely dense (> 75% fibroglandular).

[c] Based on women who underwent axillary node surgery or dissection.

ADH, atypical ductal hyperplasia; CBE, clinical breast examination; CNB, core needle biopsy; DCIS, ductal carcinoma in situ; FHBC, family history of breast cancer; FNB, fine-needle biopsy; LCIS, lobular carcinoma in situ; M, mammography; mo, month or months; NR, not reported; PHBC, personal history of breast cancer; US, ultrasonography; yr, year or years.

Adapted from *Preventive Medicine*, Volume 53, issue 3, Houssami & Ciatto (2011). The evolving role of new imaging methods in breast screening, pages 123–126, Copyright (2011), with permission from Elsevier; and from Houssami et al. (2009). Breast cancer screening: emerging role of new imaging techniques as adjuncts to mammography. *The Medical Journal of Australia*, 2009; volume 190, issue 9, pages 493–498. © Copyright 2009 *The Medical Journal of Australia* – reproduced with permission.

cancer detection (as an indicator of potential effectiveness) within screened subjects; none of these studies were designed to assess screening benefit in terms of mortality reduction or using a surrogate for effectiveness of screening, such as a reduction in interval cancer rates. Incremental detection of breast cancer by ultrasonography was in the range of 0.19% to 0.52% of all screens. The highest estimate (Kelly et al., 2010) included women at an increased risk, including some women with a history of breast cancer, and reported a modest cancer detection rate for mammography. Therefore, the incremental detection of breast cancer by ultrasonography was substantial but heterogeneous, representing approximately 14% to 48% of the detected cancers (Corsetti et al., 2008; Venturini et al., 2013). [These data should be interpreted taking into account that several studies included, among women with dense breasts, subgroups of women at increased risk due to other risk factors (i.e. dense breasts plus other risk factors), and many studies included young women, and therefore the evidence may not be generalizable to population screening of women with dense breasts.] The two prospective studies reported the lowest incremental detection rates for ultrasonography, of 0.19% (Brem et al., 2014) and 0.24% (Venturini et al., 2013) of screens. Ultrasonography-only detected cancers were frequently early-stage cancers, generally at a comparable or earlier stage than cancers detected with mammography, although comparative data on cancer characteristics were not comprehensively reported.

Giuliano & Giuliano (2013) examined detection measures for automated breast ultrasonography screening in women with dense (density > 50%) breast tissue (test group) and used a different cohort of women with dense breasts from an earlier time frame as a control group for mammography screening. [This study is limited by the comparison of two cohorts with different underlying breast cancer prevalence (test group, 1.25%; control group, 0.60%).] For the test group (n = 3418; median age, 57 years) screened with mammography and ultrasonography, the screening sensitivity was 97.7%, the specificity was 99.7%, the cancer detection rate was 12.3 per 1000 screens, and the mean tumour size of detected cancers was 14.3 mm. For the control group (n = 4076; median age, 54 years) screened with digital mammography alone, the screening sensitivity was 76.0%, the specificity was 98.2%, the cancer detection rate was 4.6 per 1000 screens, and the mean tumour size of detected cancers was 21.3 mm. [This mean size is larger than expected for a screened population. The inferred 2.6-fold increase in the cancer detection rate, which represents one additional detection in approximately 0.70% of screens, was attributed to ultrasonography. This is well above estimates from all the other reviewed studies and is probably due to the comparison of cohorts with different underlying breast cancer risk. In addition, the relatively high specificity in the test group, based on the combined screening approach, is unusual and is inconsistent with all the other studies. Because of these limitations, this study was considered uninformative.]

One prospective screening study of ultrasonography in a multimodality setting (CBE, mammography, and ultrasonography) included 3028 Chinese women aged 25 years and older (Huang et al., 2012), not restricted to women with dense breasts. The sensitivity was higher for mammography (84.8%) than for ultrasonography (72.7%); however, ultrasonography detected 3 cancers not detected with mammography (all were in women with dense breasts). Ultrasonography yielded an incremental cancer detection rate of [0.99 per 1000] screens of *all* screening participants. Mammography-detected cancers were more frequently smaller than 20 mm and node-negative than those detected with ultrasonography or CBE.

Two non-randomized studies of adjunct ultrasonography for screening dense breasts reported data on interval cancers (Kelly et al.,

2010; Weigert & Steenbergen, 2012). [Given that these studies did not have a comparison estimate and had a relatively short follow-up period (12 months), it is difficult to interpret the estimated interval cancer rates.] Corsetti et al. (2008, 2011) reported indirect comparisons based on follow-up for first-year interval cancers in a cohort of self-referring women attending a breast service in Italy. The estimated first-year interval cancer rate was 1.1 per 1000 screens (from 7172 negative screens with follow-up) in women who underwent adjunct ultrasonography and had dense breasts, compared with 1.0 per 1000 screens (from 12 438 negative screens with follow-up) in women who received mammography only and did not have dense breasts.

(b) Digital breast tomosynthesis/ three-dimensional mammography

Digital breast tomosynthesis is a derivative of digital mammography that produces quasi three-dimensional images, which reduces the effect of tissue superimposition and can therefore improve mammography interpretation (see Section 2.1.4 for details). A recent systematic review (Houssami & Skaane, 2013) examined the available evidence on the accuracy of digital breast tomosynthesis. The studies identified were relatively small (n = 14), comprised mostly test-set observer (reader) studies or clinical series that included symptomatic and screen-recalled cases, and were generally enriched with breast cancer cases. Taking into consideration the limitations of the studies, the evidence can be summed up as follows (Houssami & Skaane, 2013): (i) two-view digital breast tomosynthesis has accuracy that is equal to or better than that of standard two-view mammography; (ii) one-view digital breast tomosynthesis does not have better accuracy than two-view mammography; (iii) the *addition* of digital breast tomosynthesis to digital mammography increases interpretive accuracy; (iv) improved accuracy from using digital breast tomosynthesis (relative to, or added to, digital mammography) was the result of increased cancer detection or reduced false-positive recalls, or both; and (v) *subjective* interpretation of cancer conspicuity consistently found that cancers were equally or more conspicuous on digital breast tomosynthesis relative to digital mammography.

A review of the literature did not identify any RCTs examining the efficacy of digital breast tomosynthesis in population breast screening; however, digital breast tomosynthesis was the only other imaging technology investigated in population-based screening programmes in women at average (population) risk (Ciatto et al., 2013; Haas et al., 2013; Rose et al., 2013; Skaane et al., 2013a, b, 2014; Friedewald et al., 2014; Houssami et al., 2014a; Table 5.16). All these studies investigated digital mammography with tomosynthesis (also referred to as integrated two-dimensional/three-dimensional [2D/3D] mammography), using various methodologies (different design and reading/recall protocols). None were designed with the aim of assessing screening benefit in terms of mortality reduction or using a surrogate for effectiveness of screening, such as a reduction in interval cancer rates. Also, none of the studies reported estimates of overdiagnosis. Two studies were prospective population-based trials embedded within organized screening programmes in Europe: the Screening with Tomosynthesis or Standard Mammography (STORM) trial in Italy (Ciatto et al., 2013) and the Oslo trial in Norway (Skaane et al., 2013a, b, 2014). Both studies used double reading according to European standards, but they used different recall protocols. Both studies performed digital mammography with tomosynthesis in all participants, and hence they reported paired data for screened women (within screening participant comparison).

The STORM trial (Ciatto et al., 2013; Houssami et al., 2014a) compared *sequential* screen-readings by the same readers for the same women: digital mammography alone and integrated 2D/3D mammography. The study reported

Table 5.16 Studies evaluating tomosynthesis for population breast cancer screening: three-dimensional mammography as adjunct to digital mammography

Reference [Study] Country	Study characteristics Design (no. of screens); screen-reading methods	Preventive or screening effect				Adverse effect	
		Cancer detection rates/1000 screens	Absolute effect of 3D M on cancer detection rate compared with 2D alone	Characteristics of cancers detected only with integrated 2D/3D M only	Interval cancers	False-positive recalls	Absolute effect of 3D M on FPR compared with 2D alone
Ciatto et al. (2013) [STORM trial] Italy	Prospective trial (n = 7292) in population-based programme, comparing 2D and integrated 2D/3D screening (paired data); sequential double reading, recall by either reader at either read	2D: 5.3 2D/3D: 8.1 $P < 0.001$	Increase of 2.7/1000	Similar stage (pT, node status) distributions; similar mean invasive cancer size: 2D-detected, 13.7 mm; 2D/3D, 13.5 mm	NR	Recall for 2D alone *or* 2D/3D: 5.5% Recall *conditional* to 2D/3D-positive: 3.5% (17% decrease in all FPR)	[Decrease of 2.0%[b]]
Houssami et al. (2014a) [STORM follow-up study] Italy	Extended analysis of STORM trial (n = 7292), comparing various screening strategies, includes follow-up for year 1 *interval cancers*	2D double reading: 5.3 2D/3D single reading: 7.5 $P < 0.001$ [other comparisons also reported]	Increase of 2.2/1000	See above	6 interval cancers at 1 yr = 0.82/1000 (95% CI, 0.30–1.79)	Various comparisons reported	[Decrease of 1.2%[b]]
Skaane et al. (2013a, b) [Oslo trial] Norway	Prospective trial (n = 12 631) in population-based programme, comparing 2D and 2D/3D screening (paired data); *randomized* readings to 4 study arms with various screen-reading strategies; data shown are for analyses of single reading or double reading of tomosynthesis	2D: 6.1 2D/3D: 8.0 27% increase $P = 0.001$ Double reading: 2D: 7.1 2D/3D: 9.4 $P < 0.001$	Increase of 1.9/1000	Cancers detected with 2D/3D only were mostly invasive and more frequently grade 2 or 3 (2 DCIS cases were detected with 2D/3D only)	3 interval cancers at 9-month follow-up	2D: 6.1% 2D/3D: 5.3% (15% decrease, $P < 0.001$) Double reading: 2D: 10.3% 2D/3D: 8.5% $P < 0.001$	Decrease of 0.8%[b] $P < 0.001$

Table 5.16 (continued)

Reference [Study] Country	Study characteristics Design (no. of screens); screen-reading methods	Preventive or screening effect				Adverse effect	
		Cancer detection rates/1000 screens	Absolute effect of 3D M on cancer detection rate compared with 2D alone	Characteristics of cancers detected only with integrated 2D/3D M only	Interval cancers	False-positive recalls	Absolute effect of 3D M on FPR compared with 2D alone
Skaane et al. (2014) [Oslo trial] Norway	See above Analysis of $2D_{syn}$/3D	2D/3D: 7.8 $2D_{syn}$/3D: 7.7 Not significantly different	Increase of 2.3/1000				Decrease of 1.8% in false-positive scores; increased *overall* recall rate by 0.8%
Rose et al. (2013) USA	Retrospective: before vs after (13 856 vs 9499) introduction of 3D as adjunct to 2D screening; single reading from readers from several radiology services	2D: 4.0 2D/3D: 5.4 $P = 0.18$ For invasive cancer: 2D: 2.8 2D/3D: 4.3 $P = 0.07$	Increase of 1.4/1000 Increase of 1.5/1000	Cancers detected with 2D/3D only comprised invasive cancer; DCIS rates, mean invasive tumour size, and node status similar for 2D and 2D/3D; more grade 2 cancers detected by 2D/3D	NR	2D: 8.7% 2D/3D: 5.5% (36% reduction; $P < 0.001$)	Decrease of 3.2%
Haas et al. (2013) USA	Retrospective: services using 2D vs services using 2D/3D (7058 vs 6100) in same year; single reading from readers from breast or radiology services	2D: 5.2 2D/3D: 5.7 $P = 0.70$	Increase of 0.5/1000	NR	NR	2D: 12.0% 2D/3D: 8.4% $P < 0.01$ (30% reduction)	Decrease of 3.6%

Table 5.16 (continued)

Reference [Study] Country	Study characteristics Design (no. of screens); screen-reading methods	Preventive or screening effect				Adverse effect	
		Cancer detection rates/1000 screens	Absolute effect of 3D M on cancer detection rate compared with 2D alone	Characteristics of cancers detected only with integrated 2D/3D M only	Interval cancers	False-positive recalls	Absolute effect of 3D M on FPR compared with 2D alone
Friedewald et al. (2014) USA	Retrospective: before vs after (281 187 vs 173 663) introduction of 3D as adjunct to 2D M screening; single reading from readers from 13 radiology services	2D: 4.2 2D/3D: 5.4 $P < 0.001$ For invasive cancer: 2D: 2.9 2D/3D: 4.1 $P < 0.001$	Increase of 1.2/1000 Increase of 1.2/1000	Cancers detected with 2D/3D only comprised invasive cancer; DCIS rates similar for 2D and 2D/3D; stage data NR	NR	Data for *all recalls*: 2D: 10.7% 2D/3D: 9.1% $P < 0.001$ For *all biopsies* (includes cancer): 2D: 1.8% 2D/3D: 1.9% $P = 0.004$	Decrease of 1.6%

[a] 2D refers to digital mammography acquisition of 2-view mammographic images, whereas $2D_{syn}$ refers to 2D mammographic images synthesized (reconstructed) from the digital breast tomosynthesis acquisition.

[b] Decrease in FPR is estimated for recall *conditional* to 3D-positivity (Ciatto et al., 2013; Houssami et al., 2014a), whereas false-positive scores from the Oslo study were based on pre-arbitration data (Skaane et al., 2013a, b).

2D, two-dimensional; 3D, three-dimensional; DCIS, ductal carcinoma in situ; FPR, false-positive recall; M, mammography; NR, not reported; STORM, Screening with Tomosynthesis or Standard Mammography; $2D_{syn}$/3D, tomosynthesis with synthetically reconstructed 2D images.

a significant incremental cancer detection rate of 2.7 per 1000 screens for integrated 2D/3D mammography versus digital mammography ($P < 0.001$). The Oslo trial (Skaane et al., 2013a, b) randomized readers to four screen-reading strategies that used digital mammography or integrated 2D/3D mammography, allowing assessment of reconstructed 2D mammography in one of the study arms (Skaane et al., 2014). The study showed a significant incremental cancer detection rate of 1.9 per 1000 screens for integrated 2D/3D mammography versus digital mammography in a reader-adjusted analysis ($P = 0.001$) (Skaane et al., 2013a) and of 2.3 per 1000 screens for double reading of integrated 2D/3D mammography versus digital mammography ($P < 0.001$) (Skaane et al., 2013b). A further analysis (Skaane et al., 2014) found that integrated 2D/3D mammography yielded a similar incremental cancer detection rate compared with digital mammography whether by *dual acquisition* of digital mammography with tomosynthesis (acquired 2D and 3D images) or by tomosynthesis acquisition with synthetic 2D mammography (3D acquisition only, and 2D images reconstructed from the 3D data).

A third prospective screening trial, also conducted within a population-based programme, was in progress in Malmö, Sweden, at the time of the Handbook Working Group Meeting, in November 2014. This trial differs from the other screening studies of this technology in that it compares screen-reading using digital mammography alone (two views) with screen-reading using tomosynthesis alone (one 3D mammography view); hence, it is the only population-based breast screening study reporting detection estimates for tomosynthesis alone. [Note added after the Meeting: The results of the trial have been published (Lång et al., 2015). The incremental cancer detection rate was 2.6 per 1000 screens using tomosynthesis alone versus digital mammography ($P < 0.0001$).]

Three retrospective studies have also examined digital mammography with tomosynthesis for population screening (Haas et al., 2013; Rose et al., 2013; Friedewald et al., 2014); all three studies were conducted in the USA and hence used single reading as practised in the USA. Two studies (Rose et al., 2013; Friedewald et al., 2014) used a before–after methodology, comparing detection measures before and after the introduction of integrated 2D/3D mammography, whereas one study (Haas et al., 2013) compared services using digital mammography with services using integrated 2D/3D mammography within the same time frame. The largest retrospective study (Friedewald et al., 2014) was a comparison of 281 187 versus 173 663 screens before and after the introduction of tomosynthesis as adjunct to digital mammography screening in 13 radiology services, and reported a significant incremental cancer detection rate of 1.2 per 1000 screens. Overall, the three studies showed a modest incremental detection rate with the use of adjunct tomosynthesis (range, 0.5–1.4 per 1000 screens) relative to the prospective trials; however, the direction of the estimated increased cancer detection is consistent across all studies.

Four out of five studies provided limited data on the characteristics of the cancers detected with integrated 2D/3D mammography compared with digital mammography. [Studies were generally not powered for such analyses.] Two studies indicated that the increased cancer detection achieved by digital mammography with tomosynthesis was mostly of invasive disease (Rose et al., 2013; Friedewald et al., 2014), whereas two studies showed incremental detection of both invasive and in situ disease (Ciatto et al., 2013; Skaane et al., 2013b).

Data on interval cancer rates for this technology are limited to the follow-up report from the STORM trial; the estimated interval cancer rate based on only 12 months of follow-up is 0.82 per 1000 (95% CI, 0.30–1.79) (Houssami et al., 2014a).

Several studies reported on the use of integrated 2D/3D mammography screening in reducing false-positive recalls (Table 5.16). The reduction in false-positive recalls is most marked in the retrospective studies reported from the USA (absolute decreases in false-positive results range from 1.6% to 3.6%), where the baseline false-positive recall rates for digital mammography alone are relatively high (range, 8.7–12.0%). The estimated reduction in false-positive recalls in the prospective studies, which were conducted in European population screening programmes and had relatively low recall rates, was modest (0.8% and 2%), and the latter was an estimate conditional to 3D mammography positivity. Furthermore, one of the studies (Skaane et al., 2013b) showed that for double reading, digital mammography with tomosynthesis reduced false-positive recalls compared with mammography alone, but increased overall recall (see Table 5.16). [It is likely that the potential for digital mammography with tomosynthesis to reduce false-positive recalls will depend on both the false-positive recall rates at digital mammography and the recall rules, which vary according to the screening programme.]

5.5.2 Adverse effects

(a) Breast ultrasonography

The adverse effects of breast ultrasonography screening have been examined in non-randomized retrospective and prospective studies in women with dense breast tissue (Buchberger et al., 2000; Kaplan, 2001; Kolb et al., 2002; Corsetti et al., 2008, 2011; Kelly et al., 2010; Hooley et al., 2012; Weigert & Steenbergen, 2012; Venturini et al., 2013; Brem et al., 2014). The main adverse effect is *additional false-positive* intervention. Ultrasonography caused additional testing (needle biopsy or imaging follow-up) in 1.2–6.3%, and also surgical biopsy (although some studies included non-surgical biopsy in this percentage) in 0.9–2.7% due to false-positives (Table 5.15). The study of Kelly et al. (2010), which included some women at an increased risk, reported an overall recall rate [not distinctly false-positive recall] of 7.2% for ultrasonography (vs 4.2% for mammography; $P < 0.01$), and the combined strategy had an overall recall rate of 9.6% in that study. Venturini et al. (2013) reported a false-positive biopsy rate for ultrasonography of 0.9% (vs 0.1% for mammography) in a cohort of young women (aged 40–49 years) with dense breast tissue and intermediate lifetime risk. Brem et al. (2014) reported an overall recall rate of 28.5% for adjunct ultrasonography with mammography (vs 15% for mammography alone; $P < 0.001$).

Given that there is substantial increased detection of breast cancer using adjunct ultrasonography in women with mammography-negative dense breasts, it seems possible that overdiagnosis could occur in this context. However, overdiagnosis has not been reported in any of the studies reviewed (Buchberger et al., 2000; Kaplan, 2001; Kolb et al., 2002; Corsetti et al., 2008, 2011; Kelly et al., 2010; Hooley et al., 2012; Weigert & Steenbergen, 2012; Venturini et al., 2013; Brem et al., 2014). [It would be difficult to attempt to estimate overdiagnosis based on the available data, due to (but not limited to) the lack of a control or comparison cohort and the heterogeneity of the screened populations, including variable underlying risk profiles.]

(b) Digital breast tomosynthesis/three-dimensional mammography

All studies reviewed reported a *reduction in false-positive recalls* using integrated 2D/3D mammography (Table 5.16). Therefore, this does not seem to be an adverse effect of this technology. [The same may not apply for 3D screening alone.]

Given that there is increased detection of breast cancer using digital mammography with tomosynthesis, it seems possible that overdiagnosis could occur in this context. Several studies (Rose et al., 2013; Skaane et al., 2013a; Friedewald et al., 2014) have suggested that digital breast tomosynthesis mostly increases detection of invasive cancers. However, none of the studies have reported on overdiagnosis. [The currently available data do not allow inferences relating to overdiagnosis from the increased cancer detection attributed to tomosynthesis.]

The main potential adverse effect of digital mammography with tomosynthesis relates to the radiation dose to the breast if dual acquisition is used. Digital breast tomosynthesis is reported to deliver on average similar doses to digital mammography (Feng & Sechopoulos, 2012; Houssami & Skaane, 2013). Thus, using dual acquisition by digital mammography with tomosynthesis approximately doubles the radiation dose. In the two population screening studies, the mean glandular dose per view was 1.58 mGy for digital mammography and 1.95 mGy for digital breast tomosynthesis in the Oslo study (Skaane et al., 2013a) and 1.22 mGy for digital mammography and 2.99 mGy (1.22 + 1.77 mGy) for integrated 2D/3D mammography in the STORM study (Bernardi et al., 2014). Recent tomosynthesis technology allows reconstruction of the 2D images from the data obtained from the tomosynthesis acquisition (also referred to as synthetic 2D mammography), eliminating the need for dual acquisition. Reconstruction of the 2D images from the tomosynthesis acquisition decreases the radiation dose by 45% compared with the dual acquisition (Skaane et al., 2014) and performs similarly to digital mammography with tomosynthesis from dual acquisition (see Section 5.5.1 and Table 5.16).

5.5.3 Cost–effectiveness analysis

(a) Breast ultrasonography

There were no studies of breast ultrasonography for population breast screening that reported on cost per life year gained or QALY saved. Cost analyses were reported by four of the studies that investigated ultrasonography in women with dense breasts. Studies conducted in the USA (Hooley et al., 2012; Weigert & Steenbergen, 2012) reported relatively higher costs than those conducted in Europe (Corsetti et al., 2008; Venturini et al., 2013). Hooley et al. (2012) estimated the cost of adjunct ultrasonography, factoring in the costs of ultrasonography and related biopsy and short-interval imaging follow-up (using the Medicare reimbursement rate), to be $US 60 267 per detected breast cancer. Weigert & Steenbergen (2012), using the average reimbursement rate for ultrasonography and related biopsy, estimated the cost of adjunct ultrasonography screening to be $US 110 241 per detected breast cancer.

In the European setting, Corsetti et al. (2008) estimated the cost of adjunct ultrasonography, factoring in the costs of ultrasonography and related testing and any form of biopsy, to be in the range of €14 618–15 234 per detected breast cancer. Venturini et al. (2013) reported the cost of screening young women with dense breasts; mammography was estimated to cost €6377 per detected breast cancer, whereas adjunct ultrasonography in the same programme was estimated to cost €19 158 per detected breast cancer.

(b) Digital breast tomosynthesis/ three-dimensional mammography

There were no studies available of the cost–effectiveness, or any cost analyses, of digital mammography with tomosynthesis in population breast screening. Digital breast tomosynthesis is more expensive than digital mammography and requires more imaging storage and display infrastructure, all of which increase the costs and the resources needed for screening implementation. Digital mammography with tomosynthesis also increases screen-reading time, resulting in an approximate doubling (Houssami & Skaane, 2013); based on the Oslo trial (Skaane et al., 2013a), the mean interpretation time was 91 seconds for integrated 2D/3D mammography versus 45 seconds for digital mammography ($P < 0.001$).

5.5.4 Other techniques

(a) Magnetic resonance imaging

Breast MRI has been shown to have superior screening sensitivity to mammography in women at an increased risk of developing breast cancer (see Section 5.6). Searches of the literature did not identify any studies of MRI for screening of women considered at average (population) risk. One recent study (Kuhl et al., 2014) of an abbreviated (fast) MRI protocol screened 443 women "referred to MRI screening on clinical grounds"; 82% of the women were considered to be at mildly or moderately increased risk, because of either dense breast tissue or a mild or moderate family history of breast cancer. The 146 women with a personal history of breast cancer were having imaging of the contralateral breast. In this selected subject group, reportedly "pre-screened" with digital mammography and ultrasonography [data not reported for either], MRI yielded an incremental cancer detection rate of 18 per 1000 screens. False-positive rates varied by the applied MRI protocol and were in the range of 5.6–29%. [The findings from this "proof-of-concept" reader study are early and do not represent population screening.]

(b) Electrical impedance imaging

The literature search did not identify any RCTs or population-based studies of electrical impedance scanning for breast screening. Studies of electrical impedance technologies for imaging of the breast have used various devices and instrumentation, operated at various frequencies and interpreted using variable methods (e.g. visual, computer algorithms, or other methods) (Malich et al., 2001; Martín et al., 2002; Wersebe et al., 2002; Diebold et al., 2005; Fuchsjaeger et al., 2005; Zheng et al., 2008, 2011; Wang et al., 2010; Lederman et al., 2011).

All these studies were relatively small clinical series or diagnostic studies of women who had suspicious or equivocal (mammography or other image-detected) findings and included both symptomatic and asymptomatic women; these studies were based on women who were undergoing biopsy (surgical or core needle biopsy), and hence the studies were highly enriched with breast cancer cases (prevalence in the range of 5–60%).

One relatively large study assessed electrical impedance imaging for "risk-stratification" and screening of asymptomatic young women (aged 30–45 years) (Stojadinovic et al., 2005, 2008). [One limitation of this study is that the study participants included women with mammographic findings or clinical abnormalities who were scheduled to undergo biopsy.] The study reported an extremely low sensitivity for screening of 26.4%, and specificity of 94.7%.

(c) Scintimammography (molecular breast imaging)

The literature search did not identify any studies evaluating the efficacy or effectiveness of this technology for breast screening of women at average (population) risk.

Scintimammography has been used and evaluated in various clinical applications for breast imaging, predominantly in small and/or highly selected clinical series and diagnostic studies highly enriched with breast cancer cases (19–100%), including, but not limited to: diagnostic workup of suspicious or indeterminate mammography-detected (or other image-detected) findings; breast assessment in women scheduled for biopsy on the basis of clinical or mammographic abnormalities; staging of a known cancerous breast lesion; monitoring response to treatment; and detecting breast cancer recurrence (Bekiş et al., 2004; Rhodes et al., 2005; Adedapo & Choudhury, 2007; Duarte et al., 2007; Gommans et al., 2007; O'Connor et al., 2007; Spanu et al., 2007, 2008, 2009; Hruska et al., 2008; Kim et al., 2009; Sharma et al., 2009; Xu et al., 2011; Lee et al., 2012; Spanu et al., 2012; Weigert et al., 2012; BlueCross

BlueShield Association, 2013). A meta-analysis (Xu et al., 2011) of 45 extremely heterogeneous diagnostic accuracy studies of scintimammography reported meta-estimates of 83% for sensitivity and 85% for specificity; in the subgroup of subjects *without* a palpable mass, meta-estimates were 59% for sensitivity and 89% for specificity.

Three studies reported screening of defined asymptomatic populations, which included women at an increased risk. Brem et al. (2005) screened with scintimammography 94 women at an increased risk who had normal mammograms and CBE. They detected 2 additional invasive (9 mm) cancers (+2%); however, this was at the trade-off of 14 additional false-positives (+15%). Rhodes et al. (2011) screened 936 women (aged 25–89 years) with dense breasts *and* at an increased risk (personal history of breast cancer or lobular carcinoma in situ [LCIS] or atypical proliferations, or *BRCA* mutations) using dedicated dual-head gamma imaging (with the radiotracer ^{99m}Tc-sestamibi). The detection yield was 3.2 per 1000 screens for mammography and 9.6 per 1000 screens for scintimammography (incremental cancer detection rate, 7.5 per 1000 screens). Most of the cancers detected on scintimammography only were node-negative invasive cancers (median size, 11 mm). [The sensitivity of mammography was extremely low (27%).] False-positive recall rates (9% for mammography, 8% for scintimammography) and specificity (91% for mammography, 93% for scintimammography) were similar for the two tests. Finally, Hruska et al. (2012) reported a study of molecular breast imaging with ^{99m}Tc-sestamibi in 306 asymptomatic women (aged 37–88 years), including some women at an increased risk, such as those with a personal history of breast cancer, who were undergoing myocardial perfusion imaging. Scintimammography had an incremental cancer detection yield of 13 per 1000 screens (4 cancers) relative to mammography in the previous 12 months, and caused additional false-positives in approximately [6%] of subjects.

The radiation dose to the whole body from this technology (see Section 2.2.4 for details) is reported to be 15–30 times the radiation dose from digital mammography (BlueCross BlueShield Association, 2013).

(d) Positron emission mammography

Literature searches did not identify any population breast screening studies of positron emission mammography. This technology has been evaluated in very specific and limited clinical applications of breast imaging, predominantly for staging of a lesion; for preoperative assessment of disease extent (generally in comparison with MRI); for "screening" of the contralateral breast in preoperative staging; for response monitoring, in very small series of women with a biopsy of suspicious findings; or in phantom studies (Raylman et al., 2000; Levine et al., 2003; Tafra et al., 2005; Berg et al., 2011, 2012a; Schilling et al., 2011; Schilling, 2012; Shkumat et al., 2011; Eo et al., 2012; Kalles et al., 2013). Positron emission mammography involves much higher doses of radiation (whole-body radiation) and a much longer acquisition time (for two views of both breasts) than mammography (see Section 2.2.3).

5.5.5 Psychosocial harm

Few studies have measured psychosocial harm from imaging techniques other than mammography. One study found that MRI screening was more distressing than X-ray mammography both shortly after and 6 weeks after the screening procedure (Hutton et al., 2011), whereas another study found no difference between MRI and mammography screening in psychological outcomes (Brédart et al., 2012). As with other screening processes, psychological harm may depend on the conduct of the technology, such as the number of false-positive and false-negative screens and the waiting time from examination to result (see also Sections 3.1.4 and 5.3.5).

5.6 Screening of women at an increased risk

In some women, the risk of developing breast cancer during their lifetime is increased compared with that of women in the general population, and usually with an earlier expected age of onset. This increased risk may be attributed to the presence of a genetic or familial predisposition to breast cancer, to a personal history of invasive breast cancer or DCIS, or to the presence of lobular neoplasia or atypical proliferations. It should be noted that a familial predisposition, if not assessed by a specialized genetic centre, should not be used as an indication for screening outside the scope of the population breast cancer screening programme.

In general, it is preferable that women at an increased risk be screened outside the scope of a population breast cancer screening programme, for two reasons. First, regular population screening programmes with mammography might be insufficient, due to the earlier age of onset of breast cancer in these women and due to the reduced sensitivity of mammography in these women. In addition, women with a *BRCA1/2* mutation are more susceptible to radiation risk. Second, these women often require additional care, assessment, counselling, and information relevant to primary prevention and risk-reduction strategies (as might be provided, for example, through specialized genetics teams/units) that are generally well outside of the health-care brief of mammography screening programmes.

Evidence on the outcomes of screening for breast cancer in the several subgroups of women at an increased risk is summarized and discussed here.

5.6.1 *High familial risk, with or without a* BRCA1 *or* BRCA2 *mutation*

This section reports evidence on the effectiveness of screening with MRI alone, adjunct MRI, adjunct ultrasonography, or adjunct CBE as compared with mammography alone in women with a high familial risk, with or without a *BRCA1* or *BRCA2* mutation. Table 5.17 presents individual prospective studies, and Table 5.18 summarizes pooled and meta-analyses, and systematic reviews. The included studies are those that were performed prospectively, in which MRI and mammography were performed in the same screening round, and in which the review of the diagnostic test was performed blinded for the outcome of the other test. Studies that were performed retrospectively or unblinded, or in which MRI, ultrasonography, or mammography were not performed in parallel were excluded.

In addition, three reports reviewing the evidence of the effectiveness of adjunct MRI in the screening of women at an increased risk of breast cancer were identified (Table 5.18). One is a systematic review of the literature (Lord et al., 2007), one is a systematic review and meta-analysis at the level of published studies (Warner et al., 2008), and one is a pooled analysis of individual patient data (Phi et al., 2014).

(a) *Adjunct magnetic resonance imaging*

(i) *Sensitivity and specificity in women with a* BRCA1/2 *mutation*

Several studies focused on the added value of MRI compared with mammography and/or ultrasonography in the screening of women with a *BRCA1* or *BRCA2* mutation (Table 5.17 and Table 5.18). In the meta-analysis (Warner et al., 2008) and the pooled analysis (Phi et al., 2014), the estimates of the sensitivity of mammography were comparable, at about 40%, and increased with mammography combined with MRI similarly in both studies, to 94% (95% CI, 90–97%) in Warner et al. (2008) and 93.4% (95% CI,

Table 5.17 Prospective studies in women with a *BRCA1/2* mutation or a familial breast cancer risk screened with magnetic resonance imaging, mammography, ultrasonography, or clinical breast examination

Reference[a] Country, study	Study period	Study design	Test results and related follow-up[b]	Risk category	No. of women in study	No. of breast cancers	MRI Sens, Spec (%)	M Sens, Spec (%)	US Sens, Spec (%)	CBE Sens, Spec (%)
Kuhl et al. (2005) Germany	1996–2002	Single centre Double reading Annual MRI and M Biannual US	BI-RADS 4, 5: biopsy BI-RADS 3: short-term follow-up	Total	529	43	90.7 97.2	32.6 96.8	39.5 90.5	—
				BRCA1/2	43	8	100 97.5	25 96.9	25 91.2	—
				FH	241	20	100 97.7	25 97.4	30 91.2	—
Leach et al. (2005) United Kingdom, MARIBS study	1997–2004	Multicentre Double reading Annual MRI and M	BI-RADS 0, 3, 4, 5: biopsy	Total	649	35	77 81	40 93	—	—
				BRCA1	82	13	92 79	23 92	—	—
				BRCA2	43	12	58 82	50 94	—	—
				FH	524	10	NR	NR	—	—
Lehman et al. (2005) USA[c]	1999–2002	Multicentre Single reading 1 screening round with MRI, M, and CBE	BI-RADS 4, 5: biopsy	Total	390	4	100	25	—	NR
Cortesi et al. (2006) Italy, Modena study[d]	1994–2000	Single centre Single reading Annual MRI and M Biannual US and CBE	NR	*BRCA1/2*	48	4	100 NR	78 NR	50 NR	8.3 NR
Hagen et al. (2007) Norway	2002–2006	Multicentre Single reading Annual MRI and MG. In dense breasts, M was extended with US	BI-RADS 4, 5: biopsy BI-RADS 3: short-term follow-up	Total	491	21	86 NR	48 NR	—	—
				BRCA1	445	19	84 NR	53 NR	—	—
				BRCA2	46	2	100 NR	0 NR	—	—
Lehman et al. (2007) USA[c]	2002–2003	Multicentre Single reading 1 screening round with MRI, M, and US	BI-RADS 4, 5: biopsy	Total	190	6	100 NR	66.7 NR	16.7 NR	—
				BRCA1/2	80	3	100 NR	0 NR	0 NR	—
				FH	110	3	100 NR	66.7 NR	33.4 NR	—

Table 5.17 (continued)

Reference[a] Country, study	Study period	Study design	Test results and related follow-up[b]	Risk category	No. of women in study	No. of breast cancers	MRI Sens, Spec (%)	M Sens, Spec (%)	US Sens, Spec (%)	CBE Sens, Spec (%)
Riedl et al. (2007) Austria	1999–2006	Single centre Single reading Annual MRI, M, and US	BI-RADS 4, 5: biopsy BI-RADS 3: 6 mo follow-up	Total	327	28	85.7 92.3	50 98.1	42.9 98	—
				BRCA1	80	6	NR	NR	NR	—
				BRCA2	13	2	NR	NR	NR	—
				FH	234	20	NR	NR	NR	—
Saunders et al. (2009) Australia	2002–2005	Single centre Single reading Annual MRI, M, and US Biannual CBE	BI-RADS 3, 4, 5: biopsy BI-RADS 0: short-term follow-up	Total	72	0	—	—	—	—
Weinstein et al. (2009) USA	2002–2007	Single centre Single reading 1 screening round with MRI, M (screen-film or digital), and US	BI-RADS 3, 4, 5: biopsy BI-RADS 0: short-term follow-up	Total	609	18	71 79	39 91[e]	17 88	—
				BRCA1	27	2	50 NR	50 NR	0 NR	—
				BRCA2	17	2	0 NR	100 NR	0 NR	—
				FH	565	14	78.6 NR	35.7 NR	21 NR	—
Kuhl et al. (2010) Germany	2002–2005	Multicentre Single reading Annual MRI, M, US, and CBE	BI-RADS 4, 5: biopsy BI-RADS 3: short-term follow-up	Total	687	27	92.6 98.4	33.3 99.1	37 98	3 99.4
				BRCA1/2	53	5	NR	NR	NR	NR
				FH	436	22	NR	NR	NR	NR
Rijnsburger et al. (2010) Netherlands, MRISC study	1999–2006	Multicentre Single reading Annual MRI and M Biannual CBE	BI-RADS 4, 5: biopsy BI-RADS 0, 3: biopsy or additional imaging After abnormal CBE: additional imaging	Total	2157	97	70.7 89.7	41.3 94.6	—	20.6 97.9
				BRCA1	422	35	66.7 91	25 94.6	—	13 96.9
				BRCA2	172	18	69.2 91	61.5 93.8	—	7.7 98.3
				FH	1563	44	73 89.2	46 94.6	—	32.2 98.1

Table 5.17 (continued)

Reference[a] Country, study	Study period	Study design	Test results and related follow-up[b]	Risk category	No. of women in study	No. of breast cancers	MRI Sens, Spec (%)	M Sens, Spec (%)	US Sens, Spec (%)	CBE Sens, Spec (%)
Trop et al. (2010) Montreal, Canada	2003–2007	Single centre Single reading Annual MRI and M Biannual US and CBE	BI-RADS 4, 5: biopsy BI-RADS 3: 6 mo follow-up	Total	184	12	83 93.6	58 95.4	42 93.8	17 95.9
				BRCA1	75	6	83.3 NR	50 NR	50 NR	33.3 NR
				BRCA2	68	5	80 NR	60 NR	20 NR	0 NR
				FH	41	1	100 NR	100 NR	100 NR	0 NR
Sardanelli et al. (2011) Italy, HIBCRIT 1 study	2000–2007	Multicentre Single reading Annual MRI, M, US, and CBE	BI-RADS 4, 5: biopsy BI-RADS 3: 4 mo follow-up	Total	501	52	91.3 96.7	50 99	52 98.4	17.6 99.3
				BRCA1	184	21	NR	NR	NR	NR
				BRCA2	146	10	NR	NR	NR	NR
				FH	171	21	NR	NR	NR	NR
Passaperuma et al. (2012) Toronto, Canada	1997–2009	Single centre Single reading Annual MRI, M, US and CBE US was stopped in 2005 due to lack of Sens and Spec	BI-RADS 0, 4, 5: biopsy BI-RADS 3: 6, 12, 24 mo follow-up If MRI was positive where no other tests were, MRI was repeated within 1 mo	Total	496	57	86 90	19 97	—	NR
				BRCA1	267	31	90 NR	19 NR	—	NR
				BRCA2	229	26	80 NR	20 NR	—	NR

[a] Data reported from the most recent publication.

[b] Based on BI-RADS (Breast Imaging Reporting and Data System; D'Orsi et al., 2013) density categories: 1, almost entirely fatty (< 25% fibroglandular); 2, scattered fibroglandular densities (25–50% fibroglandular); 3, heterogeneously dense (51–75% fibroglandular); 4, extremely dense (> 75% fibroglandular).

[c] Due to the design of the Lehman et al. (2005) and Lehman et al. (2007) studies, only sensitivity could be reported.

[d] Only data for the *BRCA1/2* mutation carriers are reported, as no MRI was performed in the other risk groups.

[e] Only the results for digital mammography are reported, as they are close to those for screen-film mammography.

BI-RADS, American College of Radiology Breast Imaging Reporting and Data System; CBE, clinical breast examination; FH, family history suspicious for an increased risk of breast cancer; HIBCRIT, High Breast Cancer Risk Italian Trial; M, mammography; MARIBS, Magnetic Resonance Imaging for Breast Screening; mo, month or months; MRI, magnetic resonance imaging; MRISC, MRI Screening; NR, not reported in the most recent publication; Sens, sensitivity; Spec, specificity; US, ultrasonography.

Table 5.18 Systematic reviews, pooled analysis, and meta-analyses of women at an increased risk of breast cancer screened with adjunct magnetic resonance imaging compared with mammography alone, with or without ultrasonography

Study	Included studies	Study design	Main outcome parameters	Results on main outcome parameters
Lord et al. (2007)	Warner et al. (2004), Kuhl et al. (2005), Leach et al. (2005), Lehman et al. (2005), Sardanelli et al. (2007)	Systematic review Results expressed as ranges	Sens M	25–59%
			Sens US and M	49–67%
			Sens MRI and M (with or without US)	93–100%
			Recall rate with MRI compared with that without MRI	Adjunct MRI may increase patient recall rates 3–5-fold due to increased false-positive findings
Warner et al. (2008)	Warner et al. (2001, 2004), Hartman et al. (2004), Kriege et al. (2004), Kuhl et al. (2005), Leach et al. (2005), Lehman et al. (2005, 2007), Trecate et al. (2006), Hagen et al. (2007), Sardanelli et al. (2007)	Systematic review with meta-analysis at study level Results expressed as percentages and 95% CI	Sens M	39% (37–41%)
			Sens M and MRI	94% (90–97%)
			Spec M	94.7% (93.0–96.5%)
			Spec M and MRI	77.2% (74.7–79.7%)
Phi et al. (2014)	Leach et al. (2005), Riedl et al. (2007), Rijnsburger et al. (2010), Trop et al. (2010), Sardanelli et al. (2011), Passaperuma et al. (2012)	Pooled analysis at individual patient level Results expressed as percentages and 95% CI	Sens M	39.6% (30.1–49.9%)
			Sens MRI	85.3% (69.1–93.8%)
			Sens M and MRI	93.4% (80.2–98.0%)
			Spec M	93.6% (88.8–96.5%)
			Spec MRI	84.7% (79.0–89.1%)
			Spec M and MRI	80.3% (72.5–86.2%)
			In women aged > 50 yr:	
			Sens M	38.1% (22.4–56.7%)
			Sens MRI	84.4% (61.8–94.8%)
			Sens M and MRI	94.1% (77.7–98.7%)
			Spec M	95.9% (92.1–97.9%)
			Spec MRI	88.5% (83.5–92.2%)
			Spec M and MRI	85.3% (78.5–90.2%)

CI, confidence interval; M, mammography; MRI, magnetic resonance imaging; Sens, sensitivity; Spec, specificity; US, ultrasonography.

80.2–98.0%) in Phi et al. (2014). The specificity of adjunct MRI was also similar in the two analyses, to 77.2% (95% CI, 74.7–79.7%) in Warner et al. (2008) and 80.3% (95% CI, 72.5–86.2%) in Phi et al. (2014). Thus, adding MRI to mammography in the screening of women with a *BRCA1/2* mutation leads to a statistically significant increase in sensitivity of the screening strategy, accompanied by a decrease in specificity that was also statistically significant (see Table 5.18).

In the pooled analysis using individual data in women with *BRCA1/2* mutations, for the screening of women aged 50 years and older, the highest sensitivity was reported for adjunct MRI (94.1%; 95% CI, 77.7–98.7%) compared with mammography alone (38.1%; 95% CI, 22.4–56.7%) and compared with MRI alone (84.4%; 95% CI, 61.8–94.8%) (Phi et al., 2014); the specificity was lowest for adjunct MRI.

(ii) Sensitivity and specificity in women without a BRCA1/2 *mutation*

Only two informative studies assessed the sensitivity and specificity of mammography and MRI separately for women with a familial risk without a known *BRCA1* or *BRCA2* mutation (Kuhl et al., 2005; Rijnsburger et al., 2010). Two other studies were considered uninformative due to the small number of breast cancers in that category (Lehman et al., 2007; Trop et al., 2010; see Table 5.17). For mammography, the reported estimates for the sensitivity were 25–46% and for the specificity were 95–97%. For MRI, the reported estimates for the sensitivity were 73–100% and for the specificity were 89–98%. [All estimates reported by the earlier study (Kuhl et al., 2005) are outside the confidence intervals of the two published meta-analyses (Warner et al., 2008; Phi et al., 2014). Given the lower expected incidence of breast cancer among women without a *BRCA1* or *BRCA2* mutation, the PPV of screening with MRI will be much lower than that among women with a *BRCA1* or *BRCA2* mutation.]

(iii) Mortality reduction

There are no randomized trials assessing the efficacy of adjunct MRI in terms of mortality reduction in women at an increased risk with or without a *BRCA* gene mutation (Nelson et al., 2013). Several prospective observational studies with long-term follow-up reported on stage distribution and mortality reduction by annual MRI plus mammography screening compared with women without intensified screening.

Three studies analysed the stage distribution of cancers detected in follow-up rounds of intensified screening programmes (Schmutzler et al., 2006; Rijnsburger et al., 2010; Passaperuma et al., 2012). In two of the studies (Schmutzler et al., 2006; Rijnsburger et al., 2010), an increase of N0 stages was reported (N0 stages of 67% vs 52% and 83% vs 56%, respectively). In the third study (Passaperuma et al., 2012), a significant reduction of late stages from 6.6% to 1.9% with intensified screening was observed.

Prospective studies assessing the effectiveness of adjunct MRI in terms of mortality reduction are summarized in Table 5.19. In a four-country study (England, the Netherlands, Norway, and Scotland), the 5-year survival was assessed for 249 women (205 non-*BRCA1/2* mutation carriers with a family history of breast cancer, 36 *BRCA1* mutation carriers, and 8 *BRCA2* mutation carriers) prospectively diagnosed with breast cancer during screening (Møller et al., 2002). All women were under breast cancer surveillance at a dedicated clinic, including annual mammography and CBE, and were diagnosed with breast cancer in this setting. The 5-year survival was 63% for women with a *BRCA1* mutation compared with 91% in the women with a family history of breast cancer and without a known *BRCA1/2* mutation.

In 2001, as part of a national initiative, women in Norway with a *BRCA1* mutation were offered annual breast screening with MRI in addition to mammography. The observed 5-year

Table 5.19 Prospective studies of 5-year and 10-year survival of women with a *BRCA1/2* mutation screened with mammography and/or magnetic resonance imaging

Reference Study period and location	Study population	Study design	Main outcome parameters	Percentage survival
Møller et al. (2002)	249 women (205 non-*BRCA1/2* mutation carriers with FHBC, 36 *BRCA1* mutation carriers, and 8 *BRCA2* mutation carriers) in 4 countries or regions (England, the Netherlands, Norway, and Scotland)	Women screened with M combined with CBE and diagnosed prospectively; comparison of 5-yr survival between *BRCA1/2* mutation carriers and non-carriers with FHBC	5-yr survival: *BRCA1* mutation carriers Non-carriers with FHBC	 63% 91% $P = 0.04$
Møller et al. (2013)	802 women with a *BRCA1* mutation	Women screened with M + MRI for a mean of 4.2 yr and diagnosed prospectively; assessment of the impact of programme on 5-yr and 10-yr survival	5-yr survival 10-yr survival	75% (95% CI, 56–86%) 69% (95% CI, 48–83%)
Rijnsburger et al. (2010) Netherlands, 1999–2006	2157 women with > 15% cumulative risk of breast cancer: gene mutation carriers ($n = 599$) and FHBC with moderate or high risk ($n = 1558$)	Women screened with biannual CBE and annual M + MRI and diagnosed prospectively; assessment of overall survival at 6 yr	6-yr survival: *BRCA1/2* mutation carriers ($n = 42$) Familial groups ($n = 43$)	 92.7% (95% CI, 79.0–97.6%) 100%
Passaperuma et al. (2012) United Kingdom, 1997–2009	496 women with a known *BRCA1/2* mutation, of whom 380 had no previous cancer history, aged 25–65 yr	Women screened with annual M + MRI and diagnosed prospectively; assessment of survival ($n = 54$)	8-yr survival	1 out of 28 *BRCA1* mutation carriers with invasive breast cancer died of breast cancer
Evans et al. (2014) 1990–2013	MRI + M cohort: two prospective cohorts of 959 (647 + 312) women with proven or likely *BRCA1/2* or *p53* mutations (25% mutation-negative) M-only cohort: prospective cohort of 1223 women with *BRCA1/2* mutation or at equivalent risk of breast cancer, aged ≤ 55 yr (24% mutation-negative) Unscreened cohort: retrospective cohort of 557 women with *BRCA1/2* mutation identified from the Manchester genetic database as having been diagnosed with breast cancer, aged ≤ 55 yr	MRI + M cohort: screened annually with MRI + M either simultaneously (cohort 1) or 6 mo apart (cohort 2) M-only cohort: screened with M only [annually] Unscreened cohort: identified retrospectively as diagnosed with breast cancer and not having undergone intensive surveillance (a subset aged 50–55 yr had received 3-yearly mammography) 10-yr survival analysis	10-yr survival among *BRCA1/2* mutation carriers only: MRI + M M No screening	Log-rank test for overall survival 95.3% 87.7% NS when compared with no screening NS when compared with MRI + M 73.7% MRI + M vs no screening: $P = 0.002$

CBE, clinical breast examination; CI, confidence interval; FHBC, family history of breast cancer; M, mammography; mo, month or months; MRI, magnetic resonance imaging; NS, not statistically significant; yr, year or years.

breast cancer-specific survival for breast cancer patients with a *BRCA1* mutation was 75% (95% CI, 56–86%) and the 10-year survival was 69% (95% CI, 48–83%) (Møller et al., 2013). These results are in contrast with those of two other recent studies (Rijnsburger et al., 2010; Passaperuma et al., 2012). In one study (Rijnsburger et al., 2010), the estimated overall survival at 6 years in *BRCA1/2* mutation carriers was 92.7% (95% CI, 79.0–97.6%). In the other study (Passaperuma et al., 2012), out of 28 previously unaffected women with a *BRCA1* mutation diagnosed with invasive breast cancer, only 1 died after relapse. [The Working Group noted that the study of Møller et al. (2013) included only women with a *BRCA1* mutation, whereas the other two studies also included women with *BRCA2* mutations, which could explain the difference in outcome.]

In a recent publication (Evans et al., 2014), a survival analysis was conducted between *BRCA1/2* mutation carriers screened with MRI plus mammography and unscreened *BRCA1/2* mutation carriers (Table 5.19). There were no differences in 10-year survival between the groups screened with MRI plus mammography and with mammography only, but survival was significantly higher in the group screened with MRI plus mammography (95.3%) compared with the unscreened cohort (73.7%; $P = 0.002$). After adjustment for age at diagnosis, this difference was still statistically significant (HR, 0.13; 95% CI, 0.032–0.53). [In this study, there were no deaths among the 21 *BRCA2* carriers who received adjunct MRI, indicating that there might be differences in growth time between *BRCA1* and *BRCA2* tumours.]

(iv) False-positive recall rates

The low specificity linked to screening with mammography plus MRI implies that after several screening rounds a significant percentage of screenees will have experienced either a recall or an image-guided (often MRI-guided) biopsy or will have undergone short-term follow-up (Hoogerbrugge et al., 2008). In one systematic review on the adverse effects of adjunct MRI in the screening of women at an increased risk of breast cancer (Lord et al., 2007), there was a 3–5-fold higher risk of patient recall for investigation of false-positive results compared with that of mammography alone.

(b) Ultrasonography

Overall, the sensitivity of ultrasonography for the screening of women at an increased risk of breast cancer is comparable to or lower than that of mammography, and it is always lower than that of MRI (Warner et al., 2004; Kuhl et al., 2005, 2010; Cortesi et al., 2006; Lehman et al., 2007; Riedl et al., 2007; Weinstein et al., 2009; Trop et al., 2010; Sardanelli et al., 2011; Berg et al., 2012b; Table 5.17).

(c) Clinical breast examination

As part of the screening programme offered to women at an increased risk of breast cancer with and without a *BRCA1* or *BRCA2* mutation, CBE is offered in some settings in addition to mammography and/or MRI. The evidence on the topic was recently reviewed (Roeke et al., 2014), including seven studies (Tilanus-Linthorst et al., 2000; Warner et al., 2001, 2004; Kuhl et al., 2010; Rijnsburger et al., 2010; Trop et al., 2010; Sardanelli et al., 2011). The percentage of breast tumours detected by CBE varies from 0 out of 120 (0%) (Warner et al., 2001, 2004; Kuhl et al., 2010; Trop et al., 2010; Sardanelli et al., 2011) to 1 out of 260 (0.04%) (Tilanus-Linthorst et al., 2000) and 3 out of 97 (3.1%) (Rijnsburger et al., 2010) screen-detected cancers. [These latter two studies reported lower screen detection by mammography and/or MRI compared with studies in which no additional cases were detected by CBE. Furthermore, it is not clear whether CBE was performed blinded for the other tests, or whether these cases were detected during the screening or between the screening rounds, as most studies had annual screening with MRI plus mammography (with or without ultrasonography) and biannual screening with CBE.]

5.6.2 Personal history of invasive breast cancer or DCIS

Women with a personal history of invasive breast cancer or DCIS are at an increased risk of developing breast cancer. This section reviews the evidence on the performance of screening with mammography and on whether adjunct ultrasonography or MRI improves screening performance in these women (Table 5.20).

Women with a personal history of breast cancer are at an increased risk of ipsilateral or contralateral breast recurrence, or of a second primary breast cancer. Several studies have shown that a follow-up surveillance programme, including annual mammography, may be considered beneficial to these patients (Ciatto et al., 2004b; Lash et al., 2007; Lu et al., 2009). Only studies that included a comparison group were considered by the Working Group.

One large multicentre cohort study affiliated with the Breast Cancer Surveillance Consortium assessed the accuracy and outcomes of mammography screening in women with a personal history of breast cancer compared with those without such a history (Houssami et al., 2011; Table 5.20). Mammography data of women with a personal history of early-stage breast cancer (58 870 mammograms in 19 078 women) were matched on age, breast density, and year of screening to women without a personal history of breast cancer (58 870 mammograms in 55 315 women). Mammography screening in women with a personal history of breast cancer had lower sensitivity and specificity and a higher interval cancer rate, but a similar proportion of detected early-stage disease, compared with that in women without such a history (Houssami et al., 2011).

In a large study on the detection of breast cancer with the addition of annual screening with ultrasonography or a single screening with MRI to mammography in women at an increased risk, about 50% of the women had a personal history of breast cancer, and at baseline, about 55% of the women had a visually estimated breast density at scan of more than 60% (Berg et al., 2012b; Table 5.20). In this study, 111 cancers were detected: 33 with mammography only, 32 with ultrasonography only, and 26 by the combination of mammography and ultrasonography. In a substudy, after three rounds of mammography and ultrasonography, 9 additional cancers were detected with MRI. Overall, adding ultrasonography to mammography gave a statistically significant increase in sensitivity of the screening (first round, 55.6% vs 94.4%; subsequent rounds, 52% vs 76%) as well as a statistically significant increase in the recall rate (first round, 11.5% vs 26.6%; subsequent rounds, 9.4% vs 16.8%) (Berg et al., 2012b). When women with a personal history of breast cancer were compared with those without such a history, there were no statistically significant differences in yield between the two groups. However, the increase in the recall rate due to adjunct ultrasonography was statistically significantly smaller in the group of women with a personal history of breast cancer compared with those without such a history.

In a substudy in which MRI was added to the combination of mammography and ultrasonography, the sensitivity increased from 43.8% to 68.8%, whereas the recall rate increased from 16.3% to 36.3% (Berg et al., 2012b; Table 5.20). [The low sensitivity of the combined mammography and ultrasonography screening compared with the whole study might indicate an overselection of women with dense breast tissue in this substudy. The change in the recall rate due to supplementary MRI was statistically significantly higher in the group of women with a personal history of breast cancer compared with those without such a history. In this study, at baseline,

Table 5.20 Studies of the effects of screening in women with at least one risk factor for breast cancer

Study	Study design	Study population (*N*)	Main outcome parameters	Results for main outcome parameters
Screening of women with a personal history of invasive breast cancer or DCIS (PHBC)				
Houssami et al. (2011)	Multicentre 1996–2007 Cohort study Annual M Breast Cancer Surveillance Consortium	58 870 screening M in 19 078 women with PHBC 58 870 screening M in 55 315 women without PHBC	Sens (%): PHBC Non-PHBC Spec (%): PHBC Non-PHBC	 65.4 (95% CI, 61.5–69.0) 76.5 (95% CI, 71.7–80.7) 98.3 (95% CI, 98.2–98.4) 99.0 (95% CI, 98.9–99.1)
Berg et al. (2012b)[a] ACRIN 6666	Multicentre 2004–2006 Single reading Annual M and US Included women with PHBC and/or dense breasts	1426 women with PHBC 1236 women without PHBC	Cancer detection (*N*): All women: M only US only M + US Screening with M + US: PHBC No PHBC Increase in cancer detection when adding US to M: Recall rate (%): M only US only M + US Increase in recall rate when adding US to M: PHBC No PHBC	 111 33 32 26 59 52 NS Similar in both PHBC and non-PHBC patients 11.5 20.9 26.6 $P < 0.001$ vs M only 8.6 11.9 $P < 0.001$

Table 5.20 (continued)

Study	Study design	Study population (*N*)	Main outcome parameters	Results for main outcome parameters
Berg et al. (2012b)[a] ACRIN 6666	Multicentre 2004–2008 Single reading Annual M + US, extended with a single MRI screening Included women with PHBC and/or dense breasts	275 women with PHBC 336 women without PHBC	Cancer detection rate (/1000 screens): PHBC No PHBC Recall rate (%): M + US M + US + MRI Increase in recall rate when adding MRI to US + M: PHBC No PHBC	9 out of 25 cancers detected with MRI, after M + US 7.3 26.7 $P = 0.063$ 16.3 36.3 $P < 0.001$ 17.1 27.3 $P = 0.002$
Screening of women with lobular neoplasia or atypical proliferations				
Houssami et al. (2014b)	Multicentre 1996–2010 Cohort study Breast Cancer Surveillance Consortium	LCIS or ALH: 2505 screens Reference population: 12 525 screens	Sens (%): LCIS or ALH Matched group Spec (%): LCIS or ALH Matched group	 76.1 (61.2–87.4) 82.3 (70.5–90.8) 85.1 (83.6–86.5) 90.7 (90.2–91.2)
Houssami et al. (2014b)	Multicentre 1996–2010 Cohort study Breast Cancer Surveillance Consortium	ADH or AH: 6225 screens Reference population: 31 125 screens	Sens (%): ADH or AH Matched group Spec (%): ADH or AH Matched group	 81.0 (70.9–88.7) 82.6 (76.0–88.1) 86.2 (85.3–87.0) 90.2 (89.9–90.6)
Sung et al. (2011)	Single centre 2003–2008 Retrospective study of women with LCIS	840 MRI in 220 women; 670 were routine screens	Cancers diagnosed (*N*): M alone MRI alone Sens M (%) Sens MRI (%) Spec M (%) Spec MRI (%)	17 cancers in 14 patients 5 12 36 (13–65) 71 (42–91) 90 (85–94) 76 (70–82)

Table 5.20 (continued)

Study	Study design	Study population (*N*)	Main outcome parameters	Results for main outcome parameters
Friedlander et al. (2011)	Single centre 1996–2009 Retrospective study of women with LCIS	307 MRI in 133 women; all were routine screens	% (*N*) of women with biopsy recall	20.3% (27/133)
			% (*N*) of women with malignant findings	4% (5/133)
Port et al. (2007)	Single centre 1999–2005 Retrospective study of women with LCIS or AH	182 women screened with annual M 196 women screened with annual M and adjunct MRI	% (*N*) of women with screen-detected and interval cancer	In both groups there were 2.5% (5) screen-detected cancers and 1% (2) interval cancers
			% (*N*) of women with biopsy recall	
			M	11% (21)
			MRI	25% (55 in 46 patients)
King et al. (2013)	Single centre 1999–2009 Prospective study of women with LCIS	4321 women screened with annual M 455 women screened with annual M and adjunct MRI	Cancer detection rate (%):	
			M only	13%
			M + MRI	13%
			Characteristics of tumours	MRI was not associated with earlier stage, smaller size, or node-negativity

[a] The study by Berg et al. (2012b) included an MRI substudy. These results are presented here separately.

ADH, atypical ductal hyperplasia; AH, atypical hyperplasia of the breast; ALH, atypical lobular hyperplasia; CI, confidence interval; DCIS, ductal carcinoma in situ; FH, family history suspicious for an increased risk of breast cancer; LCIS, lobular carcinoma in situ; M, mammography; MRI, magnetic resonance imaging; NS, not significant; PHBC, personal history of breast cancer; Sens, sensitivity; Spec, specificity; US, ultrasonography.

about 55% of the women had a visually estimated breast density at scan of more than 60%.]

5.6.3 Lobular neoplasia or atypical proliferations

Women with lobular neoplasia or atypical proliferations are estimated to be at an increased risk of developing breast cancer (Collins et al., 2007; Tice et al., 2013). One large study affiliated with the Breast Cancer Surveillance Consortium assessed the accuracy and outcomes of screening women with LCIS, atypical lobular hyperplasia, atypical ductal hyperplasia, or atypical hyperplasia compared with those without such lesions (Houssami et al., 2014b; Table 5.20). The cancer rates in the cohorts of women with LCIS or with atypical lobular hyperplasia were 2–3 times that in the reference cohort, and the cancer rate in the cohort of women with atypical ductal hyperplasia was 3–4 times that in the reference cohort. There were no statistically significant differences in sensitivity between the four cohorts. However, mammography screening of women with LCIS, atypical lobular hyperplasia, atypical ductal hyperplasia, or atypical hyperplasia resulted in lower specificities and higher interval cancers rates compared with their referent population. [The higher interval cancer rates partly reflect the higher underlying breast cancer risk.]

A few studies have examined the sensitivity of MRI in screening women with LCIS (Friedlander et al., 2011; Sung et al., 2011; King et al., 2013) and those with LCIS or atypical hyperplasia (Port et al., 2007). In the two studies that did not have a comparison group, high sensitivities were reported for MRI screening in women with LCIS (Friedlander et al., 2011; Sung et al., 2011). [The Working Group noted that in the study of Sung et al. (2011), only 80% of the screens were routine screens; the remaining 20% had non-specified indications, and the indications for the routine screens were not specified. Similarly, the study of Friedlander et al. (2011) reported only results from routine breast MRI screens, but the indications for the routine screens were not specified. The estimated sensitivities are thus likely to be biased in both studies.]

In the other two studies (Port et al., 2007; King et al., 2013), women with high-risk lesions (LCIS and/or atypical hyperplasia) screened annually with mammography plus MRI were compared with women with high-risk lesions screened with annual mammography only. [In both studies, women with high-risk lesions selected to undergo adjunct MRI screening were younger and had stronger family histories of breast cancer compared with those screened by mammography only.] In both studies, adjunct MRI screening generated more follow-up biopsies compared with mammography alone.

5.7 Clinical breast examination

5.7.1 Preventive effects of clinical breast examination

Randomized trials of CBE versus no screening have shown a significant shift from late-stage (T3/T4) to early-stage (T1/T2) breast cancers in the intervention arm (Pisani et al., 2006; Mittra et al., 2010; Sankaranarayanan et al., 2011; see Section 4.3). Compliance with screening is one of the factors that determine effectiveness. In all three trials of CBE, the compliance with screening was high (> 85%), indicating acceptance of the procedure and ease of administering CBE. Access to care after recall and diagnosis is of paramount importance in the success of any screening trial, as is evident in the two randomized trials in India of CBE versus no screening (Mittra et al., 2010; Sankaranarayanan et al., 2011). This was the major reason that the study in the Philippines was discontinued (Pisani et al., 2006). The active intervention was stopped after the first screening round due to poor compliance (35% of screen-positive women) of participants with clinical follow-up for confirmation of diagnosis and treatment.

5.7.2 Adverse effects

In the Mumbai study, the recall rate after CBE was 0.71%. Out of 153 130 screens by CBE, 1539 women were recalled for diagnostic investigations and 81 were confirmed to have invasive cancers (Mittra et al., 2010).

Some harm of CBE may be attributed to pain or discomfort. Baines et al. (1990) carried out a survey of women who participated in the CNBSS to document women's attitudes to screening by CBE and mammography. Of those who underwent CBE, 8.4% reported moderate discomfort and 2.1% extreme discomfort, whereas of those who underwent mammography, 36.2% reported moderate discomfort and 8.7% extreme discomfort.

5.7.3 Cost–effectiveness analysis

Determining the cost–effectiveness of CBE alone is difficult because no trial has reported independent efficacy of CBE versus no screening. There have been many reports of cost–effectiveness analyses (Okonkwo et al., 2008; Ahern & Shen, 2009) on screening with reference to CBE. [The Working Group noted that most reports made assumptions about mortality reductions to simulate or estimate cost–effectiveness that were not realistic. It may be appropriate to look at cost analysis instead.] The cost of delivering breast cancer screening by CBE is less than one third that of mammography (Sarvazyan et al., 2008).

5.8 Breast self-examination

5.8.1 Preventive effects of teaching breast self-examination

Randomized trials and multiple observational studies have generally shown little or no reduction in mortality from breast cancer in women who practised BSE (see Section 4.4). If BSE is to have an effect on breast cancer mortality, it will have to be practised competently, and more frequently than in the Shanghai trial (see Section 4.4). Table 5.21 shows results of 11 surveys on BSE practice, based on self-reports, conducted primarily in countries with limited resources. Proficiency of BSE practice was not assessed in any of the studies. [It is unlikely that the proportion of women who reported practising BSE in any of the studies was sufficiently high to result in a meaningful reduction in breast cancer mortality rates in the populations surveyed.]

Results of two studies of BSE practice before and after BSE instruction have been reported. Approximately 1000 women aged 30–50 years in Madhya Pradesh, India, attended BSE instruction sessions in which a film was shown, reinforced by a lecture with flip charts showing proper technique, and including a question-and-answer period (Gupta et al., 2009). None of the women were practising BSE before the instruction. Two months after the instruction, 53% reported practising BSE regularly. [It is uncertain what regular practice means in just 2 months of alleged practice.] In Lower Saxony, Germany, women invited to instruction sessions received a lecture on BSE techniques followed by individual BSE training by a gynaecologist (Funke et al., 2008). The self-reported prevalence of monthly BSE practice was 21% before the instruction and 62% 1 year after the instruction. Proficiency of BSE practice was not assessed in either of these studies. [It is therefore unclear whether a sufficient number of women in either study practised BSE with sufficient competence and frequency to result in a reduction in mortality from breast cancer.]

In three studies, BSE practice after BSE instruction was compared with BSE practice in a control group that did not receive instruction. In a study in rural women in the Republic of Korea (Lee et al., 2003), women were given BSE instruction after appraisal of their individual risk on the basis of a questionnaire. Three months after the

Table 5.21 Percentage of women who reported practising breast self-examination in surveys conducted in selected countries

Country Reference	Age of participants (years)	Definition of sample	Definition of BSE practice	Number of women	Percentage practising BSE
Africa					
Ethiopia Azage et al. (2013)	16–37	Health extension workers	Regularly	390	14.4%
Nigeria Obaji et al. (2013)	20–65	Market workers	Regularly	238	0.4%
East and South Asia					
Malaysia Rosmawati (2010)	Mean, 40.5 (SD, 15.5)	Rural women	Classified as good	86	7.0%
Malaysia Parsa et al. (2011)	Not given	Teachers	Regular	425	19.0%
Pakistan Sobani et al. (2012)	Mean, 32.4 (SD, 10.9)	Outpatients	Regularly	373	25.9%
Thailand Satitvipawee et al. (2009)	20–64	Rural women	Monthly in past year	705	49.3%
West Asia					
Iraq Alwan et al. (2012)	18–62	Women affiliated with universities	Ever practised	858	53.9%
Islamic Republic of Iran Khalili & Shahnazi (2010)	20–50	Clinic enrollees	Ever practised	400	18.8%
Turkey Güleser et al. (2009)	Mean, 29 (SD, 5.6)	Health-care workers	Monthly	246	17.0%
West Bank and Gaza Strip Azaiza et al. (2010)	30–65	Residents of West Bank	Monthly or more	397	62%
Europe					
Poland Lepecka-Klusek et al. (2007)	22–45	Nursing students, hospital workers, and gynaecological outpatients	Regularly	492	33.7%

BSE, breast self-examination; SD, standard deviation.

instruction, 30.5% of the women reported practising BSE regularly, compared with 10.2% in a control group. In a study of Latinas in the USA (Jandorf et al., 2008), women were randomized to a group receiving information on BSE and CBE or to a control group. Telephone interviews 2 months after the instruction revealed that 45% of the women in the instruction group practised BSE compared with 27% in the control group. [Proficiency was not assessed in either of these studies.] In a BSE instruction programme in Ribe County, Denmark, up to 20 women at a time attended an intensive BSE training session lasting up to 2 hours that included videos as well as individual instruction on breast models and on the women's own breasts (Sørensen et al., 2005). An unreported number of years later (< 5 years), a questionnaire was mailed to the women who had participated and to a sample of women in the county who had not participated; 485 (77%) and 313 (53%) responded, respectively. Women were asked about frequency of BSE practice and whether they practised the various components of the BSE technique that was taught (positioning, use of mirror, and palpation pattern). On the basis of their answers, women were classified as performing BSE correctly, nearly correctly, or partly correctly. A higher percentage of women in the intervention group than in the control group practised BSE monthly (30.7% vs 21.1%) and practised it correctly or nearly correctly (27.6% vs 10.2%).

[The level of BSE practice in women taught BSE in all five of the evaluations of BSE instruction summarized in this section was lower than that in the trial in Shanghai, which showed no reduction in breast cancer mortality from BSE instruction. It is therefore reasonable to conclude that the level of BSE activity that was probably achieved in these studies was insufficient to have a meaningful impact on breast cancer mortality rates in the populations in which they were conducted. All of these studies except one were conducted in developed countries in which women, like the women in the Shanghai trial, had reasonable access to care, and in which women would be expected to seek medical attention for breast symptoms suggestive of breast cancer early in the course of the disease. The study in India may be an exception. In that country, many women with breast cancer typically present with advanced disease. It is unknown whether breast cancer mortality would be reduced if women in that country could be motivated to practise BSE on a regular basis, as was reported in the study by Gupta et al. (2009), and to do so competently.]

5.8.2 Adverse effects

In both randomized trials of BSE, more women in the instruction group than in the control group found breast lumps that required further evaluation and that were subsequently confirmed as not being breast cancer (Section 4.4). In the trial in St Petersburg (Semiglazov et al., 2003), nearly twice as many women were referred for further evaluation in the instruction group than in the control group; in the Shanghai trial, 80% more women in the intervention group than in the control group were found to have a histologically confirmed benign lesion (Thomas et al., 2002). Such false-positives on screening can produce considerable anxiety, and the further evaluation of suspicious findings is not a trivial expense. Given that there is no proven benefit of BSE in reducing mortality from breast cancer, the risk–benefit ratio is very high.

5.8.3 Cost–effectiveness analysis

Given that there is no good evidence that BSE, as it has been reported to be practised in studies to date, contributes to a reduction in mortality from breast cancer, there can be no estimate of the cost per life year gained by practising BSE. Based on data from the study in Ribe County, Denmark, Sørensen & Hertz (2003) estimated the cost per avoided cancer with spread to lymph nodes to be €15 410 and the cost of avoiding a cancerous tumour larger than 20 mm to be €16 318. [In their model, they assumed that there was considerable shift to a lower stage as a result of BSE practice, but as discussed in Section 4.4, the evidence for this is questionable and inconsistent, and the results of their estimates are highly dependent on the assumptions that they made as to the magnitude of the stage shift. They used only the cost of the BSE programme in their model. Their estimates did not take into account the costs of diagnostic confirmation or of changes in treatment if there is a stage shift at the time of diagnosis by BSE practice. If there truly is a stage shift, then this could result in less aggressive and less costly treatment, which would be a benefit even in the absence of a reduction in mortality. However, given the uncertainties as to any beneficial effects of BSE, no meaningful cost–effectiveness estimates are possible.]

References

Aarts MJ, Voogd AC, Duijm LE, Coebergh JW, Louwman WJ (2011). Socioeconomic inequalities in attending the mass screening for breast cancer in the south of the Netherlands – associations with stage at diagnosis and survival. *Breast Cancer Res Treat*, 128(2):517–25. doi:10.1007/s10549-011-1363-z PMID:21290176

Absetz P, Aro AR, Sutton SR (2003). Experience with breast cancer, pre-screening perceived susceptibility and the psychological impact of screening. *Psychooncology*, 12(4):305–18. doi:10.1002/pon.644 PMID:12748969

Adedapo KS, Choudhury PS (2007). Scintimammography screening for recurrent breast cancer in women. *Afr J Med Med Sci*, 36(3):279–82. PMID:18390069

Ahern CH, Shen Y (2009). Cost-effectiveness analysis of mammography and clinical breast examination strategies: a comparison with current guidelines. *Cancer Epidemiol Biomarkers Prev*, 18(3):718–25. doi:10.1158/1055-9965.EPI-08-0918 PMID:19258473

Alderete E, Juarbe TC, Kaplan CP, Pasick R, Pérez-Stable EJ (2006). Depressive symptoms among women with an abnormal mammogram. *Psychooncology*, 15(1):66–78. doi:10.1002/pon.923 PMID:15816053

Alexander FE, Anderson TJ, Brown HK, Forrest AP, Hepburn W, Kirkpatrick AE et al. (1999). 14 years of follow-up from the Edinburgh randomised trial of breast-cancer screening. *Lancet*, 353(9168):1903–8. doi:10.1016/S0140-6736(98)07413-3 PMID:10371567

Allgood PC, Warwick J, Warren RML, Day NE, Duffy SW (2008). A case-control study of the impact of the East Anglian breast screening programme on breast cancer mortality. *Br J Cancer*, 98(1):206–9. doi:10.1038/sj.bjc.6604123 PMID:18059396

Altman DG, Bland JM (2003). Interaction revisited: the difference between two estimates. *BMJ*, 326(7382):219. doi:10.1136/bmj.326.7382.219 PMID:12543843

Alwan N, Al Attar W, Eliessa R, Al-Madfaie Z, Nedal F (2012). Knowledge and practices of women in Iraqi universities on breast self-examination [in Arabic] *East Mediterr Health J*, 18(7):742–8. PMID:22891523

Anttila A, Koskela J, Hakama M (2002). Programme sensitivity and effectiveness of mammography service screening in Helsinki, Finland. *J Med Screen*, 9(4):153–8. doi:10.1136/jms.9.4.153 PMID:12518004

Anttila A, Sarkeala T, Hakulinen T, Heinävaara S (2008). Impacts of the Finnish service screening programme on breast cancer rates. *BMC Public Health*, 8(1):38. doi:10.1186/1471-2458-8-38 PMID:18226204

Aro AR, Pilvikki Absetz S, van Elderen TM, van der Ploeg E, van der Kamp LJ (2000). False-positive findings in mammography screening induces short-term distress – breast cancer-specific concern prevails longer. *Eur J Cancer*, 36(9):1089–97. doi:10.1016/S0959-8049(00)00065-4 PMID:10854941

Ascunce EN, Moreno-Iribas C, Barcos Urtiaga A, Ardanaz E, Ederra Sanz M, Castilla J et al. (2007). Changes in breast cancer mortality in Navarre (Spain) after introduction of a screening programme. *J Med Screen*, 14(1):14–20. doi:10.1258/096914107780154558 PMID:17362566

Austoker J, Ong G (1994). Written information needs of women who are recalled for further investigation of breast screening: results of a multicentre study. *J Med Screen*, 1(4):238–44. PMID:8790528

Autier P, Boniol M (2012). The incidence of advanced breast cancer in the West Midlands, United Kingdom. *Eur J Cancer Prev*, 21(3):217–21. doi:10.1097/CEJ.0b013e328350b107 PMID:22314850

Autier P, Boniol M, Middleton R, Doré JF, Héry C, Zheng T et al. (2011). Advanced breast cancer incidence following population-based mammographic screening. *Ann Oncol*, 22(8):1726–35. doi:10.1093/annonc/mdq633 PMID:21252058

Azage M, Abeje G, Mekonnen A (2013). Assessment of factors associated with breast self-examination among health extension workers in West Gojjam Zone, Northwest Ethiopia. *Int J Breast Cancer*, 2013:814395. doi:10.1155/2013/814395 PMID:24298389

Azaiza F, Cohen M, Awad M, Daoud F (2010). Factors associated with low screening for breast cancer in the Palestinian Authority: relations of availability, environmental barriers, and cancer-related fatalism. *Cancer*, 116(19):4646–55. doi:10.1002/cncr.25378 PMID:20589933

Baines CJ, To T, Wall C (1990). Women's attitudes to screening after participation in the National Breast Screening Study. A questionnaire survey. *Cancer*, 65(7):1663–9. doi:10.1002/1097-0142(19900401)65:7<1663::AID-CNCR2820650735>3.0.CO;2-A PMID:2311075

Baker LH (1982). Breast Cancer Detection Demonstration Project: five-year summary report. *CA Cancer J Clin*, 32(4):194–225. doi:10.3322/canjclin.32.4.194 PMID:6805867

Barratt AL, Les Irwig M, Glasziou PP, Salkeld GP, Houssami N (2002). Benefits, harms and costs of screening mammography in women 70 years and over: a systematic review. *Med J Aust*, 176(6):266–71. PMID:11999259

Barton MB, Morley DS, Moore S, Allen JD, Kleinman KP, Emmons KM et al. (2004). Decreasing women's anxieties after abnormal mammograms: a controlled trial. *J Natl Cancer Inst*, 96(7):529–38. doi:10.1093/jnci/djh083 PMID:15069115

Bassett LW, Hendrick RE, Bassford TL, Butler PF, Carter D, DeBor M et al. (1994). Clinical practice guideline number 13: quality determinants of mammography. AHCPR publication 95-0632. Rockville (MD), USA: Agency for Health Care Policy and Research, US Department of Health and Human Services.

Beahrs OH, Shapiro S, Smart C (1979). Report of the Working Group to Review the National Cancer Institute-American Cancer Society Breast Cancer Detection Demonstration Projects. *J Natl Cancer Inst*, 62(3):639–709. PMID:283293

Beck AT, Ward CH, Mendelson M, Mock J, Erbaugh J (1961). An inventory for measuring depression. *Arch Gen Psychiatry*, 4(6):561–71. doi:10.1001/archpsyc.1961.01710120031004 PMID:13688369

Beckmann KR, Lynch JW, Hiller JE, Farshid G, Houssami N, Duffy SW et al. (2015). A novel case-control design to estimate the extent of over-diagnosis of breast cancer due to organised population-based mammography screening. *Int J Cancer*, 136(6):1411–21. doi:10.1002/ijc.29124 PMID:25098753

Beckmann KR, Roder DM, Hiller JE, Farshid G, Lynch JW (2013). Do breast cancer risk factors differ among those who do and do not undertake mammography screening? *J Med Screen*, 20(4):208–19. doi:10.1177/0969141313510293 PMID:24153439

Beemsterboer PM, Warmerdam PG, Boer R, Borras JM, Moreno V, Viladiu P et al. (1998b). Screening for breast cancer in Catalonia. Which policy is to be preferred? *Eur J Public Health*, 8(3):241–6. doi:10.1093/eurpub/8.3.241

Beemsterboer PM, Warmerdam PG, Boer R, de Koning HJ (1998a). Radiation risk of mammography related to benefit in screening programmes: a favourable balance? *J Med Screen*, 5(2):81–7. doi:10.1136/jms.5.2.81 PMID:9718526

Bekiş R, Derebek E, Balci P, Koçdor MA, Değirmenci B, Canda T et al. (2004). ^{99m}Tc sestamibi scintimammography. Screening mammographic non-palpable suspicious breast lesions: preliminary results. *Nuklearmedizin*, 43(1):16–20. PMID:14978536

Bennett RL, Sellars SJ, Moss SM (2011). Interval cancers in the NHS breast cancer screening programme in England, Wales and Northern Ireland. *Br J Cancer*, 104(4):571–7. doi:10.1038/bjc.2011.3 PMID:21285989

Berg WA, Blume JD, Cormack JB, Mendelson EB, Lehrer D, Böhm-Vélez M et al.; ACRIN 6666 Investigators (2008). Combined screening with ultrasound and mammography vs mammography alone in women at elevated risk of breast cancer. *JAMA*, 299(18):2151–63. doi:10.1001/jama.299.18.2151 PMID:18477782

Berg WA, Madsen KS, Schilling K, Tartar M, Pisano ED, Larsen LH et al. (2011). Breast cancer: comparative effectiveness of positron emission mammography and MR imaging in presurgical planning for the ipsilateral breast. *Radiology*, 258(1):59–72. doi:10.1148/radiol.10100454 PMID:21076089

Berg WA, Madsen KS, Schilling K, Tartar M, Pisano ED, Larsen LH et al. (2012a). Comparative effectiveness of positron emission mammography and MRI in the contralateral breast of women with newly diagnosed breast cancer. *AJR Am J Roentgenol*, 198(1):219–32. doi:10.2214/AJR.10.6342 PMID:22194501

Berg WA, Zhang Z, Lehrer D, Jong RA, Pisano ED, Barr RG et al.; ACRIN 6666 Investigators (2012b). Detection of breast cancer with addition of annual screening ultrasound or a single screening MRI to mammography in women with elevated breast cancer risk. *JAMA*, 307(13):1394–404. doi:10.1001/jama.2012.388 PMID:22474203

Bernardi D, Caumo F, Macaskill P, Ciatto S, Pellegrini M, Brunelli S et al. (2014). Effect of integrating 3D-mammography (digital breast tomosynthesis) with 2D-mammography on radiologists' true-positive and false-positive detection in a population breast screening trial. *Eur J Cancer*, 50(7):1232–8. doi:10.1016/j.ejca.2014.02.004 PMID:24582915

Berrington de González A, Berg CD, Visvanathan K, Robson M (2009). Estimated risk of radiation-induced breast cancer from mammographic screening for young *BRCA* mutation carriers. *J Natl Cancer Inst*, 101(3):205–9. doi:10.1093/jnci/djn440 PMID:19176458

Berrington de González A, Reeves G (2005). Mammographic screening before age 50 years in the UK: comparison of the radiation risks with the mortality benefits. *Br J Cancer*, 93(5):590–6. doi:10.1038/sj.bjc.6602683 PMID:16136033

Berry DA, Cronin KA, Plevritis SK, Fryback DG, Clarke L, Zelen M et al.; Cancer Intervention and Surveillance Modeling Network (CISNET) Collaborators (2005). Effect of screening and adjuvant therapy on mortality from breast cancer. *N Engl J Med*, 353(17):1784–92. doi:10.1056/NEJMoa050518 PMID:16251534

Biesheuvel C, Barratt A, Howard K, Houssami N, Irwig L (2007). Effects of study methods and biases on estimates of invasive breast cancer overdetection with mammography screening: a systematic review. *Lancet Oncol*, 8(12):1129–38. doi:10.1016/S1470-2045(07)70380-7 PMID:18054882

Bijwaard H, Brenner A, Dekkers F, van Dillen T, Land CE, Boice JD Jr (2010). Breast cancer risk from different mammography screening practices. *Radiat Res*, 174(3):367–76. doi:10.1667/RR2067.1 PMID:20726723

Bijwaard H, Dekkers F, van Dillen T (2011). Modelling breast cancer in a TB fluoroscopy cohort: implications for the Dutch mammography screening. *Radiat Prot Dosimetry*, 143(2–4):370–4. doi:10.1093/rpd/ncq468 PMID:21217135

Bjurstam N, Björneld L, Warwick J, Sala E, Duffy SW, Nyström L et al. (2003). The Gothenburg Breast Screening Trial. *Cancer*, 97(10):2387–96. doi:10.1002/cncr.11361 PMID:12733136

Blanks RG, Bennett RL, Patnick J, Cush S, Davison C, Moss SM (2005). The effect of changing from one to two views at incident (subsequent) screens in the NHS breast screening programme in England: impact on cancer detection and recall rates. *Clin Radiol*, 60(6):674–80. doi:10.1016/j.crad.2005.01.008 PMID:16038694

Blanks RG, Bennett RL, Wallis MG, Moss SM (2002). Does individual programme size affect screening performance? Results from the United Kingdom NHS breast screening programme. *J Med Screen*, 9(1):11–4. doi:10.1136/jms.9.1.11 PMID:11943791

Blanks RG, Moss SM, McGahan CE, Quinn MJ, Babb PJ (2000). Effect of NHS breast screening programme on mortality from breast cancer in England and Wales, 1990–8: comparison of observed with predicted mortality. *BMJ*, 321(7262):665–9. doi:10.1136/bmj.321.7262.665 PMID:10987769

Bleyer A, Welch HG (2012). Effect of three decades of screening mammography on breast-cancer incidence. *N Engl J Med*, 367(21):1998–2005. doi:10.1056/NEJMoa1206809 PMID:23171096

Bloom JR, Stewart SL, Napoles AM, Hwang ES, Livaudais JC, Karliner L et al. (2013). Quality of life of Latina and Euro-American women with ductal carcinoma in situ. *Psychooncology*, 22(5):1008–16. doi:10.1002/pon.3098 PMID:22678743

BlueCross BlueShield Association (2013). Breast-specific gamma imaging (BSGI), molecular breast imaging (MBI), or scintimammography with breast-specific gamma camera. *Technol Eval Cent Assess Program Exec Summ*, 28(2):14. PMID:23865107

Bobo JK, Lee NC, Thames SF (2000). Findings from 752,081 clinical breast examinations reported to a national screening program from 1995 through 1998. *J Natl Cancer Inst*, 92(12):971–6. doi:10.1093/jnci/92.12.971 PMID:10861308

Boer R, de Koning HJ, van Oortmarssen GJ, van der Maas PJ (1995). In search of the best upper age limit for breast cancer screening. *Eur J Cancer*, 31(12):2040–3. doi:10.1016/0959-8049(95)00457-2 PMID:8562162

Bolejko A, Zackrisson S, Hagell P, Wann-Hansson C (2013). A roller coaster of emotions and sense – coping with the perceived psychosocial consequences of a false-positive screening mammography. *J Clin Nurs*, PMID:24313329

Bond M, Pavey T, Welch K, Cooper C, Garside R, Dean S et al. (2013a). Systematic review of the psychological consequences of false-positive screening mammograms. *Health Technol Assess*, 17(13):1–170, v–vi. PMID:23540978

Bond M, Pavey T, Welch K, Cooper C, Garside R, Dean S et al. (2013b). Psychological consequences of false-positive screening mammograms in the UK. *Evid Based Med*, 18(2):54–61. doi:10.1136/eb-2012-100608 PMID:22859786

Brédart A, Kop JL, Fall M, Pelissier S, Simondi C, Dolbeault S et al.; Magnetic Resonance Imaging study group (STIC IRM 2005) (2012). Anxiety and specific distress in women at intermediate and high risk of breast cancer before and after surveillance by magnetic resonance imaging and mammography versus standard mammography. *Psychooncology*, 21(11):1185–94. doi:10.1002/pon.2025 PMID:21812069

Brem RF, Rapelyea JA, Zisman G, Mohtashemi K, Raub J, Teal CB et al. (2005). Occult breast cancer: scintimammography with high-resolution breast-specific gamma camera in women at high risk for breast cancer. *Radiology*, 237(1):274–80. doi:10.1148/radiol.2371040758 PMID:16126919

Brem RF, Tabár L, Duffy SW, Inciardi MF, Guingrich JA, Hashimoto BE et al. (2014). Assessing improvement in detection of breast cancer with three-dimensional automated breast US in women with dense breast tissue: the SomoInsight Study. *Radiology*, 274(3):663–73. doi:10.1148/radiol.14132832 PMID:25329763

Brett J, Austoker J (2001). Women who are recalled for further investigation for breast screening: psychological consequences 3 years after recall and factors affecting re-attendance. *J Public Health Med*, 23(4):292–300. doi:10.1093/pubmed/23.4.292 PMID:11873891

Brett J, Austoker J, Ong G (1998). Do women who undergo further investigation for breast screening suffer adverse psychological consequences? A multi-centre follow-up study comparing different breast screening result groups five months after their last breast screening appointment. *J Public Health Med*, 20(4):396–403. doi:10.1093/oxfordjournals.pubmed.a024793 PMID:9923945

Brett J, Bankhead C, Henderson B, Watson E, Austoker J (2005). The psychological impact of mammographic screening. A systematic review. *Psychooncology*, 14(11):917–38. doi:10.1002/pon.904 PMID:15786514

Brewer NT, Salz T, Lillie SE (2007). Systematic review: the long-term effects of false-positive mammograms. *Ann Intern Med*, 146(7):502–10. PMID:17404352

Brewer NT, Weinstein ND, Cuite CL, Herrington JE (2004). Risk perceptions and their relation to risk behavior. *Ann Behav Med*, 27(2):125–30. doi:10.1207/s15324796abm2702_7 PMID:15026296

Brodersen J, Siersma VD (2013). Long-term psychosocial consequences of false-positive screening mammography. *Ann Fam Med*, 11(2):106–15. doi:10.1370/afm.1466 PMID:23508596

Brodersen J, Thorsen H, Cockburn J (2004). The adequacy of measurement of short and long-term consequences of false-positive screening mammography. *J Med Screen*, 11(1):39–44. doi:10.1258/096914104772950745 PMID:15006113

Broeders M, Moss S, Nyström L, Njor S, Jonsson H, Paap E et al.; EUROSCREEN Working Group (2012). The impact of mammographic screening on breast cancer mortality in Europe: a review of observational studies. *J Med Screen*, 19(Suppl 1):14–25. doi:10.1258/jms.2012.012078 PMID:22972807

Broeders MJ, Verbeek AL, Straatman H, Peer PG, Jong PC, Beex LV et al. (2002). Repeated mammographic screening reduces breast cancer mortality along the continuum of age. *J Med Screen*, 9(4):163–7. doi:10.1136/jms.9.4.163 PMID:12518006

Brown ML, Fintor L (1993). Cost-effectiveness of breast cancer screening: preliminary results of a systematic review of the literature. *Breast Cancer Res Treat*, 25(2):113–8. doi:10.1007/BF00662136 PMID:8347843

Bucchi L, Ravaioli A, Foca F, Colamartini A, Falcini F, Naldoni C; Emilia-Romagna Breast Screening Programme (2008). Incidence of interval breast cancers after 650,000 negative mammographies in 13 Italian health districts. *J Med Screen*, 15(1):30–5. doi:10.1258/jms.2008.007016 PMID:18416953

Buchberger W, Niehoff A, Obrist P, DeKoekkoek-Doll P, Dünser M (2000). Clinically and mammographically occult breast lesions: detection and classification with high-resolution sonography. *Semin Ultrasound CT MR*, 21(4):325–36. doi:10.1016/S0887-2171(00)90027-1 PMID:11014255

Buist DS, Porter PL, Lehman C, Taplin SH, White E (2004). Factors contributing to mammography failure in women aged 40–49 years. *J Natl Cancer Inst*, 96(19):1432–40. doi:10.1093/jnci/djh269 PMID:15467032

Bull AR, Campbell MJ (1991). Assessment of the psychological impact of a breast screening programme. *Br J Radiol*, 64(762):510–5. doi:10.1259/0007-1285-64-762-510 PMID:2070180

Bulliard JL, Ducros C, Jemelin C, Arzel B, Fioretta G, Levi F (2009). Effectiveness of organised versus opportunistic mammography screening. *Ann Oncol*, 20(7):1199–202. doi:10.1093/annonc/mdn770 PMID:19282467

Burnside ES, Lin Y, Munoz del Rio A, Pickhardt PJ, Wu Y, Strigel RM et al. (2014). Addressing the challenge of assessing physician-level screening performance: mammography as an example. *PLoS ONE*, 9(2):e89418. doi:10.1371/journal.pone.0089418 PMID:24586763

Carbonaro LA, Azzarone A, Paskeh BB, Brambilla G, Brunelli S, Calori A et al. (2014). Interval breast cancers: absolute and proportional incidence and blinded review in a community mammographic screening program. *Eur J Radiol*, 83(2):e84–91. doi:10.1016/j.ejrad.2013.11.025 PMID:24369953

Carles M, Vilaprinyo E, Cots F, Gregori A, Pla R, Román R et al. (2011). Cost-effectiveness of early detection of breast cancer in Catalonia (Spain). *BMC Cancer*, 11(1):192. doi:10.1186/1471-2407-11-192 PMID:21605383

Carney PA, Miglioretti DL, Yankaskas BC, Kerlikowske K, Rosenberg R, Rutter CM et al. (2003). Individual and combined effects of age, breast density, and hormone replacement therapy use on the accuracy of screening mammography. *Ann Intern Med*, 138(3):168–75. doi:10.7326/0003-4819-138-3-200302040-00008 PMID:12558355

Chen CC, David A, Thompson K, Smith C, Lea S, Fahy T (1996). Coping strategies and psychiatric morbidity in women attending breast assessment clinics. *J Psychosom Res*, 40(3):265–70. doi:10.1016/0022-3999(95)00529-3 PMID:8861122

Chiu SY, Duffy S, Yen AM, Tabár L, Smith RA, Chen HH (2010). Effect of baseline breast density on breast cancer incidence, stage, mortality, and screening parameters: 25-year follow-up of a Swedish mammographic screening. *Cancer Epidemiol Biomarkers Prev*, 19(5):1219–28. doi:10.1158/1055-9965.EPI-09-1028 PMID:20406961

Ciatto S, Houssami N, Bernardi D, Caumo F, Pellegrini M, Brunelli S et al. (2013). Integration of 3D digital mammography with tomosynthesis for population breast-cancer screening (STORM): a prospective comparison study. *Lancet Oncol*, 14(7):583–9. doi:10.1016/S1470-2045(13)70134-7 PMID:23623721

Ciatto S, Miccinesi G, Zappa M (2004b). Prognostic impact of the early detection of metachronous contralateral breast cancer. *Eur J Cancer*, 40(10):1496–501. doi:10.1016/j.ejca.2004.03.010 PMID:15196532

Ciatto S, Visioli C, Paci E, Zappa M (2004a). Breast density as a determinant of interval cancer at mammographic screening. *Br J Cancer*, 90(2):393–6. doi:10.1038/sj.bjc.6601548 PMID:14735182

Cockburn J, De Luise T, Hurley S, Clover K (1992). Development and validation of the PCQ: a questionnaire to measure the psychological consequences of screening mammography. *Soc Sci Med*, 34(10):1129–34. doi:10.1016/0277-9536(92)90286-Y PMID:1641674

Cockburn J, Staples M, Hurley SF, De Luise T (1994). Psychological consequences of screening mammography. *J Med Screen*, 1(1):7–12. PMID:8790480

Coldman A, Phillips N (2013). Incidence of breast cancer and estimates of overdiagnosis after the initiation of a population-based mammography screening program. *CMAJ*, 185(10):E492–8. doi:10.1503/cmaj.121791 PMID:23754101

Coldman A, Phillips N, Wilson C, Decker K, Chiarelli AM, Brisson J et al. (2014). Pan-Canadian study of mammography screening and mortality from breast cancer. *J Natl Cancer Inst*, 106(11):dju261. doi:10.1093/jnci/dju261 PMID:25274578

Collette HJ, Day NE, Rombach JJ, de Waard F (1984). Evaluation of screening for breast cancer in a non-randomised study (the DOM project) by means of a case-control study. *Lancet*, 1(8388):1224–6. doi:10.1016/S0140-6736(84)91704-5 PMID:6144934

Collins LC, Baer HJ, Tamimi RM, Connolly JL, Colditz GA, Schnitt SJ (2007). Magnitude and laterality of breast cancer risk according to histologic type of atypical hyperplasia: results from the Nurses' Health Study. *Cancer*, 109(2):180–7. doi:10.1002/cncr.22408 PMID:17154175

Connor RJ, Boer R, Prorok PC, Weed DL (2000). Investigation of design and bias issues in case-control studies of cancer screening using microsimulation. *Am*

J Epidemiol, 151(10):991–8. doi:10.1093/oxfordjournals.aje.a010143 PMID:10853638

Corsetti V, Houssami N, Ferrari A, Ghirardi M, Bellarosa S, Angelini O et al. (2008). Breast screening with ultrasound in women with mammography-negative dense breasts: evidence on incremental cancer detection and false positives, and associated cost. *Eur J Cancer*, 44(4):539–44. doi:10.1016/j.ejca.2008.01.009 PMID:18267357

Corsetti V, Houssami N, Ghirardi M, Ferrari A, Speziani M, Bellarosa S et al. (2011). Evidence of the effect of adjunct ultrasound screening in women with mammography-negative dense breasts: interval breast cancers at 1 year follow-up. *Eur J Cancer*, 47(7):1021–6. doi:10.1016/j.ejca.2010.12.002 PMID:21211962

Cortesi L, Turchetti D, Marchi I, Fracca A, Canossi B, Rachele B et al. (2006). Breast cancer screening in women at increased risk according to different family histories: an update of the Modena Study Group experience. *BMC Cancer*, 6(1):210. doi:10.1186/1471-2407-6-210 PMID:16916448

CPAC (2013). Report from the Evaluation Indicators Working Group: guidelines for monitoring breast cancer screening program performance, 3rd edition. Toronto: Canadian Partnership Against Cancer. Available from: http://www.cancerview.ca/idc/groups/public/documents/webcontent/guideline_monitoring_breast.pdf.

Cuzick J, Edwards R, Segnan N (1997). Adjusting for non-compliance and contamination in randomized clinical trials. *Stat Med*, 16(9):1017–29. doi:10.1002/(SICI)1097-0258(19970515)16:9<1017::AID-SIM508>3.0.CO;2-V PMID:9160496

D'Orsi CJ, Sickles EA, Mendelson EB, Morris EA et al. (2013). ACR BI-RADS: Breast imaging reporting and data system, Breast Imaging Atlas, 5th edition. Reston (VA), USA: American College of Radiology.

Das B, Feuer EJ, Mariotto A (2005). Geographic association between mammography use and mortality reduction in the US. *Cancer Causes Control*, 16(6):691–9. doi:10.1007/s10552-005-1991-x PMID:16049808

Day N, McCann J, Camilleri-Ferrante C, Britton P, Hurst G, Cush S et al.; Quality Assurance Management Group of the East Anglian Breast Screening Programme (1995). Monitoring interval cancers in breast screening programmes: the East Anglian experience. *J Med Screen*, 2(4):180–5. PMID:8719145

Day NE (1985). Estimating the sensitivity of a screening test. *J Epidemiol Community Health*, 39(4):364–6. doi:10.1136/jech.39.4.364 PMID:4086970

Day NE, Williams DR, Khaw KT (1989). Breast cancer screening programmes: the development of a monitoring and evaluation system. *Br J Cancer*, 59(6):954–8. doi:10.1038/bjc.1989.203 PMID:2736233

de Gelder R, Bulliard JL, de Wolf C, Fracheboud J, Draisma G, Schopper D et al. (2009). Cost-effectiveness of opportunistic versus organised mammography screening in Switzerland. *Eur J Cancer*, 45(1):127–38. doi:10.1016/j.ejca.2008.09.015 PMID:19038540

de Gelder R, Draisma G, Heijnsdijk EA, de Koning HJ (2011b). Population-based mammography screening below age 50: balancing radiation-induced vs prevented breast cancer deaths. *Br J Cancer*, 104(7):1214–20. doi:10.1038/bjc.2011.67 PMID:21364575

de Gelder R, Heijnsdijk EA, van Ravesteyn NT, Fracheboud J, Draisma G, de Koning HJ (2011a). Interpreting overdiagnosis estimates in population-based mammography screening. *Epidemiol Rev*, 33(1):111–21. doi:10.1093/epirev/mxr009 PMID:21709144

de Gelder R, Heijnsdijk EAM, Fracheboud J, Draisma G, de Koning HJ (2015). The effects of population-based mammography screening starting between age 40 and 50 in the presence of adjuvant systemic therapy. *Int J Cancer*, 137(1):165–72. doi:10.1002/ijc.29364 PMID:25430053

de Koning HJ (2000). Breast cancer screening; cost-effective in practice? *Eur J Radiol*, 33(1):32–7. doi:10.1016/S0720-048X(99)00105-9 PMID:10674787

de Koning HJ, Boer R, Warmerdam PG, Beemsterboer PM, van der Maas PJ (1995). Quantitative interpretation of age-specific mortality reductions from the Swedish breast cancer-screening trials. *J Natl Cancer Inst*, 87(16):1217–23. doi:10.1093/jnci/87.16.1217 PMID:7563167

de Koning HJ, van Ineveld BM, de Haes JC, van Oortmarssen GJ, Klijn JG, van der Maas PJ (1992). Advanced breast cancer and its prevention by screening. *Br J Cancer*, 65(6):950–5. doi:10.1038/bjc.1992.199 PMID:1377485

de Koning HJ, van Ineveld BM, van Oortmarssen GJ, de Haes JC, Collette HJ, Hendriks JH et al. (1991). Breast cancer screening and cost-effectiveness; policy alternatives, quality of life considerations and the possible impact of uncertain factors. *Int J Cancer*, 49(4):531–7. doi:10.1002/ijc.2910490410 PMID:1917154

de Moor JS, Partridge AH, Winer EP, Ligibel J, Emmons KM (2010). The role of socioeconomic status in adjustment after ductal carcinoma in situ. *Cancer*, 116(5):1218–25. doi:10.1002/cncr.24832 PMID:20143325

De Morgan S, Redman S, D'Este C, Rogers K (2011). Knowledge, satisfaction with information, decisional conflict and psychological morbidity amongst women diagnosed with ductal carcinoma in situ (DCIS). *Patient Educ Couns*, 84(1):62–8. doi:10.1016/j.pec.2010.07.002 PMID:20696544

De Morgan S, Redman S, White KJ, Cakir B, Boyages J (2002). "Well, have I got cancer or haven't I?" The psycho-social issues for women diagnosed with ductal carcinoma in situ. *Health Expect*, 5(4):310–8. doi:10.1046/j.1369-6513.2002.00199.x PMID:12460220 de Waard F, Collette HJ, Rombach JJ, Baanders-van Halewijn EA, Honing C (1984a). The DOM project for the early detection of breast cancer, Utrecht, The Netherlands. *J Chronic Dis*, 37(1):1–44. doi:10.1016/0021-9681(84)90123-1 PMID:6690457

Demissie K, Mills OF, Rhoads GG (1998). Empirical comparison of the results of randomized controlled trials and case-control studies in evaluating the effectiveness of screening mammography. *J Clin Epidemiol*, 51(2):81–91. doi:10.1016/S0895-4356(97)00243-6 PMID:9474068

Department of Health (2013). Public Health functions to be exercised by NHS England. Service Specification No. 24, Breast Screening Programme. London, UK: Department of Health. Available from: https://www.gov.uk/government/uploads/system/uploads/attachment_data/file/192975/24_Breast_Screening_Programme__service_specification_VARIATION__130422_-NA.pdf.

Derogatis LR, Morrow GR, Fetting J, Penman D, Piasetsky S, Schmale AM et al. (1983). The prevalence of psychiatric disorders among cancer patients. *JAMA*, 249(6):751–7. doi:10.1001/jama.1983.03330300035030 PMID:6823028

DeSantis C, Ma J, Bryan L, Jemal A (2014). Breast cancer statistics, 2013. *CA Cancer J Clin*, 64(1):52–62. doi:10.3322/caac.21203 PMID:24114568

Devi BC, Tang TS, Corbex M (2007). Reducing by half the percentage of late-stage presentation for breast and cervix cancer over 4 years: a pilot study of clinical downstaging in Sarawak, Malaysia. *Ann Oncol*, 18(7):1172–6. doi:10.1093/annonc/mdm105 PMID:17434897

Dibden A, Offman J, Parmar D, Jenkins J, Slater J, Binysh K et al. (2014). Reduction in interval cancer rates following the introduction of two-view mammography in the UK breast screening programme. *Br J Cancer*, 110(3):560–4. doi:10.1038/bjc.2013.778 PMID:24366303

Diebold T, Jacobi V, Scholz B, Hensel C, Solbach C, Kaufmann M et al. (2005). Value of electrical impedance scanning (EIS) in the evaluation of BI-RADS III/IV/V-lesions. *Technol Cancer Res Treat*, 4(1):93–7. PMID:15649092

Dolan NC, Feinglass J, Priyanath A, Haviley C, Sorensen AV, Venta LA (2001). Measuring satisfaction with mammography results reporting. *J Gen Intern Med*, 16(3):157–62. doi:10.1111/j.1525-1497.2001.00509.x PMID:11318910

Domingo L, Blanch J, Servitja S, Corominas JM, Murta-Nascimento C, Rueda A et al. (2013a). Aggressiveness features and outcomes of true interval cancers: comparison between screen-detected and symptom-detected cancers. *Eur J Cancer Prev*, 22(1):21–8. doi:10.1097/CEJ.0b013e328354d324 PMID:22584215

Domingo L, Jacobsen KK, von Euler-Chelpin M, Vejborg I, Schwartz W, Sala M et al. (2013b). Seventeen-years overview of breast cancer inside and outside screening in Denmark. *Acta Oncol*, 52(1):48–56. doi:10.3109/0284186X.2012.698750 PMID:22943386

Doré C, Gallagher F, Saintonge L, Hébert M (2013). Breast cancer screening program: experiences of Canadian women and their unmet needs. *Health Care Women Int*, 34(1):34–49. doi:10.1080/07399332.2012.673656 PMID:23216095

Drossaert CH, Boer H, Seydel ER (2002). Monitoring women's experiences during three rounds of breast cancer screening: results from a longitudinal study. *J Med Screen*, 9(4):168–75. doi:10.1136/jms.9.4.168 PMID:12518007

Duarte GM, Cabello C, Torresan RZ, Alvarenga M, Telles GH, Bianchessi ST et al. (2007). Fusion of magnetic resonance and scintimammography images for breast cancer evaluation: a pilot study. *Ann Surg Oncol*, 14(10):2903–10. doi:10.1245/s10434-007-9476-7 PMID:17632758

Duffy SW (2007). Case-control studies to evaluate the effect of mammographic service screening on mortality from breast cancer. *Semin Breast Dis*, 10(2):61–3. doi:10.1053/j.sembd.2007.09.001

Duffy SW, Agbaje O, Warwick J, Olsen AH, Gabe R, Fielder H et al. (2008). Screening opportunity bias in case-control studies of cancer screening. *J Appl Stat*, 35(5):537–46. doi:10.1080/02664760701835755

Duffy SW, Chen TH, Smith RA, Yen MF, Tabár L (2013). Real and artificial controversies in breast cancer screening. *Breast Cancer Manag*, 2(6):519–28. doi:10.2217/bmt.13.53

Duffy SW, Cuzick J, Tabar L, Vitak B, Chen H-HT, Yen M-F et al. (2002a). Correcting for non-compliance bias in case control studies to evaluate cancer screening programmes. *J R Stat Soc Ser C Appl Stat*, 51(2):235–43. doi:10.1111/1467-9876.00266

Duffy SW, Gabe R (2005). What should the detection rates of cancers be in breast screening programmes? *Br J Cancer*, 92(3):597–600. PMID:15668711

Duffy SW, Parmar D (2013). Overdiagnosis in breast cancer screening: the importance of length of observation period and lead time. *Breast Cancer Res*, 15(3):R41. doi:10.1186/bcr3427 PMID:23680223

Duffy SW, Tabár L, Chen HH, Holmqvist M, Yen MF, Abdsalah S et al. (2002b). The impact of organized mammography service screening on breast carcinoma mortality in seven Swedish counties. *Cancer*, 95(3):458–69. doi:10.1002/cncr.10765 PMID:12209737

Duffy SW, Tabár L, Chen THH, Yen AMF, Gabe R, Smith RA (2007). Methodologic issues in the evaluation of service screening. *Semin Breast Dis*, 10(2):68–71. doi:10.1053/j.sembd.2007.09.003

Duffy SW, Tabar L, Fagerberg G, Gad A, Gröntoft O, South MC et al. (1991). Breast screening, prognostic factors and survival – results from the Swedish two county study. *Br J Cancer*, 64(6):1133–8. doi:10.1038/bjc.1991.477 PMID:1764377

Duffy SW, Tabár L, Olsen AH, Vitak B, Allgood PC, Chen TH et al. (2010). Absolute numbers of lives saved and overdiagnosis in breast cancer screening, from a randomized trial and from the Breast Screening Programme in England. *J Med Screen*, 17(1):25–30. doi:10.1258/jms.2009.009094 PMID:20356942

Duncan AA, Wallis MG (1995). Classifying interval cancers. *Clin Radiol*, 50(11):774–7. doi:10.1016/S0009-9260(05)83218-0 PMID:7489628

Early Breast Cancer Trialists' Collaborative Group (2005). Effects of chemotherapy and hormonal therapy for early breast cancer on recurrence and 15-year survival: an overview of the randomised trials. *Lancet*, 365(9472):1687–717. doi:10.1016/S0140-6736(05)66544-0 PMID:15894097

Eisemann N, Waldmann A, Katalinic A (2013). Epidemiology of breast cancer - current figures and trends. *Geburtshilfe Frauenheilkd*, 73(2):130–5. doi:10.1055/s-0032-1328075 PMID:24771909

Ekeberg Ø, Skjauff H, Kåresen R (2001). Screening for breast cancer is associated with a low degree of psychological distress. *Breast*, 10(1):20–4. doi:10.1054/brst.2000.0177 PMID:14965553

Ellman R, Angeli N, Christians A, Moss S, Chamberlain J, Maguire P (1989). Psychiatric morbidity associated with screening for breast cancer. *Br J Cancer*, 60(5):781–4. doi:10.1038/bjc.1989.359 PMID:2803955

Elmore JG, Armstrong K, Lehman CD, Fletcher SW (2005). Screening for breast cancer. *JAMA*, 293(10):1245–56. doi:10.1001/jama.293.10.1245 PMID:15755947

Elmore JG, Barton MB, Moceri VM, Polk S, Arena PJ, Fletcher SW (1998). Ten-year risk of false positive screening mammograms and clinical breast examinations. *N Engl J Med*, 338(16):1089–96. doi:10.1056/NEJM199804163381601 PMID:9545356

Elting LS, Cooksley CD, Bekele BN, Giordano SH, Shih YCT, Lovell KK et al. (2009). Mammography capacity impact on screening rates and breast cancer stage at diagnosis. *Am J Prev Med*, 37(2):102–8. doi:10.1016/j.amepre.2009.03.017 PMID:19524392

Engholm G, Ferlay J, Christensen N, Bray F, Gjerstorff ML, Klint A et al. (2010). NORDCAN–a Nordic tool for cancer information, planning, quality control and research. *Acta Oncol*, 49(5):725–36. doi:10.3109/02841861003782017 PMID:20491528

Eo JS, Chun IK, Paeng JC, Kang KW, Lee SM, Han W et al. (2012). Imaging sensitivity of dedicated positron emission mammography in relation to tumor size. *Breast*, 21(1):66–71. doi:10.1016/j.breast.2011.08.002 PMID:21871801

Eriksson L, Czene K, Rosenberg L, Humphreys K, Hall P (2013). Possible influence of mammographic density on local and locoregional recurrence of breast cancer. *Breast Cancer Res*, 15(4):R56. doi:10.1186/bcr3450 PMID:23844592

Ernster VL, Ballard-Barbash R, Barlow WE, Zheng Y, Weaver DL, Cutter G et al. (2002). Detection of ductal carcinoma in situ in women undergoing screening mammography. *J Natl Cancer Inst*, 94(20):1546–54. doi:10.1093/jnci/94.20.1546 PMID:12381707

Espasa R, Murta-Nascimento C, Bayés R, Sala M, Casamitjana M, Macià F et al. (2012). The psychological impact of a false-positive screening mammogram in Barcelona. *J Cancer Educ*, 27(4):780–5. doi:10.1007/s13187-012-0349-9 PMID:22477233

Etzioni R, Gulati R, Mallinger L, Mandelblatt J (2013). Influence of study features and methods on overdiagnosis estimates in breast and prostate cancer screening. *Ann Intern Med*, 158(11):831–8. doi:10.7326/0003-4819-158-11-201306040-00008 PMID:23732716

Evans DG, Kesavan N, Lim Y, Gadde S, Hurley E, Massat NJ et al.; MARIBS Group (2014). MRI breast screening in women at an increased risk: cancer detection and survival analysis. *Breast Cancer Res Treat*, 145(3):663–72. doi:10.1007/s10549-014-2931-9 PMID:24687378

Falk RS, Hofvind S, Skaane P, Haldorsen T (2013). Overdiagnosis among women attending a population-based mammography screening program. *Int J Cancer*, 133(3):705–12. doi:10.1002/ijc.28052 PMID:23355313

Feig SA (2007). Auditing and benchmarks in screening and diagnostic mammography. *Radiol Clin North Am*, 45(5):791–800, vi. doi:10.1016/j.rcl.2007.07.001 PMID:17888769

Feig SA, Hendrick RE (1997). Radiation risk from screening mammography of women aged 40–49 years. *J Natl Cancer Inst Monogr*, 22(22):119–24. PMID:9709287

Feinleib M, Zelen M (1969). Some pitfalls in the evaluation of screening programs. *Arch Environ Health*, 19(3):412–5. doi:10.1080/00039896.1969.10666863 PMID:5807744

Feng SS, Sechopoulos I (2012). Clinical digital breast tomosynthesis system: dosimetric characterization. *Radiology*, 263(1):35–42. doi:10.1148/radiol.11111789 PMID:22332070

Ferlay J, Bray F, Steliarova-Foucher E, Forman D (2014). Cancer Incidence in Five Continents, CI5plus. IARC CancerBase No. 9. Lyon, France: International Agency for Research on Cancer. Available from: http://ci5.iarc.fr.

Fielder HM, Warwick J, Brook D, Gower-Thomas K, Cuzick J, Monypenny I et al. (2004). A case-control study to estimate the impact on breast cancer death of the breast screening programme in Wales. *J Med Screen*, 11(4):194–8. doi:10.1258/0969141042467304 PMID:15563774

Fischerman K, Mouridsen HT (1988). Danish Breast Cancer Cooperative Group (DBCG) Structure and results of the organization. *Acta Oncol (Madr)*, 27:593–6. doi:10.3109/02841868809091756

Fisher B, Anderson S, Bryant J, Margolese RG, Deutsch M, Fisher ER et al. (2002). Twenty-year follow-up of a randomized trial comparing total mastectomy, lumpectomy, and lumpectomy plus irradiation for the treatment of invasive breast cancer. *N Engl J Med*, 347(16):1233–41. doi:10.1056/NEJMoa022152 PMID:12393820

Foca F, Mancini S, Bucchi L, Puliti D, Zappa M, Naldoni C et al.; IMPACT Working Group (2013). Decreasing incidence of late-stage breast cancer after the introduction of organized mammography screening in Italy. *Cancer*, 119(11):2022–8. doi:10.1002/cncr.28014 PMID:23504860

Friedewald SM, Rafferty EA, Rose SL, Durand MA, Plecha DM, Greenberg JS et al. (2014). Breast cancer screening using tomosynthesis in combination with digital mammography. *JAMA*, 311(24):2499–507. doi:10.1001/jama.2014.6095 PMID:25058084

Friedlander LC, Roth SO, Gavenonis SC (2011). Results of MR imaging screening for breast cancer in high-risk patients with lobular carcinoma in situ. *Radiology*, 261(2):421–7. doi:10.1148/radiol.11103516 PMID:21900618

Fuchsjaeger MH, Flöry D, Reiner CS, Rudas M, Riedl CC, Helbich TH (2005). The negative predictive value of electrical impedance scanning in BI-RADS category IV breast lesions. *Invest Radiol*, 40(7):478–85. doi:10.1097/01.rli.0000167425.34577.d1 PMID:15973141

Funke L, Krause-Bergmann B, Pabst R, Nave H (2008). Prospective analysis of the long-term effect of teaching breast self-examination and breast awareness. *Eur J Cancer Care (Engl)*, 17(5):477–82. doi:10.1111/j.1365-2354.2007.00889.x PMID:18616506

Gabe R, Tryggvadóttir L, Sigfússon BF, Olafsdóttir GH, Sigurdsson K, Duffy SW (2007). A case-control study to estimate the impact of the Icelandic population-based mammography screening program on breast cancer death. *Acta Radiol*, 48(9):948–55. doi:10.1080/02841850701501725 PMID:18080359

Ganry OF, Peng J, Raverdy NL, Dubreuil AR (2001). Interval cancers in a French breast cancer-screening programme (Somme Department). *Eur J Cancer Prev*, 10(3):269–74. doi:10.1097/00008469-200106000-00011 PMID:11432715

Ganz PA (2010). Quality-of-life issues in patients with ductal carcinoma in situ. *J Natl Cancer Inst Monogr*, 41:218–22. doi:10.1093/jncimonographs/lgq029 PMID:20956834

Gartlehner G, Thaler K, Chapman A, Kaminski-Hartenthaler A, Berzaczy D, Van Noord MG et al. (2013). Mammography in combination with breast ultrasonography versus mammography for breast cancer screening in women at average risk. *Cochrane Database Syst Rev*, 4:CD009632. doi:10.1002/14651858.CD009632.pub2 PMID:23633376

Gierach GL, Ichikawa L, Kerlikowske K, Brinton LA, Farhat GN, Vacek PM et al. (2012). Relationship between mammographic density and breast cancer death in the Breast Cancer Surveillance Consortium. *J Natl Cancer Inst*, 104(16):1218–27. doi:10.1093/jnci/djs327 PMID:22911616

Gilbert FJ, Cordiner CM, Affleck IR, Hood DB, Mathieson D, Walker LG (1998). Breast screening: the psychological sequelae of false-positive recall in women with and without a family history of breast cancer. *Eur J Cancer*, 34(13):2010–4. doi:10.1016/S0959-8049(98)00294-9 PMID:10070302

Giordano L, von Karsa L, Tomatis M, Majek O, de Wolf C, Lancucki L et al.; Eunice Working Group (2012). Mammographic screening programmes in Europe: organization, coverage and participation. *J Med Screen*, 19(Suppl 1):72–82. doi:10.1258/jms.2012.012085 PMID:22972813

Giuliano V, Giuliano C (2013). Improved breast cancer detection in asymptomatic women using 3D-automated breast ultrasound in mammographically dense breasts. *Clin Imaging*, 37(3):480–6. doi:10.1016/j.clinimag.2012.09.018 PMID:23116728

Goldberg D (1978). *Manual of the General Health Questionnaire*. Windsor, UK: National Foundation for Educational Research, Nelson Publishing.

Goldoni CA, Bonora K, Ciatto S, Giovannetti L, Patriarca S, Sapino A et al.; IMPACT Working Group (2009). Misclassification of breast cancer as cause of death in a service screening area. *Cancer Causes Control*, 20(5):533–8. doi:10.1007/s10552-008-9261-3 PMID:19015942

Gommans GM, van der Zant FM, van Dongen A, Boer RO, Teule GJ, de Waard JW (2007). ^{99m}Technetium-sestamibi scintimammography in non-palpable breast lesions found on screening X-ray mammography. *Eur J Surg Oncol*, 33(1):23–7. doi:10.1016/j.ejso.2006.10.025 PMID:17126524

Gøtzsche PC, Jørgensen KJ (2013). Screening for breast cancer with mammography. *Cochrane Database Syst Rev*, 6:CD001877. doi:10.1002/14651858.CD001877.pub5 PMID:23737396

Gøtzsche PC, Nielsen M (2009). Screening for breast cancer with mammography. *Cochrane Database Syst Rev*, 4:CD001877. doi:10.1002/14651858.CD001877.pub3 PMID:19821284

Gram IT, Lund E, Slenker SE (1990). Quality of life following a false positive mammogram. *Br J Cancer*, 62(6):1018–22. doi:10.1038/bjc.1990.430 PMID:2257206

Greenland S, Thomas DC (1982). On the need for the rare disease assumption in case-control studies. *Am J Epidemiol*, 116(3):547–53. PMID:7124721

Groenewoud JH, Otten JD, Fracheboud J, Draisma G, van Ineveld BM, Holland R et al. ; NETB(2007). Cost-effectiveness of different reading and referral strategies in mammography screening in the Netherlands. *Breast*

Cancer Res Treat, 102(2):211–8. doi:10.1007/s10549-006-9319-4 PMID:17004116

Grosse SD (2008). Assessing cost-effectiveness in healthcare: history of the $50,000 per QALY threshold. *Expert Rev Pharmacoecon Outcomes Res*, 8(2):165–78. doi:10.1586/14737167.8.2.165 PMID:20528406

Güleser GN, Unalan D, Akyldz HY (2009). The knowledge and practice of breast self-examination among healthcare workers in Kayseri, Turkey. *Cancer Nurs*, 32(5):E1–7. doi:10.1097/NCC.0b013e3181a2dbd2 PMID:19661791

Gunsoy NB, Garcia-Closas M, Moss SM (2014). Estimating breast cancer mortality reduction and overdiagnosis due to screening for different strategies in the United Kingdom. *Br J Cancer*, 110(10):2412–9. doi:10.1038/bjc.2014.206 PMID:24762956

Gupta SK, Pal DK, Garg R, Tiwari R, Shrivastava AK, Bansal M (2009). Impact of a health education intervention program regarding breast self examination by women in a semi-urban area of Madhya Pradesh, India. *Asian Pac J Cancer Prev*, 10(6):1113–7. PMID:20192594

Haas BM, Kalra V, Geisel J, Raghu M, Durand M, Philpotts LE (2013). Comparison of tomosynthesis plus digital mammography and digital mammography alone for breast cancer screening. *Radiology*, 269(3):694–700. doi:10.1148/radiol.13130307 PMID:23901124

Haas J, Kaplan C, McMillan A, Esserman LJ (2001). Does timely assessment affect the anxiety associated with an abnormal mammogram result? *J Womens Health Gend Based Med*, 10(6):599–605. doi:10.1089/15246090152543184 PMID:11559457

Habbema JD, Wilt TJ, Etzioni R, Nelson HD, Schechter CB, Lawrence WF et al. (2014). Models in the development of clinical practice guidelines. *Ann Intern Med*, 161(11):812–8. doi:10.7326/M14-0845 PMID:25437409

Hafslund B,, Nortvedt MW (2009). Mammography screening from the perspective of quality of life: a review of the literature. *Scand J Caring Sci*, 23(3):539–48. doi:10.1111/j.1471-6712.2008.00634.x PMID:19170959

Hagen AI, Kvistad KA, Maehle L, Holmen MM, Aase H, Styr B et al. (2007). Sensitivity of MRI versus conventional screening in the diagnosis of BRCA-associated breast cancer in a national prospective series. *Breast*, 16(4):367–74. doi:10.1016/j.breast.2007.01.006 PMID:17317184

Hakama M, Auvinen A, Day NE, Miller AB (2007). Sensitivity in cancer screening. *J Med Screen*, 14(4):174–7. doi:10.1258/096914107782912077 PMID:18078561

Hakama M, Holli K, Isola J, Kallioniemi OP, Kärkkäinen A, Visakorpi T et al. (1995). Aggressiveness of screen-detected breast cancers. *Lancet*, 345(8944):221–4. doi:10.1016/S0140-6736(95)90223-6 PMID:7741862

Hakama M, Pukkala E, Heikkilä M, Kallio M (1997). Effectiveness of the public health policy for breast cancer screening in Finland: population based cohort study. *BMJ*, 314(7084):864–7. doi:10.1136/bmj.314.7084.864 PMID:9093096

Hall P, Easton D (2013). Breast cancer screening: time to target women at risk. *Br J Cancer*, 108(11):2202–4. doi:10.1038/bjc.2013.257 PMID:23744280

Hartman AR, Daniel BL, Kurian AW, Mills MA, Nowels KW, Dirbas FM et al. (2004). Breast magnetic resonance image screening and ductal lavage in women at high genetic risk for breast carcinoma. *Cancer*, 100(3):479–89. doi:10.1002/cncr.11926 PMID:14745863

Hauge IH, Pedersen K, Olerud HM, Hole EO, Hofvind S (2014). The risk of radiation-induced breast cancers due to biennial mammographic screening in women aged 50–69 years is minimal. *Acta Radiol*, 55(10):1174–9. doi:10.1177/0284185113514051 PMID:24311702

Haukka J, Byrnes G, Boniol M, Autier P (2011). Trends in breast cancer mortality in Sweden before and after implementation of mammography screening. *PLoS ONE*, 6(9):e22422. doi:10.1371/journal.pone.0022422 PMID:21966354

Heckman BD, Fisher EB, Monsees B, Merbaum M, Ristvedt S, Bishop C (2004). Coping and anxiety in women recalled for additional diagnostic procedures following an abnormal screening mammogram. *Health Psychol*, 23(1):42–8. doi:10.1037/0278-6133.23.1.42 PMID:14756602

Heijnsdijk EA, Warner E, Gilbert FJ, Tilanus-Linthorst MM, Evans G, Causer PA et al. (2012). Differences in natural history between breast cancers in *BRCA1* and *BRCA2* mutation carriers and effects of MRI screening – MRISC, MARIBS, and Canadian studies combined. *Cancer Epidemiol Biomarkers Prev*, 21(9):1458–68. doi:10.1158/1055-9965.EPI-11-1196 PMID:22744338

Heinävaara S, Sarkeala T, Anttila A (2014). Overdiagnosis due to breast cancer screening: updated estimates of the Helsinki service study in Finland. *Br J Cancer*, 111(7):1463–8. doi:10.1038/bjc.2014.413 PMID:25121953

Hellquist BN, Duffy SW, Abdsaleh S, Björneld L, Bordás P, Tabár L et al. (2011). Effectiveness of population-based service screening with mammography for women ages 40 to 49 years: evaluation of the Swedish Mammography Screening in Young Women (SCRY) cohort. *Cancer*, 117(4):714–22. doi:10.1002/cncr.25650 PMID:20882563

Helvie MA, Chang JT, Hendrick RE, Banerjee M (2014). Reduction in late-stage breast cancer incidence in the mammography era: implications for overdiagnosis of invasive cancer. *Cancer*, 120(17):2649–56. doi:10.1002/cncr.28784 PMID:24840597

Hendrick RE (2010). Radiation doses and cancer risks from breast imaging studies. *Radiology*, 257(1):246–53. doi:10.1148/radiol.10100570 PMID:20736332

Hendrick RE, Pisano ED, Averbukh A, Moran C, Berns EA, Yaffe MJ et al. (2010). Comparison of acquisition parameters and breast dose in digital mammography and screen-film mammography in the American

College of Radiology Imaging Network digital mammographic imaging screening trial. *AJR Am J Roentgenol*, 194(2):362–9. doi:10.2214/AJR.08.2114 PMID:20093597

Heyes GJ, Mill AJ, Charles MW (2009). Mammography – oncogenecity at low doses. *J Radiol Prot*, 29:2A: A123–32. doi:10.1088/0952-4746/29/2A/S08 PMID:19454801

Hislop TG, Harris SR, Jackson J, Thorne SE, Rousseau EJ, Coldman AJ et al. (2002). Satisfaction and anxiety for women during investigation of an abnormal screening mammogram. *Breast Cancer Res Treat*, 76(3):245–54. doi:10.1023/A:1020820103126 PMID:12462385

Hofvind S, Bjurstam N, Sørum R, Bjørndal H, Thoresen S, Skaane P (2006). Number and characteristics of breast cancer cases diagnosed in four periods in the screening interval of a biennial population-based screening programme. *J Med Screen*, 13(4):192–6. PMID:17217608

Hofvind S, Geller BM, Skelly J, Vacek PM (2012b). Sensitivity and specificity of mammographic screening as practised in Vermont and Norway. *Br J Radiol*, 85(1020):e1226–32. doi:10.1259/bjr/15168178 PMID:22993383

Hofvind S, Lee CI, Elmore JG (2012c). Stage-specific breast cancer incidence rates among participants and non-participants of a population-based mammographic screening program. *Breast Cancer Res Treat*, 135(1):291–9. doi:10.1007/s10549-012-2162-x PMID:22833199

Hofvind S, Ponti A, Patnick J, Ascunce N, Njor S, Broeders M et al.; EUNICE Project and Euroscreen Working Groups (2012a). False-positive results in mammographic screening for breast cancer in Europe: a literature review and survey of service screening programmes. *J Med Screen*, 19(Suppl 1): 57–66. doi:10.1258/jms.2012.012083 PMID:22972811

Hofvind S, Ursin G, Tretli S, Sebuødegård S, Møller B (2013). Breast cancer mortality in participants of the Norwegian Breast Cancer Screening Program. *Cancer*, 119(17):3106–12. doi:10.1002/cncr.28174 PMID:23720226

Holmberg L, Duffy SW, Yen AMF, Tabár L, Vitak B, Nyström L et al. (2009). Differences in endpoints between the Swedish W-E (two county) trial of mammographic screening and the Swedish overview: methodological consequences. *J Med Screen*, 16(2):73–80. doi:10.1258/jms.2009.008103 PMID:19564519

Hoogerbrugge N, Kamm YJ, Bult P, Landsbergen KM, Bongers EM, Brunner HG et al. (2008). The impact of a false-positive MRI on the choice for mastectomy in *BRCA* mutation carriers is limited. *Ann Oncol*, 19(4):655–9. doi:10.1093/annonc/mdm537 PMID:18096566

Hooley RJ, Greenberg KL, Stackhouse RM, Geisel JL, Butler RS, Philpotts LE (2012). Screening US in patients with mammographically dense breasts: initial experience with Connecticut Public Act 09-41. *Radiology*, 265(1):59–69. doi:10.1148/radiol.12120621 PMID:22723501

Hou N, Huo D (2013). A trend analysis of breast cancer incidence rates in the United States from 2000 to 2009 shows a recent increase. *Breast Cancer Res Treat*, 138(2):633–41. doi:10.1007/s10549-013-2434-0 PMID:23446808

Houssami N, Abraham LA, Miglioretti DL, Sickles EA, Kerlikowske K, Buist DS et al. (2011). Accuracy and outcomes of screening mammography in women with a personal history of early-stage breast cancer. *JAMA*, 305(8):790–9. doi:10.1001/jama.2011.188 PMID:21343578

Houssami N, Abraham LA, Onega T, Collins LC, Sprague BL, Hill DA et al. (2014b). Accuracy of screening mammography in women with a history of lobular carcinoma in situ or atypical hyperplasia of the breast. *Breast Cancer Res Treat*, 145(3):765–73. doi:10.1007/s10549-014-2965-z PMID:24800915

Houssami N, Ciatto S (2011). The evolving role of new imaging methods in breast screening. *Prev Med*, 53(3):123–6. doi:10.1016/j.ypmed.2011.05.003 PMID:21605590

Houssami N, Irwig L, Ciatto S (2006). Radiological surveillance of interval breast cancers in screening programmes. *Lancet Oncol*, 7(3):259–65. doi:10.1016/S1470-2045(06)70617-9 PMID:16510335

Houssami N, Lord SJ, Ciatto S (2009). Breast cancer screening: emerging role of new imaging techniques as adjuncts to mammography. *Med J Aust*, 190(9):493–7. PMID:19413520

Houssami N, Macaskill P, Bernardi D, Caumo F, Pellegrini M, Brunelli S et al. (2014a). Breast screening using 2D-mammography or integrating digital breast tomosynthesis (3D-mammography) for single-reading or double-reading – evidence to guide future screening strategies. *Eur J Cancer*, 50(10):1799–807. doi:10.1016/j.ejca.2014.03.017 PMID:24746887

Houssami N, Skaane P (2013). Overview of the evidence on digital breast tomosynthesis in breast cancer detection. *Breast*, 22(2):101–8. doi:10.1016/j.breast.2013.01.017 PMID:23422255

Howe GR, Sherman GJ, Semenciw RM, Miller AB (1981). Estimated benefits and risks of screening for breast cancer. *Can Med Assoc J*, 124(4):399–403. PMID:7011526

HPA (2011). Risk of solid cancers following radiation exposure: estimates for the UK population. Report of the independent Advisory group on Ionising Radiation. Document HPA RCE-19. London, UK: Health Protection Agency. Available from: http://www.hpa.org.uk.

Hruska CB, Phillips SW, Whaley DH, Rhodes DJ, O'Connor MK (2008). Molecular breast imaging: use of a dual-head dedicated gamma camera to detect small breast tumors. *AJR Am J Roentgenol*, 191(6):1805–15. doi:10.2214/AJR.07.3693 PMID:19020253

Hruska CB, Rhodes DJ, Collins DA, Tortorelli CL, Askew JW, O'Connor MK (2012). Evaluation of molecular breast imaging in women undergoing myocardial perfusion imaging with Tc-99m sestamibi. *J Womens Health (Larchmt)*, 21(7):730–8. doi:10.1089/jwh.2011.3267 PMID:22404787

Huang Y, Kang M, Li H, Li JY, Zhang JY, Liu LH et al. (2012). Combined performance of physical examination, mammography, and ultrasonography for breast cancer screening among Chinese women: a follow-up study. *Curr Oncol*, 19(Suppl 2):eS22–30. doi:10.3747/co.19.1137 PMID:22876165

Hubbard RA, Miglioretti DL, Smith RA (2010). Modelling the cumulative risk of a false positive screening test. *Stat Methods Med Res*, 19(5):429–49. doi:10.1177/0962280209359842 PMID:20356857

Hutton J, Walker LG, Gilbert FJ, Evans DG, Eeles R, Kwan-Lim GE et al.; UK Study Group for MRI Screening in Women at High Risk Study (2011). Psychological impact and acceptability of magnetic resonance imaging and X-ray mammography: the MARIBS Study. *Br J Cancer*, 104(4):578–86. doi:10.1038/bjc.2011.1 PMID:21326245

ICRP (2007). The 2007 recommendations of the International Commission on Radiological Protection. ICRP Publication 103. Ann ICRP. 37(2–4):1–332. doi:10.1016/j.icrp.2007.10.003 PMID:18082557

Independent UK Panel on Breast Cancer Screening (2012). The benefits and harms of breast cancer screening: an independent review. *Lancet*, 380(9855):1778–86. doi:10.1016/S0140-6736(12)61611-0 PMID:23117178

Irvin VL, Kaplan RM (2014). Screening mammography & breast cancer mortality: meta-analysis of quasi-experimental studies. *PLoS ONE*, 9(6):e98105. doi:10.1371/journal.pone.0098105 PMID:24887150

Ishida T, Suzuki A, Kawai M, Narikawa Y, Saito H, Yamamoto S et al. (2014). A randomized controlled trial to verify the efficacy of the use of ultrasonography in breast cancer screening aged 40–49 (J-START): 76 196 women registered. *Jpn J Clin Oncol*, 44(2):134–40. doi:10.1093/jjco/hyt199 PMID:24407835

Jandorf L, Bursac Z, Pulley L, Trevino M, Castillo A, Erwin DO (2008). Breast and cervical cancer screening among Latinas attending culturally specific educational programs. *Prog Community Health Partnersh*, 2(3):195–204. doi:10.1353/cpr.0.0034 PMID:20208198

Jatoi I, Zhu K, Shah M, Lawrence W (2006). Psychological distress in U.S. women who have experienced false-positive mammograms. *Breast Cancer Res Treat*, 100(2):191–200. doi:10.1007/s10549-006-9236-6 PMID:16773439

Jonsson H, Bordás P, Wallin H, Nyström L, Lenner P (2007). Service screening with mammography in Northern Sweden: effects on breast cancer mortality – an update. *J Med Screen*, 14(2):87–93. doi:10.1258/096914107781261918 PMID:17626708

Jonsson H, Johansson R, Lenner P (2005). Increased incidence of invasive breast cancer after the introduction of service screening with mammography in Sweden. *Int J Cancer*, 117(5):842–7. doi:10.1002/ijc.21228 PMID:15957172

Jonsson H, Nyström L, Törnberg S, Lenner P (2001). Service screening with mammography of women aged 50–69 years in Sweden: effects on mortality from breast cancer. *J Med Screen*, 8(3):152–60. doi:10.1136/jms.8.3.152 PMID:11678556

Jonsson H, Nyström L, Törnberg S, Lundgren B, Lenner P (2003a). Service screening with mammography. Long-term effects on breast cancer mortality in the county of Gävleborg, Sweden. *Breast*, 12(3):183–93. doi:10.1016/S0960-9776(03)00031-6 PMID:14659325

Jonsson H, Törnberg S, Nyström L, Lenner P (2000). Service screening with mammography in Sweden – evaluation of effects of screening on breast cancer mortality in age group 40–49 years. *Acta Oncol*, 39(5):617–23. doi:10.1080/028418600750013302 PMID:11093370

Jonsson H, Törnberg S, Nyström L, Lenner P (2003b). Service screening with mammography of women aged 70–74 years in Sweden. Effects on breast cancer mortality. *Cancer Detect Prev*, 27(5):360–9. doi:10.1016/S0361-090X(03)00131-4 PMID:14585323

Jørgensen KJ, Gøtzsche PC (2009). Overdiagnosis in publicly organised mammography screening programmes: systematic review of incidence trends. *BMJ*, 339(1):b2587. doi:10.1136/bmj.b2587 PMID:19589821

Jørgensen KJ, Zahl PH, Gøtzsche PC (2009). Overdiagnosis in organised mammography screening in Denmark. A comparative study. *BMC Womens Health*, 9(1):36. doi:10.1186/1472-6874-9-36 PMID:20028513

Jørgensen KJ, Zahl PH, Gøtzsche PC (2010). Breast cancer mortality in organised mammography screening in Denmark: comparative study. *BMJ*, 340:c1241. doi:10.1136/bmj.c1241 PMID:20332505

José Bento M, Gonçalves G, Aguiar A, Antunes L, Veloso V, Rodrigues V (2014). Clinicopathological differences between interval and screen-detected breast cancers diagnosed within a screening programme in Northern Portugal. *J Med Screen*, 21(2):104–9. doi:10.1177/0969141314534406 PMID:24803482

Junod B, Zahl PH, Kaplan RM, Olsen J, Greenland S (2011). An investigation of the apparent breast cancer epidemic in France: screening and incidence trends in birth cohorts. *BMC Cancer*, 11(1):401. doi:10.1186/1471-2407-11-401 PMID:21936933

Kalager M (2011). Regression of screening-detected breast cancer. *Lancet Oncol*, 12(12):1083–4. doi:10.1016/S1470-2045(11)70262-5 PMID:21996167

Kalager M, Adami HO, Bretthauer M, Tamimi RM (2012). Overdiagnosis of invasive breast cancer due to mammography screening: results from the Norwegian screening program. *Ann Intern Med*, 156(7):491–9. doi:10.7326/0003-4819-156-7-201204030-00005 PMID: 22473436

Kalager M, Zelen M, Langmark F, Adami H-O (2010). Effect of screening mammography on breast-cancer mortality in Norway. *N Engl J Med*, 363(13):1203–10. doi:10.1056/NEJMoa1000727 PMID:20860502

Kalles V, Zografos GC, Provatopoulou X, Koulocheri D, Gounaris A (2013). The current status of positron emission mammography in breast cancer diagnosis. *Breast Cancer*, 20(2):123–30. doi:10.1007/s12282-012-0433-3 PMID:23239242

Kaplan SS (2001). Clinical utility of bilateral whole-breast US in the evaluation of women with dense breast tissue. *Radiology*, 221(3):641–9. doi:10.1148/radiol.2213010364 PMID:11719658

Kelly KM, Dean J, Comulada WS, Lee SJ (2010). Breast cancer detection using automated whole breast ultrasound and mammography in radiographically dense breasts. *Eur Radiol*, 20(3):734–42. doi:10.1007/s00330-009-1588-y PMID:19727744

Kennedy F, Harcourt D, Rumsey N (2008). The challenge of being diagnosed and treated for ductal carcinoma in situ (DCIS). *Eur J Oncol Nurs*, 12(2):103–11. doi:10.1016/j.ejon.2007.09.007 PMID:18023255

Kennedy F, Harcourt D, Rumsey N (2012). The shifting nature of women's experiences and perceptions of ductal carcinoma in situ. *J Adv Nurs*, 68(4):856–67. doi:10.1111/j.1365-2648.2011.05788.x PMID:21790736

Kerlikowske K, Hubbard RA, Miglioretti DL, Geller BM, Yankaskas BC, Lehman CD et al.; Breast Cancer Surveillance Consortium (2011). Comparative effectiveness of digital versus film-screen mammography in community practice in the United States: a cohort study. *Ann Intern Med*, 155(8):493–502. doi:10.7326/0003-4819-155-8-201110180-00005 PMID:22007043

Kerlikowske K, Salzmann P, Phillips KA, Cauley JA, Cummings SR (1999). Continuing screening mammography in women aged 70 to 79 years: impact on life expectancy and cost-effectiveness. *JAMA*, 282(22):2156–63. doi:10.1001/jama.282.22.2156 PMID: 10591338

Kerlikowske K, Zhu W, Hubbard RA, Geller B, Dittus K, Braithwaite D et al.; Breast Cancer Surveillance Consortium (2013). Outcomes of screening mammography by frequency, breast density, and postmenopausal hormone therapy. *JAMA Intern Med*, 173(9):807–16. doi:10.1001/jamainternmed.2013.307 PMID:23552817

Keyzer-Dekker CM, De Vries J, van Esch L, Ernst MF, Nieuwenhuijzen GA, Roukema JA et al. (2012). Anxiety after an abnormal screening mammogram is a serious problem. *Breast*, 21(1):83–8. doi:10.1016/j.breast.2011.08.137 PMID:21924905

Khalili AF, Shahnazi M (2010). Breast cancer screening (breast self-examination, clinical breast exam, and mammography) in women referred to health centers in Tabriz, Iran. *Indian J Med Sci*, 64(4):149–62. doi:10.4103/0019-5359.97355 PMID:22718010

Kim IJ, Kim YK, Kim SJ (2009). Detection and prediction of breast cancer using double phase Tc-99m MIBI scintimammography in comparison with MRI. *Onkologie*, 32(10):556–60. doi:10.1159/000232316 PMID:19816071

King TA, Muhsen S, Patil S, Koslow S, Oskar S, Park A et al. (2013). Is there a role for routine screening MRI in women with LCIS? *Breast Cancer Res Treat*, 142(2):445–53. doi:10.1007/s10549-013-2725-5 PMID:24141896

Klabunde C, Bouchard F, Taplin S, Scharpantgen A, Ballard-Barbash R; International Breast Cancer Screening Network (IBSN) (2001). Quality assurance for screening mammography: an international comparison. *J Epidemiol Community Health*, 55(3):204–12. doi:10.1136/jech.55.3.204 PMID:11160176

Kolb TM, Lichy J, Newhouse JH (2002). Comparison of the performance of screening mammography, physical examination, and breast US and evaluation of factors that influence them: an analysis of 27,825 patient evaluations. *Radiology*, 225(1):165–75. doi:10.1148/radiol.2251011667 PMID:12355001

Korfage IJ, de Koning HJ, Roobol M, Schröder FH, Essink-Bot ML (2006). Prostate cancer diagnosis: the impact on patients' mental health. *Eur J Cancer*, 42(2):165–70. doi:10.1016/j.ejca.2005.10.011 PMID:16326098

Kriege M, Brekelmans CT, Boetes C, Besnard PE, Zonderland HM, Obdeijn IM et al.; Magnetic Resonance Imaging Screening Study Group (2004). Efficacy of MRI and mammography for breast-cancer screening in women with a familial or genetic predisposition. *N Engl J Med*, 351(5):427–37. doi:10.1056/NEJMoa031759 PMID:15282350

Kuhl C, Weigel S, Schrading S, Arand B, Bieling H, König R et al. (2010). Prospective multicenter cohort study to refine management recommendations for women at elevated familial risk of breast cancer: the EVA trial. *J Clin Oncol*, 28(9):1450–7. doi:10.1200/JCO.2009.23.0839 PMID:20177029

Kuhl CK, Schrading S, Leutner CC, Morakkabati-Spitz N, Wardelmann E, Fimmers R et al. (2005). Mammography, breast ultrasound, and magnetic resonance imaging for surveillance of women at high familial risk for breast cancer. *J Clin Oncol*, 23(33):8469–76. doi:10.1200/JCO.2004.00.4960 PMID:16293877

Kuhl CK, Schrading S, Strobel K, Schild HH, Hilgers RD, Bieling HB (2014). Abbreviated breast magnetic resonance imaging (MRI): first postcontrast subtracted images and maximum-intensity projection – a novel approach to breast cancer screening with MRI. *J Clin Oncol*, 32(22):2304–10. doi:10.1200/JCO.2013.52.5386 PMID:24958821

Lampic C, Thurfjell E, Bergh J, Sjödén PO (2001). Short- and long-term anxiety and depression in women recalled after breast cancer screening. *Eur J Cancer*, 37(4):463–9. doi:10.1016/S0959-8049(00)00426-3 PMID:11267855

Lampic C, Thurfjell E, Sjödén PO (2003). The influence of a false-positive mammogram on a woman's subsequent behaviour for detecting breast cancer. *Eur J Cancer*, 39(12):1730–7. doi:10.1016/S0959-8049(02)00451-3 PMID:12888368

Lång K, Andersson I, Rosso A, Tingberg A, Timberg P, Zackrisson S (2015). Performance of one-view breast tomosynthesis as a stand-alone breast cancer screening modality: results from the Malmö Breast Tomosynthesis Screening Trial, a population-based study. *Eur Radiol*, 26(1):184–90. doi:10.1007/s00330-015-3803-3 PMID:25929946

Lash TL, Fox MP, Buist DS, Wei F, Field TS, Frost FJ et al. (2007). Mammography surveillance and mortality in older breast cancer survivors. *J Clin Oncol*, 25(21):3001–6. doi:10.1200/JCO.2006.09.9572 PMID:17548838

Law J, Faulkner K (2001). Cancers detected and induced, and associated risk and benefit, in a breast screening programme. *Br J Radiol*, 74(888):1121–7. doi:10.1259/bjr.74.888.741121 PMID:11777770

Law J, Faulkner K (2002). Two-view screening and extending the age range: the balance of benefit and risk. *Br J Radiol*, 75(899):889–94. doi:10.1259/bjr.75.899.750889 PMID:12466254

Law J, Faulkner K (2006). Radiation benefit and risk at the assessment stage of the UK Breast Screening Programme. *Br J Radiol*, 79(942):479–82. doi:10.1259/bjr/33577478 PMID:16714749

Law J, Faulkner K, Young KC (2007). Risk factors for induction of breast cancer by X-rays and their implications for breast screening. *Br J Radiol*, 80(952):261–6. doi:10.1259/bjr/20496795 PMID:17038413

Lawrence G, O'Sullivan E, Kearins O, Tappenden N, Martin K, Wallis M (2009). Screening histories of invasive breast cancers diagnosed 1989–2006 in the West Midlands, UK: variation with time and impact on 10-year survival. *J Med Screen*, 16(4):186–92. doi:10.1258/jms.2009.009040 PMID:20054093

Leach MO, Boggis CR, Dixon AK, Easton DF, Eeles RA, Evans DG et al.; MARIBS study group (2005). Screening with magnetic resonance imaging and mammography of a UK population at high familial risk of breast cancer: a prospective multicentre cohort study (MARIBS). *Lancet*, 365(9473):1769–78. doi:10.1016/S0140-6736(05)66481-1 PMID:15910949

Lederman D, Zheng B, Wang X, Sumkin JH, Gur D (2011). A GMM-based breast cancer risk stratification using a resonance-frequency electrical impedance spectroscopy. *Med Phys*, 38(3):1649–59. doi:10.1118/1.3555300 PMID:21520878

Lee A, Chang J, Lim W, Kim BS, Lee JE, Cha ES et al. (2012). Effectiveness of breast-specific gamma imaging (BSGI) for breast cancer in Korea: a comparative study. *Breast J*, 18(5):453–8. doi:10.1111/j.1524-4741.2012.01280.x PMID:22897514

Lee CY, Kim HS, Ko IS, Ham OK (2003). Evaluation of a community-based program for breast self-examination offered by the community health nurse practitioners in Korea. *Taehan Kanho Hakhoe Chi*, 33(8):1119–26. PMID:15314358

Lehman CD, Blume JD, Weatherall P, Thickman D, Hylton N, Warner E et al.; International Breast MRI Consortium Working Group (2005). Screening women at high risk for breast cancer with mammography and magnetic resonance imaging. *Cancer*, 103(9):1898–905. doi:10.1002/cncr.20971 PMID:15800894

Lehman CD, Isaacs C, Schnall MD, Pisano ED, Ascher SM, Weatherall PT et al. (2007). Cancer yield of mammography, MR, and US in women at an increased risk: prospective multi-institution breast cancer screening study. *Radiology*, 244(2):381–8. doi:10.1148/radiol.2442060461 PMID:17641362

Leivo T, Sintonen H, Tuominen R, Hakama M, Pukkala E, Heinonen OP (1999). The cost-effectiveness of nationwide breast carcinoma screening in Finland, 1987–1992. *Cancer*, 86(4):638–46. doi:10.1002/(SICI)1097-0142(19990815)86:4<638::AID-CNCR12>3.0.CO;2-H PMID:10440691

León A, Verdú G, Cuevas MD, Salas MD, Villaescusa JI, Bueno F (2001). Study of radiation induced cancers in a breast screening programme. *Radiat Prot Dosimetry*, 93(1):19–30. doi:10.1093/oxfordjournals.rpd.a006407 PMID:11548322

Lepecka-Klusek C, Jakiel G, Krasuska ME, Stanisławek A (2007). Breast self-examination among Polish women of procreative age and the attached significance. *Cancer Nurs*, 30(1):64–8. doi:10.1097/00002820-200701000-00012 PMID:17235223

Lerman C, Daly M, Sands C, Balshem A, Lustbader E, Heggan T et al. (1993). Mammography adherence and psychological distress among women at risk for breast cancer. *J Natl Cancer Inst*, 85(13):1074–80. doi:10.1093/jnci/85.13.1074 PMID:8515494

Lerman C, Trock B, Rimer BK, Boyce A, Jepson C, Engstrom PF (1991a). Psychological and behavioral implications of abnormal mammograms. *Ann Intern Med*, 114(8):657–61. doi:10.7326/0003-4819-114-8-657 PMID:2003712

Lerman C, Trock B, Rimer BK, Jepson C, Brody D, Boyce A (1991b). Psychological side effects of breast cancer screening. *Health Psychol*, 10(4):259–67. doi:10.1037/0278-6133.10.4.259 PMID:1915212

Levine EA, Freimanis RI, Perrier ND, Morton K, Lesko NM, Bergman S et al. (2003). Positron emission mammography: initial clinical results. *Ann Surg Oncol*, 10(1):86–91. doi:10.1245/ASO.2003.03.047 PMID:12513966

Lidbrink E, Levi L, Pettersson I, Rosendahl I, Rutqvist LE, de la Torre B et al. (1995). Single-view screening mammography: psychological, endocrine and immunological effects of recalling for a complete three-view examination. *Eur J Cancer*, 31A(6):932–3. doi:10.1016/0959-8049(95)00017-8 PMID:7646925

Lidgren M, Wilking N, Jönsson B, Rehnberg C (2007). Health related quality of life in different states of breast cancer. *Qual Life Res*, 16(6):1073–81. doi:10.1007/s11136-007-9202-8 PMID:17468943

Lightfoot N, Steggles S, Wilkinson D, Bissett R, Bakker D, Darlington G et al. (1994). The short-term psychological impact of organised breast screening *Curr Oncol*, 1:206–11.

Lindfors KK, O'Connor J, Parker RA (2001). False-positive screening mammograms: effect of immediate versus later work-up on patient stress. *Radiology*, 218(1):247–53. doi:10.1148/radiology.218.1.r01ja35247 PMID:11152810

Lipkus IM, Halabi S, Strigo TS, Rimer BK (2000). The impact of abnormal mammograms on psychosocial outcomes and subsequent screening. *Psychooncology*, 9(5):402–10. doi:10.1002/1099-1611(200009/10)9:5<402::AID-PON475>3.0.CO;2-U PMID:11038478

Lord SJ, Lei W, Craft P, Cawson JN, Morris I, Walleser S et al. (2007). A systematic review of the effectiveness of magnetic resonance imaging (MRI) as an addition to mammography and ultrasound in screening young women at high risk of breast cancer. *Eur J Cancer*, 43(13):1905–17. doi:10.1016/j.ejca.2007.06.007 PMID:17681781

Lowe JB, Balanda KP, Del Mar C, Hawes E (1999). Psychologic distress in women with abnormal findings in mass mammography screening. *Cancer*, 85(5):1114–8. doi:10.1002/(SICI)1097-0142(19990301)85:5<1114::AID-CNCR15>3.0.CO;2-Y PMID:10091796

Lu W, Schaapveld M, Jansen L, Bagherzadegan E, Sahinovic MM, Baas PC et al. (2009). The value of surveillance mammography of the contralateral breast in patients with a history of breast cancer. *Eur J Cancer*, 45(17):3000–7. doi:10.1016/j.ejca.2009.08.007 PMID:19744851

Lund E, Mode N, Waaseth M, Thalabard JC (2013). Overdiagnosis of breast cancer in the Norwegian Breast Cancer Screening Program estimated by the Norwegian Women and Cancer cohort study. *BMC Cancer*, 13(1):614. doi:10.1186/1471-2407-13-614 PMID:24377727

Lynge E, Ponti A, James T, Májek O, von Euler-Chelpin M, Anttila A et al.; ICSN DCIS Working group (2014). Variation in detection of ductal carcinoma in situ during screening mammography: a survey within the International Cancer Screening Network. *Eur J Cancer*, 50(1):185–92. doi:10.1016/j.ejca.2013.08.013 PMID:24041876

Malich A, Boehm T, Facius M, Freesmeyer MG, Fleck M, Anderson R et al. (2001). Differentiation of mammographically suspicious lesions: evaluation of breast ultrasound, MRI mammography and electrical impedance scanning as adjunctive technologies in breast cancer detection. *Clin Radiol*, 56(4):278–83. doi:10.1053/crad.2000.0621 PMID:11286578

Mandelblatt J, Saha S, Teutsch S, Hoerger T, Siu AL, Atkins D et al.; Cost Work Group of the U.S. Preventive Services Task Force (2003). The cost-effectiveness of screening mammography beyond age 65 years: a systematic review for the U.S. Preventive Services Task Force. *Ann Intern Med*, 139(10):835–42. doi:10.7326/0003-4819-139-10-200311180-00011 PMID:14623621

Mandelblatt JS, Cronin KA, Bailey S, Berry DA, de Koning HJ, Draisma G et al.; Breast Cancer Working Group of the Cancer Intervention and Surveillance Modeling Network (2009). Effects of mammography screening under different screening schedules: model estimates of potential benefits and harms. *Ann Intern Med*, 151(10):738–47. doi:10.7326/0003-4819-151-10-200911170-00010 PMID:19920274

Mandelson MT, Oestreicher N, Porter PL, White D, Finder CA, Taplin SH et al. (2000). Breast density as a predictor of mammographic detection: comparison of interval- and screen-detected cancers. *J Natl Cancer Inst*, 92(13):1081–7. doi:10.1093/jnci/92.13.1081 PMID:10880551

Marmot MG, Altman DG, Cameron DA, Dewar JA, Thompson SG, Wilcox M; Independent UK Panel on Breast Cancer Screening (2013). The benefits and harms of breast cancer screening: an independent review. *Br J Cancer*, 108(11):2205–40. doi:10.1038/bjc.2013.177 PMID:23744281

Martín G, Martín R, Brieva MJ, Santamaría L (2002). Electrical impedance scanning in breast cancer imaging: correlation with mammographic and histologic diagnosis. *Eur Radiol*, 12(6):1471–8. doi:10.1007/s00330-001-1275-0 PMID:12042956

Martinez-Alonso M, Vilaprinyo E, Marcos-Gragera R, Rue M (2010). Breast cancer incidence and overdiagnosis in Catalonia (Spain). *Breast Cancer Res*, 12(4):R58. doi:10.1186/bcr2620 PMID:20682042

Mattsson A, Leitz W, Rutqvist LE (2000). Radiation risk and mammographic screening of women from 40 to 49 years of age: effect on breast cancer rates and years of life. *Br J Cancer*, 82(1):220–6. PMID:10638993

McCormack VA, dos Santos Silva I (2006). Breast density and parenchymal patterns as markers of breast cancer risk: a meta-analysis. *Cancer Epidemiol Biomarkers Prev*, 15(6):1159–69. doi:10.1158/1055-9965.EPI-06-0034 PMID:16775176

Meystre-Agustoni G, Paccaud F, Jeannin A, Dubois-Arber F (2001). Anxiety in a cohort of Swiss women participating in a mammographic screening programme.

J Med Screen, 8(4):213–9. doi:10.1136/jms.8.4.213 PMID:11743038

Miltenburg GA, Peeters PH, Fracheboud J, Collette HJ (1998). Seventeen-year evaluation of breast cancer screening: the DOM project, The Netherlands. *Br J Cancer*, 78(7):962–5. doi:10.1038/bjc.1998.609 PMID:9764591

Mittra I, Mishra GA, Singh S, Aranke S, Notani P, Badwe R et al. (2010). A cluster randomized, controlled trial of breast and cervix cancer screening in Mumbai, India: methodology and interim results after three rounds of screening. *Int J Cancer*, 126(4):976–84. PMID:19697326

Møller B, Weedon-Fekjaer H, Hakulinen T, Tryggvadóttir L, Storm HH, Talbäck M et al. (2005). The influence of mammographic screening on national trends in breast cancer incidence. *Eur J Cancer Prev*, 14(2):117–28. doi:10.1097/00008469-200504000-00007 PMID:15785315

Møller P, Borg A, Evans DG, Haites N, Reis MM, Vasen H et al. (2002). Survival in prospectively ascertained familial breast cancer: analysis of a series stratified by tumour characteristics, *BRCA* mutations and oophorectomy. *Int J Cancer*, 101(6):555–9. doi:10.1002/ijc.10641 PMID:12237897

Møller P, Stormorken A, Jonsrud C, Holmen MM, Hagen AI, Clark N et al. (2013). Survival of patients with *BRCA1*-associated breast cancer diagnosed in an MRI-based surveillance program. *Breast Cancer Res Treat*, 139(1):155–61. doi:10.1007/s10549-013-2540-z PMID:23615785

Morrell S, Barratt A, Irwig L, Howard K, Biesheuvel C, Armstrong B (2010). Estimates of overdiagnosis of invasive breast cancer associated with screening mammography. *Cancer Causes Control*, 21(2):275–82. doi:10.1007/s10552-009-9459-z PMID:19894130

Morrison AS, Brisson J, Khalid N (1988). Breast cancer incidence and mortality in the breast cancer detection demonstration project [published erratum appears in J Natl Cancer Inst 1989 Oct 4;81(19):1513]. *J Natl Cancer Inst*, 80(19):1540–7. doi:10.1093/jnci/80.19.1540 PMID:3193469

Moss SM, Cuckle H, Evans A, Johns L, Waller M, Bobrow L; Trial Management Group (2006). Effect of mammographic screening from age 40 years on breast cancer mortality at 10 years' follow-up: a randomised controlled trial. *Lancet*, 368(9552):2053–60. doi:10.1016/S0140-6736(06)69834-6 PMID:17161727

Moss SM, Nyström L, Jonsson H, Paci E, Lynge E, Njor S et al.; Euroscreen Working Group (2012). The impact of mammographic screening on breast cancer mortality in Europe: a review of trend studies. *J Med Screen*, 19(Suppl 1): 26–32. doi:10.1258/jms.2012.012079 PMID:22972808

Mukhtar TK, Yeates DRG, Goldacre MJ (2013). Breast cancer mortality trends in England and the assessment of the effectiveness of mammography screening: population-based study. *J R Soc Med*, 106(6):234–42. doi:10.1177/0141076813486779 PMID:23761583

Munoz D, Near AM, van Ravesteyn NT, Lee SJ, Schechter CB, Alagoz O et al. (2014). Effects of screening and systemic adjuvant therapy on ER-specific US breast cancer mortality. *J Natl Cancer Inst*, 106(11):dju289. doi:10.1093/jnci/dju289 PMID:25255803

Mushlin AI, Kouides RW, Shapiro DE (1998). Estimating the accuracy of screening mammography: a meta-analysis. *Am J Prev Med*, 14(2):143–53. doi:10.1016/S0749-3797(97)00019-6 PMID:9631167

Nagtegaal ID, Allgood PC, Duffy SW, Kearins O, Sullivan EO, Tappenden N et al. (2011). Prognosis and pathology of screen-detected carcinomas: how different are they? *Cancer*, 117(7):1360–8. doi:10.1002/cncr.25613 PMID:21425135

Nagtegaal ID, Duffy SW (2013). Reduction in rate of node metastases with breast screening: consistency of association with tumor size. *Breast Cancer Res Treat*, 137(3):653–63. doi:10.1007/s10549-012-2384-y PMID:23263739

National Quality Management Committee of BreastScreen Australia (2008). BreastScreen Australia National Accreditation Standards. Canberra: BreastScreen Australia.

National Research Council (2006). Health risks from exposure to low levels of ionizing radiation: BEIR VII Phase 2. Washington (DC), USA: National Academies Press.

Nederend J, Duijm LE, Voogd AC, Groenewoud JH, Jansen FH, Louwman MW (2012). Trends in incidence and detection of advanced breast cancer at biennial screening mammography in The Netherlands: a population based study. *Breast Cancer Res*, 14(1):R10. doi:10.1186/bcr3091 PMID:22230363

Nelson HD, Fu R, Goddard K, Mitchell JP, Okinaka-Hu L, Pappas M et al. (2013). Risk assessment, genetic counseling, and genetic testing for BRCA-related cancer: systematic review to update the U.S. Preventive Services Task Force recommendation [Internet]. AHRQ Publication No. 12-05164-EF-1. Rockville (MD), USA: Agency for Healthcare Research and Quality. PMID:24432435

NETB (2014). National evaluation of breast cancer screening in the Netherlands 1990–2011/2012. National Evaluation Team for Breast cancer screening, Thirteenth evaluation report. Erasmus MC, University Medical Center Rotterdam and Radboud University Medical Centre, Nijmegen.

Neumann PJ, Cohen JT, Weinstein MC (2014). Updating cost-effectiveness – the curious resilience of the $50,000-per-QALY threshold. *N Engl J Med*, 371(9):796–7. doi:10.1056/NEJMp1405158 PMID:25162885

NHS (2005). Monitoring NHSBSP standards: a guide for quality assurance reference centres. Version 3.

Available from: http://www.cancerscreening.nhs.uk/breastscreen/publications/monitoring-standards.html.

NHSBSP (2009). NHS Breast Screening Programme Annual Review 2009: Expanding Our Reach. Sheffield, UK: NHS Cancer Screening Programmes.

NICE (2014). National Institute for Health and Care Excellence. Available from: http://www.nice.org.uk/.

Nickson C, Mason KE, English DR, Kavanagh AM (2012). Mammographic screening and breast cancer mortality: a case-control study and meta-analysis. *Cancer Epidemiol Biomarkers Prev*, 21(9):1479–88. doi:10.1158/1055-9965.EPI-12-0468 PMID:22956730

Niëns LM, Zelle SG, Gutiérrez-Delgado C, Rivera Peña G, Hidalgo Balarezo BR, Rodriguez Steller E et al. (2014). Cost-effectiveness of breast cancer control strategies in Central America: the cases of Costa Rica and Mexico. *PLoS ONE*, 9(4):e95836. doi:10.1371/journal.pone.0095836 PMID:24769920

Njor S, Nyström L, Moss S, Paci E, Broeders M, Segnan N et al.; Euroscreen Working Group (2012). Breast cancer mortality in mammographic screening in Europe: a review of incidence-based mortality studies. *J Med Screen*, 19(Suppl 1):33–41. doi:10.1258/jms.2012.012080 PMID:22972809

Njor SH, Garne JP, Lynge E (2013a). Over-diagnosis estimate from The Independent UK Panel on Breast Cancer Screening is based on unsuitable data. *J Med Screen*, 20(2):104–5. doi:10.1177/0969141313495190 PMID:24065032

Njor SH, Olsen AH, Blichert-Toft M, Schwartz W, Vejborg I, Lynge E (2013b). Overdiagnosis in screening mammography in Denmark: population based cohort study. *BMJ*, 346(1):f1064. doi:10.1136/bmj.f1064 PMID:23444414

Norman SA, Russell Localio A, Weber AL, Coates RJ, Zhou L, Bernstein L et al. (2007). Protection of mammography screening against death from breast cancer in women aged 40–64 years. *Cancer Causes Control*, 18(9):909–18. doi:10.1007/s10552-007-9006-8 PMID:17665313

Nyström L, Andersson I, Bjurstam N, Frisell J, Nordenskjöld B, Rutqvist LE (2002). Long-term effects of mammography screening: updated overview of the Swedish randomised trials. *Lancet*, 359(9310):909–19. doi:10.1016/S0140-6736(02)08020-0 PMID:11918907

O'Connor MK, Li H, Rhodes DJ, Hruska CB, Clancy CB, Vetter RJ (2010). Comparison of radiation exposure and associated radiation-induced cancer risks from mammography and molecular imaging of the breast. *Med Phys*, 37(12):6187–98. doi:10.1118/1.3512759 PMID:21302775

O'Connor MK, Phillips SW, Hruska CB, Rhodes DJ, Collins DA (2007). Molecular breast imaging: advantages and limitations of a scintimammographic technique in patients with small breast tumors. *Breast J*, 13(1):3–11. doi:10.1111/j.1524-4741.2006.00356.x PMID:17214787

Obaji N, Elom H, Agwu U, Nwigwe C, Ezeonu P, Umeora O (2013). Awareness and practice of breast self-examination among market women in Abakaliki, South East Nigeria. *Ann Med Health Sci Res*, 3(1):7–12. doi:10.4103/2141-9248.109457 PMID:23634322

Offman J, Duffy SW (2012). National Collation of Breast Interval Cancer Data: Screening years 1st April 2003–31st March 2005. Sheffield, UK: NHS Cancer Screening Programmes. Available from: http://www.cancerscreening.nhs.uk/breastscreen/publications/nhsbsp-occasional-report1203.pdf.

Okonkwo QL, Draisma G, der Kinderen A, Brown ML, de Koning HJ (2008). Breast cancer screening policies in developing countries: a cost-effectiveness analysis for India. *J Natl Cancer Inst*, 100(18):1290–300. doi:10.1093/jnci/djn292 PMID:18780864

Olsen AH, Agbaje OF, Myles JP, Lynge E, Duffy SW (2006). Overdiagnosis, sojourn time, and sensitivity in the Copenhagen mammography screening program. *Breast J*, 12(4):338–42. doi:10.1111/j.1075-122X.2006.00272.x PMID:16848843

Olsen AH, Bihrmann K, Jensen MB, Vejborg I, Lynge E (2009). Breast density and outcome of mammography screening: a cohort study. *Br J Cancer*, 100(7):1205–8. doi:10.1038/sj.bjc.6604989 PMID:19293800

Olsen AH, Lynge E, Njor SH, Kumle M, Waaseth M, Braaten T et al. (2013). Breast cancer mortality in Norway after the introduction of mammography screening. *Int J Cancer*, 132(1):208–14. doi:10.1002/ijc.27609 PMID:22532175

Olsen AH, Njor SH, Vejborg I, Schwartz W, Dalgaard P, Jensen MB et al. (2005). Breast cancer mortality in Copenhagen after introduction of mammography screening: cohort study. *BMJ*, 330(7485):220 doi:10.1136/bmj.38313.639236.82 PMID:15649904

Olsson P, Armelius K, Nordahl G, Lenner P, Westman G (1999). Women with false positive screening mammograms: how do they cope? *J Med Screen*, 6(2):89–93. doi:10.1136/jms.6.2.89 PMID:10444727

Ong G, Austoker J (1997). Recalling women for further investigation of breast screening: women's experiences at the clinic and afterwards. *J Public Health Med*, 19(1):29–36. doi:10.1093/oxfordjournals.pubmed.a024582 PMID:9138214

Ong G, Austoker J, Brett J (1997). Breast screening: adverse psychological consequences one month after placing women on early recall because of a diagnostic uncertainty. A multicentre study. *J Med Screen*, 4(3):158–68. PMID:9368874

Osterø J, Siersma V, Brodersen J (2014). Breast cancer screening implementation and reassurance. *Eur J Public Health*, 24(2):258–63. doi:10.1093/eurpub/ckt074 PMID:23788014

Otten JD, Broeders MJ, Fracheboud J, Otto SJ, de Koning HJ, Verbeek AL (2008). Impressive time-related influence of the Dutch screening programme on breast cancer incidence and mortality, 1975–2006. *Int J Cancer*, 123(8):1929–34. doi:10.1002/ijc.23736 PMID:18688863

Otto SJ, Fracheboud J, Looman CWN, Broeders MJ, Boer R, Hendriks JH et al.; National Evaluation Team for Breast Cancer Screening (2003). Initiation of population-based mammography screening in Dutch municipalities and effect on breast-cancer mortality: a systematic review. *Lancet*, 361(9367):1411–7. doi:10.1016/S0140-6736(03)13132-7 PMID:12727393

Otto SJ, Fracheboud J, Verbeek AL, Boer R, Reijerink-Verheij JC, Otten JD et al.; National Evaluation Team for Breast Cancer Screening (2012b). Mammography screening and risk of breast cancer death: a population-based case-control study. *Cancer Epidemiol Biomarkers Prev*, 21(1):66–73. doi:10.1158/1055-9965.EPI-11-0476 PMID:22147362

Otto SJ, Fracheboud J, Verbeek ALM, Boer R, Reijerink-Verheij JCIY, Otten JDM et al. (2012a). Mammography screening and breast cancer mortality – Response. *Cancer Epidemiol Biomarkers Prev*, 21(5):870–1. doi:10.1158/1055-9965.EPI-12-0235

Paap E, Holland R, den Heeten GJ, van Schoor G, Botterweck AA, Verbeek AL et al. (2010). A remarkable reduction of breast cancer deaths in screened versus unscreened women: a case-referent study. *Cancer Causes Control*, 21(10):1569–73. doi:10.1007/s10552-010-9585-7 PMID:20512656

Paap E, Verbeek AL, Botterweck AA, van Doorne-Nagtegaal HJ, Imhof-Tas M, de Koning HJ et al. (2014). Breast cancer screening halves the risk of breast cancer death: a case-referent study. *Breast*, 23(4):439–44. doi:10.1016/j.breast.2014.03.002 PMID:24713277

Paap E, Verbeek AL, Puliti D, Paci E, Broeders MJ (2011). Breast cancer screening case-control study design: impact on breast cancer mortality. *Ann Oncol*, 22(4):863–9. doi:10.1093/annonc/mdq447 PMID:20924073

Paci E, Duffy SW, Giorgi D, Zappa M, Crocetti E, Vezzosi V et al. (2002). Are breast cancer screening programmes increasing rates of mastectomy? Observational study. *BMJ*, 325(7361):418 doi:10.1136/bmj.325.7361.418 PMID:12193357

Paci E; EUROSCREEN Working Group (2012). Summary of the evidence of breast cancer service screening outcomes in Europe and first estimate of the benefit and harm balance sheet. *J Med Screen*, 19(Suppl 1): 5–13. doi:10.1258/jms.2012.012077 PMID:22972806

Paci E, Giorgi Rossi P (2010). Tailored screening for breast cancer in premenopausal women: not just looking at sensitivity, but aiming to reduce burden. *Womens Health (Lond Engl)*, 6(4):477–9. doi:10.2217/whe.10.32 PMID:20597608

Paci E, Miccinesi G, Puliti D, Baldazzi P, De Lisi V, Falcini F et al. (2006). Estimate of overdiagnosis of breast cancer due to mammography after adjustment for lead time. A service screening study in Italy. *Breast Cancer Res*, 8(6):R68. doi:10.1186/bcr1625 PMID:17147789

Paci E, Warwick J, Falini P, Duffy SW (2004). Overdiagnosis in screening: is the increase in breast cancer incidence rates a cause for concern? *J Med Screen*, 11(1):23–7. doi:10.1258/096914104772950718 PMID:15006110

Padgett DK, Yedidia MJ, Kerner J, Mandelblatt J (2001). The emotional consequences of false positive mammography: African-American women's reactions in their own words. *Women Health*, 33(3–4):1–15. doi:10.1300/J013v33n03_01 PMID:11527098

Palli D, Del Turco MR, Buiatti E, Carli S, Ciatto S, Toscani L et al. (1986). A case-control study of the efficacy of a non-randomized breast cancer screening program in Florence (Italy). *Int J Cancer*, 38(4):501–4. doi:10.1002/ijc.2910380408 PMID:3093391

Palli D, Rosselli del Turco M, Buiatti E, Ciatto S, Crocetti E, Paci E (1989). Time interval since last test in a breast cancer screening programme: a case-control study in Italy. *J Epidemiol Community Health*, 43(3):241–8. doi:10.1136/jech.43.3.241 PMID:2607303

Parsa P, Kandiah M, Parsa N (2011). Factors associated with breast self-examination among Malaysian women teachers. *East Mediterr Health J*, 17(6):509–16. PMID:21796969

Parvinen I, Helenius H, Pylkkänen L, Anttila A, Immonen-Räihä P, Kauhava L et al. (2006). Service screening mammography reduces breast cancer mortality among elderly women in Turku. *J Med Screen*, 13(1):34–40. doi:10.1258/096914106776179845 PMID:16569304

Passaperuma K, Warner E, Causer PA, Hill KA, Messner S, Wong JW et al. (2012). Long-term results of screening with magnetic resonance imaging in women with *BRCA* mutations. *Br J Cancer*, 107(1):24–30. doi:10.1038/bjc.2012.204 PMID:22588560

Pataky R, Phillips N, Peacock S, Coldman AJ (2014). Cost-effectiveness of population-based mammography screening strategies by age range and frequency. *J Cancer Policy*, 2(4):97–102. doi:10.1016/j.jcpo.2014.09.001

Peer PG, Werre JM, Mravunac M, Hendriks JH, Holland R, Verbeek AL (1995). Effect on breast cancer mortality of biennial mammographic screening of women under age 50. *Int J Cancer*, 60(6):808–11. doi:10.1002/ijc.2910600614 PMID:7896450

Peeters PH, Verbeek AL, Hendriks JH, van Bon MJ (1989a). Screening for breast cancer in Nijmegen. Report of 6 screening rounds, 1975–1986. *Int J Cancer*, 43(2):226–30. doi:10.1002/ijc.2910430209 PMID:2917799

Peeters PH, Verbeek AL, Straatman H, Holland R, Hendriks JH, Mravunac M et al. (1989b). Evaluation of overdiagnosis of breast cancer in screening with mammography: results of the Nijmegen programme.

Int J Epidemiol, 18(2):295–9. doi:10.1093/ije/18.2.295 PMID:2788627

Perry N, Broeders M, de Wolf C, Törnberg S, Holland R, von Karsa L (2008). European guidelines for quality assurance in breast cancer screening and diagnosis. Fourth edition - summary document. *Ann Oncol*, 19(4):614–22. doi:10.1093/annonc/mdm481 PMID:18024988

Perry N, Broeders M, de Wolf C, Törnberg S, Holland R, von Karsa L et al., editors (2006). European guidelines for quality assurance in breast cancer screening and diagnosis. Fourth edition. Luxembourg: European Commission, Office for Official Publications of the European Communities; pp. 15–56. Available from: http://ec.europa.eu/health/ph_projects/2002/cancer/cancer_2002_01_en.htm.

Peto R, Davies C, Godwin J, Gray R, Pan HC, Clarke M et al.; Early Breast Cancer Trialists' Collaborative Group (EBCTCG) (2012). Comparisons between different polychemotherapy regimens for early breast cancer: meta-analyses of long-term outcome among 100,000 women in 123 randomised trials. *Lancet*, 379(9814):432–44. doi:10.1016/S0140-6736(11)61625-5 PMID:22152853

Phi X-A, Houssami N, Obdeijn I-M, Warner E, Sardanelli F, Leach MO et al. (2014). Magnetic resonance imaging improves breast screening sensitivity in *BRCA* mutation carriers age ≥ 50 years: evidence from an individual patient data meta-analysis. *J Clin Oncol*, 33(4):349–56. doi:10.1200/JCO.2014.56.6232 PMID:25534390

Pijpe A, Andrieu N, Easton DF, Kesminiene A, Cardis E, Noguès C et al.; GENEPSO; EMBRACE; HEBON (2012). Exposure to diagnostic radiation and risk of breast cancer among carriers of *BRCA1/2* mutations: retrospective cohort study (GENE-RAD-RISK). *BMJ*, 345:e5660. doi:10.1136/bmj.e5660 PMID:22956590

Pisani P, Parkin DM, Ngelangel C, Esteban D, Gibson L, Munson M et al. (2006). Outcome of screening by clinical examination of the breast in a trial in the Philippines. *Int J Cancer*, 118(1):149–54. doi:10.1002/ijc.21343 PMID:16049976

Pisano ED, Earp JA, Gallant TL (1998). Screening mammography behavior after a false positive mammogram. *Cancer Detect Prev*, 22(2):161–7. doi:10.1046/j.1525-1500.1998.CDOA21.x PMID:9544437

Pisano ED, Hendrick RE, Yaffe MJ, Baum JK, Acharyya S, Cormack JB et al.; DMIST Investigators Group (2008). Diagnostic accuracy of digital versus film mammography: exploratory analysis of selected population subgroups in DMIST. *Radiology*, 246(2):376–83. doi:10.1148/radiol.2461070200 PMID:18227537

Port ER, Park A, Borgen PI, Morris E, Montgomery LL (2007). Results of MRI screening for breast cancer in high-risk patients with LCIS and atypical hyperplasia. *Ann Surg Oncol*, 14(3):1051–7. doi:10.1245/s10434-006-9195-5 PMID:17206485

Preston DL, Ron E, Tokuoka S, Funamoto S, Nishi N, Soda M et al. (2007). Solid cancer incidence in atomic bomb survivors: 1958–1998. *Radiat Res*, 168(1):1–64. doi:10.1667/RR0763.1 PMID:17722996

Prinjha S, Evans J, McPherson A (2006). Women's information needs about ductal carcinoma in situ before mammographic screening and after diagnosis: a qualitative study. *J Med Screen*, 13(3):110–4. doi:10.1258/096914106778440581 PMID:17007650

Puliti D, Duffy SW, Miccinesi G, de Koning H, Lynge E, Zappa M et al.; EUROSCREEN Working Group (2012). Overdiagnosis in mammographic screening for breast cancer in Europe: a literature review. *J Med Screen*, 19(Suppl 1):42–56. doi:10.1258/jms.2012.012082 PMID:22972810

Puliti D, Miccinesi G, Collina N, De Lisi V, Federico M, Ferretti S et al.; IMPACT Working Group (2008). Effectiveness of service screening: a case-control study to assess breast cancer mortality reduction. *Br J Cancer*, 99(3):423–7. doi:10.1038/sj.bjc.6604532 PMID:18665188

Puliti D, Zappa M (2012). Breast cancer screening: are we seeing the benefit? *BMC Med*, 10(1):106. doi:10.1186/1741-7015-10-106 PMID:22995098

Puliti D, Zappa M, Miccinesi G, Falini P, Crocetti E, Paci E (2009). An estimate of overdiagnosis 15 years after the start of mammographic screening in Florence. *Eur J Cancer*, 45(18):3166–71. doi:10.1016/j.ejca.2009.06.014 PMID:19879130

Ramos M, Ferrer S, Villaescusa JI, Verdú G, Salas MD, Cuevas MD (2005). Use of risk projection models to estimate mortality and incidence from radiation-induced breast cancer in screening programs. *Phys Med Biol*, 50(3):505–20. doi:10.1088/0031-9155/50/3/008 PMID:15773726

Raylman RR, Majewski S, Wojcik R, Weisenberger AG, Kross B, Popov V et al. (2000). The potential role of positron emission mammography for detection of breast cancer. A phantom study. *Med Phys*, 27(8):1943–54. doi:10.1118/1.1287439 PMID:10984240

Renart-Vicens G, Puig-Vives M, Albanell J, Castañer F, Ferrer J, Carreras M et al. (2014). Evaluation of the interval cancer rate and its determinants on the Girona Health Region's early breast cancer detection program. *BMC Cancer*, 14(1):558. doi:10.1186/1471-2407-14-558 PMID:25085350

Rhodes DJ, Hruska CB, Phillips SW, Whaley DH, O'Connor MK (2011). Dedicated dual-head gamma imaging for breast cancer screening in women with mammographically dense breasts. *Radiology*, 258(1):106–18. doi:10.1148/radiol.10100625 PMID:21045179

Rhodes DJ, O'Connor MK, Phillips SW, Smith RL, Collins DA (2005). Molecular breast imaging: a new technique using technetium Tc 99m scintimammography to detect small tumors of the breast. *Mayo Clin Proc*, 80(1):24–30. doi:10.1016/S0025-6196(11)62953-4 PMID:15667025

Rickels K, Garcia CR, Lipman RS, Derogatis LR, Fisher EL (1976). The Hopkins Symptom Checklist. Assessing emotional distress in obstetric-gynecologic practice. *Prim Care*, 3(4):751–64. PMID:1051525

Riedl CC, Ponhold L, Flöry D, Weber M, Kroiss R, Wagner T et al. (2007). Magnetic resonance imaging of the breast improves detection of invasive cancer, preinvasive cancer, and premalignant lesions during surveillance of women at high risk for breast cancer. *Clin Cancer Res*, 13(20):6144–52. doi:10.1158/1078-0432.CCR-07-1270 PMID:17947480

Rijnsburger AJ, Obdeijn IM, Kaas R, Tilanus-Linthorst MM, Boetes C, Loo CE et al. (2010). *BRCA1*-associated breast cancers present differently from *BRCA2*-associated and familial cases: long-term follow-up of the Dutch MRISC Screening Study. *J Clin Oncol*, 28(36):5265–73. doi:10.1200/JCO.2009.27.2294 PMID: 21079137

Rijnsburger AJ, van Oortmarssen GJ, Boer R, Draisma G, To T, Miller AB et al. (2004). Mammography benefit in the Canadian National Breast Screening Study-2: a model evaluation. *Int J Cancer*, 110(5):756–62. doi:10.1002/ijc.20143 PMID:15146566

Rimer BK, Bluman LG (1997). The psychosocial consequences of mammography. *J Natl Cancer Inst Monogr*, (22):131–8. PMID:9709289

Roder D, Houssami N, Farshid G, Gill G, Luke C, Downey P et al. (2008). Population screening and intensity of screening are associated with reduced breast cancer mortality: evidence of efficacy of mammography screening in Australia. *Breast Cancer Res Treat*, 108(3):409–16. doi:10.1007/s10549-007-9609-5 PMID:18351455

Roeke T, van Bommel AC, Gaillard-Hemmink MP, Hartgrink HH, Mesker WE, Tollenaar RA (2014). The additional cancer yield of clinical breast examination in screening of women at hereditary increased risk of breast cancer: a systematic review. *Breast Cancer Res Treat*, 147(1):15–23. doi:10.1007/s10549-014-3074-8 PMID:25104440

Román M, Hubbard RA, Sebuodegard S, Miglioretti DL, Castells X, Hofvind S (2013). The cumulative risk of false-positive results in the Norwegian Breast Cancer Screening Program: updated results. *Cancer*, 119(22):3952–8. doi:10.1002/cncr.28320 PMID:23963877

Román R, Sala M, Salas D, Ascunce N, Zubizarreta R, Castells X; Cumulative False Positive Risk Group (2012). Effect of protocol-related variables and women's characteristics on the cumulative false-positive risk in breast cancer screening. *Ann Oncol*, 23(1):104–11. doi:10.1093/annonc/mdr032 PMID:21430183

Rose SL, Tidwell AL, Bujnoch LJ, Kushwaha AC, Nordmann AS, Sexton R Jr (2013). Implementation of breast tomosynthesis in a routine screening practice: an observational study. *AJR Am J Roentgenol*, 200(6):1401–8. doi:10.2214/AJR.12.9672 PMID:23701081

Rosmawati NH (2010). Knowledge, attitudes and practice of breast self-examination among women in a suburban area in Terengganu, Malaysia. *Asian Pac J Cancer Prev*, 11(6):1503–8. PMID:21338188

Salz T, Richman AR, Brewer NT (2010). Meta-analyses of the effect of false-positive mammograms on generic and specific psychosocial outcomes. *Psychooncology*, 19(10):1026–34. doi:10.1002/pon.1676 PMID:20882572

Sandin B, Chorot P, Valiente RM, Lostao L, Santed MA (2002). Adverse psychological effects in women attending a second-stage breast cancer screening. *J Psychosom Res*, 52(5):303–9. doi:10.1016/S0022-3999(01)00227-6 PMID:12023127

Sankaranarayanan R, Ramadas K, Thara S, Muwonge R, Prabhakar J, Augustine P et al. (2011). Clinical breast examination: preliminary results from a cluster randomized controlled trial in India. *J Natl Cancer Inst*, 103(19):1476–80. doi:10.1093/jnci/djr304 PMID:21862730

Sardanelli F, Podo F, D'Agnolo G, Verdecchia A, Santaquilani M, Musumeci R et al.; High Breast Cancer Risk Italian Trial (2007). Multicenter comparative multimodality surveillance of women at genetic-familial high risk for breast cancer (HIBCRIT study): interim results. *Radiology*, 242(3):698–715. doi:10.1148/radiol.2423051965 PMID:17244718

Sardanelli F, Podo F, Santoro F, Manoukian S, Bergonzi S, Trecate G et al.; High Breast Cancer Risk Italian 1 (HIBCRIT-1) Study (2011). Multicenter surveillance of women at high genetic breast cancer risk using mammography, ultrasonography, and contrast-enhanced magnetic resonance imaging (the High Breast Cancer Risk Italian 1 study): final results. *Invest Radiol*, 46(2):94–105. doi:10.1097/RLI.0b013e3181f3fcdf PMID:21139507

Sarkeala T, Heinävaara S, Anttila A (2008a). Organised mammography screening reduces breast cancer mortality: a cohort study from Finland. *Int J Cancer*, 122(3):614–9. doi:10.1002/ijc.23070 PMID:17847022

Sarkeala T, Heinävaara S, Anttila A (2008b). Breast cancer mortality with varying invitational policies in organised mammography. *Br J Cancer*, 98(3):641–5. doi:10.1038/sj.bjc.6604203 PMID:18231108

Sarvazyan A, Egorov V, Son JS, Kaufman CS (2008). Cost-effective screening for breast cancer worldwide: current state and future directions. *Breast Cancer (Auckl)*, 1:91–9. PMID:19578481

Satitvipawee P, Promthet SS, Pitiphat W, Kalampakorn S, Parkin DM (2009). Factors associated with breast self-examination among Thai women living in rural areas in Northeastern Thailand. *J Med Assoc Thai*, 92(Suppl 7):S29–35. PMID:20235356

Saunders CM, Peters G, Longman G, Thomson J, Taylor D, Hua J et al. (2009). A pilot study of trimodality breast imaging surveillance in young women at high risk of breast cancer in Western Australia. *Med J Aust*, 191(6):330–3. PMID:19769556

Scaf-Klomp W, Sanderman R, van de Wiel HB, Otter R, van den Heuvel WJ (1997). Distressed or relieved? Psychological side effects of breast cancer screening in The Netherlands. *J Epidemiol Community Health*, 51(6):705–10. doi:10.1136/jech.51.6.705 PMID:9519137

Schilling K (2012). Positron emission mammography: better than magnetic resonance mammography? *Eur J Radiol*, 81(Suppl 1):S139–41. doi:10.1016/S0720-048X(12)70058-X PMID:23083565

Schilling K, Narayanan D, Kalinyak JE, The J, Velasquez MV, Kahn S et al. (2011). Positron emission mammography in breast cancer presurgical planning: comparisons with magnetic resonance imaging. *Eur J Nucl Med Mol Imaging*, 38(1):23–36. doi:10.1007/s00259-010-1588-9 PMID:20871992

Schmutzler RK, Rhiem K, Breuer P, Wardelmann E, Lehnert M, Coburger S et al. (2006). Outcome of a structured surveillance programme in women with a familial predisposition for breast cancer. *Eur J Cancer Prev*, 15(6):483–9. doi:10.1097/01.cej.0000220624.70234.14 PMID:17106326

Schou Bredal I, Kåresen R, Skaane P, Engelstad KS, Ekeberg Ø (2013). Recall mammography and psychological distress. *Eur J Cancer*, 49(4):805–11. doi:10.1016/j.ejca.2012.09.001 PMID:23021930

Schousboe JT, Kerlikowske K, Loh A, Cummings SR (2011). Personalizing mammography by breast density and other risk factors for breast cancer: analysis of health benefits and cost-effectiveness. *Ann Intern Med*, 155(1):10–20. doi:10.7326/0003-4819-155-1-201107050-00003 PMID:21727289

Seigneurin A, François O, Labarère J, Oudeville P, Monlong J, Colonna M (2011). Overdiagnosis from non-progressive cancer detected by screening mammography: stochastic simulation study with calibration to population based registry data. *BMJ*, 343:d7017. doi:10.1136/bmj.d7017 PMID:22113564

Semiglazov VF, Manikhas AG, Moiseenko VM, Protsenko SA, Kharikova RS, Seleznev IK et al. (2003). Results of a prospective randomized investigation [Russia (St Petersburg)/WHO] to evaluate the significance of self-examination for the early detection of breast cancer [in Russian]. *Vopr Onkol*, 49(4):434–41. PMID:14569932

Sharma R, Tripathi M, Panwar P, Chuttani K, Jaimini A, Maitra S et al. (2009). ^{99m}Tc-methionine scintimammography in the evaluation of breast cancer. *Nucl Med Commun*, 30(5):338–42. doi:10.1097/MNM.0b013e32832999dc PMID:19282793

Shkumat NA, Springer A, Walker CM, Rohren EM, Yang WT, Adrada BE et al. (2011). Investigating the limit of detectability of a positron emission mammography device: a phantom study. *Med Phys*, 38(9):5176–85. doi:10.1118/1.3627149 PMID:21978062

Skaane P (2009). Studies comparing screen-film mammography and full-field digital mammography in breast cancer screening: updated review. *Acta Radiol*, 50(1):3–14. doi:10.1080/02841850802563269 PMID:19037825

Skaane P, Bandos AI, Eben EB, Jebsen IN, Krager M, Haakenaasen U et al. (2014). Two-view digital breast tomosynthesis screening with synthetically reconstructed projection images: comparison with digital breast tomosynthesis with full-field digital mammographic images. *Radiology*, 271(3):655–63. doi:10.1148/radiol.13131391 PMID:24484063

Skaane P, Bandos AI, Gullien R, Eben EB, Ekseth U, Haakenaasen U et al. (2013a). Comparison of digital mammography alone and digital mammography plus tomosynthesis in a population-based screening program. *Radiology*, 267(1):47–56. doi:10.1148/radiol.12121373 PMID:23297332

Skaane P, Bandos AI, Gullien R, Eben EB, Ekseth U, Haakenaasen U et al. (2013b). Prospective trial comparing full-field digital mammography (FFDM) versus combined FFDM and tomosynthesis in a population-based screening programme using independent double reading with arbitration. *Eur Radiol*, 23(8):2061–71. doi:10.1007/s00330-013-2820-3 PMID:23553585

Smith RA, Duffy SW, Gabe R, Tabár L, Yen AM, Chen TH (2004). The randomized trials of breast cancer screening: what have we learned? *Radiol Clin North Am*, 42(5):793–806, v. doi:10.1016/j.rcl.2004.06.014 PMID:15337416

Smith-Bindman R, Ballard-Barbash R, Miglioretti DL, Patnick J, Kerlikowske K (2005). Comparing the performance of mammography screening in the USA and the UK. *J Med Screen*, 12(1):50–4. doi:10.1258/0969141053279130 PMID:15814020

Sobani ZU, Saeed Z, Baloch HN, Majeed A, Chaudry S, Sheikh A et al. (2012). Knowledge attitude and practices among urban women of Karachi, Pakistan, regarding breast cancer. *J Pak Med Assoc*, 62(11):1259–64. PMID:23866428

Solbjør M, Forsmo S, Skolbekken JA, Sætnan AR (2011). Experiences of recall after mammography screening – a qualitative study. *Health Care Women Int*, 32(11):1009–27. doi:10.1080/07399332.2011.565530 PMID:21978146

Sørensen J, Hertz A (2003). Cost-effectiveness of a systematic training programme in breast self-examination. *Eur J Cancer Prev*, 12(4):289–94. doi:10.1097/00008469-200308000-00008 PMID:12883381

Sørensen J, Hertz A, Gudex C (2005). Evaluation of a Danish teaching program in breast self-examination. *Cancer Nurs*, 28(2):141–7. PMID:15815184

Spanu A, Chessa F, Meloni GB, Sanna D, Cottu P, Manca A et al. (2008). The role of planar scintimammography with high-resolution dedicated breast camera in the diagnosis of primary breast cancer. *Clin Nucl Med*, 33(11):739–42. doi:10.1097/RLU.0b013e318187ee75 PMID:18936602

Spanu A, Chessa F, Sanna D, Cottu P, Manca A, Nuvoli S et al. (2009). Scintimammography with a high resolution dedicated breast camera in comparison with SPECT/CT in primary breast cancer detection. *Q J Nucl Med Mol Imaging*, 53(3):271–80. PMID:18596669

Spanu A, Cottu P, Manca A, Chessa F, Sanna D, Madeddu G (2007). Scintimammography with dedicated breast camera in unifocal and multifocal/multicentric primary breast cancer detection: a comparative study with SPECT. *Int J Oncol*, 31(2):369–77. PMID:17611694

Spanu A, Sanna D, Chessa F, Manca A, Cottu P, Fancellu A et al. (2012). The clinical impact of breast scintigraphy acquired with a breast specific γ-camera (BSGC) in the diagnosis of breast cancer: incremental value versus mammography. *Int J Oncol*, 41(2):483–9. PMID:22641247

Spielberger C, Gorsuch R, Luchene R (1970). *Manual for the State Trait Anxiety Inventory*. Palo Alto (CA), USA: Consulting Psychologists Press.

Sprague BL, Stout NK, Schechter C, van Ravesteyn NT, Cevik M, Alagoz O et al. (2015). Benefits, harms, and cost-effectiveness of supplemental ultrasonography screening for women with dense breasts. *Ann Intern Med*, 162(3):157–66. doi:10.7326/M14-0692 PMID:25486550

Steffens RF, Wright HR, Hester MY, Andrykowski MA (2011). Clinical, demographic, and situational factors linked to distress associated with benign breast biopsy. *J Psychosoc Oncol*, 29(1):35–50. doi:10.1080/07347332.2011.534024 PMID:21240724

Steggles S, Lightfoot N, Sellick SM (1998). Psychological distress associated with organized breast cancer screening. *Cancer Prev Control*, 2(5):213–20. PMID:10093635

Stojadinovic A, Nissan A, Gallimidi Z, Lenington S, Logan W, Zuley M et al. (2005). Electrical impedance scanning for the early detection of breast cancer in young women: preliminary results of a multicenter prospective clinical trial. *J Clin Oncol*, 23(12):2703–15. doi:10.1200/JCO.2005.06.155 PMID:15837985

Stojadinovic A, Nissan A, Shriver CD, Mittendorf EA, Akin MD, Dickerson V et al. (2008). Electrical impedance scanning as a new breast cancer risk stratification tool for young women. *J Surg Oncol*, 97(2):112–20. doi:10.1002/jso.20931 PMID:18050282

Stout NK, Lee SJ, Schechter CB, Kerlikowske K, Alagoz O, Berry D et al. (2014). Benefits, harms, and costs for breast cancer screening after US implementation of digital mammography. *J Natl Cancer Inst*, 106(6):dju092. doi:10.1093/jnci/dju092 PMID:24872543

Stout NK, Rosenberg MA, Trentham-Dietz A, Smith MA, Robinson SM, Fryback DG (2006). Retrospective cost-effectiveness analysis of screening mammography. *J Natl Cancer Inst*, 98(11):774–82. doi:10.1093/jnci/djj210 PMID:16757702

Suhrke P, Mæhlen J, Schlichting E, Jørgensen KJ, Gøtzsche PC, Zahl PH (2011). Effect of mammography screening on surgical treatment for breast cancer in Norway: comparative analysis of cancer registry data. *BMJ*, 343:d4692. doi:10.1136/bmj.d4692 PMID:21914765

Sung JS, Malak SF, Bajaj P, Alis R, Dershaw DD, Morris EA (2011). Screening breast MR imaging in women with a history of lobular carcinoma in situ. *Radiology*, 261(2):414–20. doi:10.1148/radiol.11110091 PMID:21900617

Sutton S, Saidi G, Bickler G, Hunter J (1995). Does routine screening for breast cancer raise anxiety? Results from a three wave prospective study in England. *J Epidemiol Community Health*, 49(4):413–8. doi:10.1136/jech.49.4.413 PMID:7650466

Swanson V, McIntosh IB, Power KG, Dobson H (1996). The psychological effects of breast screening in terms of patients' perceived health anxieties. *Br J Clin Pract*, 50(3):129–35. PMID:8733330

Swedish Organised Service Screening Evaluation Group (2006a). Reduction in breast cancer mortality from organized service screening with mammography: 1. Further confirmation with extended data. *Cancer Epidemiol Biomarkers Prev*, 15(1):45–51. doi:10.1158/1055-9965.EPI-05-0349 PMID:16434585

Swedish Organised Service Screening Evaluation Group (2006b). Reduction in breast cancer mortality from the organised service screening with mammography: 2. Validation with alternative analytic methods. *Cancer Epidemiol Biomarkers Prev*, 15(1):52–6. doi:10.1158/1055-9965.EPI-05-0953 PMID:16434586

Swedish Organised Service Screening Evaluation Group (2007). Effect of mammographic service screening on stage at presentation of breast cancers in Sweden. *Cancer*, 109(11):2205–12. doi:10.1002/cncr.22671 PMID:17471486

Tabár L, Fagerberg G, Duffy SW, Day NE, Gad A, Gröntoft O (1992). Update of the Swedish two-county program of mammographic screening for breast cancer. *Radiol Clin North Am*, 30(1):187–210. PMID:1732926

Tabár L, Vitak B, Chen HH, Duffy SW, Yen MF, Chiang CF et al. (2000). The Swedish Two-County Trial twenty years later. Updated mortality results and new insights from long-term follow-up. *Radiol Clin North Am*, 38(4):625–51. doi:10.1016/S0033-8389(05)70191-3 PMID:10943268

Tabár L, Vitak B, Chen HH, Yen MF, Duffy SW, Smith RA (2001). Beyond randomized controlled trials: organized mammographic screening substantially reduces breast carcinoma mortality. *Cancer*, 91(9):1724–31. doi:10.1002/1097-0142(20010501)91:9<1724::AID-CNCR1190>3.0.CO;2-V PMID:11335897

Tafra L, Cheng Z, Uddo J, Lobrano MB, Stein W, Berg WA et al. (2005). Pilot clinical trial of ^{18}F-fluorodeoxyglucose positron-emission mammography in the surgical management of breast cancer. *Am J Surg*, 190(4):628–32. doi:10.1016/j.amjsurg.2005.06.029 PMID:16164937

Tan SY, van Oortmarssen GJ, de Koning HJ, Boer R, Habbema JD (2006). The MISCAN-Fadia continuous tumor growth model for breast cancer. *J Natl Cancer Inst Monogr*, 2006(36):56–65. doi:10.1093/jncimonographs/lgj009 PMID:17032895

Taylor R, Page A, Bampton D, Estoesta J, Rickard M (2004). Age-specific interval breast cancers in New South Wales and meta-analysis of studies of women aged 40–49 years. *J Med Screen*, 11(4):199–206. doi:10.1258/0969141042467403 PMID:15563775

Taylor R, Supramaniam R, Rickard M, Estoesta J, Moreira C (2002). Interval breast cancers in New South Wales, Australia, and comparisons with trials and other mammographic screening programmes. *J Med Screen*, 9(1):20–5. doi:10.1136/jms.9.1.20 PMID:11943793

Thierry-Chef I, Simon SL, Weinstock RM, Kwon D, Linet MS (2012). Reconstruction of absorbed doses to fibroglandular tissue of the breast of women undergoing mammography (1960 to the present). *Radiat Res*, 177(1):92–108. doi:10.1667/RR2241.1 PMID:21988547

Thomas DB, Gao DL, Ray RM, Wang WW, Allison CJ, Chen FL et al. (2002). Randomized trial of breast self-examination in Shanghai: final results. *J Natl Cancer Inst*, 94(19):1445–57. doi:10.1093/jnci/94.19.1445 PMID:12359854

Thompson RS, Barlow WE, Taplin SH, Grothaus L, Immanuel V, Salazar A et al. (1994). A population-based case-cohort evaluation of the efficacy of mammographic screening for breast cancer. *Am J Epidemiol*, 140(10):889–901. PMID:7977276

Thorne SE, Harris SR, Hislop TG, Vestrup JA (1999). The experience of waiting for diagnosis after an abnormal mammogram. *Breast J*, 5(1):42–51. doi:10.1046/j.1524-4741.1999.005001042.x PMID:11348255

Tice JA, O'Meara ES, Weaver DL, Vachon C, Ballard-Barbash R, Kerlikowske K (2013). Benign breast disease, mammographic breast density, and the risk of breast cancer. *J Natl Cancer Inst*, 105(14):1043–9. doi:10.1093/jnci/djt124 PMID:23744877

Tilanus-Linthorst MM, Obdeijn IM, Bartels KC, de Koning HJ, Oudkerk M (2000). First experiences in screening women at high risk for breast cancer with MR imaging. *Breast Cancer Res Treat*, 63(1):53–60. doi:10.1023/A:1006480106487 PMID:11079159

Törnberg S, Kemetli L, Ascunce N, Hofvind S, Anttila A, Sèradour B et al. (2010). A pooled analysis of interval cancer rates in six European countries. *Eur J Cancer Prev*, 19(2):87–93. doi:10.1097/CEJ.0b013e32833548ed PMID:20010429

Törnberg S, Kemetli L, Lynge E, Helene Olsen A, Hofvind S, Wang H et al. (2006). Breast cancer incidence and mortality in the Nordic capitals, 1970–1998. Trends related to mammography screening programmes. *Acta Oncol*, 45(5):528–35. doi:10.1080/02841860500501610 PMID:16864165

Tosteson AN, Stout NK, Fryback DG, Acharyya S, Herman BA, Hannah LG et al.; DMIST Investigators (2008). Cost-effectiveness of digital mammography breast cancer screening. *Ann Intern Med*, 148(1):1–10. doi:10.7326/0003-4819-148-1-200801010-00002 PMID:18166758

Trecate G, Vergnaghi D, Manoukian S, Bergonzi S, Scaperrotta G, Marchesini M et al. (2006). MRI in the early detection of breast cancer in women with high genetic risk. *Tumori*, 92(6):517–23. PMID:17260493

Trop I, Lalonde L, Mayrand MH, David J, Larouche N, Provencher D (2010). Multimodality breast cancer screening in women with a familial or genetic predisposition. *Curr Oncol*, 17(3):28–36. doi:10.3747/co.v17i3.494 PMID:20567624

Tyndel S, Austoker J, Henderson BJ, Brain K, Bankhead C, Clements A et al. (2007). What is the psychological impact of mammographic screening on younger women with a family history of breast cancer? Findings from a prospective cohort study by the PIMMS Management Group. *J Clin Oncol*, 25(25):3823–30. doi:10.1200/JCO.2007.11.0437 PMID:17761970

Uhry Z, Hédelin G, Colonna M, Asselain B, Arveux P, Exbrayat C et al. (2011). Modelling the effect of breast cancer screening on related mortality using French data. *Cancer Epidemiol*, 35(3):235–42. doi:10.1016/j.canep.2010.10.009 PMID:21159568

UK Trial of Early Detection of Breast Cancer Group (1999). 16-year mortality from breast cancer in the UK Trial of Early Detection of Breast Cancer. *Lancet*, 353(9168):1909–14. doi:10.1016/S0140-6736(98)07412-1 PMID:10371568

van de Velde CJ, Verma S, van Nes JG, Masterman C, Pritchard KI (2010). Switching from tamoxifen to aromatase inhibitors for adjuvant endocrine therapy in postmenopausal patients with early breast cancer. *Cancer Treat Rev*, 36(1):54–62. doi:10.1016/j.ctrv.2009.10.003 PMID:19944537

Van Dijck JA, Verbeek AL, Beex LV, Hendriks JH, Holland R, Mravunac M et al. (1996). Mammographic screening after the age of 65 years: evidence for a reduction in breast cancer mortality. *Int J Cancer*, 66(6):727–31. doi:10.1002/(SICI)1097-0215(19960611)66:6<727::AID-IJC3>3.0.CO;2-1 PMID:8647640

Van Dijck JA, Verbeek AL, Beex LV, Hendriks JH, Holland R, Mravunac M et al. (1997). Breast-cancer mortality in a non-randomized trial on mammographic screening in women over age 65. *Int J Cancer*, 70(2):164–8. doi:10.1002/(SICI)1097-0215(19970117)70:2<164::AID-IJC5>3.0.CO;2-V PMID:9009155

van Gils CH, Otten JD, Verbeek AL, Hendriks JH, Holland R (1998). Effect of mammographic breast density on breast cancer screening performance: a study in Nijmegen, The Netherlands. *J Epidemiol Community*

Health, 52(4):267–71. doi:10.1136/jech.52.4.267 PMID: 9616416

van Ineveld BM, van Oortmarssen GJ, de Koning HJ, Boer R, van der Maas PJ (1993). How cost-effective is breast cancer screening in different EC countries? *Eur J Cancer*, 29(12):1663–8. doi:10.1016/0959-8049(93)90100-T PMID:8398290

van Ravesteyn NT, Stout NK, Schechter CB, Heijnsdijk EA, Alagoz O, Trentham-Dietz A et al. (2015). Benefits and harms of mammography screening after age 74 years: model estimates of overdiagnosis. *J Natl Cancer Inst*, 107(7):djv103. PMID:25948872

van Schoor G, Moss SM, Otten JDM, Donders R, Paap E, den Heeten GJ et al. (2010). Effective biennial mammographic screening in women aged 40–49. *Eur J Cancer*, 46(18):3137–40. doi:10.1016/j.ejca.2010.09.041 PMID:21036034

van Schoor G, Moss SM, Otten JDM, Donders R, Paap E, den Heeten GJ et al. (2011). Increasingly strong reduction in breast cancer mortality due to screening. *Br J Cancer*, 104(6):910–4. doi:10.1038/bjc.2011.44 PMID:21343930

Venturini E, Losio C, Panizza P, Rodighiero MG, Fedele I, Tacchini S et al. (2013). Tailored breast cancer screening program with microdose mammography, US, and MR imaging: short-term results of a pilot study in 40–49-year-old women. *Radiology*, 268(2):347–55. doi:10.1148/radiol.13122278 PMID:23579052

Verbeek AL, Broeders MJ (2010). Evaluation of cancer service screening: case referent studies recommended. *Stat Methods Med Res*, 19(5):487–505. doi:10.1177/0962280209359856 PMID:20356858

Verbeek AL, Hendriks JH, Holland R, Mravunac M, Sturmans F (1985). Mammographic screening and breast cancer mortality: age-specific effects in Nijmegen Project, 1975–82. *Lancet*, 1(8433):865–6. doi:10.1016/S0140-6736(85)92223-8 PMID:2858721

Verbeek AL, Hendriks JH, Holland R, Mravunac M, Sturmans F, Day NE (1984). Reduction of breast cancer mortality through mass screening with modern mammography. First results of the Nijmegen project, 1975–1981. *Lancet*, 1(8388):1222–4. doi:10.1016/S0140-6736(84)91703-3 PMID:6144933

Veronesi U, Cascinelli N, Mariani L, Greco M, Saccozzi R, Luini A et al. (2002). Twenty-year follow-up of a randomized study comparing breast-conserving surgery with radical mastectomy for early breast cancer. *N Engl J Med*, 347(16):1227–32. doi:10.1056/NEJMoa020989 PMID:12393819

Veronesi U, Paganelli G, Viale G, Luini A, Zurrida S, Galimberti V et al. (2003). A randomized comparison of sentinel-node biopsy with routine axillary dissection in breast cancer. *N Engl J Med*, 349(6):546–53. doi:10.1056/NEJMoa012782 PMID:12904519

Vilaprinyo E, Forné C, Carles M, Sala M, Pla R, Castells X et al.; Interval Cancer (INCA) Study Group (2014). Cost-effectiveness and harm-benefit analyses of risk-based screening strategies for breast cancer. *PLoS ONE*, 9(2):e86858. doi:10.1371/journal.pone.0086858 PMID:24498285

Vinnicombe S, Pinto Pereira SM, McCormack VA, Shiel S, Perry N, Dos Santos Silva IM (2009). Full-field digital versus screen-film mammography: comparison within the UK breast screening program and systematic review of published data. *Radiology*, 251(2):347–58. doi:10.1148/radiol.2512081235 PMID:19401569

Waller M, Moss S, Watson J, Møller H (2007). The effect of mammographic screening and hormone replacement therapy use on breast cancer incidence in England and Wales. *Cancer Epidemiol Biomarkers Prev*, 16(11):2257–61. doi:10.1158/1055-9965.EPI-07-0262 PMID:18006913

Wallis MG, Lawrence G, Brenner RJ (2008). Improving quality outcomes in a single-payer system: lessons learned from the UK National Health Service Breast Screening Programme. *J Am Coll Radiol*, 5(6):737–43. doi:10.1016/j.jacr.2008.02.004 PMID:18514953

Walter SD (2003). Mammographic screening: case-control studies. *Ann Oncol*, 14(8):1190–2. doi:10.1093/annonc/mdg320 PMID:12881374

Wang H, Bjurstam N, Bjørndal H, Braaten A, Eriksen L, Skaane P et al. (2001). Interval cancers in the Norwegian breast cancer screening program: frequency, characteristics and use of HRT. *Int J Cancer*, 94(4):594–8. doi:10.1002/ijc.1511 PMID:11745450

Wang T, Wang K, Yao Q, Chen JH, Ling R, Zhang JL et al. (2010). Prospective study on combination of electrical impedance scanning and ultrasound in estimating risk of development of breast cancer in young women. *Cancer Invest*, 28(3):295–303. doi:10.3109/07357900802203658 PMID:19857040

Warner E, Messersmith H, Causer P, Eisen A, Shumak R, Plewes D (2008). Systematic review: using magnetic resonance imaging to screen women at high risk for breast cancer. *Ann Intern Med*, 148(9):671–9. doi:10.7326/0003-4819-148-9-200805060-00007 PMID:18458280

Warner E, Plewes DB, Hill KA, Causer PA, Zubovits JT, Jong RA et al. (2004). Surveillance of *BRCA1* and *BRCA2* mutation carriers with magnetic resonance imaging, ultrasound, mammography, and clinical breast examination. *JAMA*, 292(11):1317–25. doi:10.1001/jama.292.11.1317 PMID:15367553

Warner E, Plewes DB, Shumak RS, Catzavelos GC, Di Prospero LS, Yaffe MJ et al. (2001). Comparison of breast magnetic resonance imaging, mammography, and ultrasound for surveillance of women at high risk for hereditary breast cancer. *J Clin Oncol*, 19(15):3524–31. PMID:11481359

Webb C, Koch T (1997). Women's experiences of non-invasive breast cancer: literature review and study report.

J Adv Nurs, 25(3):514–25. doi:10.1046/j.1365-2648.1997.t01-1-1997025514.x PMID:9080278

Weedon-Fekjær H, Romundstad PR, Vatten LJ (2014). Modern mammography screening and breast cancer mortality: population study. *BMJ*, 348:g3701. doi:10.1136/bmj.g3701 PMID:24951459

Weigert J, Steenbergen S (2012). The Connecticut experiment: the role of ultrasound in the screening of women with dense breasts. *Breast J*, 18(6):517–22. doi:10.1111/tbj.12003 PMID:23009208

Weigert JM, Bertrand ML, Lanzkowsky L, Stern LH, Kieper DA (2012). Results of a multicenter patient registry to determine the clinical impact of breast-specific gamma imaging, a molecular breast imaging technique. *AJR Am J Roentgenol*, 198(1):W69–W75. doi:10.2214/AJR.10.6105 PMID:22194518

Weinstein MC, Stason WB (1977). Foundations of cost-effectiveness analysis for health and medical practices. *N Engl J Med*, 296(13):716–21. doi:10.1056/NEJM197703312961304 PMID:402576

Weinstein SP, Localio AR, Conant EF, Rosen M, Thomas KM, Schnall MD (2009). Multimodality screening of women at an increased risk: a prospective cohort study. *J Clin Oncol*, 27(36):6124–8. doi:10.1200/JCO.2009.24.4277 PMID:19884532

Wersebe A, Siegmann K, Krainick U, Fersis N, Vogel U, Claussen CD et al. (2002). Diagnostic potential of targeted electrical impedance scanning in classifying suspicious breast lesions. *Invest Radiol*, 37(2):65–72. doi:10.1097/00004424-200202000-00003 PMID:11799329

WHO (2001). WHO Commission on Macroeconomics and Health. Available from: http://www.who.int/macrohealth/en/.

WHO (2014). Cost-effectiveness and strategic planning (WHO-CHOICE): threshold values for intervention cost-effectiveness by region. Available from: www.who.int/choice/costs/CER_levels/en/.

Wilson R, Liston J, editors (2011). Quality assurance guidelines for breast cancer screening radiology, 2nd edition. NHSBSP Publication No. 59. Sheffield, UK: NHS Cancer Screening Programmes. Available from: http://www.cancerscreening.nhs.uk/breastscreen/publications/nhsbsp59.pdf.

Wrixon AD (2008). New ICRP recommendations. *J Radiol Prot*, 28(2):161–8. doi:10.1088/0952-4746/28/2/R02 PMID:18495983

Xu HB, Li L, Xu Q (2011). Tc-99m sestamibi scintimammography for the diagnosis of breast cancer: meta-analysis and meta-regression. *Nucl Med Commun*, 32(11):980–8. doi:10.1097/MNM.0b013e32834b43a9 PMID:21956488

Yaffe MJ, Mainprize JG (2011). Risk of radiation-induced breast cancer from mammographic screening. *Radiology*, 258(1):98–105. doi:10.1148/radiol.10100655 PMID:21081671

Zahl PH, Mæhlen J (2012). Overdiagnosis of breast cancer after 14 years of mammography screening. *Tidsskr Nor Laegeforen*, 132(4):414–7. doi:10.4045/tidsskr.11.0195 PMID:22353833

Zahl PH, Strand BH, Maehlen J (2004). Incidence of breast cancer in Norway and Sweden during introduction of nationwide screening: prospective cohort study. *BMJ*, 328(7445):921–4. doi:10.1136/bmj.38044.666157.63 PMID:15013948

Zelle SG, Nyarko KM, Bosu WK, Aikins M, Niëns LM, Lauer JA et al. (2012). Costs, effects and cost-effectiveness of breast cancer control in Ghana. *Trop Med Int Health*, 17(8):1031–43. doi:10.1111/j.1365-3156.2012.03021.x PMID:22809238

Zelle SG, Vidaurre T, Abugattas JE, Manrique JE, Sarria G, Jeronimo J et al. (2013). Cost-effectiveness analysis of breast cancer control interventions in Peru. *PLoS ONE*, 8(12):e82575. doi:10.1371/journal.pone.0082575 PMID:24349314

Zhang S, Ivy JS, Diehl KM, Yankaskas BC (2013). The association of breast density with breast cancer mortality in African American and white women screened in community practice. *Breast Cancer Res Treat*, 137(1):273–83. doi:10.1007/s10549-012-2310-3 PMID:23143213

Zheng B, Lederman D, Sumkin JH, Zuley ML, Gruss MZ, Lovy LS et al. (2011). A preliminary evaluation of multi-probe resonance-frequency electrical impedance based measurements of the breast. *Acad Radiol*, 18(2):220–9. doi:10.1016/j.acra.2010.09.017 PMID:21126888

Zheng B, Zuley ML, Sumkin JH, Catullo VJ, Abrams GS, Rathfon GY et al. (2008). Detection of breast abnormalities using a prototype resonance electrical impedance spectroscopy system: a preliminary study. *Med Phys*, 35(7):3041–8. doi:10.1118/1.2936221 PMID:18697526

Zigmond AS, Snaith RP (1983). The Hospital Anxiety and Depression Scale. *Acta Psychiatr Scand*, 67(6):361–70. doi:10.1111/j.1600-0447.1983.tb09716.x PMID:6880820

Zorzi M, Guzzinati S, Puliti D, Paci E; IMPACT Working Group (2010). A simple method to estimate the episode and programme sensitivity of breast cancer screening programmes. *J Med Screen*, 17(3):132–8. doi:10.1258/jms.2010.009060 PMID:20956723

Zorzi M, Puliti D, Vettorazzi M, De Lisi V, Falcini F, Federico M et al.; IMPACT Working Group (2006). Mastectomy rates are decreasing in the era of service screening: a population-based study in Italy (1997-2001). *Br J Cancer*, 95(9):1265–8. doi:10.1038/sj.bjc.6603405 PMID:17043685

6. SUMMARY

6.1 Breast cancer

Breast cancer is the most commonly diagnosed cancer in women and the most common cause of cancer death in women worldwide. Globally, it is estimated that in 2012 there were 1.68 million new diagnoses (25% of all new cancer diagnoses in women) and 0.52 million deaths (15% of all cancer deaths in women) from breast cancer, corresponding to age-standardized incidence and mortality rates of 43.3 and 12.9 per 100 000, respectively. Thus, in 2012 there were an estimated 6.3 million women alive who had had a diagnosis of breast cancer in the previous 5 years (more than one third of all 5-year prevalent cancer cases in women). The largest contributor to the global burden was East and Central Asia (including China and India), where more than one third of the cases and more than 40% of the deaths occurred. In 2012, more than a 3-fold variation in the age-standardized breast cancer incidence rates was recorded between countries in North America and western Europe (rates > 90 per 100 000) and countries in Central Africa and East and South-Central Asia (rates < 30 per 100 000). In many high-income countries, 5-year survival rates now reach 80–90% (with 10-year survival rates of 60–70%), whereas in low- and middle-income countries (LMICs), 5-year survival rates may be less than 60% and as low as 12%. Globally, about one third of breast cancer cases are diagnosed in women younger than 50 years, and about one half in women aged 50–74 years; however, the mean age of diagnosis is lower in LMICs. In most countries, an increase in incidence rates and a decrease in mortality rates were evident over recent decades, beginning in many countries before the implementation of mammography screening programmes. In those countries where screening was introduced in the 1980s and 1990s, the increase in incidence rates has been most evident in the age group of invited women.

Invasive adenocarcinoma of the breast is a malignant tumour that penetrates the basement membrane and spreads via both the blood and lymphatic systems, progressing to regional lymph node and systemic metastasis. Invasive breast cancers vary in morphological and molecular genetic characteristics, clinical features, and prognosis. The main non-invasive form of breast carcinoma in situ, ductal carcinoma in situ, has at least a 40% likelihood of progression to invasive cancer when untreated. Most benign breast lesions have no known relationship to the development of invasive breast cancer. However, some forms of breast epithelial proliferation, such as usual epithelial hyperplasia and atypical hyperplasia, are associated with an increased risk of subsequent breast cancer (by 1.5–2.0-fold and 2.5–4-fold, respectively).

Established breast cancer risk factors include early menarche, late menopause, later age at first pregnancy, nulliparity and low parity, little or no breastfeeding, higher body mass index at postmenopausal ages, and tall stature. Other factors associated with an increased risk include low physical activity levels, alcohol consumption, certain exogenous hormone therapies, mammographic density, a history of proliferative benign breast conditions, and a family history of breast cancer. Exposure to ionizing radiation is linearly associated with an increased breast cancer risk. The risk shows an inverse relationship with age at exposure, with very low or no risk for women exposed after age 50 years and an increase in risk for women exposed before age 40 years. In addition to the above-mentioned breast cancer risk factors, genetic factors are of particular importance. The risk increases with the number of affected first-degree relatives and is most pronounced in young adults. Mutations in the high-penetrance genes *BRCA1* and *BRCA2*, together with mutations in additional cancer susceptibility genes, account for approximately 27% of all hereditary breast cancer cases and 5% of all breast cancer cases. The majority of cancer susceptibility genes code for tumour suppressor proteins involved in critical DNA repair pathways, which may increase the radiosensitivity of women in this population.

In LMICs, breast cancer cases are frequently diagnosed at more advanced stages than those in high-income countries, mostly due to the lack of effective diagnostic services. The mortality and morbidity associated with advanced disease may be reduced through early diagnosis of symptomatic breast cancer or early detection of breast cancer by screening in asymptomatic women. Promotion of breast cancer awareness may be a feasible option for early detection in settings with limited resources where screening is not feasible.

Comprehensive quality assurance, via evaluation and monitoring of performance indicators, is essential to maintain an appropriate balance between the benefits (mainly reduced mortality from breast cancer) and harms of screening. Quality assurance of breast cancer screening requires appropriate, sustainable resources for planning, coordination, and training.

6.2 Implementation of breast cancer screening worldwide

There is a social gradient to participation in breast cancer screening. Income, education level, place of residence, age, health, access to general health services (including screening), and cultural factors are among the factors that influence participation. Knowledge about breast cancer and screening is associated with higher participation. Worry about breast cancer and perceived risk of breast cancer are also associated with higher participation, but fatalism about cancer is associated with lower participation. Acculturation among minority women and immigrant women in settings with access to screening is usually associated with higher rates of screening.

Informed decision-making is a principle that underpins participation in screening; however, laypeople may conceptualize informed choice differently from policy-makers. Professionals debate about what constitutes appropriate information to provide to women, especially about overdiagnosis and false-positive test results (see Section 6.3.3a, b).

Participation in breast cancer screening can have psychological or psychosocial consequences for women, either from the invitation to screening or from the outcome, which may in turn affect further participation in screening (see also Section 6.3.3d).

6.2.1 Europe

Breast cancer screening is well established in western Europe and is delivered according to a common pattern, which has been guided by the activity of projects funded by the European Union. Some countries, particularly those in central and eastern Europe, have less well developed programmes or have not yet implemented screening. Breast cancer screening is delivered mainly by organized programmes, as encouraged by the European Commission, which has published quality assurance guidelines, now in their fourth edition.

Participation rates vary across Europe, from less than 20% in Poland to more than 85% in Finland, with an estimated average of just less than 50%. Commonly, participation rates are higher among more affluent and more educated women and lower among women of lower socio-economic status or from a minority or immigrant background.

6.2.2 North America

Breast cancer screening has been widely available in parts of Canada and the USA since the late 1980s or early 1990s and typically achieves population attendance rates of about 50%, varying from 30% to 60%. In Canada, breast cancer screening is delivered primarily through organized programmes, whereas in the USA, screening is opportunistic. Both countries have well-developed quality assurance programmes. In the USA, management of quality assurance is mandated by federal regulations. Both Canada and the USA have programmes to raise awareness. Women in Canada and the USA face similar barriers to breast cancer screening, including living in a rural area, low income, low education level, and minority status.

6.2.3 Latin America

In Latin America, there has been increasing activity in breast cancer screening during the past decade. Currently, almost all Latin American countries in which breast cancer is the leading cause of cancer mortality among women have national recommendations or guidelines; however, no country in the region has a screening system that meets all the criteria of organized screening programmes. Most countries use mammography screening combined with clinical breast examination (CBE) and breast self-examination (BSE); half of the countries recommend mammography for women younger than 50 years. Screening participation rates vary enormously across and within countries, with large differences between urban and rural areas and by income level. There is intensive advocacy activity, and information is provided by governments, NGOs, and the media, which appear to have induced a good level of breast awareness, although in a non-coordinated manner.

6.2.4 Sub-Saharan Africa

With the exception of South Africa, no country in sub-Saharan Africa has developed national recommendations or guidelines for breast cancer screening; however, relevant activity by NGOs is present throughout the region, and a few governments have carried out periodic campaigns to promote breast awareness. No population-based data on screening participation were available for most countries, and the only available national survey from South Africa found that 15.5% of women reported having had a mammogram during their lifetime. Accordingly, diagnosis occurs at a late stage of the disease. Despite several initiatives to increase breast awareness and provide health education, poverty, the lack of governmental support, and sociocultural influences represent relevant barriers to breast cancer awareness and screening.

6.2.5 Central and West Asia and North Africa

Countries located in Central and West Asia and North Africa are heterogeneous, and this is reflected in terms of access to breast cancer screening. While high-income countries such as Israel, Kuwait, and Qatar have well-developed health services, most countries in this area are classified as LMICs, with limited resources allocated to health care. Recent and current emergencies in several countries in this area have exacerbated previous problems, and screening is not available to women in these circumstances and is not a priority.

Some screening is available in the more affluent countries, and there is NGO activity in some areas. A few pilot and exploratory projects have taken place. Both awareness and participation rates are low. Israel has a well-developed breast cancer screening system, and participation is high.

6.2.6 South-East Asia

Among the four countries or areas that have national programmes based on cancer screening guidelines, organized screening is present in the Republic of Korea, Singapore, and Taiwan, China, but not in Japan. The age group younger than 50 years has been included in the target population for breast cancer screening, except in Singapore. Some countries, such as China and Indonesia, have local community-based screening programmes. In several countries, such as India, screening is performed only within research studies. For the efficient use of limited resources, Thailand is developing risk-prediction models to target only women at an increased risk. National programmes for cancer control and prevention of noncommunicable diseases have promoted breast cancer awareness in Asian countries.

6.2.7 Oceania

Australia and New Zealand provide organized screening programmes for breast cancer. The target age groups were expanded in the past decade, in Australia to women in their early seventies and in New Zealand to women in their late forties. In the past decade, the participation rate has remained about 50% in Australia and has increased from 50% to more than 70% in New Zealand. Australia, Fiji, and New Zealand have national programmes for breast care awareness. Because minority groups have low participation rates in breast cancer screening, they have been the major target of programmes to promote breast cancer awareness.

6.3 Mammography screening

The technology, technique, and interpretation skills of mammography have advanced enormously since its early development, leading, chiefly, to improved sensitivity and specificity, and reduced radiation doses. Digital mammography provides improved sensitivity in moderately dense breasts. Digital breast tomosynthesis produces three-dimensional mammographic images, allowing better visualization and localization of potential lesions. The radiation dose of digital mammography with tomosynthesis is approximately twice that of mammography alone, but is significantly reduced by reconstruction of two-dimensional images from the three-dimensional images. Many countries have developed detailed guidelines for quality control in mammography screening.

6.3.1 Efficacy of mammography screening from randomized controlled trials

Efficacy of a specific intervention generally refers to its beneficial effect under ideal circumstances. In practice, it is rarely possible to assess true efficacy. Randomized controlled trials (RCTs), which have been designed initially to assess whether mammography screening may reduce breast cancer mortality, increase life expectancy, and reduce the number of women undergoing aggressive treatments, may suffer from a low compliance rate, contamination in the control arm, long screening intervals, or suboptimal quality.

The Working Group considered all 10 randomized trials of breast cancer screening that have been conducted to be eligible for evaluation. These trials, initiated from 1963 until

1991, are: the Health Insurance Plan trial (USA); the Malmö I and Malmö II trials (Sweden); the Two-County trial (Sweden); the Stockholm trial (Sweden); the Gothenburg trial (Sweden); the Canadian National Breast Screening Study trials, CNBSS 1 and CNBSS 2 (Canada); the Edinburgh trial (United Kingdom); and the United Kingdom Age trial (United Kingdom). Individual randomization was performed in the Health Insurance Plan, Malmö, CNBSS, and Gothenburg trials (the latter only in women aged 39–49 years), and cluster randomization in the other trials. The mean duration of follow-up for breast cancer mortality ranged from 9 years for the Malmö II trial to 25–29 years for the Two-County trial. All but two RCTs, which had screening of the control group by design, showed breast cancer mortality reductions of between 10% and 35% for women invited to screening (across the ages 39–74 years at entry); however, the reduction was statistically significant in only two trials (the Two-County and Edinburgh trials). Meta-analyses of the RCTs showed a statistically significant reduction in breast cancer mortality of about 23% in women invited to screening aged 50–69 years at entry. Concerns have been raised that cluster randomization may not achieve balance in critical risk factors for breast cancer. This effect was demonstrated as a bias in the Edinburgh trial; in the Two-County trial, substantial bias was found to be unlikely. For only the Health Insurance Plan and CNBSS trials were data obtained to confirm balance in the distribution of conventional risk factors for breast cancer in women in the compared arms.

Evidence from the RCTs for the efficacy of mammography screening of women starting at age 40 years and continuing to age 74 years in reducing breast cancer mortality is less extensive. The United Kingdom Age trial, which included women aged 39–41 years at entry, was the only trial aimed at answering the question of whether mammography screening at age 40–41 years is effective in reducing breast cancer mortality in women diagnosed during their forties; a 17% statistically non-significant reduction in breast cancer mortality was found in the trial. For women aged 70–74 years, only in the Two-County trial was screening offered to this age group, and a 24% non-significant reduction in breast cancer mortality was reported.

The CNBSS trials incorporated screening by CBE and the teaching and reinforcement of BSE in both the mammography and the control arms. The CNBSS 2 trial for women aged 50–59 years specifically addressed the question of whether adding mammography screening to CBE leads to additional benefits, and found no difference in breast cancer mortality. By modelling of the individual data, it was estimated that a reduction of more than 20% in breast cancer mortality could have been derived from the CBE if compared with a no-screening arm.

Eight of the RCTs had reported cumulative incidence of advanced breast cancers (the Health Insurance Plan, Malmö, Two-County, CNBSS 1 and CNBSS 2, Stockholm, Gothenburg, and United Kingdom Age trials), with reductions varying from 3% to 31% in the individual trials.

It was not possible to estimate the average overdiagnosis in women screened from age 50 years to age 69 years (or 74 years), because many trials had provided screening also for the control group or had not reported data specifically for the screening of women in the age range 50–69 years.

Screening intervals were 12 months in the Health Insurance Plan, CNBSS, and United Kingdom Age trials, 18 months in the Gothenburg trial, 18–24 months in the Malmö trials, 28 months in the Stockholm trial, and 24 months for women aged 40–49 years and 33 months for those aged 50–69 years in the Two-County trial. However, the different designs of the trials preclude an assessment of the comparative efficacy of screening by different intervals. One additional trial in the United Kingdom was specifically designed to evaluate the effects of varying screening frequency; reduction in breast cancer mortality was modelled based on results of tumour size, nodal status, and histological grade. No statistically significant difference was found between a 3-year and a 1-year interval for women aged 50–64 years.

6.3.2 Effectiveness of mammography screening

Evaluation of the effectiveness of screening on breast cancer mortality can use various design and analytical approaches. Incidence-based mortality (IBM) cohort studies and nested case–control studies are the most robust designs for evaluating the effectiveness of service mammography screening, when they achieve a sufficient follow-up time. All of the studies currently available for evaluation were performed in high-income countries.

(a) Incidence-based mortality cohort studies

(i) Women aged 50–69 years

Nineteen separate IBM cohort study analyses have estimated the overall effects on breast cancer mortality of invitation to mammography screening, with or without CBE, in women aged 50–69 years or in a wider age group including this range (beginning at < 50 years in eight analyses and ending at > 69 years in five analyses).

Given substantial overlaps in space and time among reports based on population-based mammography screening programmes in Sweden, Finland, and Norway, the Working Group considered only the more extensive studies for each country (two of the six analyses based on the Swedish mammography screening programme, one of the five analyses based on the Finnish breast cancer screening programme, and two of the three analyses based on the Norwegian breast cancer screening programme).

The relative risks from IBM studies for invitation to screening ranged from 0.58 (95% confidence interval [CI], 0.44–0.75), for year 8 to year 12 of screening in Navarre, Spain, to 0.94 (95% CI, 0.68–1.29), for the first 15 years of screening in Nijmegen, the Netherlands. The median relative risk of all studies considered was 0.77, between the values of 0.76 (95% CI, 0.53–1.09), based on the first 6 years of screening in Finland, and 0.78 (95% CI, 0.70–0.87), based on 12 years of screening in Finland (1992–2003). If all Norwegian studies are removed from the analysis, because of the introduction of multidisciplinary breast cancer care centres in parallel with the roll-out of the organized screening programme, the median relative risk is 0.76. The remaining analyses included one each from Denmark, Italy, and the United Kingdom. The study in the United Kingdom, which included CBE (annual) with mammography (biennial), reported a relative risk of 0.73 (95% CI, 0.63–0.84). Lead-time bias was the most common residual bias and would be expected to be conservative.

Eleven independent informative IBM cohort study analyses of effects of participation in mammography screening on breast cancer mortality were considered, after exclusion of studies reporting a relative risk based on an analysis of invitation to screening multiplied by an estimate of the participation rate.

Two of the four analyses based on the Swedish mammography screening programme substantially overlapped in space and time, and thus the Working Group considered only the more extensive study. Two further studies, one in Sweden and one in Italy, were not, or were probably only partially, adjusted for self-selection bias. A third study, in Canada, although it was not adjusted for self-selection bias, provided an analysis of a small component of the data that suggested that self-selection bias (in populations in which only one third to one half of women had been screened) was small and conservative. The remaining five analyses included one each in Denmark, Finland, and Norway, and two in the USA. The relative risks for attendance to screening from these studies ranged from 0.57

(95% CI, 0.53–0.62), based on 11–22 years of screening in Sweden, to 0.80 (95% CI, 0.34–1.85), based on 3.5 years of organized screening in a health maintenance organization in the USA. The median relative risk was 0.60, from both the Danish programme (95% CI, 0.49–0.74) and the Canadian programme (95% CI, 0.52–0.67). The Norwegian study, on attendance in the breast cancer screening programme, is methodologically probably the best of the studies considered, since it was based on individually linked data for all women studied; the relative risk was 0.57 (95% CI, 0.51–0.64) for screening in the period 1996–2009. The two studies in the USA included CBE as part of the screening offered.

Overall, IBM cohort studies indicate reductions in breast cancer mortality of about 20% for women invited to screening and of about 40% for women who attend screening, in this age range.

(ii) Women younger than 50 years or older than 69 years

IBM analyses can provide evidence on the effectiveness of screening in women younger than 50 years if they are based on women who were only offered screening while they were younger than 50 years or are limited to women whose breast cancer was diagnosed while they were younger than 50 years. Similarly, to provide evidence on the effectiveness of screening in women older than 69 years, IBM analyses must be based on women first offered screening after age 69 years and limited to breast cancer deaths that followed a diagnosis of breast cancer when the women were older than 69 years.

Based on screening experience for most of Sweden in the period 1986–2005, the relative risk for invitation to screening at age 40–49 years was estimated to be 0.74 (95% CI, 0.66–0.83); it was 0.83 (95% CI, 0.70–1.00) for invitation at age 40–44 years, and 0.68 (95% CI, 0.59–0.78) for invitation at age 45–49 years.

Three studies provided evidence on the effectiveness of screening in women older than 69 years. One study in the Netherlands reported an odds ratio of 0.89 (95% CI, 0.56–1.40) for women first invited to screening at age 68–83 years. One study in Sweden reported an odds ratio of 0.96 (95% CI, 0.73–1.25) for women first invited to screening at age 65–74 years. One study in Canada reported an odds ratio of 0.65 (95% CI, 0.56–0.74) for women first attending organized screening at age 70–79 years. An alternative analysis of the Swedish data, using estimated excess mortality from breast cancer instead of the number of breast cancers that were registered as the underlying cause of death, gave an estimated relative risk of 0.84 (95% CI, 0.59–1.19); this alternative could be justifiable if there was material error in assignment of underlying cause of death in older women in this study. The Canadian study was limited by lack of adjustment for self-selection bias and lack of consideration of probable opportunistic screening before acceptance of an invitation to organized screening at age 70 years or older.

(b) Case–control studies

(i) Women aged 50–69 years

Eleven separate case-control studies conducted in Europe and Australia provided relevant data on the effectiveness of mammography in service screening programmes. Most of these studies enrolled women invited for screening at ages 50–69 years; two included women younger than 50 years at invitation, and four included women older than 69 years at invitation. Although some studies were conducted in the same geographical area, the studies were judged to have no effective overlap and hence to be independent. In these case-control studies, odds ratios for all ages ranged from 0.24 (with correction for self-selection bias) to 0.75.

Eight additional case-control studies conducted in Europe and the USA provided relevant data on the effectiveness of mammography screening conducted in other settings. Three of the studies included women younger than 50 years at invitation, and none included women older than 70 years. Odds ratios for the largest range of ages included in these studies ranged from 0.30 to 0.91.

Case–control studies typically provide estimates of the effect of screening for women who participated in screening compared with women who had been invited or to whom screening was otherwise offered but who did not participate. Non-participating women may have a different risk of dying from breast cancer, so this may result in selection bias in the absence of appropriate adjustment. Information bias can be considered minimal if the case–control study is based on systematic historical databases on screening, but may be larger in other types of case–control studies. Self-selection bias can be assessed by comparing breast cancer mortality rates in unscreened women with those in screened women just before service screening started; in practice, self-selection bias has been shown to be limited in service screening programmes with high attendance rates. The results of case–control studies indicate that breast cancer mortality is reduced by about 48% in screened women.

(ii) Women younger than 50 years or older than 69 years

Case–control study analyses can provide evidence on the effectiveness of screening in women younger than 50 years if they are based only on deaths from breast cancer of women whose cancer was diagnosed when they were younger than 50 years or whose last screening or invitation to screening before diagnosis of breast cancer was while they were younger than 50 years. Similarly, to provide evidence on the effectiveness of screening in women older than 69 years, analyses must be based on women first offered screening after age 69 years and limited to breast cancer deaths that followed a diagnosis of breast cancer when the women were older than 69 years.

Six case–control study analyses estimated the effectiveness of invitation to or attendance of screening at ages 40–49 years (five studies) or below age 50 years (one study) in reducing breast cancer mortality. Odds ratios for invitation or attendance ranged from 0.50 to 1.18, with only one greater than 1.0. The two studies in women invited to attend the screening programme in Nijmegen, the Netherlands, analysed some of the same breast cancer deaths.

One case–control study provided a potentially valid estimate of the effectiveness of first attendance of screening at age 65–74 years, with an odds ratio of 0.54 (95% CI, 0.31–0.95) in women ever screened in that age range. (The breast cancer deaths included as cases in this study probably include most of those in the Dutch cohort study of women first invited to screening at age 68–83 years referred to above.)

(c) Ecological studies

Despite their lower value, ecological studies may be appropriate for evaluating population-level interventions, such as screening, when geographical areas or population groups are expected to be similar in cancer risk except for the introduction of screening. The Working Group considered that accurate information on standards of breast cancer treatment in different regions analysed and careful matching of regions by treatment standards or adjustment for differences between regions in treatment standards are minimum criteria for validity of ecological studies. Of the 87 studies considered, 5 studies were included in the review. Of those, three found benefits from mammography screening and two did not. Thus, evidence from the small number of informative studies was consistent with that from cohort studies and case–control studies.

(d) Stage-specific incidence

Overall, studies that compared incidence rates of advanced breast cancer in screened versus unscreened populations showed significantly lower rates of advanced cancers in screened women. Ecological studies, which are based on cancer registries, without distinction between breast cancer cases detected by screening or otherwise (intention to screen), reported smaller differences.

(e) *Effect of adjuvant therapy on effectiveness of screening*

Adjuvant systemic therapy has been increasingly used since the late 1980s, and has thus probably affected the effects of screening. Two important studies have recently reported on this issue. A study using micro-simulation modelling reported that in 2008, adjuvant treatment was estimated to have reduced the breast cancer mortality rate in the simulated population by 13.9%, compared with a situation without treatment; biennial screening between age 50 years and age 74 years further reduced the mortality rate by 15.7%. Another modelling study, which included six natural history models for the population in the USA and used very similar techniques, reported that in 2000, screening and adjuvant treatment were estimated to have reduced breast cancer mortality by 34.8%, compared with a situation with no screening or adjuvant treatment; a reduction by 15.9% was estimated to have been a result of screening, and 23.4% as a result of treatment.

6.3.3 *Adverse effects of mammography screening*

Early detection of breast cancer by mammography screening is associated with harms, of which the most important are false-positive results of the screening test, overdiagnosis, and possibly risk of radiation-induced breast cancer.

(a) *Cumulative risk of false-positive recall*

The cumulative risk of a false-positive recall, an important harm of screening, is defined as the cumulative risk of recall for further assessment at least once during the screening period (usually 10 biennial screening episodes in organized programmes) minus the cancer detection rate over the same period. There is a similar definition for the cumulative risk of recall with a subsequent invasive procedure (needle biopsy or surgical biopsy) and a benign outcome. There are large differences in estimates of the cumulative risk between organized breast cancer screening programmes and opportunistic screening. The modelled estimate of cumulative risk of false-positive recall in organized screening programmes in Europe is about 20% for a woman who had 10 screenings between the ages of 50 years and 70 years; less than 5% have an invasive procedure. In opportunistic screening, such as in the USA, rates of recall are higher, and the protocols for assessment are different; the cumulative risk of having at least one false-positive recall after 10 years of screening has been estimated to be about 40% with biennial screening and about 60% with annual screening, and these rates are similar for women starting screening at age 40 years and at age 50 years.

(b) *Overdiagnosis*

Overdiagnosis refers to the detection by screening of breast cancers (ductal carcinoma in situ and invasive) that would never have been diagnosed clinically if the women had not been screened. Overdiagnosed breast cancers are treated because they cannot be distinguished from cancers that would progress if not treated; therefore, treatment is the main component of the harm of overdiagnosis. The epidemiological quantification of overdiagnosis in observational studies is important because estimates may be influenced by local screening practice and technological innovations.

The Working Group noted and endorsed the classification of measures of overdiagnosis suggested by the Independent United Kingdom Panel (measures A to D). Use of this classification when reporting overdiagnosis estimates will enhance the prospects of valid comparison between overdiagnosis estimates made in different studies and in different screening programmes.

RCTs have shown that after the drop in incidence that follows the end of regular screening has occurred, there is a persistent excess of diagnosed cases, which can give an estimate of the number of overdiagnosed cases. Based on a start of screening at age 40–69 years and a follow-up time of at least 10 years after the end of the screening period, two RCTs with long follow-up periods estimated overdiagnosis to be 4–12% of all cancers detected in control (unscreened) women over the same follow-up period (measure A). As a proportion of screen-detected cancers only, the estimate was 22–29% (measure D). To obtain a truly valid estimate of overdiagnosis in RCTs, there should be no screening after the trial has ended in either the study or the control arm. It is doubtful whether any RCT has met this requirement. Moreover, the RCT estimates relate to screening performed in the 1980s, and there are no pooled age-specific estimates (e.g. for women aged 40–49 years or 50–69 years).

The methodology for evaluating overdiagnosis in observational studies, based mainly on organized programmes, has varied widely across studies. Two main approaches, aided by modelling, are currently proposed. The cumulative incidence approach follows a population (cohort or dynamic) over time, including over the period of the compensatory drop in incidence after the end of screening. Models have estimated that breast cancers may be screen-detectable up to 10 years before they would present clinically (i.e. screening has a lead time of up to 10 years), although the issue is controversial and others have argued for shorter lead times. Assuming a lead time of up to 10 years, a follow-up period of at least 5–10 years after the end of screening attendance is needed to include the compensatory drop. The second approach involves statistical adjustment for the lead time that has produced the excess of cases initially. A further challenge in estimating overdiagnosis is proper allowance for any underlying trend in incidence with time or adjustment for exposure to factors confounded with screening (e.g. hormone replacement therapy) that may cause such a trend. Studies evaluate incidence rates in populations invited and not invited to screening, or screened and not screened, and in the latter case bias from self-selection for screening should be taken into account.

The Working Group considered 30 observational studies that reported estimates of overdiagnosis. Their results varied widely; estimates of the overdiagnosis risk, principally the Independent United Kingdom Panel's measure A, ranged from −0.7% to 76% for invasive cancer only and from 1% to 57% for in situ and invasive cancers together. For 13 of these studies that were considered to be adequately adjusted for underlying trend in breast cancer incidence and for lead time, the measure A estimates ranged from 2% to 25% for invasive cancer only and from 2% to 22% for in situ and invasive cancers together.

(c) Risk of radiation-induced breast cancer

The low dose of X-ray photon radiation received during mammography is a potential adverse effect of breast cancer screening, since exposure of the breast to ionizing radiation may induce breast cancer. The number of breast cancers induced by mammography is estimated through risk assessment approaches, which use a range of hypotheses about risk model, latency time, correction factor for low dose and dose rate, mean glandular dose to the breast during mammography, targeted population, and screening modalities. For biennial screening from age 50 years to age 74 or 80 years (with follow-up until age 85 years or older), the estimated number of breast cancer deaths induced by mammography screening ranges from 1 to 7 per 100 000 women screened. These estimates are smaller than estimates of breast cancer deaths prevented by mammography screening by a factor of at least 100. For 10 years of annual screening from age 40 years to age 49 years (with follow-up until age 85 years or older), the estimated number of breast cancer deaths induced by mammography screening ranges from 8 to 20 per 100 000 women screened.

(d) Psychosocial consequences

Studies of the psychological impact of false-positive mammography, which were summarized in seven reviews, showed varied results. Some studies reported that women who have further investigations after a routine mammogram experience anxiety in the short term, and possibly in the long term. Also, some studies reported that some women with false-positive results conducted more frequent BSE and had higher levels of distress and anxiety, although not apparently pathologically so, and thought more about breast cancer than did those with normal results; in other studies, the effects were limited to breast cancer-specific outcomes. Two of the reviews concluded that the process decreased women's quality of life for weeks and even months.

6.3.4 Cost–effectiveness of mammography screening

Decisions about implementation of health-care interventions are based primarily on health benefits and a favourable harm–benefit ratio, but – to use limited resources efficiently – are also often based on cost–effectiveness analyses. A cost–effectiveness analysis compares different policies, including the current one, with no intervention (average cost–effectiveness) or compares a more-intensive programme with a less-intensive programme (incremental cost–effectiveness). Effects are often defined as disease-specific deaths prevented and life years gained but are ideally adjusted for quality of life, resulting in quality-adjusted life years.

Ideally, all possible screening policies that are of relevance are compared in a cost–effectiveness analysis. However, it is not feasible to compare all scenarios of interest in an RCT or observational study. By the use of mathematical models, findings from screening trials and observational studies are extrapolated to simulated populations. Numerous cost–effectiveness analyses showed that organized mammography screening, often biennially, is cost-effective. Despite their greater effectiveness, screening strategies that consist of annual screening are often found to be less efficient and less cost-effective, due to a disproportionate increase in costs or due to diminishing returns; about 80% of the effect of annual screening is retained when screening is performed every 2 years.

Several studies have assessed the cost–effectiveness of CBE, mass media awareness-raising campaigns, limited mammography screening, and increasing the coverage level of treatment in LMICs. However, evidence on the effectiveness of these approaches in these countries is still absent.

6.4 Other imaging techniques

6.4.1 Techniques

Ultrasonography is performed using handheld ultrasonography (also called two-dimensional [2D] ultrasonography) or automated breast ultrasonography (also called three-dimensional [3D] ultrasonography). Since with handheld ultrasonography only a very small selection of images seen during acquisition is recorded for interpretation, image acquisition requires high diagnostic skills to minimize selection error. This problem may be eliminated by using automated breast ultrasonography, in which all images are recorded. Screening with ultrasonography has been used mostly as an adjunct to mammography in women with dense breasts. In addition, use of ultrasonography as a primary tool for breast cancer screening has been reported recently in China. Knowledge about quality assurance of image acquisition or reading of breast ultrasonography is still limited.

Digital breast tomosynthesis, a three-dimensional approach to digital mammography, is described in Section 6.3.

Magnetic resonance imaging (MRI) without contrast agent and MRI spectroscopy have not been applied or validated for screening use, and their application is being tested for diagnostic use. Contrast-enhanced MRI has been evaluated as an adjunct to mammography in studies of women at an increased risk (see Section 6.5). Potential side-effects of the magnetic field (in women with metallic devices) must be considered. Contrast-enhanced MRI screening also leads to risk of severe kidney disease and severe allergy. Costly equipment, false-positive test results, and the expensive assessment of MRI-only detected lesions result in high costs for this technique. No quality assurance programme has yet been established for MRI screening.

Positron emission tomography (PET) and positron emission mammography (PEM) involve intravenous application of radioactively marked [^{18}F]-fluorodeoxyglucose to measure glucose metabolism, which is assumed to be higher in tumours. Other metabolites could be measured but have not been validated for clinical use. PET has a lower resolution and signal-to-noise ratio than PEM. No study has evaluated screening by PET or PEM. In the diagnostic situation, PEM has sensitivity and specificity comparable to those of MRI. Due to the slow clearance time of the radioactive marker from the body, PEM (like PET) is associated with a radiation dose to the whole body 16 times that for mammography.

Scintimammography measures the uptake of radioactively marked ^{99}Tc-sestamibi, which binds to mitochondria. The density of mitochondria is assumed to be increased in tumours. A single study assessed the validity of scintimammography for screening, but it included a high percentage of women at an increased risk of breast cancer. In that study, sensitivity and specificity were comparable to those of MRI. The radiation dose received for scintimammography and similar technologies is 9–20 times that for mammography.

Infrared spectroscopy measures spectral differences in the examined tissue, and the proportions of haemoglobin and deoxyhaemoglobin have been suggested to differ between benign and malignant tissue. Thermography measures temperature distribution in the examined tissue, assuming that malignant tissue has a higher temperature. Electrical impedance imaging measures conductivity and impedance, relying on the assumption that cancer cells have increased conductivity and thus decreased impedance. Initial clinical experience and/or attempts to use these methods for screening have generally yielded lower sensitivity and specificity than those of standard imaging technologies. None of these methods has been validated for screening.

Molecular imaging uses vectors that emit a fluoroscopic or scintigraphic signal attached to targeting agents, which might identify molecules within the cell membrane or cellular matrix of tumours. Development of such agents is in the preclinical stage.

6.4.2 Effectiveness in screening

(a) Ultrasonography

Nine observational studies (the majority retrospective) conducted in Austria, Italy, and the USA assessed ultrasonography as an adjunct to mammography for breast cancer screening in women with dense breast tissue and negative mammography. The incremental breast cancer detection rate ranged from 1.9 per 1000 screens to 4.0 per 1000 screens. In one additional prospective study in China in women screened with mammography and ultrasonography without restriction to those with dense breasts, adjunct ultrasonography detected additional cancers in 1 per 1000 screened women. However, none of the studies had a comparison or control group, and some included women at an increased risk of developing breast cancer. Ultrasonography-only detected cancers were frequently early-stage cancers, generally at a comparable or earlier stage than cancers detected by mammography. Two of these studies reported estimates of interval cancer rates of 1.1 per 1000 screens and 1.7 per 1000 screens at 12 months of follow-up, but interpretation of these estimates is limited due to the lack of a comparison group and to substantial heterogeneity in the underlying breast cancer incidence rates in study populations.

All available studies consistently showed that adjunct ultrasonography substantially increases rates of false-positive recall or testing. Five studies reported incremental rates of false-positive biopsy (mostly surgical biopsy) of between 1.2% and 2.8%, and seven studies reported additional false-positive testing or follow-up in 1.7% to 7.5% of screens.

There were no observational studies assessing screening efficacy in terms of mortality reduction or assessing screening impact using surrogate end-points for screening efficacy.

(b) Digital breast tomosynthesis

In five non-randomized studies of digital mammography with tomosynthesis (also referred to as integrated 2D/3D mammography), two of which were prospective trials within population-based programmes, the incremental breast cancer detection rate relative to digital mammography ranged from 0.5 per 1000 screens to 2.7 per 1000 screens. Two of four observational studies reporting cancer stage distribution showed that the incremental detection was of invasive tumours, whereas the other two studies showed incremental detection of in situ and invasive tumours. One observational study reported an estimated interval cancer rate of 0.8 per 1000 screens at 12 months of follow-up, but interpretation of this estimate is limited due to the lack of a comparison group.

Digital mammography with tomosynthesis reduced rates of false-positive recalls in four informative observational studies, with absolute decreases in false-positive recalls ranging from 0.8% to 3.6% of screened women, representing reductions of 15% to 36% in false-positive recalls.

Given the dual acquisition of images, digital mammography with tomosynthesis increases the radiation dose received by approximately doubling the mean glandular dose; however, this will depend on the exact technology used and the number of acquisitions. Based on one observational study, reconstruction of the 2D images from the tomosynthesis acquisition decreases the radiation dose by 45% compared with the dual acquisition and yields similar incremental cancer detection to that from the dual acquisition.

6.5 Screening of women at an increased risk

6.5.1 Women with a BRCA1/2 *mutation*

Fourteen prospective cohort studies of women with a *BRCA1* or *BRCA2* mutation assessed the screening performance of MRI plus mammography performed in the same screening round, with a review of the diagnostic test performed. The sensitivity and specificity of mammography in this population of women were about 40% and 95%, respectively; corresponding values for MRI plus mammography were about 95% and 80%, respectively, showing a clear increase in sensitivity and decrease in specificity compared with mammography alone.

Four prospective cohort studies assessed reduction in breast cancer mortality in women with a *BRCA1* or *BRCA2* mutation screened with mammography. The studies reported varying results, from a 5-year all-cause survival of 63% in *BRCA1* mutation carriers to a 6-year all-cause survival of 93% in *BRCA1/2* mutation carriers. In the only study in which the breast cancer-specific survival of women with a *BRCA1* mutation screened annually with MRI plus mammography was compared with that in unscreened women with a *BRCA1* mutation, a significant difference in 10-year breast cancer-specific survival was found (95.3% in the screened group vs 73.7% in the unscreened group).

6.5.2 *Women with a high familial risk without a* BRCA1/2 *mutation*

Two prospective cohort studies of women with a high familial risk without a *BRCA1* or *BRCA2* mutation assessed the screening performance of MRI plus mammography performed in the same screening round, with a review of the diagnostic test performed. The reported estimates for the sensitivity and specificity of mammography were 25–46% and 95–97%, respectively; corresponding values for adjunct MRI were 73–100% and 89–98%, respectively.

6.5.3 *Women with a high familial risk with or without a* BRCA1/2 *mutation*

One observational study with long-term follow-up reported a shift to a lower stage of the tumours detected in women with annual MRI and mammography screening compared with women without intensified screening.

In the 10 studies that evaluated the sensitivity of ultrasonography in women with a high familial risk with or without a *BRCA1* or *BRCA2* mutation, the sensitivity was comparable to or lower than that of mammography and was always lower than that of MRI. No study assessed the specificity of ultrasonography.

Seven prospective cohort studies assessed the incremental cancer detection rate of CBE in women with an increased familial risk screened with MRI plus mammography, with or without ultrasonography. None of the studies addressed the effect of CBE alone. Five of the studies did not detect any additional cancers; in the remaining two studies, which reported a lower screen detection rate, a total of 4 out of 243 cancers (1.6%) were found by CBE only.

6.5.4 *Women with a personal history of breast cancer (invasive or in situ)*

One large multicentre study assessed mammography screening in women with a personal history of breast cancer compared with those without such a history (58 870 screens in each group). The sensitivity and the specificity of mammography were significantly lower in women with a personal history of breast cancer compared with those without such a history.

One comparative study assessed the value of adding ultrasonography to annual mammography in women with a personal history of breast cancer versus women with various types of risk factors for breast cancer. The incremental cancer detection rate was comparable between the two groups; when ultrasonography was added to mammography, the recall rate increased significantly, from 11.5% to 26.6%.

In a small substudy that assessed the value of adding MRI to annual mammography plus ultrasonography in women with a personal history of breast cancer versus those without such a history, the recall rate increased significantly, from 16.3% to 36.3%.

6.5.5 *Women with lobular neoplasia or atypical proliferations*

One large multicentre comparative study assessed mammography screening in women with lobular carcinoma in situ (LCIS) or atypical proliferations compared with women without such lesions (2505 and 12 525 screens, respectively). The sensitivity of mammography in women with LCIS or atypical proliferations was not statistically significantly lower than that in matched controls; however, the specificity was lower. Four studies (two comparative and two non-comparative) evaluated a series of patients to examine the sensitivity of MRI in screening women with LCIS or atypical hyperplasia. In the non-comparative studies, high sensitivities were reported for the MRI screening in women with LCIS. In the comparative studies, women with such lesions selected to undergo MRI screening were younger and had stronger family histories of breast cancer. In addition, MRI screening generated more recall biopsies compared with mammography.

6.6 Clinical breast examination

CBE is a simple technique involving visual inspection and systematic palpation of both breasts and nipples by a trained health-care provider. This technique has a moderate sensitivity (range, 50–60%) and a specificity of more than 85%.

Three RCTs, two conducted in India and one in the Philippines, assessed the efficacy of CBE alone versus no screening. All three studies reported a significant shift to a lower stage of the tumours detected (early detection). Although the study in the Philippines was stopped after one round of screening, the two studies in India are currently under way and the effect of CBE on breast cancer mortality in these studies is awaited.

Two RCTs showed that CBE in combination with mammography reduced breast cancer mortality compared with no intervention in women older than 50 years. In the earlier study, conducted in 1963 in the USA, 67% of the tumours were detected by CBE and mammography, and 45% were detected by CBE alone. In the other study, conducted in 1979 in the United Kingdom, 74% of the tumours were detected by CBE and mammography, and 3% by CBE alone. In an RCT conducted in Canada, CBE plus mammography screening did not show a significant mortality benefit compared with CBE alone. In addition, five observational studies, conducted mostly in the 1970s, reported that CBE contributed 5–10% in incremental detection rate over and above mammography.

CBE is a low-cost intervention and thus a feasible screening modality in LMICs.

6.7 Breast self-examination

Several techniques for BSE have been described, with the number of steps ranging from 21 to 34. Women are unlikely to perform such elaborate techniques, and hence simpler techniques have been recommended. Structured training and individual instruction have been shown to improve compliance with BSE practice. Sensitivity, specificity, and positive predictive value of 58.3%, 87.4%, and 29.2%, respectively, have been reported for BSE. Breast cancer awareness, socioeconomic status, level of education, and availability of privacy are the principal determinants of BSE practice.

Two RCTs of BSE have been conducted. A study in St Petersburg, Russian Federation, compared women who received intensive instruction in BSE and annual reinforcement sessions, plus annual CBE, with women who received only annual CBE. A study in Shanghai, China, compared women who received intensive BSE instruction, periodic reminders, two reinforcement sessions 2 years and 4 years after initial instruction, and periodic practice sessions under the supervision of a medical worker, with women who received no BSE instruction or any other type of breast cancer screening. In both studies, after about 10 years of follow-up, there were no differences between the instruction and control arms in breast cancer mortality rates, in breast cancer incidence rates, in the size or stage of the breast cancers, or in survival rates in the cancer cases. In both RCTs, more benign lesions were detected in the instruction arms than in the control arms. In the St Petersburg trial, the frequency of BSE practice declined with time after initial instruction and after a re-education programme; in the Shanghai trial, no information on compliance was collected. One possible explanation for the trial results is poor compliance. Both trials were conducted in populations with easy access to diagnostic and treatment facilities, and the women in the control groups of both studies presented with relatively small tumours.

Two of three observational cohort studies showed reduced mortality from breast cancer in women who received BSE instruction, but the results are likely to be due to factors unrelated to BSE practice. Results of four case–control studies provided inconsistent results with regard to the relationship between the frequency of BSE practice and the risk of fatal or advanced breast cancer (as a surrogate for breast cancer death). However, two studies showed weak decreasing trends in the risk of fatal or advanced disease with increasing level of proficiency of BSE. In a study at Duke University, USA, women at moderate to high risk of breast cancer who received annual screening by mammography and MRI were given detailed BSE instruction in conjunction with CBE two or three times a year. All 12 interval cancers were detected in women who reported practising BSE competently and regularly, and 6 of the cancers were initially detected by BSE.

Surveys of BSE practice in the general population in LMICs as well as surveys in women before and after receiving BSE instruction have generally shown that the percentages of women who report practising BSE are too low to be likely to have a meaningful impact on mortality from breast cancer.

7. EVALUATION

7.1 Mammography screening

7.1.1 Mammography screening: preventive effects

There is *sufficient evidence* that screening women aged 50–69 years by mammography reduces breast cancer mortality. This evaluation is supported by randomized controlled trials of efficacy of mammography screening and by observational studies of effectiveness of both invitation to and attendance at service mammography screening. Women aged 50–69 years invited to service mammography screening have, on average, a 24% reduced risk of mortality from breast cancer. Women aged 50–69 years who attend service mammography screening have, on average, about a 40% reduced risk of mortality from breast cancer.

There is *limited evidence* that screening women aged 45–49 years by mammography reduces breast cancer mortality. There is *limited evidence* that screening women aged 40–44 years by mammography reduces breast cancer mortality. These evaluations are supported by observational studies of service mammography screening and are consistent with the one relevant randomized controlled trial. Invitation or attendance of women aged 40–49 years to service mammography screening have been associated with a reduction of about 20% in risk of breast cancer mortality; this reduction may be greater in women aged 45–49 years (~32%) than in women aged 40–44 years (~17%).

There is *sufficient evidence* that screening women aged 70–74 years by mammography reduces breast cancer mortality. This evaluation is supported by observational studies of service mammography screening.

7.1.2 Mammography screening: adverse effects

There is *sufficient evidence* that mammography screening of women aged 50–69 years detects breast cancers that would never have been diagnosed or never have caused harm if the women had not been screened (overdiagnosis). The percentage of overdiagnosis ranges from 1% to 10% when estimated by comparing the cumulative incidence of breast cancer in women screened from age 50–69 years and followed up for about 10 years after the last screen with the cumulative incidence of breast cancer in similar but unscreened women over the same period of time.

There is *sufficient evidence* that the risk of radiation-induced cancer from mammography in women aged 50–74 years is substantially outweighed by the reduction in breast cancer mortality from mammography screening.

There is *sufficient evidence* that mammography screening produces short-term negative psychological consequences when the result is false-positive.

7.1.3 Mammography screening: cost–effectiveness

There is *sufficient evidence* that mammography screening has a net benefit for women aged 50–69 years who are invited to attend organized mammography screening programmes.

There is *sufficient evidence* that mammography screening can be cost-effective among women aged 50–69 years in countries with a high incidence of breast cancer.

There is *limited evidence* that breast cancer screening can be cost-effective in low- and middle-income countries.

7.2 Other imaging techniques

7.2.1 Breast ultrasonography

There is *inadequate evidence* that ultrasonography as adjunct to screening by mammography in women with dense breasts and negative mammography reduces breast cancer mortality.

There is *limited evidence* that ultrasonography as adjunct to screening by mammography in women with dense breasts and negative mammography increases the detection rate of breast cancer.

There is *inadequate evidence* that ultrasonography as adjunct to screening by mammography in women with dense breasts and negative mammography reduces the rate of interval cancers.

There is *sufficient evidence* that ultrasonography as adjunct to screening by mammography in women with dense breasts and negative mammography increases the rate of false-positive screening outcomes.

7.2.2 Digital breast tomosynthesis/ three-dimensional mammography

There is *inadequate evidence* that screening by digital mammography with tomosynthesis reduces breast cancer mortality compared with mammography alone.

There is *sufficient evidence* that screening by digital mammography with tomosynthesis increases detection rates of breast cancers compared with mammography alone.

There is *limited evidence* that the incremental detection from mammography with tomosynthesis is mostly of invasive cancers.

There is *limited evidence* that screening by digital mammography with tomosynthesis reduces the rate of false-positive screening outcomes compared with mammography alone.

There is *inadequate evidence* that screening by digital mammography with tomosynthesis reduces the rate of interval cancers compared with mammography alone.

There is *sufficient evidence* that screening by digital mammography with tomosynthesis (from dual acquisition) increases the radiation dose received compared with that of mammography alone. Reconstructing the two-dimensional images from the tomosynthesis acquisition substantially reduces the radiation dose received compared with that of dual acquisition by mammography and tomosynthesis.

7.3 Screening of women at an increased risk

There is *sufficient evidence* that in women with a high familial risk and with a *BRCA1/2* mutation, magnetic resonance imaging (MRI) as adjunct to screening by mammography increases the sensitivity and decreases the specificity of screening.

There is *limited evidence* that in women with a high familial risk and without a known *BRCA1/2* mutation, MRI as adjunct to screening by mammography increases the sensitivity and decreases the specificity of screening.

There is *inadequate evidence* that in women with a *BRCA1/2* mutation, MRI as adjunct to screening by mammography reduces breast cancer mortality.

There is *sufficient evidence* that in women with a high familial risk, with or without a *BRCA1/2* mutation, screening with ultrasonography alone yields sensitivity similar to or lower than that obtained with mammography alone, and lower than that obtained with MRI alone.

There is *inadequate evidence* that in women with a high familial risk screened with MRI and mammography, clinical breast examination detects additional cancers.

There is *limited evidence* that in women with a personal history of breast cancer, the sensitivity and the specificity of mammography are lower than those in women without such a history.

There is *inadequate evidence* that in women with a personal history of breast cancer, ultrasonography as adjunct to mammography detects additional cancers.

There is *inadequate evidence* that in women with a personal history of breast cancer, ultrasonography as adjunct to mammography increases the rate of false-positive screening outcomes compared with women without such a history.

There is *inadequate evidence* that in women with a personal history of breast cancer, MRI added to mammography plus ultrasonography increases the rate of false-positive screening outcomes compared with women without such a history.

There is *limited evidence* that in women with lobular neoplasia or atypical proliferations, the sensitivity of mammography is equal to and the specificity of mammography is lower than that in women without such lesions.

There is *inadequate evidence* that in women with lobular neoplasia or atypical proliferations, MRI as adjunct to mammography detects additional cancers.

There is *limited evidence* that in women with lobular neoplasia or atypical proliferations, MRI as adjunct to mammography increases the rate of false-positive screening outcomes compared with mammography alone.

7.4 Clinical breast examination

There is *sufficient evidence* that screening by clinical breast examination alone shifts the stage distribution of tumours detected towards a lower stage.

There is *inadequate evidence* that screening by clinical breast examination alone reduces breast cancer mortality.

7.5 Breast self-examination

There is *inadequate evidence* that teaching breast self-examination reduces breast cancer mortality.

There is *inadequate evidence* that teaching breast self-examination reduces the rate of interval cancers.

There is *inadequate evidence* that breast self-examination reduces breast cancer mortality in women who practise it competently and regularly.